Recent Advances in Implant Dentistry

Recent Advances in Implant Dentistry

Editor: Jonathan Lewis

MURPHY & MOORE
www.murphy-moorepublishing.com

www.murphy-moorepublishing.com

MURPHY & MOORE

Cataloging-in-Publication Data

Recent advances in implant dentistry / edited by Jonathan Lewis.
p. cm.
Includes bibliographical references and index.
ISBN 978-1-63987-476-7
1. Dental implants. 2. Dentures. 3. Implants, Artificial. 4. Dentistry. I. Lewis, Jonathan.
RK667.I45 R43 2022
617.693--dc23

Murphy & Moore Publishing,
1 Rockefeller Plaza,
New York City, NY 10020, USA

ISBN 978-1-63987-476-7 (Hardback)

Contents

Preface

The world is advancing at a fast pace like never before. Therefore, the need is to keep up with the latest developments. This book was an idea that came to fruition when the specialists in the area realized the need to coordinate together and document essential themes in the subject. That's when I was requested to be the editor. Editing this book has been an honour as it brings together diverse authors researching on different streams of the field. The book collates essential materials contributed by veterans in the area which can be utilized by students and researchers alike.

Dental implants refer to the surgical components which interface with the bone of the skull or jaw in order to support a dental prosthesis. Dental implants function through a biological process known as osseointegration, wherein certain substances such as Titanium, form a bond with the bone. The success of implant dentistry procedures depend on various factors, like the drugs used to assist in osseointegration, health of the person and the health of the tissues present in the mouth. The implant can be either removable or fixed. Major types of implants are small diameter implants, implant supported bridge, implant-supported overdenture and single tooth implant restoration. This book discusses the fundamentals as well as modern approaches of implant dentistry. It elucidates new techniques and their applications in a multidisciplinary manner. As this field is emerging at a rapid pace, the contents of this book will help the readers understand the recent advances in this field.

Each chapter is a sole-standing publication that reflects each author´s interpretation. Thus, the book displays a multi-facetted picture of our current understanding of application, resources and aspects of the field. I would like to thank the contributors of this book and my family for their endless support.

Editor

1

Bisphosphonate-Related Osteonecrosis of the Jaw Around Dental Implants

Tatsuo Shirota[1], Atsushi Nakamura[2], Yoshiro Matsui[3], Masashi Hatori[1], Masanori Nakamura[1] and Satoru Shintani[1]
[1]*Showa University,*
[2]*Yamato Tokushukai Hospital,*
[3]*Kagawa University,*
Japan

1. Introduction

Bisphosphonate is the collective name for compounds in which the backbone of pyrophosphoric acid, a P-O-P structure, is converted to chemically stable P-C-P, and this structure shows the affinity of bisphosphonate for bone hydroxyapatite in the body (Fleisch et al. 2002). Administered bisphosphonate preparations (BPs) transfer to and deposit in bone, exhibiting a bone resorption-inhibitory effect. The chemical structure of the side chain bound to the carbon atom of P-C-P markedly influences bisphosphonate activity, and, particularly, side chains containing nitrogen molecules not only markedly increase the affinity for HA but also bone resorption-inhibitory activity (Migliorati et al. 2005). Because of this potent bone resorption-inhibitory effect, BPs are the first-choice treatment for osteoporosis worldwide (Russell et al. 2007), and their efficacy for malignant tumor-associated hypercalcemia (Body et al.1999), ostealgia complicating bone metastasis of solid tumors (Hortobagyi et al. 1998), and multiple myeloma accompanied by bone destruction (Berenson et al. 1996) has been shown. Adverse effects of BPs were previously considered to be relatively mild, such as digestive symptoms induced by oral preparations and fever induced by injections (Berenson et al. 1996), but the association of BPs with osteonecrosis of the jaw has been frequently described since Marx (2003) initially reported it (Ruggiero et al. 2004; Marx et al. 2005; Khosla et al. 2007)

Bisphosphonate-related osteonecrosis of the jaw (BRONJ) is clinically diagnosed when the following 3 conditions are met: 1) current or previous treatment with BPs, 2) persistent exposure of necrotized bone in the maxillofacial region for 8 weeks or longer, 3) no past medical history of radiotherapy for the jaw bone (AAOMS 2007; Ruggiero et al. 2009). BPs inducing BRONJ mostly contain nitrogen (NBPs). BRONJ frequently develops in patients under NBP treatment upon dental treatment, such as tooth extraction, implant placement, and surgical periodontal treatment accompanied by bone invasion, and inflammatory diseases, such as periodontal disease and abscess (Ruggieri et al. 2009; Vahtsevanos et al. 2009; Yoneda et al. 2010). BRONJ shows poor responses to the standard treatment for common osteomyelitis of the jaw, such as curettage/resection of necrotized tissue and antimicrobial drugs, and its intractability is the most serious problem.

Stack & Epker (1995) initially reported the influence of BPs on dental implant treatment. They introduced a case in which all 5 favorably functioning implants in the lower anterior tooth region were lost after the 5-month administration of a BP containing no nitrogen, etidronatedisodium (Didronel; Procter and Gamble, Cincinnati, OH), for osteoporosis. The details of the bone wound healing process after implant loss or whether BRONJ developed were not described, but the author concluded that Didronel administration is a risk factor for implant treatment. However, several recent studies reported that implant treatment in the presence of NBPs was possible when the NBPs were oral drugs. Fugazzotto et al (2007) evaluated that a retrospective analysis of case records of patients with a history of oral BPs therapy treated as part of routine periodontal and implant treatment. They reported that no osteonecrosis was noted immediately postoperatively or during follow-up period 61 patients, and all implants were functioning successfully 12 to 24 months post-insertion.Grant et al. (2008) evaluated the clinical results of 115 patients who received oral BPs during implant treatment. They showed that there was no significant difference in treatment results between patients with and without oral BPs during implant treatment. It was also reported that no patients developed ONJ after implant treatment. Bell & Bell (2008) reported that bone grafting for implant treatment in 42 patients who received oral BPs for osteoporosis treatment was conducted safely. Therefore, no conclusion has been reached regarding whether oral BPs are contraindicated for implant treatment. On the other hand, it has been clarified that the risk of developing BRONJ upon open dental treatment rises in patients treated with NBP intravenous injection showing a potent bone adsorption-inhibitory action, and implant treatment is considered contraindicated for such cases (Khan et al. 2008; Ruggiero et al. 2009). However, there have been fewer reports on the influence of intravenous BPs on implants which have already acquired osseointegration and are favorably functioning, and the actual state is unclear.

We experienced the case of a patient who developed ONJ around implants in the maxilla, considered to be caused by intravenous BP administration for osteometastasis treatment of breast cancer, and underwent partial maxillectomy to relieve inflammation (Shirota et al. 2009). This chapter introduces clinical findings, the treatment and its outcome, and peri-implant histopathological findings in the patient, and the developmental mechanism of peri-implant BRONJ is discussed with a literature review.

2. Patient and methods

2.1 Outline of the patient

The patient was a 54-year-old female who visited our hospital for chief complaints of peri-implant pain in the upper left molar region and bone exposure. The patient developed breast cancer about 6 years ago and underwent left mastectomy followed by irradiation and chemotherapy. However, multiple cancer metastases occurred about 2 years ago, and the patient underwent cancer chemotherapy and intravenous BPs injection.

The patient underwent implant treatment for the upper left molar region at a dental clinic immediately before the development of breast cancer, in which 2 implants were placed. These implants functioned without a problem for about 6 years, but peri-implant gingival recession, bone exposure, and pain appeared about one month ago, and the patient received antimicrobial drug administration, irrigation, and disinfection at a clinic, but the symptoms did not improve. Thus, the patient visited our department. On the first examination, brown-colored necrotized bone was exposed in the upper left first molar region on the buccal side.

The peri-implant gingiva was painful and swollen with slight flare, but no implant mobility was observed (Fig.1). On panoramic radiography, mild bone resorption was noted in alveolar bone in the implant neck. Computed tomography (CT) revealed sequestration with an irregular trabecular bone structure around the implant (Fig.2). Biopsy was performed in consideration of metastasis of breast cancer to the oral cavity, but only inflammatory cell infiltration was observed without tumor cells.

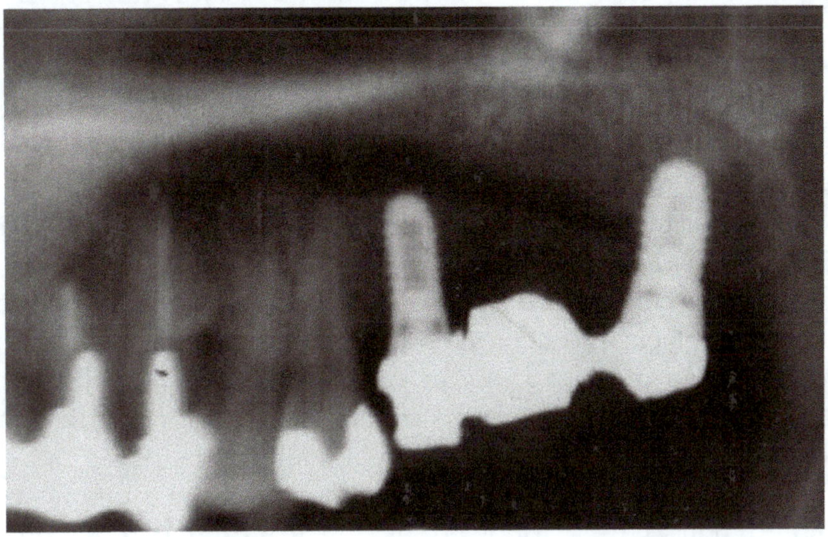

Fig. 1. Radiograph showing slight bone resorption around the implants.

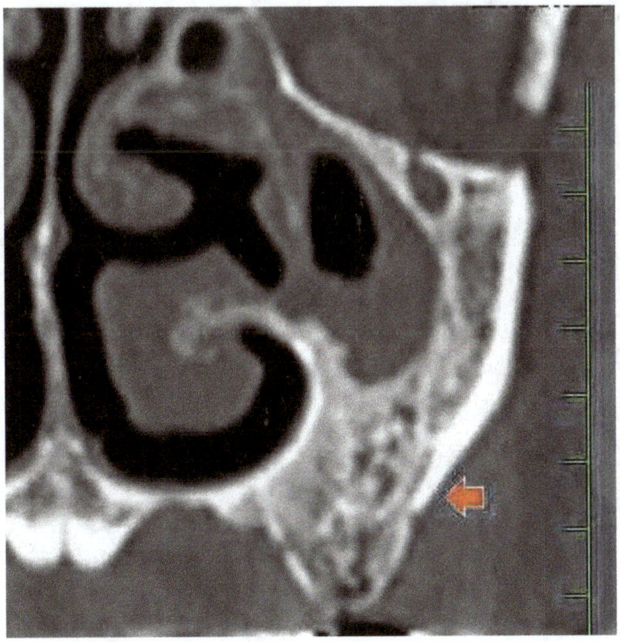

Fig. 2. Computed tomography (CT) image around the implants (arrow).

2.2 Diagnosis and treatment

It is well-known that curative chemotherapy or long-term adrenocortical steroid administration for lymphoblastic leukemia and Hodgkin and non-Hodgkin lymphomas induces osteonecrosis of the femoral head (Kubo et al. 2001; Bojko et al 2003; Karimova et al.

2008). Many anticancer drugs were administered for breast cancer metastasis in this patient, but no osteonecrosis of the jaw caused by these drugs has been reported. In addition, the clinical symptoms of this patient met all diagnostic criteria of BRONJ proposed by AAOMS (AAOMS 2007; Ruggiero et al. 2009). Based on these findings, BP-induced osteonecrosis was diagnosed.

In the treatment, morbid bone tissue including implants was resected in consideration of the following 3 conditions: 1) early chemotherapy for metastatic cancer was necessary, for which removal of the infected lesion was necessary, 2) there was a possibility that continuation of the withdrawal of BPs would aggravate metastatic cancer-associated bone destruction and hypercalcemia, and 3) it was difficult to remit inflammation by employing conservative treatment proposed by the American Association of Oral and Maxillofacial Surgeons (AAOMS 2007; Ruggiero et al. 2009). After considering these points, sequestrectomy of the left maxilla was selected. The gingival margin was incised between the upper left first premolar and implant towards the maxillary tuberosity, and the lesion area was exposed by forming a buccal and palatal mucoperiosteal flap. The bone cortex of the lesion was brownish black, and necrotic bone was confirmed between the distal surface of the second premolar and mesial surface of the implant placed in the second molar area, but particularly around the implant placed in the first molar area (Fig.3a). The area for resection around the living bone in the lesion was determined after the extraction of the second premolar, and the pathological bone tissue including the implant was removed with a Lindeman bar and bone chisel, followed by the grinding of the bone surface of the resection stump until bleeding was confirmed. As a result, the instrument partially perforated the maxillary sinus floor, and the thickened maxillary sinus mucosa was exposed. This sinus mucosa was spared, and the surgical wound was completely closed by suturing the mucoperiosteal flaps (Fig.3b)

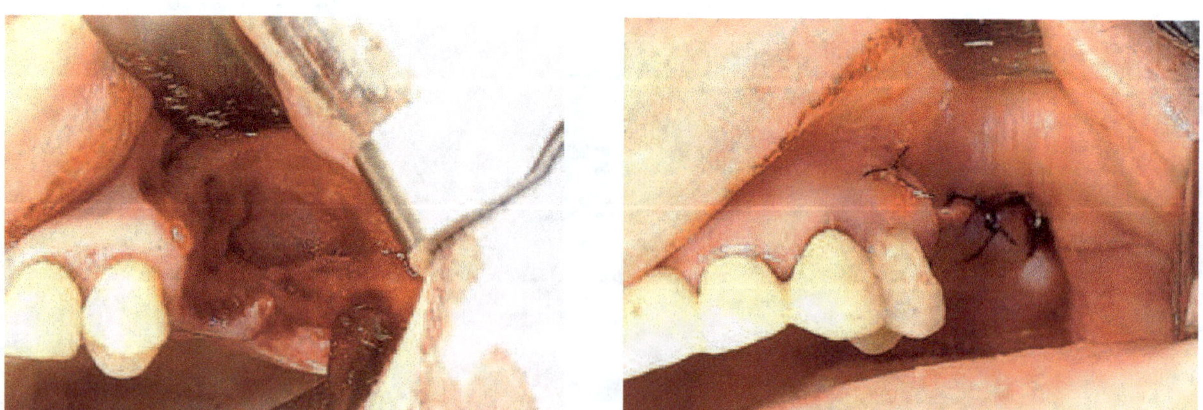

(a) Pathological bone including the implants was removed, and maxillary sinus mucosa was exposed.

(b) The surgical wound was completely closed by suturing the mucoperiosteal flap.

Fig. 3. Intraoperative view of the sequestomy of the left maxilla.

After surgery, antibiotic was intravenously administered for 3 days and oral antibiotic was administered for 3 days. In addition, hyperbaric oxygen therapy was performed. The efficacy of hyperbaric oxygen therapy for BRONJ is controversial (Ruggiero et al. 2004; Freiberger et al 2009), but, at least, it may be effective to promote mucoepithelial wound healing in the sequestration-resected region. The wound was completely covered with healthy mucosa 2 weeks after surgery (Fig.4.). Since the remission of inflammation could be confirmed, anticancer drug and BP administration was initiated for metastatic cancer and bone metastasis-associated bone destruction. The patient died of multiorgan failure associated with multiple cancer metastasis 8 months after surgery, but BRONJ did not recur before death.

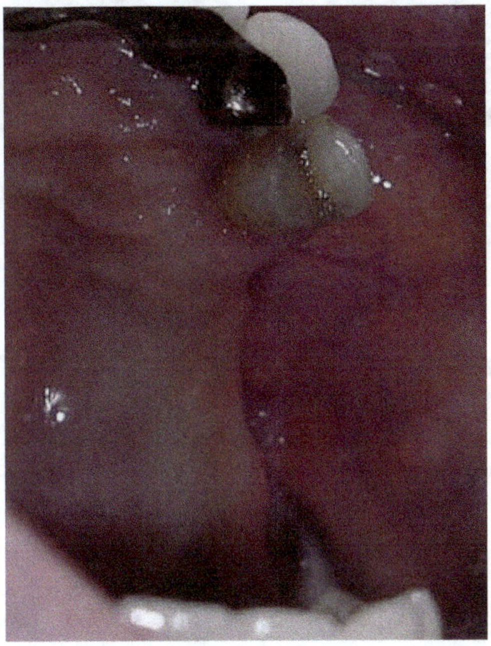

Fig. 4. Intraoral view at 4 weeks after surgery.

2.3 Macroscopic and μCT findings of the resected specimen

Implants were strongly fixed to the bone, and areas of brown sequestration were observed around them (Fig.5.). On μCT, no apparent abnormality, such as trabecular destruction, was observed, and the implant surface was in direct contact with the trabecula at various sites (Fig.6.).

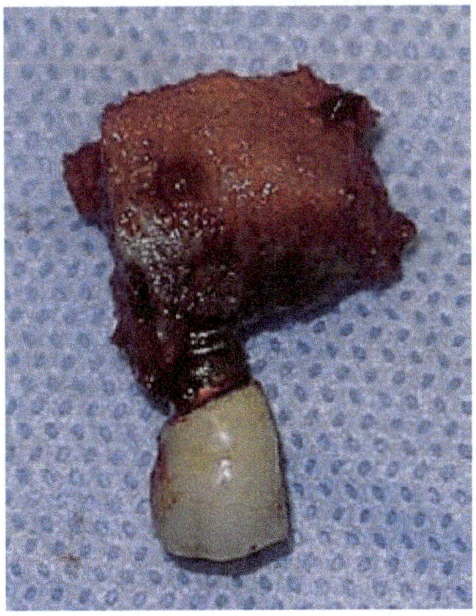

Fig. 5. The resected specimen shows a portion of the left maxilla including two implants.

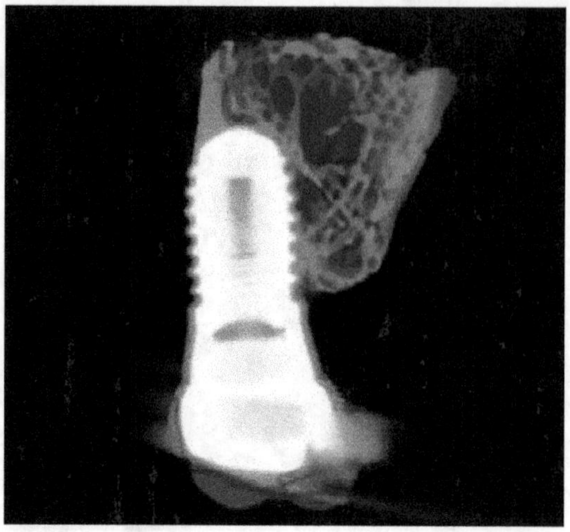

Fig. 6. μCT findings of the resected specimen.

2.4 Histopathological analysis

2.4.1 Histologic preparation

The resected specimen was divided into the lesion including the implants and peri-lesion, i.e., healthy tissue in the resected stump. The bone tissue around the implants was fixed, dehydrated, and embedded in polyester resin (Ligorac®, Wako Pure Chemical Industries, Ltd., Tokyo, Japan). Undecalcified ground sections 15 μm in thickness were cut along the long axis of the implant using the EXAKT Cutting-Grinding System (EXAKT, Norderstedt, Germany) and stained with 1% toluidine blue (pH 7.2), then the bone tissue around the implant was observed under light microscopy. Meanwhile, the bone tissue around the lesion was dehydrated and embedded in paraffin according to the conventional procedure. Some of the sections were stained with hematoxylin-eosin (HE) and AZAAN. Other sections were processed for immunohistochemical analysis by immunostaining with anti-human CD3, CD20, CD45 and CD68 (Daco, Carpinteria, CA).

2.4.2 Peri-implant histopathological findings in undecalcified ground sections

The implant surface was mostly in direct contact with bone tissue, suggesting that osseointegration was maintained until BRONJ development (Fig.7a). No osteocyte was present in the cavity of bone contacting implants or the surrounding trabeculae, nor were there cellular components on the bone surface, and bone tissue mostly showed sequestration (Fig.7b). The marrow cavity was filled with aggregates of actinomycete-like microorganisms, neutrophils, and other necrotized soft tissue (Fig.8a). In addition, adsorption cavities with a worm-eaten appearance were widely present. Normally, bone tissue necrotized in the body is absorbed by osteoclasts, shows sequestration, and is naturally excreted. However, no osteoclasts were present in the resorption cavity, suggesting that active resorption of the bone occurred in the BRONJ developmental process, rather than the resorption of necrotized bone by osteoclasts (Fig.8b).

2.4.3 Histopathological findings around lesions in decalcified sections

Osteocytes were present in the bone cavity (Fig.9a,b). The trabecular surface was smooth, and osteoid formation and osteoblast arrangement were observed. Reactive bone formation was also observed at various trabecular sites. Granulation tissue rich in capillary blood

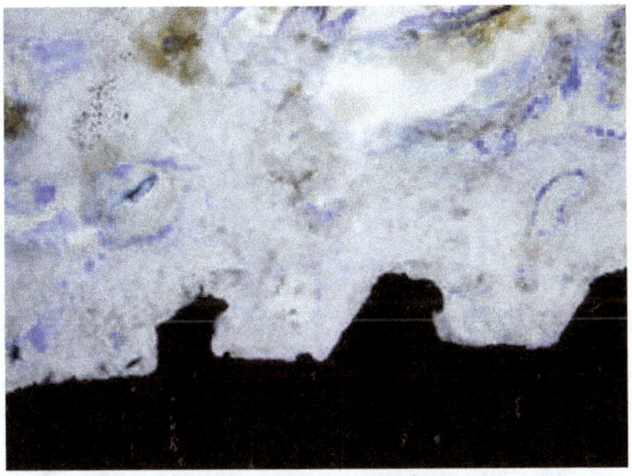

(a) Most of the implant surfaces are in direct contact with the bone (× 40).

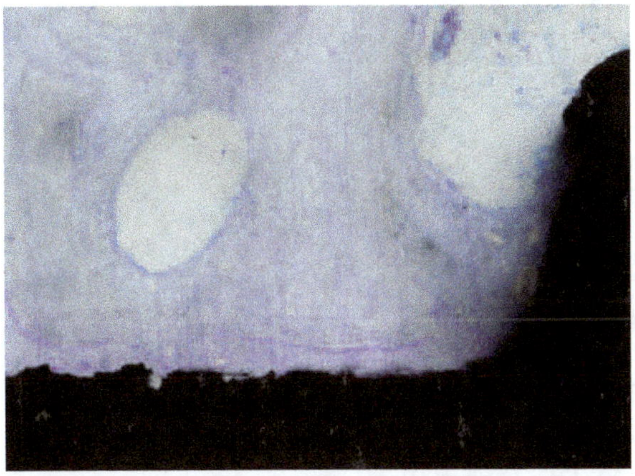

(b) The bone in contact with the implant sureface is necrotic (× 200).

Fig. 7. Histological findings of the tissue from the implants in an undecalcofied sections stained with toluidine blue.

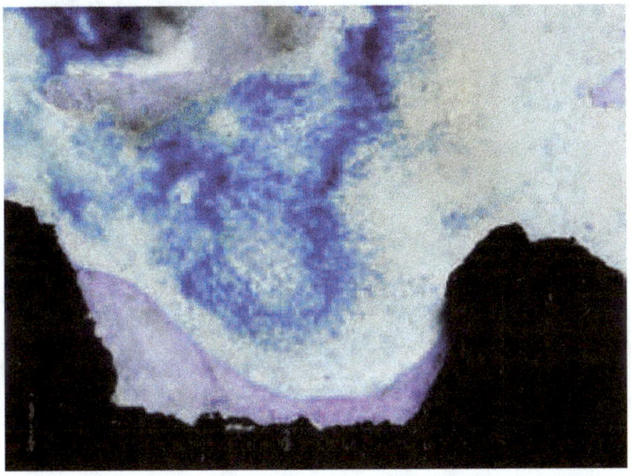

(a) Growth of a bacterial colony into the marrow cavity is observed (× 200).

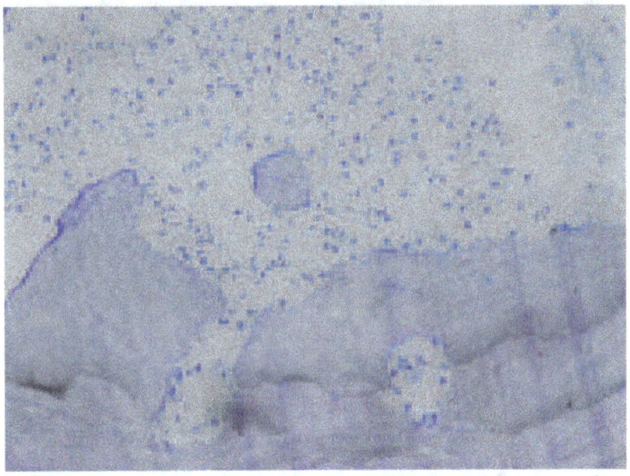

(b) Marked bone destruction with a moth eaten appearance is observed on the necrotic trabecular bone surface (× 200).

Fig. 8. Histological findings of the tissue from the implants in an undecalcofied sections stained with toluidine blue.

vessels invaded the bone marrow region (Fig.10a,b). On immunohistological staining, lymphocytes infiltrating the bone marrow were mostly CD3-positive, showing that the cells were derived from T cells. In contrast, only a few lymphoctyes were positive for CD20 and CD45 (Fig.11a,b), but they were considered not to be significant. Multinucleated giant cells strongly positive for CD68, assumed to be osteoclasts, were present at various sites on the trabecular surface (Fig.12a,b).

3. Discussion on the peri-implant BRONJ developmental mechanism

No viewpoint regarding the pathogenesis of BRONJ has been established. Based on clinical experience, mucosal injuries caused by poorly fitting dentures and oral surgical treatment, such as that for periodontal disease and tooth extraction, have been reported as local risk factors, but this patient received no surgical dental treatment during the BP administration

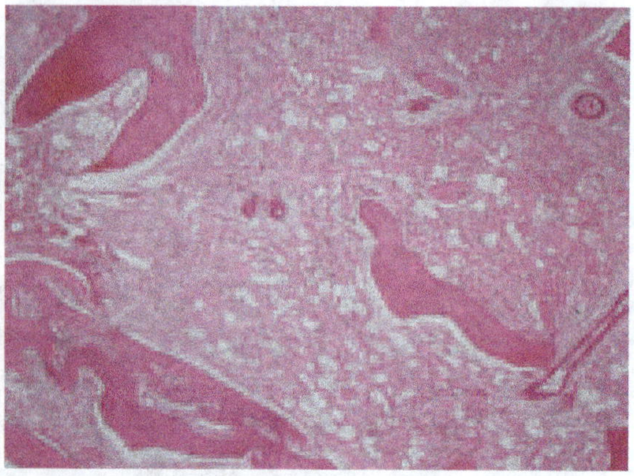

(a) The trabecular bone surface are smooth (HE stain; × 40)

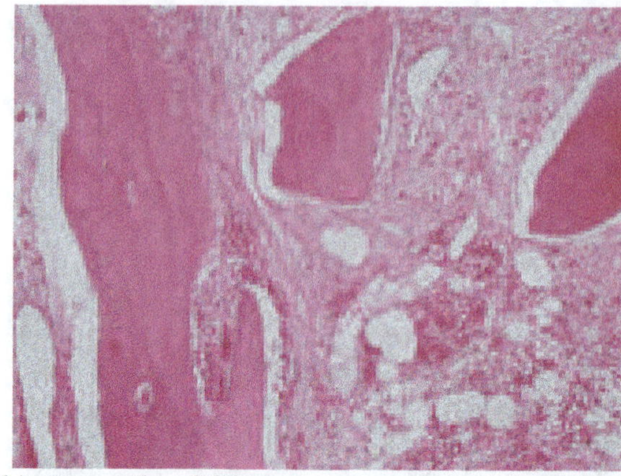

b) Growth of fibrous connective tissue and vascular formation are observed in the marrow(HE stain, × 100).

Fig. 9. Histological findings of the tissue around the lesion in a decalcified thin section.

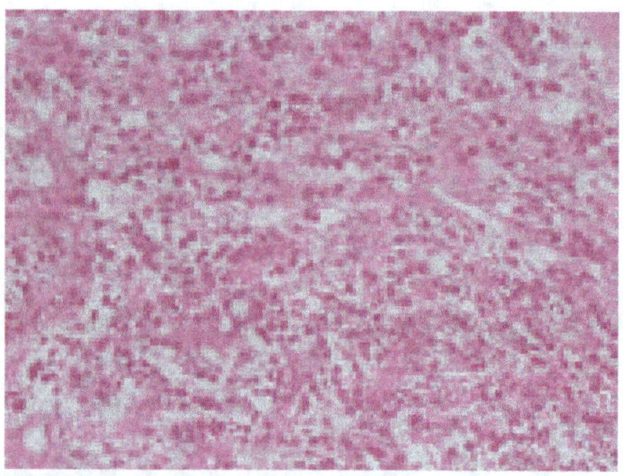

(a) Numerous lymphoid cells are observed in the marrow (HE stain; × 200).

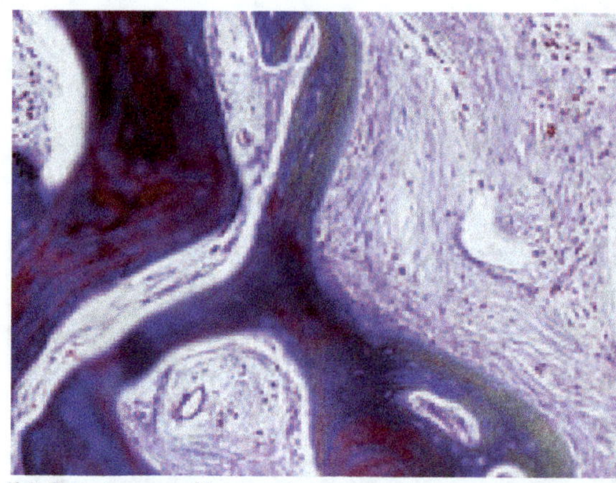

(b) Lining cells and osteoid formation are observed (AZAN; × 100).

Fig. 10. Histological findings of the tissue around the lesion in a decalcified thin section.

(a) Many lymphoid cells are positive for anti-human CD3 (× 200).

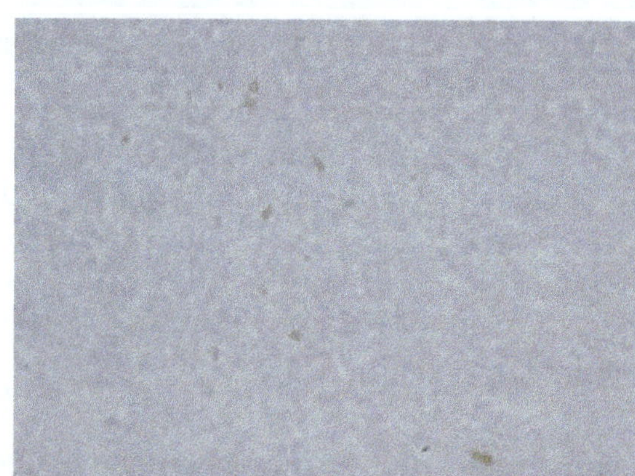

(b) Only a few lymphoctyes are positive for CD20 (× 200).

Fig. 11. Immunohistological staining ot hte tissue around the lesion in a decalcified thin section.

(a) Only a few lymphoctyes are positive for CD45 (× 200).

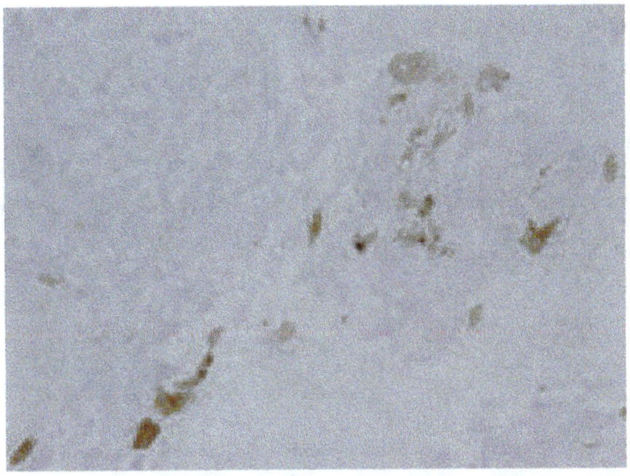

(b) Multinuclear cells are strongly positive for anti-human CD68 antibody (× 200).

Fig. 12. Immunohistological staining ot hte tissue around the lesion in a decalcified thin section.

period, and no implant mobility was observed in the BRONJ site. Histologically, oseointegration was widely maintained on the implant surface, and no deep overgrowth of gingival epithelium was noted, suggesting that BRONJ in this patient suddenly occurred around favorably functioning implants, and was not induced by peri-implant inflammation.

Necrosis of the femoral head (Kerachian et al. 2006) and irradiation-induced osteonecrosis of the jaw (Marx 1983) are widely known as osteonecrotic lesions, and the cause is insufficiency of vascular formation in both diseases. Reportedly, zoledronate exhibits a potent vascularization-inhibitory effect (Giraudo et al. 2004), and the BP-induced obstruction of blood vessels in bone and necrosis of osteocytes around them have been reported (Hansen et al. 2007). Based on these findings, it is hypothesized that insufficiency of the blood supply is also involved in BRONJ, but, histologically, the absence of vascularization inhibition in BRONJ has been reported (Bedogni et al. 2008). Another important hypothesis suggests an influence of reduced bone remodeling due to the BP-induced inhibition of bone resorption by osteoclasts. It has been reported that osteocyte mortality increases when bone remodeling declines, i.e., BPs reduce bone remodeling, increasing osteocyte death, which is involved in BRONJ (Allen et al. 2009). However, many resorption cavities were present on the peri-implant-sequestered bone surface, and the growth of granulation tissue containing abundant capillary blood vessels and reactive bone formation in the resected stump were confirmed in this patient. Thus, it is difficult to explain the cause of BRONJ with insufficient blood supply and the bone remodeling-inhibitory effect of BPs alone.

Pamidronate and zoledronate administered intravenously to this patient are BPs that incorporate nitrogen. BPs containing nitrogen (NBPs) induce an inflammatory reaction by stimulating cells (Hewit et al. 2005; Endo et al. 1993; Nakamura et al. 1996). NBPs also exist on the surface of gram-negative cell walls, and increase inflammatory reactions to lipopolysaccharide (LPS), which has a strong inflammatory effect (Yamaguchi et al. 2000). Therefore, BRONJ may be caused by interactions among several factors differing among cases, not by a single cause. For example, in this patient, the following conditions may have influenced each other and caused BRONJ: 1) the excessive inhibition of bone turnover due to the NBP-related inhibition of bone resorption; 2) the occlusal force loaded on implants was directly transmitted to the bone, which activated local bone metabolism in the surrounding region, releasing BP accumulated in the bone at a high level; 3) free NBP-induced inflammatory reactions, induction of osteoclast apoptosis (Roelofs et al. 2006), and inhibition of epithelial activity (Landesberg et al. 2009); 4) increased risk of bacterial infection due to suppression of the immune system; 5) enhanced inflammatory reactions due to interactions between gram-negative bacterial lipopolysaccharides and NBPs and 6) reduced local blood flow by vascularization inhibition and vascular obstruction (Fig.13).

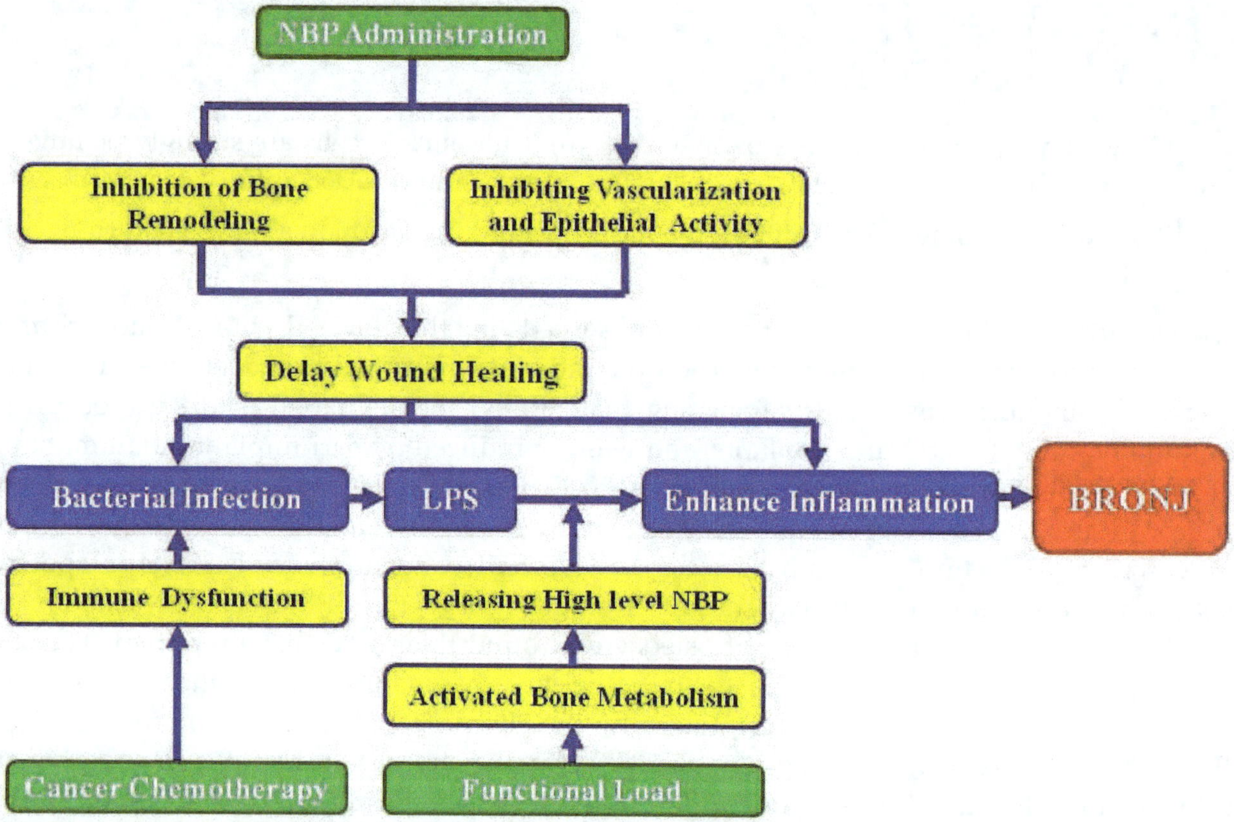

Fig. 13. Hypothetical mechanism of BRONJ aroud the implants.

4. Conclusion

BRONJ is intractable, and no treatment method has been established. Only guidelines mainly concerning prevention and conservative treatment have been proposed. When peri-implant BRONJ occurs, firstly, conservative treatment should be selected following the AAOMS treatment guidelines, placing great importance on the prevention of exacerbation of BRONJ, but when NBPs are administered to control bone metastasis, it should be a priority to re-start BP administration and prevent any delay in cancer chemotherapy. Accordingly, although the appropriateness and timing of sequestration site resection should be carefully investigated, active surgical treatment may be one choice for some patients. Implant treatment is no longer special treatment. It is widely introduced into routine dental practice as a method to recover the occlusal function of defective teeth. Therefore, NBP intravenous injections will be increasingly administered to patients with a past medical history of implant treatment, for which the establishment of a practical clinical policy for the prevention and treatment of BRONJ is strongly desired.

5. References

AAOMS. (2007) American association of oral and maxillofacial surgeons position paper on bisphosphonate-related osteonecrosis of the jaws. *The Journal of Oral and Maxillofacial Surgery*, Vol. 67, No.3, (March 2007), pp. 943-950, ISSN 0278-2391

Allen, M.R. & Burr, D.B. (2009). The pathogenesis of bisphosphonate-related osteonecrosis of the jaw: so many hypotheses, so few data. *The Journal of Oral and Maxillofacial surgaery*, Vol.67 No.5 Supplement 1, (May 2009), pp. 61-70, ISSN 0278-2391

Bedogni, A., Blandamura, S., Lokmic, Z., Palumbo, C., Ragazzo, M., Ferrari, F., Tregnaghi, A., Pietrogrande, F., Procopio, O., Saia, G., Ferretti, M., Bedogni, G., Chiarini, L., Ferronato, G., Ninfo, V., Lo Russo, L., Lo Muzio, L. & Nocini P.F. (2008). Bisphosphonate-associated jawbone osteonecrosis: a correlation between imaging techniques and histopathology. *Oral Surgery, Oral Medicine, Oral Pathology, Oral Radiology and Endodontology*, Vol. 105, No. 3, (March 2009), pp.358-364, ISSN 1079-2104

Bell, B.M., & Bell, R.E. (2008). Oral bisphosphonates and dental implants: a retrospective study. *The Journal of Oral and Maxillofacial Surgaery*, Vol. 66, No.5, (May 2008), pp.1022-1024, ISSN 1079-2104

Berenson, J. R., Lichtenstein, A., Porter, L., Dimopoulos, M.A., Bordoni, R., George, S., Lipton, A., Keller, A., Ballester, O., Kovacs, M. J., Blacklock H.A., Bell, R., Simeone, J., Reitsma, D. J., Hefferman, M., Seaman, J. & Knight, R. D. (1996). Efficacy of pamidronate in reducing skeletal event in patients with advanced multiple myeloma. Myeloma Aredia Study Group. *The New England Journal of Medicine*, Vol. 334, No. 8, (Feburuary 1996), pp.488-493, ISSN 0028-4793

Body, J. J., Lortholary, A., Romieu, G., Vigneron, A. M. & Ford, J. (1999). A dose-finding sudy of zoledronate in hypercalcemic cancer patients. *Journal of Bone and Mineral Research*, Vol.14, No.19, (September 1999), pp.1557-61, ISSN 1523-4681

Bojko, P., Hilger, R.A., Ruehm, S.G., Dirsch, O., Seeber, S. & Scheulen, M.E. (2003). Femoral head necrosis in three patients with relapsed ovarian cancer receiving high-dose chemotherapy followed by autologous peripheral blood stem cell transplantation. *Bone Marrow Teansplantation*, Vol. 31, No.6, (March 2003), pp.487-491, ISSN 0268-3369

Endo, Y., Nakamura, M., Kikuchi, T., Shinoda, H., Takeda. Y., Nitta, Y. & Kumagai, K. (1993) Aminoalkylbisphosphonates, potent inhibitors of bone resorption, induce a prolonged stimulation of histamine synthesis and increase macrophages, granulocytes, and osteoclasts in vivo. *Calcified Tissue International* Vol.52, No.3, (March 1993), pp.248-254, ISSN 0171-967X

Fleisch, H., Reszka, A., Rodan, G. & Rogers, M. (2002). Bisphosphonates: Mechanisms of action, *Principles of Bone Biology*, Bilezikian, J. P., Raisz, L. G. & Rodan, G.A., pp. 13161-1385, Academic Press, ISBN 012-0986-523, San Diego

Freiberger, J.J. (2009). Utility of hyperbaric oxygen in treatment of bisphosphonate-related osteonecrosis of the jaws. *The Journal of Oral Maxillofacial Surgery*. Vol.67, No.5 Supplement 1, (March 2009), pp.96-106, ISSN 1079-2104

Fugazzotto, P.A., Lightfoot, W.S., Jaffin, R. & Kumar, A. (2007). Implant placement with or without simultaneous tooth extraction in patients taking oral bisphosphonates: postoperative healing, early follow-up, and the incidence of complications in two private practices. *Journal of Periodontology*, Vol.78, No.9, (September 2007), pp.1664-1669 ISSN 0022-3492

Giraudo, E., Inoue, M. & Hanahan, D. (2004). An amino-bisphosphonate targets MMP-9-expressing macrophages and angiogenesis to impair cervical carcinogenesis. *The Journal of Clinical Investigation*, Vol.114, No.5, (September 1 2004), pp.623-633, ISSN, 0021-9738

Grant, B.T., Amenedo, C., Freeman, K. & Kraut RA. (2008). Outcomes of placing dental implants in patients taking oral bisphosphonates: a review of 115 cases. *The Journal of Oral and Maxillofacial Surgery*, Vol. 66, No.2, (February 2008), pp.223-230, ISSN 0278-2391

Hansen, T., Kunkel, M., Springer, E., Walter, C., Weber, A., Siegel, E. & Kirkpatrick, C.J. (2007). Actinomycosis of the jaws--histopathological study of 45 patients shows significant involvement in bisphosphonate-associated osteonecrosis and infected osteoradionecrosis *Virchows Archiv* Vol.451, No.6, (December 2007), pp.1009-1017, ISSN 0945-6317

Hewit, R.E., Lissina, A., Green, A.E., Slay, E.S., Price, D.A. & Sewell, D.A. (2005) The bisphosphonate acute phase response: rapid and copious production of proinflammatory cytokines by peripheral blood gd T cells in response to aminobisphosphonates is inhibited by statins. *Clinical Experimental Immunology*, Vol.139, No.1, (January 2005), pp.101-111, ISSN 0009-9104

Hortobagyi, G. N., Theriault, R. L., Lipton, A., Porter, L., Blayney, D., Sinoff, C., Wheeler, H., Simeone, J. F., Seaman, J. J., Knight, R. D., Heffernan, M., Mellars, K. & Reitsma, D. J. (1998). Long-term prevention of skeletal complications of metastatic brest cancer with pamidronate. Protocol 19 Aredia Brest Cancer Study Group. *Journal of Clinical Oncology*, Vol.16, No.6, (June 1998), pp.2038-2044, ISSN 0732-183X

Karimova, E.J., Rai, S.N., Wu, J., Britton, L., Kaste, S.C. & Neel, M.D. (2008). Femoral resurfacing inyoung patients with hematologic cancer and osteonecrosis. *Clinical Orthopaedics Related Research*, Vol. 466, No. 12, (December 2008), pp.3044-3050, ISSN 1528-1132

Kerachian, M.A., Harvey, E. J., Cournoyer, D., Chow, T.Y. & Séguin C. (2006). A vascular necrosis of the femoral head: vascular hypotheses. *Journal of Endothelial Cell Research*, Vol.23, No. 4, (July-August 2006), pp.237-244, ISSN 1062-3329

Khan, A.A., Sándor, G.K., Dore, E., Morrison, A.D., Alsahli, M., Amin, F., Peters, E., Hanley, D.A., Chaudry, S.R., Dempster, D.W., Glorieux, F.H., Neville, A.J., Talwar, R.M., Clokie, C.M., Al Mardini, M., Paul, T., Khosla, S., Josse, R. G., Sutherland, S., Lam, D.K., Carmichael, R.P., Blanas, N., Kendler, D., Petak, S., St-Marie, L.G., Brown, J., Evans, A.W., Rios L. & Compston, J.E.; Canadian Association of Oral and Maxillofacial Surgeons. (2008). Canadian consensus practice guidelines for bisphosphonate associated osteonecrosis of the jaw. *The Journal of Rheumatology*, Vol.35, No.7, (July 2008), pp.1391-1397, ISSN 0315-162X

Khosla, S., Burr, D., Cauley, J., Dempster, D.W., Ebeling, P.R., Felsenberg, D., Gagel, R.F., Gilsanz , V., Guise, T., Koka, S., McCauley, L.K., McGowan, J., McKee, M.D., Mohla, S., Pendrys, D.G., Raisz, L.G., Ruggiero, S.L., Shafer, D.M., Shum, L., Silverman, S.L., Van Poznak, C.H., Watts, N., Woo, S.B. & Shane, E.; American Society for Bone and Mineral Research. (2007). Bisphosphonate-associated osteonecrosis of the jaw: Report of a task force of the American Society for Bone and Mineral Research. *Journal of Bone and Mineral Research*, Vol.22, No. 10, (October 2007), pp.1479-1491, ISSN 1523-4681

Kubo, T., Kojima, A., Yamazoe, S., Ueshima, K., Yamamoto, T. & Hirasawa, Y. (2001). Osteonecrosis of the femoral head that developed after long-term topical application. *Journal of Orthopaedic Science*, Vol.6, No.1, (January 2001), pp.92-94, ISSN 0949-2658

Landesberg, R., Eisig, S., Fennoy, I. & Siris, E. (2009). Alternative indications for bisphosphonate therapy. *The Journal of Oral and Maxillofacial Surgery*, Vol.67, No.5 Supplement 1, (May 2009), pp.27-34, ISSN 1079-2104

Marx, R. E. (1983). Osteonecrosis: a new concept of its pathophysiology. J *The Journal of Oral and Maxillofacial Surgery*, Vol.41, No.5, (May 1983), pp. 283-288, ISSN 1079-2104

Marx, R. E. (2003). Pamidronate (Aredia) and Zoledronate (Zometa) Induced Avascular Necrosis of the Jaws: A growing epidemic. *Journal of Oral and Maxillofacial Surgery*, Vol.61, No.9, (September 2003), pp.1115-1117, ISSN 1079-2104

Marx, R. E., Sawatari, Y., Fortin, M. & Broumand, N. (2005). Bisphosphonate-induced exposed bone (osteonecrosis/osteopetrosis) of the jaws. Journal of Oral and Maxillofacial Surgery, Vol.63, No.11, (November 2005), pp.1567-1575, ISSN 1079-2104

Migliorati, C.A., Casiglia, J., Epstein, J., Jacobsen, P.L., Siegel, M.A. & Woo, S.B. (2005). Managing the care of patients with bisphosphonate-associated osteonecrosis: an American Academy of Oral Medicine position paper. *Journal of the American Dental Association*, Vol.136, No.12, (December 2005), pp.1658-68, ISSN 0002-8177

Nakamura, M., Ando, T., Abe, M., Kumagai, K & Endo, Y. (1996) Contrast between effects of aminobisphosphonates and non-aminobisphosphonates on collagen-induced arthritis in mice. *British Journal of Pharmacology*, Vol.119, No.2, (September 1996), pp.205-212, ISSN 1476-5381

Roelofs, A.J., Thompson, K., Gordon, S. & Rogers, M.J. (2006). Molecular mechanisms of action of bisphosphonates: current status. *Clinical Cancer Research*, Vol.12, No.20 Pt 2, (October 2006), pp.6222s-6230s, ISSN1557-3265

Ruggiero, S. L., Mehrotra, B., Rosenberg, T.J. & Engroff, S. L. (2004). Osteonecrosis of the Jaws associated with the use of bisphosphonates: a review of 63 cases. *The Journal of Oral and Maxillofacial Surgery*, Vol.62, No.5, pp.527-534, ISSN 1079-2104

Ruggiero, S.L., Dodson, T.B., Assael, L.A., Landesberg, R., Marx, R.E. & Mehrotra, B.; American Association of oral and Maxillofacial Surgeons. (2009). American Association of Oral and Maxillofacial Surgeons Position Paper on Bisphosphonate-Related Osteonecrosis of the Jaws – 2009 update. *The Journal of Oral and Maxillofacial Surgery*, Vol.67, No.5 Supplement, pp.2-12, ISSN 1079-2104

Russell, R.G., Xia, Z., Dunford, J.E., Oppermann, U., Kwaasi, A., Hulley, P.A., Kavanagh, K.L., Triffitt, J.T., Lundy, M.W., Phipps, R.J., Barnet, B.L., Coxon, F.P., Rogers, M.J., Wattss, N.B. & Ebetino, F.H. (2007). Bisphosphonates an update on mechanisms of action and how these relate to clinical efficacy. *Annals of the New York Academy of Sciences* Vol.1117, (November 2007), pp.209-257, ISSN 1749-6632

Shirota, T., Nakamura, A., Matsui, Y., Hatori, M., Nakamura, M. & Shintani, S. (2009) Bisphosphonate-related osteonecrosis of the jaw around dental implants in the maxilla: report of a case. *Clinical Oral Implants Ressearch*, Vol.20, No.12, (December 2009), pp. 1402-1408, ISSN 0905-7161

Starck, W.J. & Epker, B.N. (1995). Failure of osseointegrated dental implants after diphosphonate therapy for osteoporosis: a case report. *The International Journal of Oral & Maxillofacacial Implants,* Vol. 10, No.1, (January-February 1995), pp.74-78, 0882-2786

Vahtsevanos, K., Kyrgidis, A., Verrou, E., Katodritou, E., Triaridis, S., Andreadis, C.G., Boukovinas, I., Koloutsos, G.E., Teleioudis, Z., Kitikidou, K., Paraskevopoulos, P., Zervas, K. & Antoniades, K. (2009). Longitudinal cohort study of risk factors in cancer patients of bisphosphonate-related osteonecrosis of the jaw. Journal of *Clinical Oncology,* Vol.27, No.32, (November 2009), pp.5356-5362, ISSN 0732-183X

Yamaguchi, K., Motegi, K., Iwakura, Y. & Endo, Y. (2000). Involvement of interleukin-1 in the inflammatory actions of aminobisphosphonates in mice. *British Journal of Pharmacology,* Vol.130, No.7, (August 2000), pp.1646-1654, ISSN 1476-5381

Yoneda, T., Hagino, H., Sugimoto, T., Ohta, H, Takahashi, S., Soen, S., Taguchi, A., Toyosawa, S., Nagata, T. & Urade, M. (2010). Bisphosphonate-related osteonecrosis of the jaw: position paper from the Allied Task Force Committee of Japanese Society for Bone and Mineral Research, Japan Osteoporosis Society, Japanese Society of Periodontology, Japanese Society for Oral and Maxillofacial Radiology, and Japanese Society of Oral and Maxillofacial Surgeons. *Journal of Bone and Mineral Metabolism,* Vol.28, No.4, pp.365-383, ISSN 1435-5604

2

Dental Implant Surface Enhancement and Osseointegration

S.Anil[1,4], P.S. Anand[2], H. Alghamdi[3,4] and J.A. Jansen[3,4]
[1]*Department of Periodontics and Community Dentistry, College of Dentistry, King Saud University, Riyadh*
[2]*People's College of Dental Sciences & Research Centre, Bhanpur, Bhopal, Madhya Pradesh,*
[3]*Radboud University Nijmegen Medical Center, HB Nijmegen,*
[4]*Dental Implant and Osseointegration Research Chair, King Saud University, Riyadh*
[1,4]*Saudi Arabia*
[2]*India*
[3]*The Netherlands*

1. Introduction

The long-term success of dental implants largely depends on rapid healing with safe integration into the jaw bone. Geometry and surface topography are crucial for the short- and long-term success of dental implants. Implant surfaces have been developed in the last decade in a concentrated effort to provide bone in a faster and improved osseointegration process. Several surface modifications have been developed and are currently used with the aim of enhancing clinical performance, including turned, blasted, acid-etched, porous-sintered, oxidized, plasma-sprayed and hydroxyapatite-coated surfaces, as well as combinations of these procedures. Among the several parameters influencing the success of the implants, implant-bone interface plays an important role in prolonging the longevity and improving the function of the implant-supported prosthesis. There are several modalities to improve implant-bone interface to promote faster and more effective osseointegration.

Osseointegration, defined as a direct structural and functional connection between ordered, living bone and the surface of a load-carrying implant, is critical for implant stability, and is considered a prerequisite for implant loading and long-term clinical success of endosseous dental implants. Osseointegration of titanium implant surfaces is dependent upon both physical and chemical properties (Sul *et al.*, 2005). This structural and functional union of the implant with living bone is strongly influenced by the surface properties of the titanium implant. As titanium and its alloys cannot directly bond with living bone, modification of the implant surface has been proposed as a method for enhancing osseointegration.

Scientific research works to assess the influence of implant surface properties on bone healing have identified several factors which are important for osseointegration. The surface characteristics of implant which influence the speed and strength of osseointegration include surface chemistry, topography, wettability, charge, surface energy, crystal structure and crystallinity, roughness, chemical potential, strain hardening, the presence of impurities, thickness of titanium oxide layer, and the presence of metal and non-metal composites. Among these, wettability and free surface energy of an implant surface are considered to be very crucial. The implant surface, including topography, chemistry, surface charge, and wettability, has been described as an important factor to influence osseointegration. The influence of physical properties such as surface topography and roughness on osseointegration have translated to shorter healing times from implant placement to restoration (Cochran *et al.*, 2002). The biologic basis underlying these clinical improvements continues to be explored (Kim *et al.*, 2005, Lossdorfer *et al.*, 2004). Albrektsson *et al.* (1981) suggested six factors that are particluary important for the establishment of reliable osseointegration: implant material, implant design, surface conditions, status of the bone, surgical technique, and implant loading conditions.

2. Biology of wound healing following implant placement

Wound healing involves a highly orchestrated sequence of events which is triggered by tissue injury involving soluble mediators, blood cells, extracellular matrix and parenchymal cells. Ultimately, it culminates in either partial or complete regeneration or repair. Fracture healing in bone occurs in four phases which include inflammation, soft and hard callus formation, and remodeling. Following a fracture, blood coagulation and hematoma formation takes place. This is followed by inflammation. Various chemical mediators such as thrombin and growth factors released by activated leukocytes and platelets in the hematoma serve as chemotactic signals to many cell types which play an important role in bone healing. Unlike soft tissue healing, bone healing does not lead to scarring. Instead it leads to restoration of the bony tissue. During successful implantation, insertion of metal implants into cortical bone eventually leads to complete healing. Following implant placement, unlike in fracture healing, implants extend into and persist in the marrow spaces and this may have a bearing on the healing process. Although implant healing must to some extent adjust to the presence of the implant, ultimately, sound bony tissues will be completely restored during wound healing. This adjustment involves imbedding the implant surface in a layer of bone, continuous with the original bone.

Wound healing around a dental implant placed into a prepared osteotomy follows three stages of repair- Initial formation of a blood clot occurs through a biochemical activation followed by a cellular activation and finally a cellular response(Stanford and Schneider, 2004). During surgery, dental implant surfaces interact with blood components from ruptured blood vessels. Within a short period of time, various plasma proteins such as fibrin get adsorbed on the material surface. Fibrinogen is converted to fibrin and the complement and kinin systems become activated. As in fracture healing, the migration of bone cells in peri-implant healing will occur through the fibrin of a blood clot. Since fibrin has the potential to adhere to almost all surfaces, it can be anticipated that the migration of osteogenic cell populations towards the implant surface will occur. However, as the migration of cells through fibrin will cause retraction of the fibrin scaffold, the ability of an implant surface to retain this fibrin scaffold during the phase of wound contraction is critical in determining whether the migrating cells will reach the implant surface. Activation of platelets occurs as a result of interaction of platelets with the implant surface as well as the fibrin scaffold and this leads to thrombus formation and blood clotting.

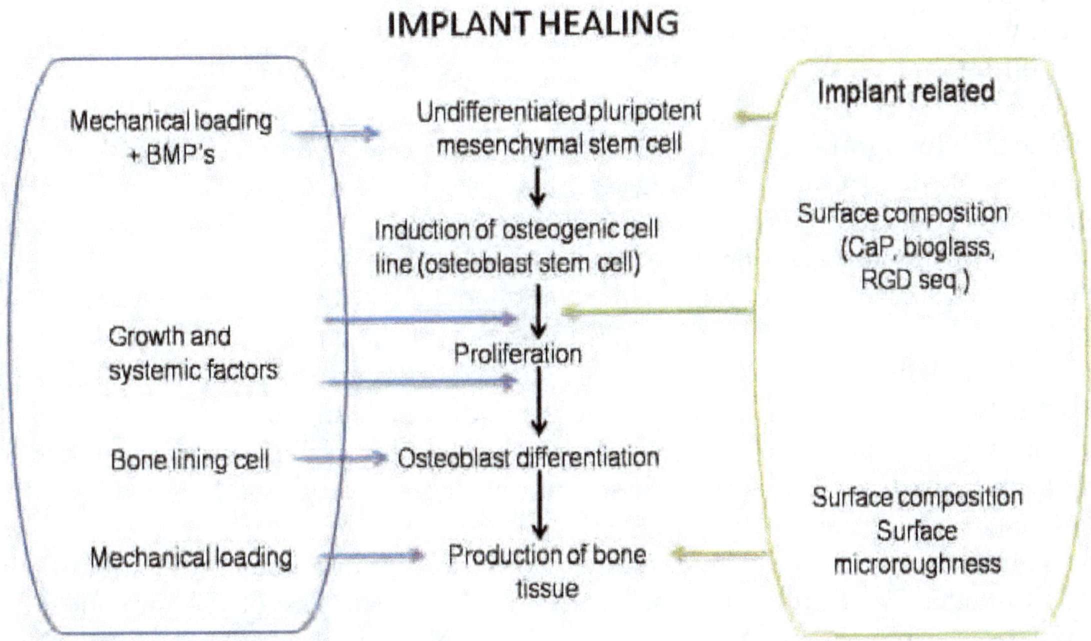

Fig. 1. The implant healing process - The surface composition, roughness and topography are interrelated surface characteristics that influence the biological response to an implant.

Moreover, platelets are a rich source of many growth and differentiation factors which play a key role in the wound healing process by acting as signaling molecules for recruitment and differentiation of the undifferentiated mesechymal stem cells at the implant surface. Plasma also contains dissolved substances such as glucose, amino acids, various ions, cholesterols, and hormones which are needed for the viability of cells and tissues. Blood interactions with implants lead to protein adsorption, which is dependent on the surface properties of the material. As hydrophilic surfaces are better for blood coagulation than hydrophobic surfaces, dental implants have been developed with high hydrophilic and rough implant surfaces which exhibit better osseointegration than conventional ones. Adsorption of proteins such as fibronectin and vitronectin on the surface of dental implants could promote cell adhesion and osseointegration. During the initial remodeling, a number of immune cells mediate early tissue response followed by migration of phagocyte macrophages. These cells initially remove the necrotic debris created by the drilling process and then undergo physiological changes which lead to expression of cell surface proteins and production of cytokines and pro-inflammatory mediators. This cytokine-regulated cellular recruitment, migration, proliferation and formation of an extracellular matrix on the implant surface can be influenced by the macrophages. These cells express growth factors such as fibroblast growth factor (FGF-1, FGF-2, FGF-4), transforming growth factors, epithelial growth factor as well as bone morphogenetic proteins (BMPs). The end result of this complex cascade is promotion of a wound healing process that includes angiogenesis.

3. Influence of implant surface topography on osseointegration

Dental implant quality depends on the chemical, physical, mechanical, and topographic characteristics of the surface (Grassi *et al.*, 2006). These different properties interact and determine the activity of the attached cells that are close to the dental implant surface.

Dental implants have been designed to provide textures and shapes that may enhance cellular activity and direct bone apposition (Huang *et al.*, 2005). Osteogenesis at the implant surface is influenced by several mechanisms. A series of coordinated events, including cell proliferation, transformation of osteoblasts and bone tissue formation might be affected by different surface topographies (Shibli *et al.*, 2007). Amount of bone-to-implant contact (BIC) is an important determinant in long-term success of dental implants. Consequently, maximizing the BIC and osseointegration has become a goal of treatment, which is enhanced by implant surface roughness (Soskolne *et al.*, 2002).

Albrektsson et al (1981) recognized that among the factors influencing BIC such as topography, chemistry, wettability and surface energy the most important is wettability. Surface wettability is largely dependent on surface energy and influences the degree of contact with the physiological environment (Kilpadi and Lemons, 1994, Zhao *et al.*, 2005). Several evaluations have demonstrated that implants with rough surfaces show better bone apposition and BIC than implants with smooth surfaces (Buser *et al.*, 1999, Cochran *et al.*, 2002).

Surface roughness also has a positive influence on cell migration and proliferation, which in turn leads to better BIC results, suggesting that the microstructure of the implant influences biomaterial–tissue interaction (Matsuo *et al.*, 1999, Novaes *et al.*, 2002). Implant surface properties are likely to be of particular relevance to the chemical and biological interface processes in the early healing stages after implantation. It is generally accepted that these early stages are likely to have an effect on the host response to the implant and, therefore, the long-term outcome and success of the treatment. Surface chemistry has the potential to alter ionic interactions, protein adsorption, and cellular activity at the implant surface (Schliephake *et al.*, 2005). These modifications may subsequently influence conformational changes in the structures and interactive natures of adsorbed proteins and cells. Furthermore, within the complexities of an *in vivo* environment containing multiple protein and cellular interactions, these alterations may differentially regulate biologic events. Modifications to the implant surface chemistry may lead to alterations in the structure of adsorbed proteins and have cascading effects that may ultimately be evident at the clinical level.

In vivo evidence has supported the use of alterations in surface chemistry to modify osseointegration events. Specifically, an investigation utilizing sandblasted, large-grit, acid-etched (SLA) surfaces that were chemically different but had the same physical properties was conducted to assess BIC as a measure of osseointegration. The chemically enhanced SLA surface demonstrated significantly enhanced BIC during the first 4 weeks of bone healing, with 60% more bone than the standard SLA surface after 2 weeks (Buser *et al.*, 2004). The chemical modifications for the test SLA surface resulted in increased wettability (ie, in a hydrophilic surface rather than a hydrophobic one). Water contact angles of zero degrees were seen with the chemically enhanced surface compared to 139.9 degrees for a standard SLA surface, and the hydrophilicity was maintained after drying. The chemical composition of the surface was also altered, including a 50% reduction in carbon concentration compared with the control implant surface (Rupp *et al.*, 2006).

4. Interaction between cells and the surface of the dental implants

Since surface properties of biomaterials are important parameters influencing cellular reactions towards artificial materials, the properties of dental implant surfaces are extremely important in influencing the healing process leading to osseointegration and ultimate clinical success of the implant. Surface morphology modulates the response of cells to a dental implant, and surfaces with defined microstructures may be useful for enhancement of the stable anchorage (Elias and Meirelles, 2010). Surface chemistry involves adhesion of proteins, bacteria, and cells on implants. Wettability and surface energy influence the adsorption of proteins, and increase adhesion of osteoblasts on the implant surface. The cell behavior on a hydrophilic surface is completely different from that on a hydrophobic one. A hydrophilic surface is better for blood coagulation than a hydrophobic surface. The expressions of bone-specific differentiation factors for osteoblasts are higher on hydrophilic surfaces. Consequently, dental implants manufacturers have developed high hydrophilic and rough implant surfaces which in turn exhibited better osseointegration than implants with smooth surfaces.

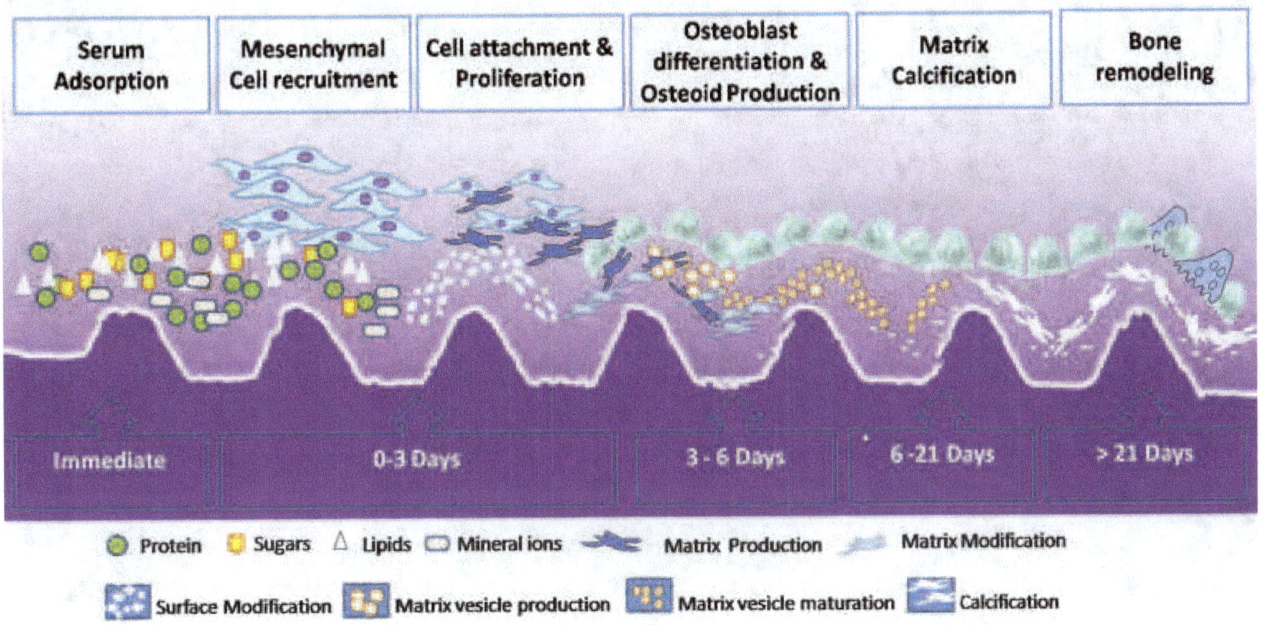

Fig. 2. Illustration showing the cellular phenomena at the implant bone interface during healing of implant

5. Implant surface topography

Implant surface topography refers to macroscopic and microscopic features of the implant surface. Although commercially pure titanium is the prime material of dental implants, the success rates of different commercially available implant systems vary. The exact reason for this is not clear. Several implant-related factors such as implant surface topography, chemical composition and surface roughness that influence osseointegration have been studied. It has been shown that titanium implants with adequate roughness may influence the primary stability of implants, enhance bone-to-implant contact, and may increase removal torque force (Wennerberg and Albrektsson, 2009).

The surface roughness of the implants can significantly alter the process of osseointegration because the cells react differently to smooth and rough surfaces. Fibroblasts and epithelial cells adhere more strongly to smooth surfaces, whereas osteoblastic proliferation and collagen synthesis are increased on rough surfaces (Boyan *et al.*, 2001). Investigators have demonstrated that while the adhesion of fibroblasts is lesser on rough surfaces, the adhesion and differentiation of osteoblastic cells are enhanced (Wennerberg and Albrektsson, 2000). It is not clear whether the height of surface irregularities is more important than the distance between them, and which combination of these factors could improve osseointegration. Although the increase in surface roughness promotes greater mechanical anchorage, the implant-bone interface strength will not increase with the continuous increase of surface roughness.

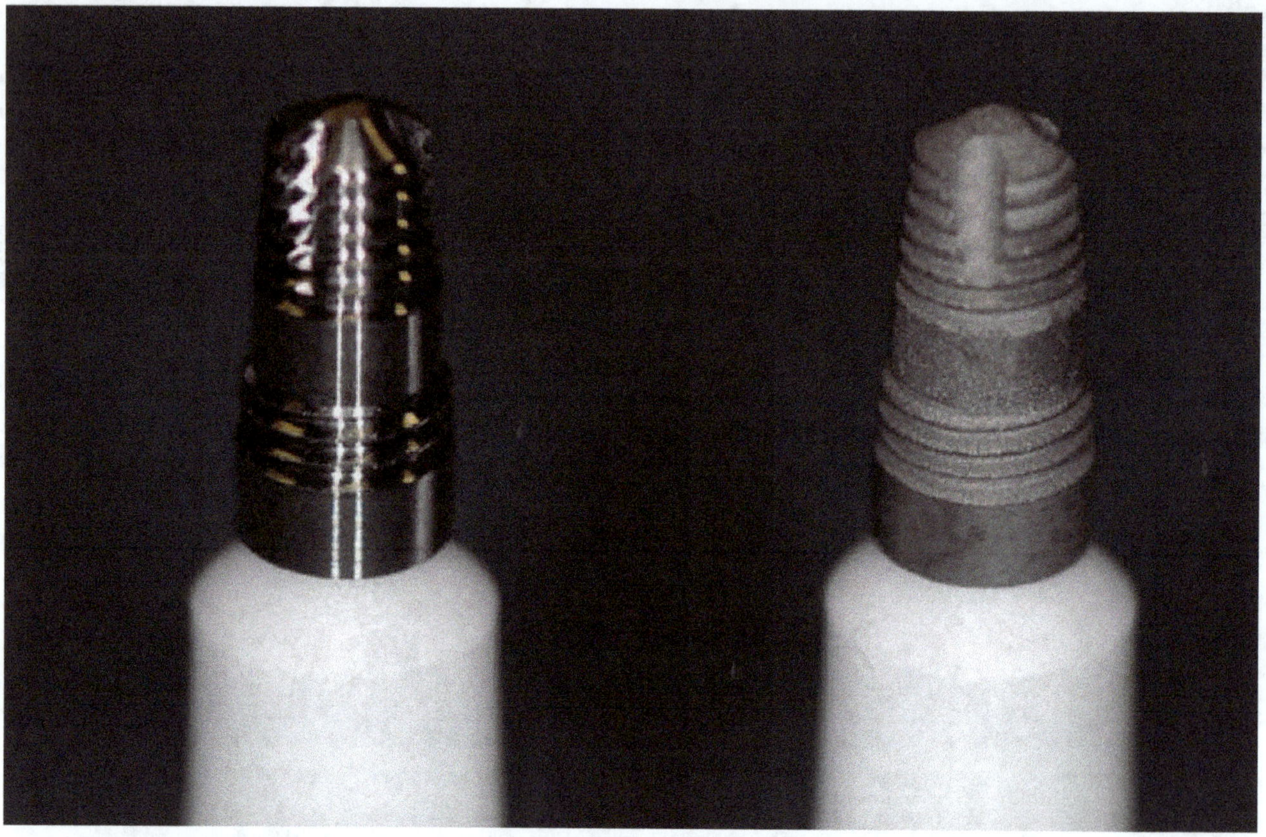

Fig. 3. The machined and nano etched implant surface

6. Surface roughness

Surface topography plays an important role in the osseointegration of titanium implants (Le Guehennec *et al.*, 2007). In vitro and *in vivo* studies have shown that titanium surface roughness influences a number of events in the behavior of cells in the osteoblastic lineage, including spreading and proliferation, differentiation, and protein synthesis (Sammons *et al.*, 2005, Zhao *et al.*, 2006). Implant surface roughness is divided, depending on the dimension of the measured surface features into **macro, micro, and nano-roughness.**

Macro roughness comprises features in the range of millimeters to tens of microns. This scale directly relates to implant geometry, with threaded screw and macro porous surface treatments. The primary implant fixation and long-term mechanical stability can be improved by an appropriate macro roughness. This will enhance the mechanical interlocking between the macro rough features of the implant surface and the surrounding bone (Wennerberg *et al.*, 1996, Shalabi *et al.*, 2006).

Micro roughness is defined as being in the range of 1–10 μm. This range of roughness maximizes the interlocking between mineralized bone and implant surface. Studies supported by some clinical evidence suggest that the micron-level surface topography results in greater accrual of bone at the implant surface (Junker *et al.*, 2009, Shalabi *et al.*, 2006). The use of surfaces provided with **nanoscale topographies** are widely used in recent years. Nanotechnology involves materials that have a nano-sized topography or are composed of nano-sized materials with a size range between 1 and 100 nm. Nanometer roughness plays an important role in the adsorption of proteins, adhesion of osteoblastic cells and thus the rate of osseointegration (Brett *et al.*, 2004).

6.1 Nanotopography

Surface properties play a key role in biological interactions between the implant surfaces and the host bone. Modifying surface roughness has been shown to enhance BIC and improve the clinical performance of implants. The nanometer-sized roughness and the chemistry have a key role in the interactions of surfaces with proteins and cells. These micromechanical features influence the process of secondary integration (bone growth, turnover and remodeling). At the nanoscale, a more textured surface topography increases the surface energy which in turn increases the wettability of the surface to blood, adhesion of cells to the surface, and facilitates binding of fibrin, matrix proteins, growth and differentiation factors. Nanotopography, by modulating cell behavior, can influence the process of cell migration, proliferation, and differentiation. These surfaces thus enhance the process of osseointegration by hastening the wound healing following implant placement (Dohan Ehrenfest *et al.*, 2010).

Various surface modification treatments create a nanometer-scale topography that allows the bone to grow into and maintain the implant surface under elevated shear forces. Grit blasting, anodisation, and acid etching, are the commonly used methods for modifying surface roughness of metal implants. Topographical features in the nanometer ranges may be helpful in the healing process as related to protein adsorption and cell adhesion as surface properties control the steps of adhesion, proliferation, and differentiation of mesenchymal stem cells and, thus, condition tissue integration.

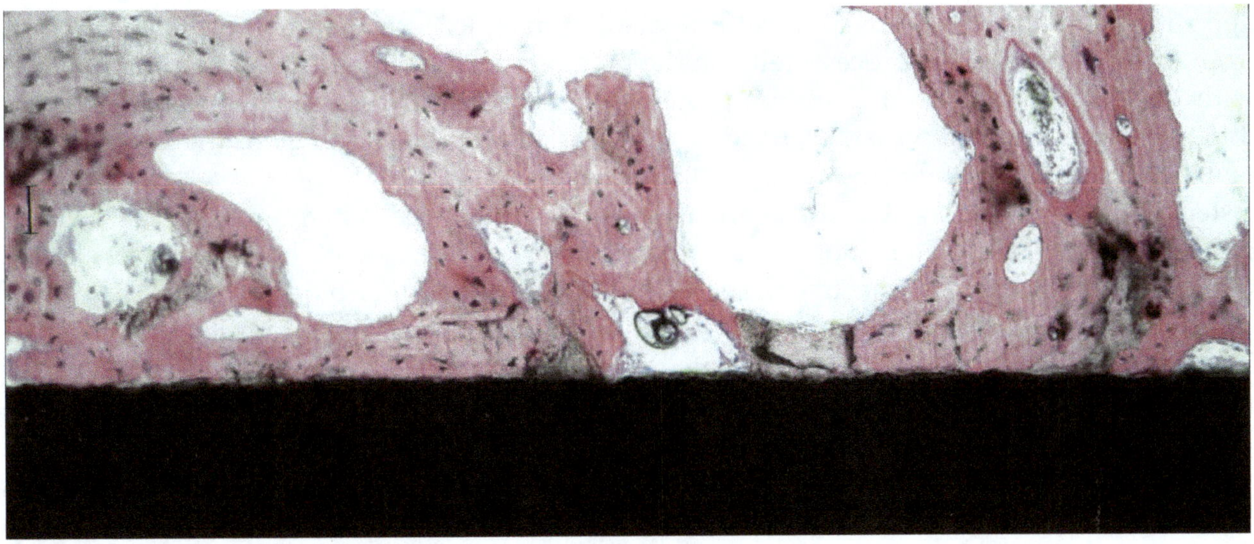

Fig. 4. Showing bone healing at the nanorough surface

Nanotopography modifications are commonly described in the literature both as nanoroughness and nanofeatures. Overall surface roughness will be modified when features are added to the surface, that is, by adding nanofeatures the surface roughness will also be modified. However, the modifications commonly used to produce the so-called nanorough materials do not intentionally produce such nanofeatures. Reproducible surface roughness in the nanometer range is difficult to obtain with chemical treatments. Although, all surfaces may show nanotopography, not all of them will have significant nanostructures. A nanostructure is an object of intermediate size between molecular and micrometre-sized structures, and often defined between 1 and 100 nm (Dohan Ehrenfest *et al.*, 2010). Nanofabricated samples have well-defined dimensions that aim to modulate cell activity, such as migration, attachment, proliferation and differentiation.

Several investigators have revealed that nanoscale topography also influences cell adhesion and osteoblastic differentiation (Dalby *et al.*, 2008, Webster *et al.*, 1999). These findings reiterate observations demonstrating that nanotopography may directly influence adherent cell behavior (Webster *et al.*, 2000). Nanotechnology can alter the implant surface at an atomic level (Oh *et al.*, 2005) and may influence the chemical composition of these surfaces. Nanorough titanium and nanostructured titanium can enhance osteoblast adhesion and differentiation compared to their nanosmooth control. Surfaces with micro- and nanopores have also been shown to greatly enhance osseointegration. The micro- and nanoscale surface properties of metal implant, including chemistry, roughness, and wettability, could affect bone formation. It has been shown that grit-blasting with biphasic calcium phosphate (BCP) ceramic particles gave a high average surface roughness and particle-free surfaces after acid etching of titanium implants. Studies have shown that BCP grit-blasted surfaces promoted an early osteoblast differentiation and bone apposition as compared to mirror-polished titanium. By the process of anodic oxidation, nanoscale oxides may be deposited on surfaces of titanium implants. The nanoscale properties can be controlled by adjusting the parameters for anodization such as voltage, time, and shaking. Osseointegration of dental implants can be improved by the application of calcium phosphate (CaP) coating by plasma spraying, biomimetic and electrophoretic deposition. While plasma-sprayed hydroxyapatite (HA)-coated dental implants have disadvantages related to coating delimitation and heterogeneous dissolution rate of deposited phases, an electrochemical process consisting of depositing CaP crystals from supersaturated solutions releases calcium and phosphate ions from these coatings. This process helps in the precipitation of biological apatite nanocrystals with the incorporation of various proteins, which in turn, promotes cell adhesion, differentiation into osteoblast, and the synthesis of mineralized collagen, the extracellular matrix of bone tissue (Sandrine *et al.*, 2010).

Osteoclast cells are also able to resorb the CaP coatings and activate osteoblast cells to produce bone tissue. Thus, these CaP coatings promote a direct bone-implant contact without an intervening connective tissue layer leading to a proper biomechanical fixation of dental implants. Currently, titanium is the standard material for dental implants because of its excellent biocompatibility and osseointegration properties. On account of the influence of surface modifications of the titanium implants on osseointegration, such modifications have been successfully exploited to influence bone integration and long-term stability of the implant.

7. Methods of surface modifications of implants

The methods employed for surface modifications of implants can be broadly classified into 3 types-mechanical; chemical; and physical. These different methods can be employed to change the implant surface chemistry, morphology, and structure. The main objective of these techniques is to improve the bio-mechanical properties of the implant such as stimulation of bone formation to enhance osseointegration, removal of surface contaminants, and improvement of wear and corrosion resistance.

7.1 Mechanical methods

The mechanical methods include grinding, blasting, machining, and polishing. These procedures involving physical treatment generally result in rough or smooth surfaces which can enhance the adhesion, proliferation, and differentiation of cells.

7.2 Chemical methods

Methods of surface modification of titanium and its alloys by chemical treatment are based on chemical reactions occurring at the interface between titanium and a solution. The chemical methods of implant surface modifications include chemical treatment with acids or alkali, hydrogen peroxide treatment, sol-gel, chemical vapor deposition, and anodization. Chemical surface modification of titanium has been widely applied to alter surface roughness and composition and enhance wettability/surface energy (Bagno and Di Bello, 2004).

The process of acid treatment serves to remove the surface oxide and contamination which leads to a clean and homogenous surface. The acids commonly used include hydrochloric acid, sulfuric acid, hydrofluoric acid, and nitric acid. Acid treatment of the surfaces of titanium implants results in uniform roughness with micro pits ranging in size from 0.5-2 μm, increase in surface area, and an improvement in bioadhesion. Acid treatment of implants enhances osseointegration as these implants can facilitate migration and retention of osteogenic cells at the implant surface (Takeuchi *et al.*, 2003).

Alkali treatment involves immersion of the implants in either sodium or potassium hydroxide followed by heat treatment by rinsing in distilled water. This results in the growth of a bioactive, nanostructured sodium titanate layer on the implant surface. The surface acts as a site for the subsequent in vitro nucleation of calcium phosphates when immersed in simulated body fluids (SBF). This involves an initial formation of Ti-OH by release of sodium ions from the sodium titanate layer by the process of ion exchange. This is followed by formation of calcium titanate as a result of reaction with the calcium ions from the fluid. Being negatively charged, Ti-OH groups react selectively with the positively charged calcium ions in the SBF to form calcium titanate. Phosphate and calcium ions get incorporated into this calcium titanate and get transformed into apatite which can provide favorable conditions for bone marrow cell differentiation.

Chemical treatment of implant surfaces with hydrogen peroxide results in chemical dissolution and oxidation of the titanium surface. When titanium surfaces react with hydrogen peroxide, Ti-peroxy gels are formed. The thickness of titania layer formed can be controlled by adjusting the treatment time and it has been demonstrated that, when immersed in SBF, thicker layers of titania gel are more favorable for the deposition of apatite (Tavares *et al.*, 2007).

Anodization is a process by which oxide films are deposited on the surface of the titanium implants by means of an electrochemical reaction. In this process, titanium surface to be oxidized serves as the anode in an electrochemical cell with diluted solution of acids serving as the electrolyte. The thickness of the oxide layer can be altered by altering the parameters

of the electrochemical process and it has been shown that these anodized surfaces demonstrate improved adhesion and bonding.
The sol-gel process used to deposit ceramic coatings can be employed to deposit HA coatings on the implant surface. This results in thin layers of less than 10 μm thickness. This process improves the biological activity of the titanium implants and contributes to enhanced bone formation and osseointegration. Materials such as TiO_2, CaP, TiO_2-CaP composite, and silica-based coatings can be deposited on the titanium surface by this technique. Chemical vapor deposition involves chemical reactions between chemicals in the gas phase and the surface of the substrate which results in the deposition of a non-volatile compound on the substrate.

7.3 Physical methods

The physical methods of implant surface modification include plasma spraying, sputtering, and ion deposition.
Plasma spraying includes atmospheric plasma spraying and vacuum plasma spraying. This is used for creating titanium and CaP coatings on the surfaces of titanium implants. One major concern in the use of plasma sprayed coatings is the resorption and degradability of HA in the case of HA (PSHA) coated implants and loosening of the titanium particles in the case of titanium plasma sprayed (TPS) implants. This can affect the stability of the implants as well as pose a health hazard.
Sputtering, a method employed to deposit thin films, has been used to deposit thin films on implant surfaces to improve their biocompatibility, biological activity, and mechanical properties such as wear resistance and corrosion resistance.

8. Surface treatment of titanium implants

8.1 Turned surface (machined dental implants)

The first generation of dental implants, termed the turned implants, had a relatively smooth surface. After being manufactured, these implants are submitted to cleaning, decontamination and sterilization procedures. Scanning electron microscopy analysis showed that the surfaces of machined implants have grooves, ridges and marks of the tools used for their manufacturing. These surface defects provide mechanical resistance through bone interlocking. The disadvantage regarding the morphology of non-treated implants (machined) is the fact that osteoblastic cells are rugophilic – that is, they are prone to grow along the grooves existing on the surface. This characteristic requires a longer waiting time between surgery and implant loading. The use of these implants follows a protocol suggested by Brånemark i.e., 3-6-month healing or waiting time prior to loading.
These are the best documented implants with several reports suggesting good long-term clinical outcomes on all indications when used in sites with good bone quality using a two-stage procedure. The success rates of turned implants in challenging situations such as low bone density has been reported to be lesser than when placed in areas with good bone quality. Studies on animal models, clinical studies, and systematic reviews have suggested a positive correlation between surface roughness and BIC (Wennerberg and Albrektsson, 2010, Junker *et al.*, 2009). With experimental studies clearly indicating that significantly greater amount of new bone is formed around HA coated, or oxidized implants, it has been suggested that these implants should be preferred over turned implants in sites with poor bone quality. Owing to

morphological characteristics and lower resistance to removal torque, machined dental implants are becoming commercially unavailable. However, clinical cases in which turned implants were placed in poor bone have reported good long-term results. Although studies have shown lower primary stability for the turned implants, they demonstrated secondary stability values and clinical success rates similar to modified implants.

8.2 Etched surface dental Implants

Etching with strong acids is another method for roughening titanium dental implants. Acid etching of titanium removes the oxide layer and parts of the underlying material. The extent of material removed depends on the acid concentration, temperature and treatment time. The most commonly used solutions for acid etching of titanium includes either a mixture of HNO_3 and HF or a mixture of HCl and H_2SO_4 (MacDonald *et al.*, 2004). Acid treatment provides homogeneous roughness, increased active surface area and improved bioadhesion (Braceras *et al.*, 2009). This yields low surface energy and reduces the possibility of contamination since no particles are encrusted in the surface. This type of surface not only facilitates retention of osteogenic cells, but also allows them to migrate towards the implant surface. The manufacturers have their own acid etching method regarding concentration, time and temperature for treating implant surfaces. Roughening of implants by acid-etching produces micro pits on titanium surfaces and has been shown to promote rapid osseointegration with long term success (Wong *et al.*, 1995, Cho and Park, 2003).

8.3 Dual acid-etched technique

Immersion of titanium implants for several minutes in a mixture of concentrated HCl and H_2SO_4 heated above 100 °C (dual acid-etching) is employed to produce a micro rough surface. The dual acid- etched surfaces enhance the osteoconductive process through the attachment of fibrin and osteogenic cells, resulting in bone formation directly on the surface of the implant (Park and Davies, 2000).

The dual acid-etched surface produces a microtexture rather than a macrotexture. It has been found that dual acid-etched surfaces enhance the osteoconductive process through the attachment of fibrin and osteogenic cells, resulting in bone formation directly on the surface of the implant (Orsini *et al.*, 2000). Advantage of the dual acid-etched technique is in higher adhesion and expression of platelet and extracellular genes, which help in colonization of osteoblasts at the site and promote osseointegration. Experimental studies have reported higher BIC and less bone resorption with dual acid-etched surfaces compared to machined or TPS surfaces (Cochran *et al.*, 1998, Cochran *et al.*, 2002). It has been hypothesized that implants treated by dual acid-etching have a specific topography which enables them to attach to the fibrin scaffold, to promote the adhesion of osteogenic cells, and thus to promote bone apposition (Trisi *et al.*, 2002). High temperature acid-etching methods produced a homogeneous micro-porous surface which showed increased cell adhesion and higher BIC than TPS surfaces. The wettability of the surface has also been proposed to promote fibrin adhesion. This fibrin adhesion provides contact guidance for the osteoblasts migrating along the surface (Buser *et al.*, 2004).

8.4 Hydroxyapatite coated implants

Hydroxyapatite is one of the materials that may form a direct and strong binding between the implant and bone tissue. The coating with hydroxyapatite (Ca10(PO4)6(OH)2) can be considered as bioactive because of the sequence of events that results in precipitation of a CaP rich layer on the implant material through a solid solution ion exchange at the implant-bone interface (Ducheyne and Cuckler, 1992). The CaP incorporated layer will gradually be developed, via octacalcium phosphate , in a biologically equivalent hydroxyapatite that will be incorporated in the developing bone (Ogiso *et al.*, 1992). Synthetic form of hydroxyapatite has also been widely investigated due to the similar chemical composition to the mineral matrix of bone, which is generally referred to as hydroxyapatite (Ducheyne and Cuckler, 1992).

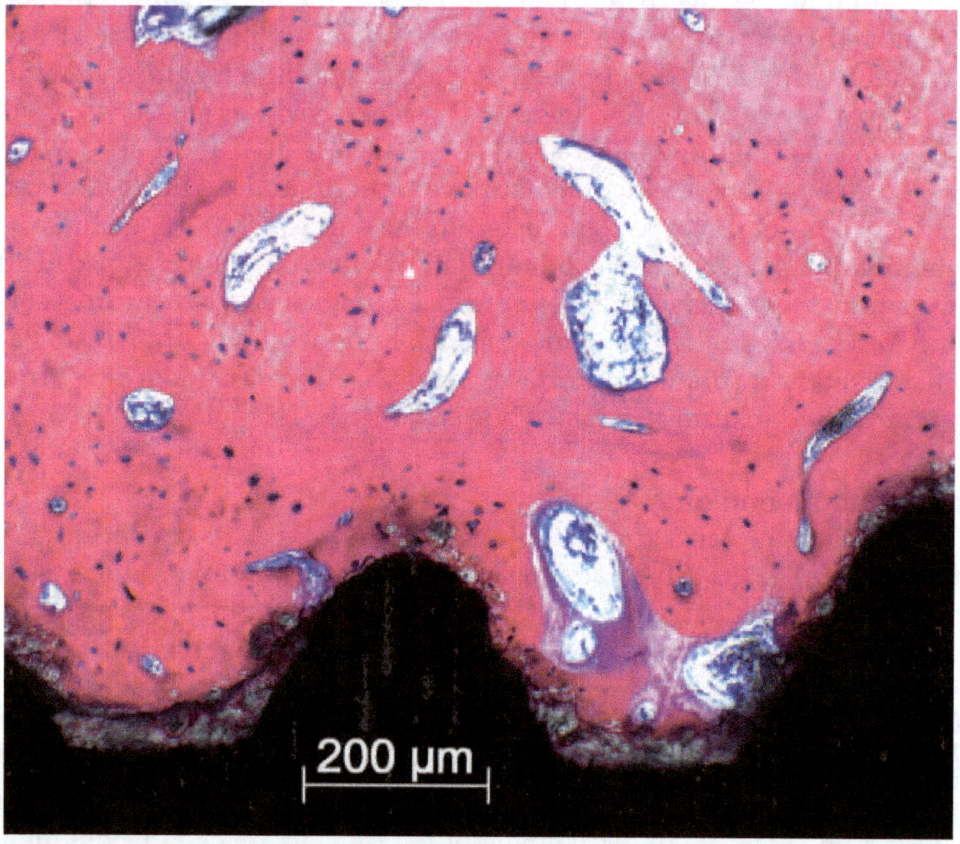

Fig. 5. Showing accelerated bone formation on the coated implant surface

Several methods have been described for applying hydroxyapatite coatings onto metals and different material properties may result from each method. Plasma-spraying is the most important commercially used technique for coating metals, especially titanium. In a so-called plasma gun, an electric arc current of high energy is struck between a cathode and an anode. Plasma spraying technique results in a coating thickness of 40-50 µm.

8.5 Sol-gel coated implants

The sol-gel method represents a simple and low cost procedure to deposit thin coatings with homogenous chemical composition onto substrates with large dimensions and complex design. The high mechanical strength and toughness of titanium alloys are the most important advantages over bioactive HA ceramics. A system that join both materials has the mechanical advantages of the underlying (metallic) substrate and biological affinity of the HA. Coating metallic implants with bioactive materials, like HA, may accelerate bone formation during initial stages of osseointegration and thereby improving implant fixation

(Vidigal *et al.*, 1999). Thin HA film on titanium substrates can be prepared using sol–gel (Xu *et al.*, 2006) or electrophoresis techniques (Wang *et al.*, 2002).
The sol-gel and electrophoresis methods are capable of improving chemical homogeneity in the resulting HA coating to a significant extent, when compared to conventional methods such as solid state reactions, wet precipitation and hydrothermal synthesis (Milev *et al.*, 2003). These methods are also simple and less expensive than the plasma spraying method that is widely used for biomedical applications. Sol-gel titania films may be prepared using a dip coating or spin coating process (Gan *et al.*, 2004). *In vivo* bone tissue evaluations of surfaces modified using the sol-gel method have shown better osseointegration with no adverse reaction (Gan *et al.*, 2004, Gil-Albarova *et al.*, 2004). However, the behavior of sol-gel modifications of loaded osseointegrated implants in the long term remains unknown.

8.6 Sandblasted and acid-etched (SLA) implants

This type of surface is produced by a large grit 250-500 µm blasting process followed by etching with hydrochloric/sulfuric acid. Sandblasting results in surface roughness and acid etching leads to microtexture and cleaning (Galli *et al.*, 2005). These surfaces are known to have better bone integration as compared to the above-stated methods (Bornstein *et al.*, 2008).

8.7 Grit-blasted surface

The grit blasting technique usually is performed with titania or alumina particles. The final surface roughness may be controlled by varying the particle size selected. Titanium implants blasted with alumina and titania particles with sizes of 25 µm and 75 µm demonstrated enhanced bone formation compared to turned implants. TioBlast implants (AstraTech) surface modification included grit blasting with titania particles. The success rate of TioBlast implants reported in a prospective study after 7 years was 96.9% with the same survival rate at 10 years. Compared to turned implants, TioBlast implants demonstrated lower bone loss and higher overall success rates (Engquist *et al.*, 2002, van Steenberghe *et al.*, 2000). Grit blasting represented the first clinically applied surface modification of titanium implants; the technique has then been further modified with acid etching, such as: SLA (Straumann) and Osseospeed (AstraTech).

8.8 Oxidized surface

Alteration of the topography and composition of the surface oxide layer of the implants can be achieved by a process of anodization. Anodic oxidation is an electrochemical process that increases the TiO_2 surface layer and roughness. The oxidation process changes the characteristic of the oxide layer and makes it more biocompatible (Gupta *et al.*, 2010). The implant is immersed in a suitable electrolyte and becomes an anode in an electrochemical cell. When a potential is applied to the sample, ionic transport of charge occurs through the cell, and an electrolytic reaction takes place at the anode, resulting in the growth of an oxide film. This results in a surface with micropores which demonstrates increased cell attachment and proliferation (Gupta *et al.*, 2010). The anodization process is rather complex and depends on various parameters such as current density, concentration of acids, composition and electrolyte temperature. The tissue healing process around anodized implants is quicker than in machined implants. In a study performed on canine models to evaluate bone healing at oxidized and turned implant surfaces, Gurgel *el al.* (2008) reported a higher percentage of BIC and bone density for anodized implants.

8.9 Plasma-spray coating

Plasma Sprayed (PS) Titanium coating is an optimized way to achieve a surface topography and morphology. The advantage of plasma coating is that these coatings give implants a porous surface that bone can penetrate more readily. Osseointegration was shown to be fastest and most effective for rough surfaces with open structure that varied between 50 to 400 μm.

Titanium plasma spraying (TPS) method consists of injecting titanium powders into a plasma torch at high temperature. The titanium particles are projected on to the surface of the implants where they condense and fuse together, forming a film about 30 μm thick. This processing results in a substantial surface area increase compared to the other commercially available surfaces. It has been shown that this three-dimensional topography increased the tensile strength at the implant-bone interface. Based on that, TPS implants have been often recommended for regions with low bone density. Studies have shown that the implant-bone interface formed faster with a TPS surface than with machined implants (Al-Nawas *et al.*, 2006, Lossdorfer *et al.*, 2004, Novaes *et al.*, 2002). Rough surfaces, obtained by TPS and grit-blasted/acid-etched have shown torque to failure values significantly higher than implants with machined profiles (Piao *et al.*, 2009, Bratu *et al.*, 2009, Schneider *et al.*, 2003).

8.10 Plasma sprayed hydroxyapatite

The addition of calcium and phosphorous based materials as coatings have received significant attention due to the fact that these elements are the same basic components of natural bone and coatings can be applied along the implant surfaces by various industrial processing methods (Kirsch, 1986). Most commercially available bio-ceramic coatings are processed as a 20–50 μm thick Plasma Sprayed Hydroxyapatite (PSHA) coatings. PSHA coatings normally rely on mechanical interlocking between a grit-blasted or etched metallic surfaces and the ceramic-like PSHA biomaterial for physical integrity during implant placement and function (Knabe *et al.*, 2002).

The osseointegration of the dental implant with plasma-sprayed HA is faster than uncoated implants. *In vivo* studies on rabbit femoral condyles have demonstrated a higher level of osseointegration for the HA-coated samples compared to the uncoated ones. Bone maturation was reported to be more significant at the bone-implant interface and coating of titanium with HA lead to improved maturation of newly formed bone tissue (Clark *et al.*, 2005). These observations were attributed to the presence of porous HA in the coated samples. Due to the high biocompatibility and osteoconduction of CaP materials, they have been widely used for different hard tissue applications such as HA-coated metallic implants and bone substitute materials.

8.11 Fluoride treatment

Titanium is very reactive to fluoride ions, forming soluble TiF_4 by treating titanium dental implants in fluoride solutions. This chemical treatment of titanium enhances the osseointegration of dental implants. An in vitro analysis of fluoride modified implants on human mesenchymal cells revealed no difference in cell attachment between the fluoride modified and control (grit-blasted) implants. Moreover, decreased cell proliferation was observed after 7 days on the fluoride modified compared to control (grit-blasted) implants. It has been shown that this chemical surface treatment enhanced osteoblastic differentiation in comparison with control samples (Ellingsen, 1995). The results of osteoblast differentiation showed increased expression of Cbfa1, osterix and bone sialoprotein to fluoridated implants (Cooper *et al.*, 2006, Isa *et al.*, 2006). Fluoridated rough implants also withstood greater push-out forces and showed a significantly higher removal torque than the control implants (Ellingsen *et al.*, 2004).

8.12 Laser deposition

The surface characteristics of titanium implants have been modified by additive methods, such as titanium and hydroxyapatite plasma spray, as well as by subtractive methods, such as acid etching and laser ablation. The laser ablation technology for surface preparation already has numerous industrial applications. This process results in titanium surface microstructures with greatly increased hardness, corrosion resistance, and a high degree of purity with a standard roughness and thicker oxide layer (Gaggl *et al.*, 2000, Hallgren *et al.*, 2003). Biological studies evaluating the role of titanium ablation topography and chemical properties showed the potential of the grooved surface to orientate osteoblast cell attachment and control the direction of ingrowth (Frenkel *et al.*, 2002).

8.13 Sputter deposition

Sputtering is a process whereby atoms or molecules of a material are ejected in a vacuum chamber by bombardment of high-energy ions. There are several sputter techniques and a common drawback inherent in all these methods is that the deposition rate is very low and the process itself is very slow (Jansen *et al.*, 1993). The deposition rate is improved by using a magnetically enhanced variant of diode sputtering, known as radio frequency magnetron sputtering.

Radio frequency sputtering (RF) : Radiofrequency (RF) magnetron sputtering is largely used to deposit thin films of CaP coatings on titanium implants. RF magnetron sputtering is a very suitable technique to deposit standardized CaP coatings on titanium substrates. The advantage of this technique is that the coating shows strong adhesion to the titanium and the Ca/P ratio and crystallinity of the deposited coating can be varied easily. Studies in animals have shown higher BIC percentages with sputter coated implants (Vercaigne *et al.*, 2000a, Vercaigne *et al.*, 2000b). Studies have shown that these coatings were more retentive, with the chemical structure being precisely controlled (Ong *et al.*, 2002).

Magnetron sputtering: Magnetron sputtering is a viable thin-film technique as it allows the mechanical properties of titanium to be preserved while maintaining the bioactivity of the coated HA. Films were deposited in a custom-built sputter deposition chamber at room temperature. This technique shows strong HA titanium bonding associated with outward diffusion of titanium into the HA layer, forming TiO_2 at the interface (Wolke *et al.*, 1994).

9. Biologically active drugs incorporated dental implants

Several attempts have been made to improve and accelerate osseointegration by modification of surface properties, such as introducing bioactive factors to titanium surfaces. Of these, some osteogenic drugs have been applied to implant surfaces. Incorporation of bone antiresorptive drugs, such as bisphosphonate, might be very relevant in clinical cases lacking bone support.

9.1 Bisphosphonates

Bisphosphate-loaded implant surfaces have been reported to improve implant osseointegration. Bisphosphates are antiresorptive agents that have beneficial effects for the patients on preventing further bone loss, and their effects on increasing the bone mass is modest (Kwak *et al.*, 2009, Yoshinari *et al.*, 2002). It has been shown that bisphosphonate incorporated on to titanium implants increased bone density locally in the peri-implant region (Josse *et al.*, 2005) with the effect of the antiresorptive drug limited to the vicinity of the implant. Experimental *in vivo* studies have demonstrated the absence of negative effects, but only a slight increase in dental implant osseointegration (Meraw and Reeve, 1999, Meraw *et al.*, 1999). Other experimental studies using PSHA-coated dental implants immersed in pamidronate or zoledronate demonstrated a significant increase in bone contact area (Yoshinari *et al.*, 2001, Kajiwara *et al.*, 2005). The main problem lies in the grafting and sustained release of antiresorptive drugs on the titanium implant surface. Due to the high chemical affinity of bisphosphonates for CaP surfaces, incorporation of the antiresorptive drug on to dental implants could be achieved by using the biomimetic coating method at room temperatures. However, the ideal dose of antiresorptive drug will have to be determined because the increase in peri-implant bone density is bisphosphonate concentration-dependent (Peter *et al.*, 2005).

9.2 Simvastatin

Statins are commonly prescribed drugs that inhibit 3-hydroxy-3-methylglutaryl coenzyme reductase to decrease cholesterol biosynthesis by the liver, thereby reducing serum cholesterol concentrations and lowering the risk of heart attack (Goldstein and Brown, 1990). Simvastatin, could induce the expression of bone morphogenetic protein (BMP) 2 mRNA that might promote bone formation (Mundy *et al.*, 1999). Simvastatin given per-orally to adult rats increased cancellous bone mass and increased cancellous bone compressive strength (Oxlund *et al.*, 2001).

Ayukawa *et al* (2009) confirmed that topical application of statins to alveolar bone increased bone formation and concurrently suppressed osteoclast activity at the bone-healing site. In addition, clinical studies reported that statin use is associated with increased bone mineral density (Edwards *et al.*, 2000, Montagnani *et al.*, 2003). Du *et al* (2009) investigated the effect of simvastatin by oral administration on implant osseointegration in osteoporotic rats and found that it significantly improved bone integration with the implant. Another animal study showed that the intra-peritoneal administration of simvastatin increased BIC ratio and bone density and implied that simvastatin might have the potential to improve the nature of osseointegration (Ayukawa *et al.*, 2004). In an in vitro study Yang *et al* (2010) showed that simvastatin-loaded porous implant surfaces promote accelerated osteogenic differentiation of preosteoblasts, which have the potential to improve the nature of osseointegration.

9.3 Antibiotic coating

Antibacterial coatings on the surface of implants that provide antibacterial activity to the implants themselves have been studied as a possible way to prevent surgical site infections associated with implants. **Gentamycin** along with the layer of HA can be coated onto the implant surface which may act as a local prophylactic agent along with the systemic antibiotics in dental implant surgery (Alt *et al.*, 2006).

Tetracycline-HCl treatment has been regarded as a practical and effective chemical modality for decontamination and detoxification of contaminated implant surfaces.

Tetracycline-HCl functions as an antimicrobial agent capable of killing microorganisms that may be present on the contaminated implant surface. It also effectively removes the smear layer as well as endotoxins from the implant surface. Further, it inhibits collagenase activity, increases cell proliferation as well as attachment and bone healing (Herr *et al.,* 2008). Tetracycline also enhances blood clot attachment and retention on the implant surface during the initial phase of the healing process and thus promotes osseointegration (Persson *et al.,* 2001).

10. Future directions in implant surface modifications

Several growth factors and cytokines have also been suggested to stimulate a deposition of cells with the capacity of regenerating the desired tissue (Liu *et al.,* 2007, Sigurdsson *et al.,* 2001). An enhanced proliferation and differentiation of undifferentiated mesenchymal cells, osteoprogenitor cells, and preosteoblasts into osteoblasts may improve bone response and subsequently osseointegration of titanium implants (Chappard *et al.,* 1999). The adhesion of plasma proteins on the surface of titanium implants has been reported to play an essential role in the process of osseointegration (Eriksson *et al.,* 2001). The specific pattern of adsorbed proteins determines the type of tissue that will develop at the interface between the implanted material and the host (Walivaara *et al.,* 1994).

Polypeptide growth and differentiation factors and cytokines have been suggested as potential candidates in this regard to stimulate a deposition of cells with the capacity of regenerating the desired tissue (Liu *et al.,* 2007, Sigurdsson *et al.,* 2001). Biologically active implants surfaces may have the potential to enhance the proliferation and differentiation of undifferentiated mesenchymal cells and osteoblasts which can improve bone response and subsequent osseointegration of titanium implants (Chappard *et al.,* 1999). Researchers have shown that growth factors released during the inflammatory phase have the potential of attracting undifferentiated mesenchymal stem cells to the injured site. These growth factors include PDGF, EGF, VEGF, TGF-β, and BMP-2 and BMP-4. These factors are released in the injured sites by cells involved in tissue healing. The surface of titanium dental implants may be coated with bone-stimulating agents such as growth factors in order to enhance the bone healing process locally. Members of the transforming growth factor (TGF-β) superfamily, and in particular bone morphogenetic proteins (BMPs), TGF-β1, platelet-derived growth factor (PDGF) and insulin-like growth factors (IGF-1 and 2) are some of the most promising candidates for this purpose. Among these, bone morphogenetic protein (BMP), has shown considerable potential to stimulate bone formation both in extra skeletal sites and in defect models in different species (Avila *et al.,* 2009, Becker *et al.,* 2006, Sigurdsson *et al.,* 2001). The effects of rhBMP-2 on the osseointegration of titanium implants have also been investigated in experimental animal studies (Sigurdsson *et al.,* 1996, Wikesjo *et al.,* 2002).

Experimental data, in which BMPs were incorporated into dental implants, have been obtained from a variety of methodologies. Besides individual growth factors, the effects of incorporating a "cocktail" of these factors have also been evaluated. In an animal study assessing the potential effects of humidifying and bioactivating titanium dental implants with liquid preparation rich in growth factors (PRGF) on implant osseointegration in the goat model, 26 implants were inserted in the tibiae of the goats. Before installation, 13 implants were carefully humidified with liquid PRGF with the aim of bioactivating the implant surface, whereas the other 13 implants were placed without PRGF treatment (Anitua *et al.,* 2009). After 8 weeks, the animals were sacrificed and histological and histomorphometric tests were performed. Histological and histomorphometric results demonstrated that application of liquid PRGF increased the percentage of BIC by 84.7%. The whole surface of the PRGF-treated implants was covered by newly formed bone, whereas only the upper half was surrounded in the control implants. This suggested that PRGF can accelerate bone regeneration in artificial defects and improve the osseointegration of titanium dental implants.

A clinical study in which 1391 implants were placed in 295 patients after bioactivating the surface with PRGF, stability and implant survival were evaluated, and it was reported that 99.6% of the implants treated with PRGF were well osseointegrated suggesting that the clinical use of this technique in oral implantology can improve the prognosis (Anitua, 2006).

Animal studies in which platelet-rich plasma in liquid form was applied to the implant surface by dipping the implant in PRP prior to placement have demonstrated that PRP in a liquid form showed a tendency to increase bone apposition to roughened titanium implants (Nikolidakis *et al.*, 2008, Nikolidakis *et al.*, 2006).

Nikolidakis *et al* (2006) investigated the effect of local application of autologous platelet-rich plasma (PRP) on bone healing in combination with the use of titanium implants with 2 different surface configurations - CaP coated and non-coated implants. PRP fractions were obtained from venous blood sample of 6 goats and applied via gel preparation and subsequent installation in the implant site or via dipping of the implant in PRP liquid before insertion. Thirty-six implants (18 non-coated and 18 CaP coated) were placed into the goat femoral condyles (trabecular bone). The animals were sacrificed at 6 weeks after implantation, and implants with surrounding tissue were processed for light microscopic evaluation. Significantly more interfacial BIC was observed for all 3 groups of CaP-coated implants and the titanium / liquid group (non-coated implant with PRP liquid) than for the other 2 non-coated titanium groups (with PRP gel or without PRP). The evaluation of the bone mass close to implant surface indicated that all the groups induced a significant increase of the bone mass except the PRP gel groups. On the basis of the observations, it was concluded that magnetron-sputtered CaP coatings can improve the integration of oral implants in trabecular bone. Although the additional use of PRP did not offer any significant effect on the bone response to the CaP-coated implants, PRP in a liquid form showed a significant effect on bone apposition to roughened titanium implants during the early post-implantation healing phase.

The role of the osteoinductive TGF-β1 application to CaP implant surfaces have been studied in animals using a goat model. It was observed that, although the BIC was highest in the TGF-β1 loaded implants, the beneficial effects of the growth factor were only marginal (Schouten *et al.*, 2009). The limiting factor regarding the use of growth factors in surface treatment of implants is that the active product has to be released progressively and not in a single burst. Although the possibility of incorporation of a plasmid containing the gene coding for a BMP exists, it is associated with disadvantages related to poor efficacy and a possible undesirable overproduction of BMPs.

11. Conclusion

The endosseous dental implant has become a scientifically accepted and well documented treatment for fully and partially edentulous patients. Titanium and its alloys are the materials of choice clinically, because of their excellent biocompatibility and superior mechanical properties. The composite effect of surface energy, composition, roughness, and topography on implant determines its ultimate ability to integrate into the surrounding tissue.

Surface modification technologies involve preparation with either an additive coating or subtractive method. Cell migration, adhesion, and proliferation on implant surfaces are important prerequisites to initiate the process of tissue regeneration, while modifications of the implant surface by incorporation of biologic mediators of growth and differentiation may be potentially beneficial in enhancing wound healing following implant placement. These topographical modifications have boosted the success rate of the implant therapy, especially in patients with poor bone quality sites, and have significantly reduced the healing period. The cellular mechanisms involved in this faster and improved osseointegration are yet to be fully determined. Further research should be directed to explore the biologic basis underlying the clinical improvement with altered implant surfaces.

12. References

Al-Nawas, B.; Wagner, W. & Grotz, K.A. (2006) Insertion torque and resonance frequency analysis of dental implant systems in an animal model with loaded implants. *The International journal of oral & maxillofacial implants,* 21, 726-732.

Albrektsson, T.; Branemark, P.I.; Hansson, H.A. & Lindstrom, J. (1981) Osseointegrated titanium implants. Requirements for ensuring a long-lasting, direct bone-to-implant anchorage in man. *Acta orthopaedica Scandinavica,* 52, 155-170.

Alt, V.; Bitschnau, A.; Osterling, J.; Sewing, A.; Meyer, C.; Kraus, R.; Meissner, S.A.; Wenisch, S.; Domann, E. & Schnettler, R. (2006) The effects of combined gentamicin-hydroxyapatite coating for cementless joint prostheses on the reduction of infection rates in a rabbit infection prophylaxis model. *Biomaterials,* 27, 4627-4634.

Anitua, E.; Orive, G.; Pla, R.; Roman, P.; Serrano, V. & Andia, I. (2009) The effects of PRGF on bone regeneration and on titanium implant osseointegration in goats: a histologic and histomorphometric study. *Journal of biomedical materials research. Part A,* 91, 158-165.

Anitua, E.A. (2006) Enhancement of osseointegration by generating a dynamic implant surface. *The Journal of oral implantology,* 32, 72-76.

Avila, G.; Misch, K.; Galindo-Moreno, P. & Wang, H.L. (2009) Implant surface treatment using biomimetic agents. *Implant dentistry,* 18, 17-26.

Ayukawa, Y.; Okamura, A. & Koyano, K. (2004) Simvastatin promotes osteogenesis around titanium implants. *Clinical oral implants research,* 15, 346-350.

Ayukawa, Y.; Yasukawa, E.; Moriyama, Y.; Ogino, Y.; Wada, H.; Atsuta, I. & Koyano, K. (2009) Local application of statin promotes bone repair through the suppression of osteoclasts and the enhancement of osteoblasts at bone-healing sites in rats. *Oral surgery, oral medicine, oral pathology, oral radiology, and endodontics,* 107, 336-342.

Bagno, A. & Di Bello, C. (2004) Surface treatments and roughness properties of Ti-based biomaterials. *Journal of materials science. Materials in medicine,* 15, 935-949.

Becker, J.; Kirsch, A.; Schwarz, F.; Chatzinikolaidou, M.; Rothamel, D.; Lekovic, V.; Laub, M. & Jennissen, H.P. (2006) Bone apposition to titanium implants biocoated with recombinant human bone morphogenetic protein-2 (rhBMP-2). A pilot study in dogs. *Clinical oral investigations,* 10, 217-224.

Bornstein, M.M.; Valderrama, P.; Jones, A.A.; Wilson, T.G.; Seibl, R. & Cochran, D.L. (2008) Bone apposition around two different sandblasted and acid-etched titanium implant surfaces: a histomorphometric study in canine mandibles. *Clinical oral implants research,* 19, 233-241.

Boyan, B.; Dean, D.; Lohmann, C.; Cochran, D.; Sylvia, V. & Schwartz, Z. (2001) The titanium-bone cell interface in vitro: The role of the surface in promoting osteointegration. *Titanium in Medicine,* 561–585.

Braceras, I.; De Maeztu, M.A.; Alava, J.I. & Gay-Escoda, C. (2009) In vivo low-density bone apposition on different implant surface materials. *International journal of oral and maxillofacial surgery,* 38, 274-278.

Bratu, E.A.; Tandlich, M. & Shapira, L. (2009) A rough surface implant neck with microthreads reduces the amount of marginal bone loss: a prospective clinical study. *Clinical oral implants research,* 20, 827-832.

Brett, P.M.; Harle, J.; Salih, V.; Mihoc, R.; Olsen, I.; Jones, F.H. & Tonetti, M. (2004) Roughness response genes in osteoblasts. *Bone,* 35, 124-133.

Buser, D.; Broggini, N.; Wieland, M.; Schenk, R.K.; Denzer, A.J.; Cochran, D.L.; Hoffmann, B.; Lussi, A. & Steinemann, S.G. (2004) Enhanced bone apposition to a chemically modified SLA titanium surface. *Journal of dental research,* 83, 529-533.

Buser, D.; Nydegger, T.; Oxland, T.; Cochran, D.L.; Schenk, R.K.; Hirt, H.P.; Snetivy, D. & Nolte, L.P. (1999) Interface shear strength of titanium implants with a sandblasted and acid-etched surface: a biomechanical study in the maxilla of miniature pigs. *Journal of biomedical materials research,* 45, 75-83.

Chappard, D.; Aguado, E.; Hure, G.; Grizon, F. & Basle, M.F. (1999) The early remodeling phases around titanium implants: a histomorphometric assessment of bone quality in a 3- and 6-month study in sheep. *The International journal of oral & maxillofacial implants,* 14, 189-196.

Cho, S.A. & Park, K.T. (2003) The removal torque of titanium screw inserted in rabbit tibia treated by dual acid etching. *Biomaterials,* 24, 3611-3617.

Clark, P.A.; Rodriguez, A.; Sumner, D.R.; Hussain, M.A. & Mao, J.J. (2005) Modulation of bone ingrowth of rabbit femur titanium implants by in vivo axial micromechanical loading. *Journal of applied physiology,* 98, 1922-1929.

Cochran, D.L.; Buser, D.; ten Bruggenkate, C.M.; Weingart, D.; Taylor, T.M.; Bernard, J.P.; Peters, F. & Simpson, J.P. (2002) The use of reduced healing times on ITI implants with a sandblasted and acid-etched (SLA) surface: early results from clinical trials on ITI SLA implants. *Clinical oral implants research,* 13, 144-153.

Cochran, D.L.; Schenk, R.K.; Lussi, A.; Higginbottom, F.L. & Buser, D. (1998) Bone response to unloaded and loaded titanium implants with a sandblasted and acid-etched surface: a histometric study in the canine mandible. *Journal of biomedical materials research,* 40, 1-11.

Cooper, L.F.; Zhou, Y.; Takebe, J.; Guo, J.; Abron, A.; Holmen, A. & Ellingsen, J.E. (2006) Fluoride modification effects on osteoblast behavior and bone formation at TiO2 grit-blasted c.p. titanium endosseous implants. *Biomaterials,* 27, 926-936.

Dalby, M.J.; Andar, A.; Nag, A.; Affrossman, S.; Tare, R.; McFarlane, S. & Oreffo, R.O. (2008) Genomic expression of mesenchymal stem cells to altered nanoscale topographies. *Journal of the Royal Society, Interface / the Royal Society,* 5, 1055-1065.

Dohan Ehrenfest, D.M.; Coelho, P.G.; Kang, B.S.; Sul, Y.T. & Albrektsson, T. (2010) Classification of osseointegrated implant surfaces: materials, chemistry and topography. *Trends in biotechnology,* 28, 198-206.

Du, Z.; Chen, J.; Yan, F. & Xiao, Y. (2009) Effects of Simvastatin on bone healing around titanium implants in osteoporotic rats. *Clinical oral implants research,* 20, 145-150.

Ducheyne, P. & Cuckler, J.M. (1992) Bioactive ceramic prosthetic coatings. *Clinical orthopaedics and related research*, 102-114.

Edwards, C.J.; Hart, D.J. & Spector, T.D. (2000) Oral statins and increased bone-mineral density in postmenopausal women. *Lancet,* 355, 2218-2219.

Elias, C.N. & Meirelles, L. (2010) Improving osseointegration of dental implants. *Expert review of medical devices,* 7, 241-256.

Ellingsen, J. (1995) Pre-treatment of titanium implants with fluoride improves their retention in bone. *Journal of Materials Science: Materials in Medicine,* 6, 749-753.

Ellingsen, J.E.; Johansson, C.B.; Wennerberg, A. & Holmen, A. (2004) Improved retention and bone-tolmplant contact with fluoride-modified titanium implants. *The International journal of oral & maxillofacial implants,* 19, 659-666.

Engquist, B.; Astrand, P.; Dahlgren, S.; Engquist, E.; Feldmann, H. & Grondahl, K. (2002) Marginal bone reaction to oral implants: a prospective comparative study of Astra Tech and Branemark System implants. *Clinical oral implants research,* 13, 30-37.

Eriksson, C.; Lausmaa, J. & Nygren, H. (2001) Interactions between human whole blood and modified TiO2-surfaces: influence of surface topography and oxide thickness on leukocyte adhesion and activation. *Biomaterials,* 22, 1987-1996.

Frenkel, S.R.; Simon, J.; Alexander, H.; Dennis, M. & Ricci, J.L. (2002) Osseointegration on metallic implant surfaces: effects of microgeometry and growth factor treatment. *Journal of biomedical materials research,* 63, 706-713.

Gaggl, A.; Schultes, G.; Muller, W.D. & Karcher, H. (2000) Scanning electron microscopical analysis of laser-treated titanium implant surfaces--a comparative study. *Biomaterials,* 21, 1067-1073.

Galli, C.; Guizzardi, S.; Passeri, G.; Martini, D.; Tinti, A.; Mauro, G. & Macaluso, G.M. (2005) Comparison of human mandibular osteoblasts grown on two commercially available titanium implant surfaces. *Journal of periodontology,* 76, 364-372.

Gan, L.; Wang, J.; Tache, A.; Valiquette, N.; Deporter, D. & Pilliar, R. (2004) Calcium phosphate sol-gel-derived thin films on porous-surfaced implants for enhanced osteoconductivity. Part II: Short-term in vivo studies. *Biomaterials,* 25, 5313-5321.

Gil-Albarova, J.; Garrido-Lahiguera, R.; Salinas, A.J.; Roman, J.; Bueno-Lozano, A.L.; Gil-Albarova, R. & Vallet-Regí, M.M. (2004) The in vivo performance of a sol-gel glass and a glass-ceramic in the treatment of limited bone defects. *Biomaterials,* 25, 4639-4645.

Goldstein, J.L. & Brown, M.S. (1990) Regulation of the mevalonate pathway. *Nature,* 343, 425-430.

Grassi, S.; Piattelli, A.; de Figueiredo, L.C.; Feres, M.; de Melo, L.; Iezzi, G.; Alba, R.C., Jr. & Shibli, J.A. (2006) Histologic evaluation of early human bone response to different implant surfaces. *J Periodontol,* 77, 1736-1743.

Gupta, A.; Dhanraj, M. & Sivagami, G. (2010) Status of surface treatment in endosseous implant: a literary overview. *Indian journal of dental research:* official publication of Indian Society for Dental Research, 21, 433-438.

Gurgel, B.C.; Goncalves, P.F.; Pimentel, S.P.; Nociti, F.H.; Sallum, E.A.; Sallum, A.W. & Casati, M.Z. (2008) An oxidized implant surface may improve bone-to-implant contact in pristine bone and bone defects treated with guided bone regeneration: an experimental study in dogs. *Journal of periodontology,* 79, 1225-1231.

Hallgren, C.; Reimers, H.; Chakarov, D.; Gold, J. & Wennerberg, A. (2003) An in vivo study of bone response to implants topographically modified by laser micromachining. *Biomaterials,* 24, 701-710.

Herr, Y.; Woo, J.; Kwon, Y.; Park, J.; Heo, S. & Chung, J. (2008) Implant Surface Conditioning with Tetracycline-HCl: A SEM Study. *Key Engineering Materials,* 361, 849-852.

Huang, Y.H.; Xiropaidis, A.V.; Sorensen, R.G.; Albandar, J.M.; Hall, J. & Wikesjo, U.M. (2005) Bone formation at titanium porous oxide (TiUnite) oral implants in type IV bone. *Clin Oral Implants Res,* 16, 105-111.

Isa, Z.M.; Schneider, G.B.; Zaharias, R.; Seabold, D. & Stanford, C.M. (2006) Effects of fluoride-modified titanium surfaces on osteoblast proliferation and gene expression. *The International journal of oral & maxillofacial implants,* 21, 203-211.

Jansen, J.A.; Wolke, J.G.; Swann, S.; Van der Waerden, J.P. & de Groot, K. (1993) Application of magnetron sputtering for producing ceramic coatings on implant materials. *Clinical oral implants research,* 4, 28-34.

Josse, S.; Faucheux, C.; Soueidan, A.; Grimandi, G.; Massiot, D.; Alonso, B.; Janvier, P.; Laïb, S.; Pilet, P. & Gauthier, O. (2005) Novel biomaterials for bisphosphonate delivery. *Biomaterials,* 26, 2073-2080.

Junker, R.; Dimakis, A.; Thoneick, M. & Jansen, J.A. (2009) Effects of implant surface coatings and composition on bone integration: a systematic review. *Clinical oral implants research,* 20 Suppl 4, 185-206.

Kajiwara, H.; Yamaza, T.; Yoshinari, M.; Goto, T.; Iyama, S.; Atsuta, I.; Kido, M.A. & Tanaka, T. (2005) The bisphosphonate pamidronate on the surface of titanium stimulates bone formation around tibial implants in rats. *Biomaterials,* 26, 581-587.

Kilpadi, D.V. & Lemons, J.E. (1994) Surface energy characterization of unalloyed titanium implants. *Journal of biomedical materials research,* 28, 1419-1425.

Kim, H.J.; Kim, S.H.; Kim, M.S.; Lee, E.J.; Oh, H.G.; Oh, W.M.; Park, S.W.; Kim, W.J.; Lee, G.J.; Choi, N.G.; Koh, J.T.; Dinh, D.B.; Hardin, R.R.; Johnson, K.; Sylvia, V.L.; Schmitz, J.P. & Dean, D.D. (2005) Varying Ti-6Al-4V surface roughness induces different early morphologic and molecular responses in MG63 osteoblast-like cells. *Journal of biomedical materials research. Part A,* 74, 366-373.

Kirsch, A. (1986) Plasma-sprayed titanium-I.M.Z. implant. *The Journal of oral implantology,* 12, 494-497.

Knabe, C.; Klar, F.; Fitzner, R.; Radlanski, R.J. & Gross, U. (2002) In vitro investigation of titanium and hydroxyapatite dental implant surfaces using a rat bone marrow stromal cell culture system. *Biomaterials,* 23, 3235-3245.

Kwak, H.B.; Kim, J.Y.; Kim, K.J.; Choi, M.K.; Kim, J.J.; Kim, K.M.; Shin, Y.I.; Lee, M.S.; Kim, H.S.; Kim, J.W.; Chun, C.H.; Cho, H.J.; Hong, G.Y.; Juhng, S.K.; Yoon, K.H.; Park, B.H.; Bae, J.M.; Han, J.K. & Oh, J. (2009) Risedronate directly inhibits osteoclast differentiation and inflammatory bone loss. *Biological & pharmaceutical bulletin,* 32, 1193-1198.

Le Guehennec, L.; Soueidan, A.; Layrolle, P. & Amouriq, Y. (2007) Surface treatments of titanium dental implants for rapid osseointegration. *Dental materials : official publication of the Academy of Dental Materials,* 23, 844-854.

Liu, Y.; Enggist, L.; Kuffer, A.F.; Buser, D. & Hunziker, E.B. (2007) The influence of BMP-2 and its mode of delivery on the osteoconductivity of implant surfaces during the early phase of osseointegration. *Biomaterials,* 28, 2677-2686.

Lossdorfer, S.; Schwartz, Z.; Wang, L.; Lohmann, C.H.; Turner, J.D.; Wieland, M.; Cochran, D.L. & Boyan, B.D. (2004) Microrough implant surface topographies increase osteogenesis by reducing osteoclast formation and activity. *Journal of biomedical materials research. Part A,* 70, 361-369.

MacDonald, D.; Rapuano, B.; Deo, N.; Stranick, M.; Somasundaran, P. & Boskey, A. (2004) Thermal and chemical modification of titanium-aluminum-vanadium implant materials: effects on surface properties, glycoprotein adsorption, and MG63 cell attachment. *Biomaterials,* 25, 3135-3146.

Matsuo, M.; Nakamura, T.; Kishi, Y. & Takahashi, K. (1999) Microvascular changes after placement of titanium implants: scanning electron microscopy observations of machined and titanium plasma-sprayed implants in dogs. *Journal of periodontology,* 70, 1330-1338.

Meraw, S.J. & Reeve, C.M. (1999) Qualitative analysis of peripheral peri-implant bone and influence of alendronate sodium on early bone regeneration. *Journal of periodontology,* 70, 1228-1233.

Meraw, S.J.; Reeve, C.M. & Wollan, P.C. (1999) Use of alendronate in peri-implant defect regeneration. *Journal of periodontology,* 70, 151-158.

Milev, A.; Kannangara, G. & Ben-Nissan, B. (2003) Morphological stability of hydroxyapatite precursor. *Materials Letters,* 57, 1960-1965.

Montagnani, A.; Gonnelli, S.; Cepollaro, C.; Pacini, S.; Campagna, M.S.; Franci, M.B.; Lucani, B. & Gennari, C. (2003) Effect of simvastatin treatment on bone mineral density and bone turnover in hypercholesterolemic postmenopausal women: a 1-year longitudinal study. *Bone,* 32, 427-433.

Mundy, G.; Garrett, R.; Harris, S.; Chan, J.; Chen, D.; Rossini, G.; Boyce, B.; Zhao, M. & Gutierrez, G. (1999) Stimulation of bone formation in vitro and in rodents by statins. *Science,* 286, 1946-1949.

Nikolidakis, D.; van den Dolder, J.; Wolke, J.G. & Jansen, J.A. (2008) Effect of platelet-rich plasma on the early bone formation around Ca-P-coated and non-coated oral implants in cortical bone. *Clinical oral implants research,* 19, 207-213.

Nikolidakis, D.; van den Dolder, J.; Wolke, J.G.; Stoelinga, P.J. & Jansen, J.A. (2006) The effect of platelet-rich plasma on the bone healing around calcium phosphate-coated and non-coated oral implants in trabecular bone. *Tissue engineering,* 12, 2555-2563.

Novaes, A.B., Jr.; Souza, S.L.; de Oliveira, P.T. & Souza, A.M. (2002) Histomorphometric analysis of the bone-implant contact obtained with 4 different implant surface treatments placed side by side in the dog mandible. *The International journal of oral & maxillofacial implants,* 17, 377-383.

Ogiso, M.; Tabata, T.; Ichijo, T. & Borgese, D. (1992) Examination of human bone surrounded by a dense hydroxyapatite dental implant after long-term use. *Journal of long-term effects of medical implants,* 2, 235-247.

Oh, S.H.; Finones, R.R.; Daraio, C.; Chen, L.H. & Jin, S. (2005) Growth of nano-scale hydroxyapatite using chemically treated titanium oxide nanotubes. *Biomaterials,* 26, 4938-4943.

Ong, J.L.; Bessho, K.; Cavin, R. & Carnes, D.L. (2002) Bone response to radio frequency sputtered calcium phosphate implants and titanium implants in vivo. *Journal of biomedical materials research,* 59, 184-190.

Orsini, G.; Assenza, B.; Scarano, A.; Piattelli, M. & Piattelli, A. (2000) Surface analysis of machined versus sandblasted and acid-etched titanium implants. *The International journal of oral & maxillofacial implants,* 15, 779-784.

Oxlund, H.; Dalstra, M. & Andreassen, T.T. (2001) Statin given perorally to adult rats increases cancellous bone mass and compressive strength. *Calcified tissue international,* 69, 299-304.

Park, J.Y. & Davies, J.E. (2000) Red blood cell and platelet interactions with titanium implant surfaces. *Clinical oral implants research,* 12, 530-539.

Persson, L.G.; Ericsson, I.; Berglundh, T. & Lindhe, J. (2001) Osseintegration following treatment of peri-implantitis and replacement of implant components. An experimental study in the dog. *Journal of clinical periodontology,* 28, 258-263.

Peter, B.; Pioletti, D.P.; Laib, S.; Bujoli, B.; Pilet, P.; Janvier, P.; Guicheux, J.; Zambelli, P.Y.; Bouler, J.M. & Gauthier, O. (2005) Calcium phosphate drug delivery system: influence of local zoledronate release on bone implant osteointegration. *Bone,* 36, 52-60.

Piao, C.M.; Lee, J.E.; Koak, J.Y.; Kim, S.K.; Rhyu, I.C.; Han, C.H.; Herr, Y. & Heo, S.J. (2009) Marginal bone loss around three different implant systems: radiographic evaluation after 1 year. *Journal of oral rehabilitation,* 36, 748-754.

Rupp, F.; Scheideler, L.; Olshanska, N.; de Wild, M.; Wieland, M. & Geis-Gerstorfer, J. (2006) Enhancing surface free energy and hydrophilicity through chemical modification of microstructured titanium implant surfaces. *Journal of biomedical materials research. Part A,* 76, 323-334.

Sammons, R.L.; Lumbikanonda, N.; Gross, M. & Cantzler, P. (2005) Comparison of osteoblast spreading on microstructured dental implant surfaces and cell behaviour in an explant model of osseointegration. A scanning electron microscopic study. *Clinical oral implants research,* 16, 657-666.

Sandrine, L.; Guy, L. & Pierre, L. (2010) Nanotechnology and Dental Implants. *International journal of biomaterials,* 2010.

Schliephake, H.; Scharnweber, D.; Dard, M.; Sewing, A.; Aref, A. & Roessler, S. (2005) Functionalization of dental implant surfaces using adhesion molecules. *Journal of biomedical materials research. Part B, Applied biomaterials,* 73, 88-96.

Schneider, G.B.; Perinpanayagam, H.; Clegg, M.; Zaharias, R.; Seabold, D.; Keller, J. & Stanford, C. (2003) Implant surface roughness affects osteoblast gene expression. *Journal of dental research,* 82, 372-376.

Schouten, C.; Meijer, G.J.; van den Beucken, J.J.; Spauwen, P.H. & Jansen, J.A. (2009) Effects of implant geometry, surface properties, and TGF-beta1 on peri-implant bone response: an experimental study in goats. *Clinical oral implants research,* 20, 421-429.

Shalabi, M.M.; Gortemaker, A.; Van't Hof, M.A.; Jansen, J.A. & Creugers, N.H. (2006) Implant surface roughness and bone healing: a systematic review. *Journal of dental research,* 85, 496-500.

Shibli, J.A.; Grassi, S.; de Figueiredo, L.C.; Feres, M.; Marcantonio, E., Jr.; Iezzi, G. & Piattelli, A. (2007) Influence of implant surface topography on early osseointegration: a histological study in human jaws. *Journal of biomedical materials research. Part B, Applied biomaterials,* 80, 377-385.

Sigurdsson, T.J.; Nguyen, S. & Wikesjo, U.M. (2001) Alveolar ridge augmentation with rhBMP-2 and bone-to-implant contact in induced bone. *The International journal of periodontics & restorative dentistry,* 21, 461-473.

Sigurdsson, T.J.; Nygaard, L.; Tatakis, D.N.; Fu, E.; Turek, T.J.; Jin, L.; Wozney, J.M. & Wikesjo, U.M. (1996) Periodontal repair in dogs: evaluation of rhBMP-2 carriers. *The International journal of periodontics & restorative dentistry,* 16, 524-537.

Soskolne, W.A.; Cohen, S.; Sennerby, L.; Wennerberg, A. & Shapira, L. (2002) The effect of titanium surface roughness on the adhesion of monocytes and their secretion of TNF-alpha and PGE2. *Clinical oral implants research,* 13, 86-93.

Stanford, C.M. & Schneider, G.B. (2004) Functional behaviour of bone around dental implants*. *Gerodontology,* 21, 71-77.

Sul, Y.T.; Johansson, C.; Wennerberg, A.; Cho, L.R.; Chang, B.S. & Albrektsson, T. (2005) Optimum surface properties of oxidized implants for reinforcement of osseointegration: surface chemistry, oxide thickness, porosity, roughness, and crystal structure. *The International journal of oral & maxillofacial implants,* 20, 349-359.

Takeuchi, M.; Abe, Y.; Yoshida, Y.; Nakayama, Y.; Okazaki, M. & Akagawa, Y. (2003) Acid pretreatment of titanium implants. *Biomaterials,* 24, 1821-1827.

Tavares, M.G.; de Oliveira, P.T.; Nanci, A.; Hawthorne, A.C.; Rosa, A.L. & Xavier, S.P. (2007) Treatment of a commercial, machined surface titanium implant with H2SO4/H2O2 enhances contact osteogenesis. *Clinical oral implants research,* 18, 452-458.

Trisi, P.; Lazzara, R.; Rao, W. & Rebaudi, A. (2002) Bone-implant contact and bone quality: evaluation of expected and actual bone contact on machined and osseotite implant surfaces. *The International journal of periodontics & restorative dentistry,* 22, 535-545.

van Steenberghe, D.; De Mars, G.; Quirynen, M.; Jacobs, R. & Naert, I. (2000) A prospective split-mouth comparative study of two screw-shaped self-tapping pure titanium implant systems. *Clinical oral implants research,* 11, 202-209.

Vercaigne, S.; Wolke, J.G.; Naert, I. & Jansen, J.A. (2000a) A histological evaluation of TiO2-gritblasted and Ca-P magnetron sputter coated implants placed into the trabecular bone of the goat: Part 2. *Clinical oral implants research,* 11, 314-324.

Vercaigne, S.; Wolke, J.G.; Naert, I. & Jansen, J.A. (2000b) A mechanical evaluation of TiO2-gritblasted and Ca-P magnetron sputter coated implants placed into the trabecular bone of the goat: Part 1. *Clinical oral implants research,* 11, 305-313.

Vidigal, G.M., Jr.; Aragones, L.C.; Campos, A., Jr. & Groisman, M. (1999) Histomorphometric analyses of hydroxyapatite-coated and uncoated titanium dental implants in rabbit cortical bone. *Implant dentistry,* 8, 295-302.

Walivaara, B.; Aronsson, B.O.; Rodahl, M.; Lausmaa, J. & Tengvall, P. (1994) Titanium with different oxides: in vitro studies of protein adsorption and contact activation. *Biomaterials,* 15, 827-834.

Wang, C.; Ma, J.; Cheng, W. & Zhang, R. (2002) Thick hydroxyapatite coatings by electrophoretic deposition. *Materials Letters,* 57, 99-105.

Webster, T.J.; Ergun, C.; Doremus, R.H.; Siegel, R.W. & Bizios, R. (2000) Enhanced functions of osteoblasts on nanophase ceramics. *Biomaterials,* 21, 1803-1810.

Webster, T.J.; Siegel, R.W. & Bizios, R. (1999) Osteoblast adhesion on nanophase ceramics. *Biomaterials,* 20, 1221-1227.

Wennerberg, A. & Albrektsson, T. (2000) Suggested guidelines for the topographic evaluation of implant surfaces. *The International journal of oral & maxillofacial implants,* 15, 331-344.

Wennerberg, A. & Albrektsson, T. (2009) Effects of titanium surface topography on bone integration: a systematic review. *Clinical oral implants research,* 20 Suppl 4, 172-184.

Wennerberg, A. & Albrektsson, T. (2010) On implant surfaces: a review of current knowledge and opinions. *The International journal of oral & maxillofacial implants,* 25, 63-74.

Wennerberg, A.; Albrektsson, T. & Andersson, B. (1996) Bone tissue response to commercially pure titanium implants blasted with fine and coarse particles of aluminum oxide. *The International journal of oral & maxillofacial implants,* 11, 38-45.

Wikesjo, U.M.; Sorensen, R.G.; Kinoshita, A. & Wozney, J.M. (2002) RhBMP-2/alphaBSM induces significant vertical alveolar ridge augmentation and dental implant osseointegration. *Clinical implant dentistry and related research,* 4, 174-182.

Wolke, J.G.; van Dijk, K.; Schaeken, H.G.; de Groot, K. & Jansen, J.A. (1994) Study of the surface characteristics of magnetron-sputter calcium phosphate coatings. *Journal of biomedical materials research,* 28, 1477-1484.

Wong, M.; Eulenberger, J.; Schenk, R. & Hunziker, E. (1995) Effect of surface topology on the osseointegration of implant materials in trabecular bone. *Journal of biomedical materials research,* 29, 1567-1575.

Xu, W.; Hu, W.; Li, M. & Wen, C. (2006) Sol-gel derived hydroxyapatite/titania biocoatings on titanium substrate. *Materials Letters,* 60, 1575-1578.

Yang, F.; Zhao, S.F.; Zhang, F.; He, F.M. & Yang, G.L. (2010) Simvastatin-loaded porous implant surfaces stimulate preosteoblasts differentiation: an in vitro study. *Oral surgery, oral medicine, oral pathology, oral radiology, and endodontics.*

Yoshinari, M.; Oda, Y.; Inoue, T.; Matsuzaka, K. & Shimono, M. (2002) Bone response to calcium phosphate-coated and bisphosphonate-immobilized titanium implants. *Biomaterials,* 23, 2879-2885.

Yoshinari, M.; Oda, Y.; Ueki, H. & Yokose, S. (2001) Immobilization of bisphosphonates on surface modified titanium. *Biomaterials,* 22, 709-715.

Zhao, G.; Zinger, O.; Schwartz, Z.; Wieland, M.; Landolt, D. & Boyan, B.D. (2006) Osteoblast-like cells are sensitive to submicron-scale surface structure. *Clinical oral implants research,* 17, 258-264.

Zhao, X.; Liu, X. & Ding, C. (2005) Acid-induced bioactive titania surface. *Journal of biomedical materials research. Part A,* 75, 888-894.

3

Oral Territorial Neurovascular Considerations in Implant Surgery

Umit Karacayli[1] and Nuket Mas[2]
[1]*Department of Oral and Maxillofacial Surgery, Gulhane School of Medicine, Ankara*
[2]*Department of Anatomy, Faculty of Medicine, Afyon Kocatepe University, Afyonkarahisar Turkey*

1. Introduction

The anatomy of the intrabony course of the inferior alveolar nerve (IAN) is very important for dentists, neurologist, radiologists and pathologists to aid in diagnosis, treatment, planning surgery, and the application of local anesthesia (Polland et al., 2001).

IAN damage negatively affects the quality of facial sensibility and the patient's ability to translate patterns of altered nerve activity into functionally meaningful motor behaviors. The sensory alteration can be attributed to anatomical or functional changes within the nerve after resolution of inflammation and edema in and surrounding the nerve (Essick, 2004; Becerra et al., 2006).

Standardization of assessment methods would facilitate the identification of diagnostic criteria for different types of neurosensory impairment. Assessment of sensory changes can be evaluated using three types of measures: (i) objective electrophysiological measures of nerve conduction, (ii) sensory testing measures and (iii) patient report (Takazakura et al., 2007).

The request of replacing missing teeth with dental implants is increasing, and as a result, incidence of postoperative complications is increasing concomitantly (Kim et al., 2009). When the height of bone between alveolar crest and inferior alveolar canal is insufficient, implant placement in the posterior mandible is limited. One of the most difficult surgical challenges to the implant surgery is severe resorption of the posterior mandible processes (Ardekian et al., 2001). Understanding of the intrabony distribution of the IAN is important in the accurate preoperative planning for the placement of mandibular implants (Kieser et al., 2002). There are several treatment options for patients with inadequate bone height superior to the inferior alveolar canal. There are lots of alternative reconstruction methods of atrophic dental arch: use of autogenous bone grafting, allografts, xenogenic, or alloplastic materials with or without guided bone regeneration, distraction osteogenesis, IAN lateralization (McAllister & Haghighat 2007; Hashemi 2010). Placing the implants to the buccal side of the IAN or lateralization of it are the two of them (Misch & Resnik 2010). An ideal alveolar ridge with adequate bone height and width is essential for a successful dental rehabilitation (McAllister & Haghighat, 2007).

The placement of dental implants to the posterior mandible with severe resorption can cause damage to the IAN. The technique of nerve repositioning has been used to create the opportunity of insertion dental implants of adequately length in those cases. In cases with atrophic posterior mandibular ridges, the IAN repositioning technique is an acceptable alternative to augmentation procedure prior to dental implants placement (Ardekian et al., 2001).

Patients often desire fixed dental implant restoration of missing posterior teeth in the mandible, defined for the present report as the region posterior to the mental foramen. Placement of implants in the posterior mandible is limited by the height of bone between the alveolar crest and IAN transposition or lateralization is a treatment option for patients with an edentulous posterior mandible with inadequate bone height superior to the IAN (Scarano et al., 2011).

Nevre lateralization carries a risk of epineurial damage or ischemic stretching. İmplant compression can cause neuropathy and drill punctures can result in neuroma formation of all types. In some cases it can cause centralized pain syndrome. Two patterns of neuropathy can be seen as a result; hypoaesthesias with impaired sensory function, often seen with phantom pain, and hyperaesthesias with minimal sensory impairment but presence of much-evoked pain phenomena (Gregg, 2000).

Damage to the alveolar nevre is largely due to insufficient information about the location of the mandibular canal and it is one of the most frequent complications. Such damage can also occur in the absence of knowledge about the traveling courses of the IAN, artery, and vein within the mandibular canal (Kim et al., 2009).

Neuropathic pain associated with implant placement is rare in literature. In the implantology literature, complications related to nevre are mentioned as 'sensory disturbances', focusing on the occurrence of paresthesia and dysesthesia, eventually accompanied by transitory pain sensations during bone drilling or implant placement (Hashemi, 2010).

The first published report of IAN replacement for the insertion of dental implants appeared in 1987. In that study, , sensory function of the IAN returned to normal 5 weeks after surgery according to subjective criteria (Jensen & Nock, 1987).

2. Anatomy of the mandibular nerve

The trigeminal nerve, which is the largest cranial nerve, is the sensory supply to the face, greater part of the scalp, the teeth, the nasal and oral cavity, the dura mater, the blood vessels of cerebrum. Additionally it gives the motor supply to the masticator muscles, and the mylohyoid and the anterior belly of digastric muscles. It has three divisions as ophthalmic, maxillary and mandibular nerves. It has been reviewed the functions of the widespread peripheral connections between the facial and trigeminal and facial nerves. The trigeminal nerve arises from the anterior surface of the pons, near its upper margin, as a large sensory and a small motor root, the latter lying ventromedial to former. On entering the pons, the fibers of the sensory root run posteromedially towards the principal sensory nucleus situated at this level before reaching the nucleus about %50 of fibers divide into ascending and descending branches. Fibers from the ophthalmic root lie posterolaterally, those from the mandibular lie posteromedially, and the maxillary fibers lie between them.

In Wallenberg's syndrome, plug of posterior inferior cerebellar branch of cranial the vertebral artery leads to loss of pain and temperature sensation in the ipsilateral half of the face with retention of common sensation. Symptomatic trigeminal neuralgia is caused by a demonstrable structural lesion other than vascular compression, typically posterior fossa tumors or multiple sclerosis (Standring et al., 2005; Ordas et al., 2011).

Fibers of sensory root are principally axons of cells in the semilunal (trigeminal) ganglion, which occupies a recess in the trigeminal cave of Meckel, in the trigeminal impression near the apex of the petrous part of temporal bone. The ganglion placed on a depth of nearly 5 cm from lateral surface of the head deep to posterior end of the zygomatic arch. Axons of unipolar cells in the trigeminal ganglion divide into central and peripheral branches, the former being grouped to from ophthalmic and maxillary nerves and the sensory part of the mandibular nerve. The central branches composed the fibers of the sensory root (Standring et al., 2005). The motor nucleus of trigeminal nerve contains characteristic large multipolar cells interspersed with smaller multipolar cells. It lies in the superior part of pons medial to the principal sensory nucleus, separated from it by fibers of the trigeminal nerve. The motor nucleus receives fibers from both corticonuclear tracts. It also receives afferents from the sensory nuclei, reticular formation, red nucleus and tectum, the medial longitudinal fasciculus and locus coeruleus.

The detailed anatomy of the trigeminal nerve and its three branches and also their course excited early clinical interest since it was known that dissociated sensory loss could occur in trigeminal region. The superior and smallest trigeminal division is the ophthalmic nerve, which is the first branch of the trigeminal, is wholly sensory. It supplies the eyeball, conjunctiva and lacrimal gland, part of nasal mucosa, skin of nose, eyelids, forehead and part of scalp. It originates from the ventromedial end of trigeminal ganglion. It divides into lachrymal, frontal and nasocilliary branches. The maxillary nerve, the intermediate division of the trigeminal, is also wholly sensory. It gives off two large branches to pterygopalatine ganglion, then gives of the branches, which distribute nose, palate and pharynx. It gives off zygomatic and posterior superior alveolar branches nearly outside the orbital periostium. About halfway between the orbital apex and the orbital rim, the nerve enters the infraorbital canal as the infraorbital nerve.

The mandibular nerve, the third and the largest branch of the trigeminal nerve which supplies the teeth and gums of mandible, the lower lip, the lower part of face and the muscles of mastication, the mucosa of both presulcal parts of tongue and oral cavity, skin of the temporal region, part of the auricle including the external meatus and tympanum. It has a large sensory root, which proceeds from lateral part of trigeminal ganglion to emerge almost at ones from the foramen ovale, and a small motor root, which passes under the ganglion to unit with the sensory root just outside the skull. The nerve immediately passes between the tensor veli palatini muscle and the lateral pterygoid. Just beyond this junction a meningeal branch and the nerve to the medial pterygoid leaves the medial side of the nerve, which then divides into a small ventral and large dorsal trunk. As it descends from the foramen ovale, the nerve is about four cm from the surface and little anterior to neck of the mandible. The ventral trunk of the mandibular nerve gives rise to the buccal nerve, which is sensory, and the masseteric, deep temporal and lateral pterygoid nerves, which are all motor. The dorsal and larger mandibular trunk is mainly sensory but receives a few filaments from the motor root to mylohyoid muscle. It divides into auriculotemporal, lingual and inferior alveolar (dental) nerves (Standring et al., 2005).

The topographic anatomic landmarks, course and the surface making of the IAN from the inside of the oral cavity is particularly significant in giving nerve blocks for maxillofacial surgeons. Dentists frequently give anesthesia to the nerve before repairing or removing the premolar or molar teeth of the mandible. The IAN might be damaged during the extraction of impacted lower third molar tooth. The roots of such teeth are commonly grooved and, very rarely, perforated by the nerve. It is also frequently damaged in fractures of the posterior tooth-bearing part of the mandible (Standring et al., 2005; Snell, 2011). So, it is important to know course of the nerve and its relation to adjacent anatomical landmarks in detailed.

The nerve descends medial to the lateral pterygoid muscle and then, at its lower margin, passes between the sphenomandibular ligament and the mandibular ramus to enter mandibular canal by the mandibular foramen.

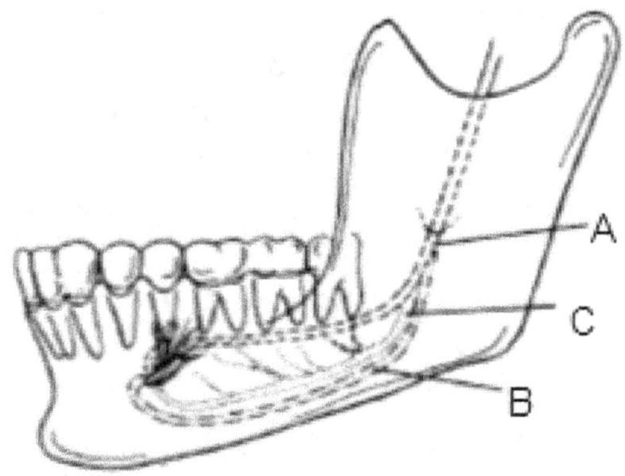

Fig. 1. Classification of the topography of the IAN. (A = the nerve has a course near the apices of the teeth, B = the main trunk is low down in the body, C = the main trunk is low down in the body of the mandible with several smaller trunks to the molar teeth.

Below the lateral pterygoid muscle it is accompanied by the inferior alveolar artery, a branch of maxillary. The artery also enters the canal. In the canal the IANlies downward and forward, usualy below the tip of the teeth until below the first and second premolars, at this point it divides into incicive and mental branches as the terminal branches. It continues forward in the canal or in a plexiform distrubition and giving off branches to the first premolar, canine and incisor teeth, and associated labial gingiva. Just before entering the mandibular canal the IAN gives off mylohyoid branch which pierces the sphenomandibular ligament and occurs a shallow groove on the medial surface of the mandible. It passes below the origin of mylohyoid muscle to lie on the surface of the muscle (Standring et al., 2005; Snell, 2011). The mandibular foramen opens into the mandibular canal, which carries the IAN. The mandibular foramen placed on midway between the ventral and dorsal magrin of ascending ramus of mandible nearly 1 cm above the occlusal surface of the lower teeth. The small triangular lingula guards the anterior border of the mandibular foramen and prvides attachments for he sphenomandibular ligament from which the mandible swings. The mylohyoid groove, immediately inferior to the lingula and lying just inferior to the mylohyoid line, carries the mylohyoid branch of the IAN. The ascending ramus diverges from the sagittal plane from front to back, once the needle engages the medial surface at this level it should be diverted laterally. At a higer level, near the base of coronoid process, the nerve is sufficiently medial to be accessible to a needle in the sagittal plane. With method the buccal and lingual nerves can be blocked (Standring et al., 2005; April, 1990; Snell, 2011). Variations in nerve architecture like these are of importance to clinicians who deal with surgery of the facial skeleton. Morphological changes of mandibular or mental foramen and variations of the nerve have also been described by many authors (Ramadhan et al., 2010;

Prado et al., 2010; Manikandhan et al., 2010; Siéssere et al., 2009; Oktem et al., 2008; Levine et al., 2007).

In many cases there is a single nerve which runs a few millimeters below the roots of teeth, nearly equal number of the nerve lies much lower in the mandible to continue near the lower border of the bone, or sometimes it is plexiform. The nerve can lie on the lingual or buccal side of the mandible (Standring et al., 2005; Snell, 2011). The MN, a branch of the IAN, when emerges through the mental foramen and then divides into three branches that supply the skin of the chin and mucous membrane of the lower lip and gum. Two of them pass upward and forward nearby the mucosal surface of the lower lip. The third one passes through the intermingled fibers of platysma and depressor anguli oris muscles to harvest the skin of the lower lip and chin. As the MN is one of the two terminal branches of the IAN, it is understandable why one's chin and lover lip on the affected side lose sensation, as well. (Standring et al., 2005; Snell, 2011).

Sensory fibers of mandibular nerve and its inferior alveolar branch transmit impulses from the teeth and gums of the lower jaw, skin of the chin and mylohyoid muscle via its mylohyoid branch (Van de Graaff, 1998).

There are numerous congenital anomalous, trauma or cancers of the oral region may affect the IAN throughout its trace. Mandibular fractures through the mandibular canal almost always produce paralysis of inferior alveolar or MNs, as well as numbness of the teeth. Injuries to the inferior alveolar or MNs can also occur during the elevation of skin or mucosal flaps in the region (Cummings et al., 1993). The tumors should be evaluated before surgical procedure or performing anesthesia with regard to size and degree of infiltration and particularly in defining the relationship to the nerve. The trigeminal nerve is the principle nerve relating to the practice of dentistry. Before teeth are filled or extracted, anesthetic is injected near the appropriate nerve to block sensation. A mandibular nerve block desensitized the lower teeth, which was performed by injecting anesthetic near the IAN as it enters the mandible through the mandibular foramen. Important complications may include damage to IAN and its branches during operation or injecting anesthetic. (Paparella et al., 1991; Van de Graaff, 1998).

An entrapment neuropathy is a nerve lesion caused by pressure or mechanical irritation from anatomic structures next to the nerve. This can occur where the nerve passes through a fibro-osseous canal or foramen like mental foramen and is relatively fixed, from impingement by an anatomic structure, or from entrapment of the nerve between the soft and hard tissues. Thus, it is important to know the anatomy of inferior alveolar nerve and its major branches with relation to their vulnerability to entrapment (Piagkou et al., 2011)

The IAN normally descends medial to the lateral pterygoid muscle passes between the sphenomandibular ligament and the mandibular ramus, and then enters the mandibular canal through the mandibular foramen. In the mandibular canal it runs downward and forward, generally below the apices of the teeth until below the first and second premolars, where it divides into the terminal incisive and mental branches (Khan et al., 2010; Krmpotic-Nemanic et al., 2001).

The mylohyoid nerve branches from the IAN, as the latter descends between the sphenomandibular ligament and the mandibular ramus. The mylohyoid nerve passes forward in a groove to reach the mylohyoid muscle and the anterior belly of the digastric muscle. (Loughner et al., 1990).

Topographically, the IAN may pass close to the medial part of the condyle. As such, a medially displaced disccould interfere mechanically with this nerve. This could explain the sharp, shooting pain felt locally in the joint with jaw movements as well as the pain and other sensations projecting to the terminal area of distribution of the nerve branches near thetemporomandibular joint, such as the ear, temple, cheek, tongue, and teeth (Piagkou et al., 2011; Johansson et al., 1990).

The MN exits the mandible through the mental foramen, divides into three branches deep to the depressor anguli, oris muscle, and supplies the skin and mucous membrane of the lower lip, the skin of the chin, and the vestibular gingiva of the mandibular incisor (Standring et al., 2005; Moore, 1983; April, 1990; Woodburne & Burkel 1994).

The MN is significant during surgical procedures of, the chin area such as genioplasty and mandibular anterior segmented osteotomy (Westermark et al.,1998; Seo et al., 2005; Gilbert & Dickerson 1981), and it can also be damaged during dental procedures such as dental implant surgery, orthodontic treatment, and endodontic treatment.

Mental neuropathy also may be caused by systemic diseases and tumors (Bodner et al., 1989; Klokkevold et al., 1989; Chand et al., 1997). Severe pain or sensation disturbance may occur when the MN is entirely or partially injuried after such applications. A relatively common problem is the use of an inappropriate attachment depth or path during the insertion of dental implant fixtures, which may injury the IAN and MN. The incidence of permanent sensory disturbance to the lower lip after dental implant insertion in the mental foramen region is reportedly 7% to 10%. (Wismeijer et al., 1997; Mardinger et al., 2000). Complications such as loss of lip and chin sensation may result in lip biting, impaired speech, and diminished salivary retention, deficits that have a significant impact on a cases' activities of daily living (Deeb et al., 2000; Smiler, 1993) . The MN can be preserved during dental implant or flap surgeries by repositioning the IAN or ridge augmentation (Hu et al., 2007).

Anatomical anomalies of the mandibular canal may have clinical implications, such as an increased risk of injury to the IAN in case of removing a mandibular third molar and inadequate local anesthetics such as bifid and trifid mandibular canal (Mizbah et al., 2010).

The IAN can be damaged secondary to the injection of a local anesthetic into the pterygomandibular space or the MN when injecting in the region of the mental foramen. Although the exact pathophysiology of this injury remains unknown, there are three possible causes as firstly direct intraneural injection with mechanical injury to the nerve such as severance of axons, partial or total, scar tissue or neuroma formation, Wallerian degeneration, and so forth, secondly interruption of vessels of the mesoneurium with perineural and intraneural hemorrhage and secondary scar formation, and thirdly chemical toxicity of the anesthetic solution from a sterilizing solution in a leaky carpule. Regardless of its cause, it is recommended that aspiration be done before all local anesthetic injections. If there is a bloody aspirate or the patient complains of a paresthesia as typically, an electric shock-like sensation, the needle is withdrawn a few millimeters and aspiration is repeated. If there is now no bloody aspirate, it can be assumed that the needle tip is no longer in contact with a blood vessel or nerve, and the injection is completed. A note of such an occurrence should be routinely entered in the cases' chart. This method may prevent direct injection into a vascular space, but does not necessarily prevent deposition of the anesthetic within the epineurium. Because the diameter of the IAN is 4–5 times greater than the associated inferior alveolar artery or vein. Nerve injury secondary to local anesthetic injection is not common. It may be difficult to differentiate from damage related to the placement of the dental implants, particularly if the case was under sedation or general anesthesia and, therefore, unable to report a paresthesia at the time of the injections (Meyer & Bagheri, 2011).

Damage to the IAN as a consequence of bone preparation or implant placement may be caused by errors in radiographic planning, drilling, or direct contact of the implant with the nerve. Drill injuries to the IAN may be difficult to diagnose. Damage caused by drilling, the extent of injury of the IAN caused by the implant itself is related to the degree of encroachment of the implant into the IAC or its direct contact with the IAN. Nerve injury caused by implant placement may occur, despite correct osseous preparation, when the implant is inserted beyond the vertical confines of the prepared bone, compressing or breaching the superior wall of the IAC and forcing bone into the canal. Consecutive, extension of drilling into the IAC may favor over insertion of the implant cylinder beyond its intended depth and into the IAC, making direct contact with the IAN (Meyer & Bagheri 2011).

The MN ranges in the mandibular buccal soft tissue and is at risk of injury during incisions. Recognition of the changing anatomy of the edentulous mandible is especially helpful in minimizing risk of damage to the MN. As the cases ages, the alveolar bone in an edentulous area resorbs, and the position of the mental foramen becomes closer to the crest of the alveolar ridge. In some cases there is actual rupture of the IAN and the MN come to lie on the alveolar ridge crest. Placement of an incision must, therefore, take these anatomic changes into gravity. During the retraction of a mucoperiosteal flap it is potential to exert continuous improper pressure on the underlying IAN and MN. Gentle soft tissue retraction with frequent short relaxation of retraction pressure is advised nerve (Meyer & Bagheri 2011).

For reconstruction of an atrophied posterior mandible, different therapeutic options have been proposed, such as autologous bone grafting, guided bone regeneration for vertical ridge augmentation, and IAN mobilization with simultaneous implant placement. The possible dehiscence of soft tissues covering the surgical zone makes the first and second techniques unpredictable. Moreover, two surgical sites are necessary and a long treatment time as nearly 12 months is required. With IAN mobilization, only one surgical intervention is required and the total treatment time is shorter as about about 6 months. However, this method risks irreversible damage to the IAN, with consequent functional alterations. Recent studies have shown extreme variability in the examination of functionality of the neurovascular bundle after its mobilization. This variability can be attributed both to the methodology used for the tests, which evoke subjective answers from the case, and to the surgical procedure, which is highly dependent on surgeon method. Nerve injury may be the result of an overstretched mucoperiosteal flap in the premolar region to achieve optimal visibility of the operative zone (Bovi, 2005).

Less common causes of nerve damage are related to placement of autologous or allogenic or also xenogenic bone grafts during simultaneous implant placement. In cases of complex implant reconstruction, the bone graft material may be placed into the donor site with additional force, thus severely compressing or even crushing the IAN. The authors have decelerated several cases of particulate bone graft material within the IAC that caused important nerve compression, and other cases of severe scarring, similar in clinical configuration to a chemical burn, when calcium hydroxyapatite came in direct contact with the nerve (Meyer & Bagheri, 2011; Ferrera & Chandler, 1994).

During surgical resection of tumors of the oral cavity, head and neck surgeons are often faced with the challenge of achieving complete resection margins while preserving a functional and anatomical features to avoid nerve injury. Injuries to peripheral branches like IAN during the removal of third molar teeth are known and accepted risks in oral and maxillofacial surgery practice. These risks might be reduced by modifications of evaluation or surgical methods depending on the operators' judgment in individual ceses. If a nerve damages, prompt recognition, subjective and objective valuing, and forming a treatment plan, if the sensory deficit fails to resolve in a rational period and is not acceptable to the cese, give the case the best chance of achieving recovery of sensory function in the distribution of the damaged nerve. Microneurosurgery may produce return of useful sensory function or complete sensory improvement if done in a timely fashion by an experienced operator, in greater than 80% of cases who prevent nerve damages during the removal of the third molar teeth (Meyer & Bagheri, 2011).

3. Mechanisms of nerve injury

3.1 Nerve morphology

The nerve trunk is surrounded of four connective tissue sheaths. These are the mesoneurium, epineurium, perineurium, and endoneurium from the outside inward (Polland et al., 2001). The mesoneurium is a connective tissue sheath which is analogous to the mesentery of the intestine. It encloses the nerve trunk within the soft tissue, contains the segmental blood supply of the nerve, it continues with the epineurium. The epineurium is the loose connective tissue sheath which protects the nerve trunk against mechanical stress. Fascicles are marked out by the perineurium, which surrounds the axons and endoneurial sheaths. The fascicular pattern can be monofascicular (one large fascicle), oligofascicular (2-10 rather large fascicles) or polyfascicular (more than 10 fascicles of different sizes). Individual nerve fibers and their Schwann cells are surrounded by the endoneurium. The perineurium and endoneurium provide elasticity together. Polyfascicular nerves with many small fascicles such as the IAN resist stretch more than monofascicular or oligofascicular nerves (Sunderland, 1951). The nerve fiber is the functional component of the peripheral nerve and it is responsible for transmitting stimuli. The nerve fiber consists of axon, a Schwann cell, and a myelin sheath in myelinated nerve fibers. The axon is a segment of a neuron and can be characterized by morphology, conduction velocity and function.

A-alpha fibers are the largest myelinated fibers. They are encoded for the transmission of muscle spindle and tendon organ afferents and skeletal muscle efferents. The A-beta fibers are the second largest myelinated axons. The sensation of touch is transmitted to these axons. The A-delta fibers are the smallest of the myelinated fibers, which transmit stimuli encoded for temperature and pain. The smallest axons are the unmyelinated C-fibers. They transmit stimuli encoded for slow or second pain, temperature, and efferent sympathetic fibers (LaBanc, 1992).

In 1943, Seddon described a triple classification of mechanical nerve injuries to characterize the morphophysiologic types. Seddon's classification includes neuropraxia, axonotmesis and neurotmesis and is based on the time course and completeness of sensory recovery (Seddon, 1943).

3.1.1 Neuropraxia

Neuropraxia represents the mildest form of nerve injury. It is characterized by a conduction block, almost complete return of sensation or function, and no degeneration of the axon. The continuity of the epineural sheat and the axons is lasts and morphologic alterations are minor. Trauma to the endoneurial capillaries causes intrafascicular edema, resulting in a conduction block. The sensation or function returns to normal within 1 to 2 days following the resolution of intrafascicular edema, generally within 1 week following nerve injury. The function deficit recovers spontaneously and usually complete within 3 to 4 weeks (LaBanc, 1992).

3.1.2 Axonotmesis

Axonotmesis is a more severe nerve injury with disruption of the neuronal axon but with maintenance of the myelin sheath. This type of nerve damage may cause paralysis of the motor, sensory, and autonomic functions.

It involves loss of the relative continuity of the axon and its covering of myelin, but preservation of the connective tissue framework of the nerve (the encapsulating tissue, the epineurium and perineurium, are preserved). Because of the loss of axonal continuity, wallerian degeneration occurs. An axonotmesis is characterized by axonal injury and continues with degeneration or regeneration. Traction and compression are the usual mechanisms of this type of injury. This may cause severe ischemia, intrafascicular edema, or demyelination. Although the axons are damaged, there is no disruption of the endoneurial sheath, perineurium, or epineurium. Complete recovery takes place in 2 to 4 months, but improvement leading to complete recovery may take as long as 12 months.

It is important to know that within 2 to 4 months following injury, signs of sensation or function begin and continue to improve over the next 8 to 10 months. Anesthesia followed by a paresthesia is the psychophysical response to an axonotmesis as recovery begins (LaBanc, 1992).

3.1.3 Neurotmesis

Neurotmesis is the most severe lesion with potential of recovering. A neurotmesis is characterized by severe disruption of the connective tissue components of the nerve trunk. The etiology of nerve injury is traction, compression, injection injury, chemical injury, local anesthetic toxicity or in a complete distruption of the nerve trunk laceration and avulsion. In this type of nerve injury, sensory and functional recovery is never complete.

The psychophysical response to these injuries is an immediate anestesia. This may be followed by paresthesia or possibly neuropathic responses such as allodynia, hyperpathia, hyperalgesia, or chronic pain. This type of nerve injury has a high probability of development of a central neuroma (LaBanc, 1992).

4. Inferior alveolar nerve lateralisation

4.1 Surgical procedure

IAN lateralisation is a new technique. In the literature of implantology, the techniques described are partial and located at the anterior part of the nerve, near the foramen mentalis. Total lateralisation technique can be used in dental prosthesis in mandibular posterior edentulism when the alveolar bone is reduced and when the prosthesis compresses the nerve in the foramen region. This technique can also be used in implantology when terminal implant restitution is needed. On patients with benign tumors when the horizontal branch of the mandible is resected total lateralisation technique is a choice.

The procedure starts with the soft tissue incision slightly buccal to the crest of the residual alveolar ridge.The incision begins at the retromolar region and continues forward to the mesial portion of the cuspid tooth area, where a vertical relaxing incision is made. A full thickness mucoperiosteal flap is elevated to the inferior border of the mandible. For performing IAN lateralization, the corticotomy starts usually 3–4 mm distal to the mental foramen. Corticotomy should be extended 4–5 mm distal to the most distal implant position. To remove the trabecular bone and gain access to the neurovascular bundle, only hand instruments such as small curettes are used. The MN is mobilized from its position. After the nerve is completely released from the canal, half a rubber piston from a dental anaesthetic cartridge or a piece of aluminum foil is inserted between the nerve bundle and the bone.

Once the drilling is completed, the implant is inserted while the nerve bundle remains retracted in situ ensuring that the apical ends of the implants are positioned inferior to the canal. Once the implants are in position, the nerve is repositioned over the lateral aspect of the implants. The surgical protocol for IAN transposition, followed by implant placement, presented excellent results, with complete recovery of the sensitivity within 6 months after the surgical procedure.

4.2 Case report

45 year-old female patient applied to Gulhane Scholl of Medicine, Department of Oral and Maxillofacial Surgery, with missing teeth in the mandibula. As she couldn't use removable partial denture, we evaluated posterior mandibular area. But mandibular posterior bone height was inadequate for implant placement. A preoperative panoramic radiograph (Fig 2) and computerized tomograhic (CT) scan revealed only 5 mm. of bone between the alveolar crest and the inferior alveolar canal.

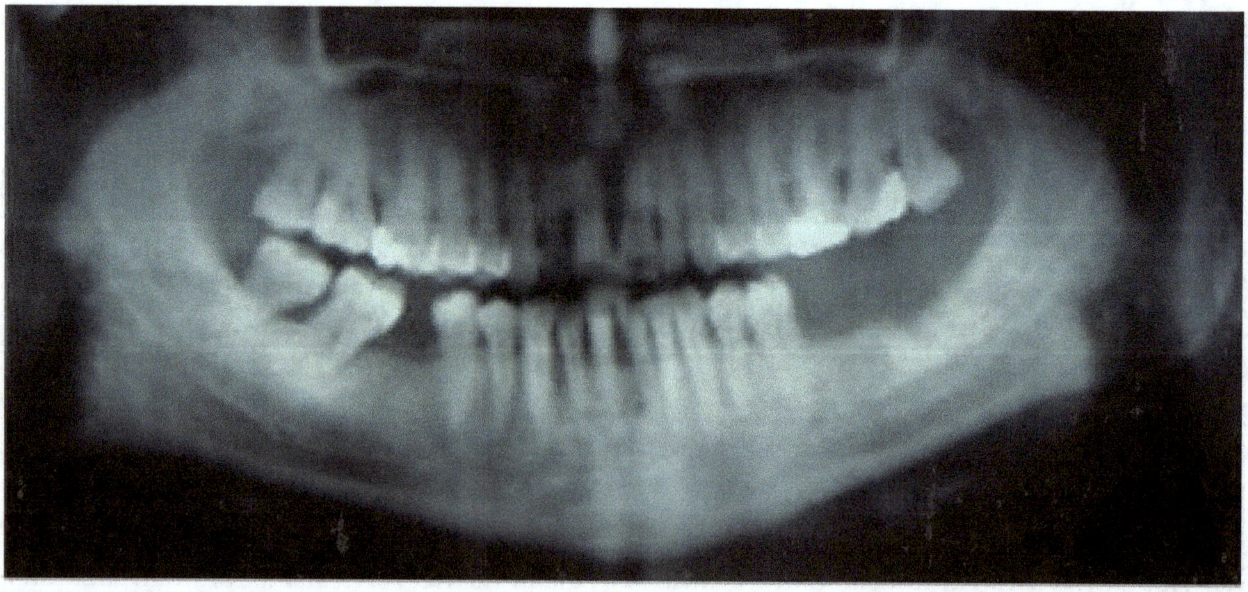

Fig. 2. Preoperatif panoramic radiograph.

We planed alternative methods including IAN lateralization technique at this place. The surgical procedure was performed under local anesthesia. A full thickness mucoperiosteal flap was elevated to the inferior border of the mandible. For performing inferior alveolar nerve lateralization, the corticotomy started 4 mm distal to the mental foramen. A small round bur in a straight hand piece with high torque and copious amount of water irrigation was used to prepare the corticotomy site. To remove the trabecular bone and gain access to the neurovascular bundle, only hand instruments (small curettes) were used. The IAN was mobilized from its position. After the nerve was completely released from the canal and before starting to drill, half a rubber piston from a dental anaesthetic cartridge or a piece of membrane was inserted between the nerve bundle and the bone where the drill was expected to reach (Fig 3). At second premolar and second molar region, we placed 3.5x12 mm. MIS implant (Fig 4).

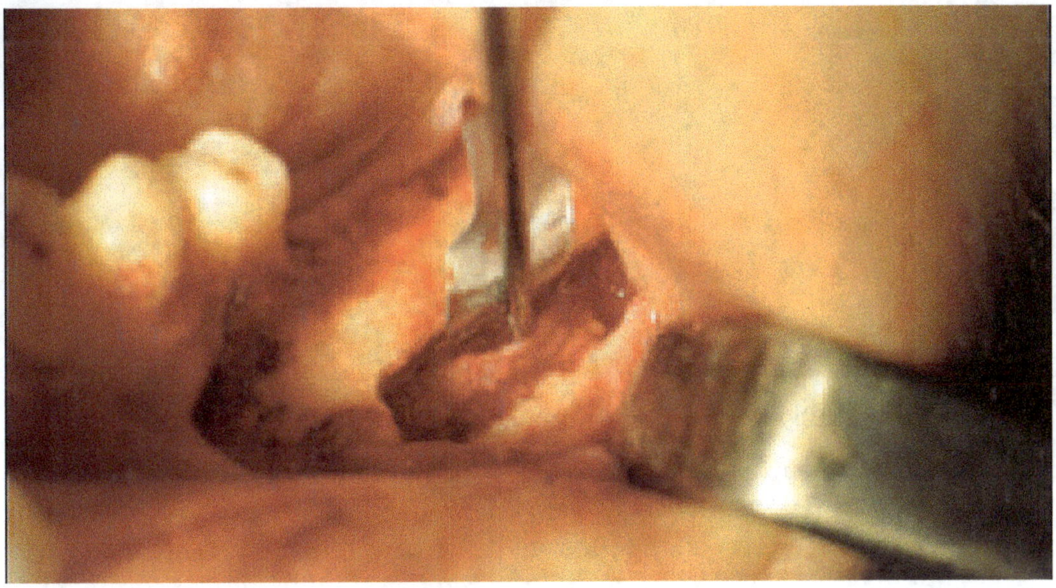

Fig. 3. Nerve retraction with a retractor.

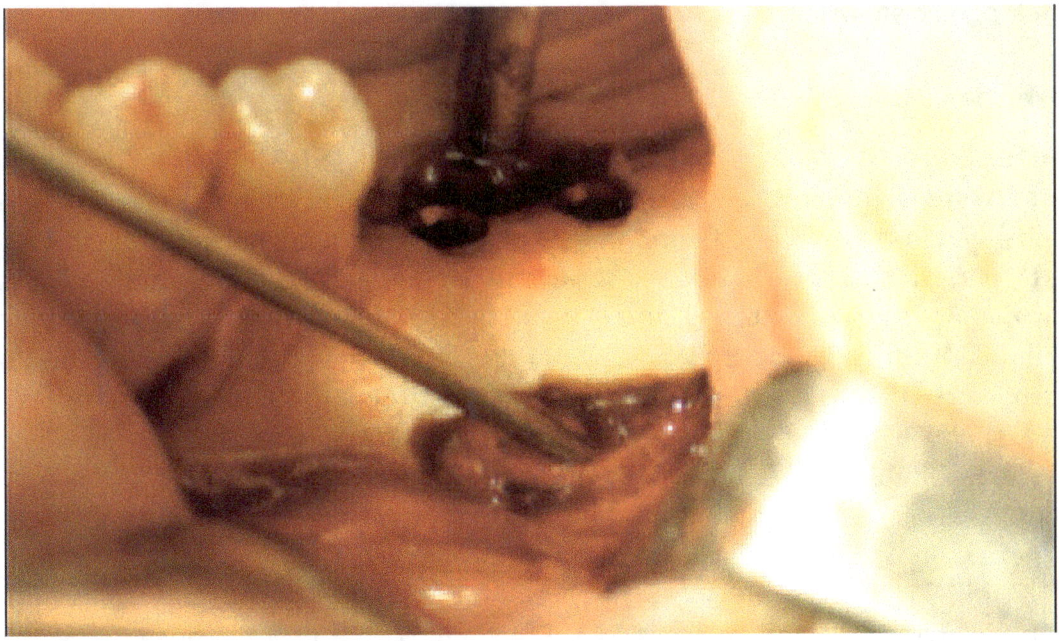

Fig. 4. Two implants was placed after nerve retractions.

The releasing incisions were carried out and mucoperiostal flap were sutured by using 3.0 silk. CT scan and panoramic radiograph (Fig 5) were taken after placing the endosseos implants. Surgical exposure and moving the nerve laterally results in a high incidence of sensory nerve disturbance and an excessive crown-to-root ratio of the prosthesis.

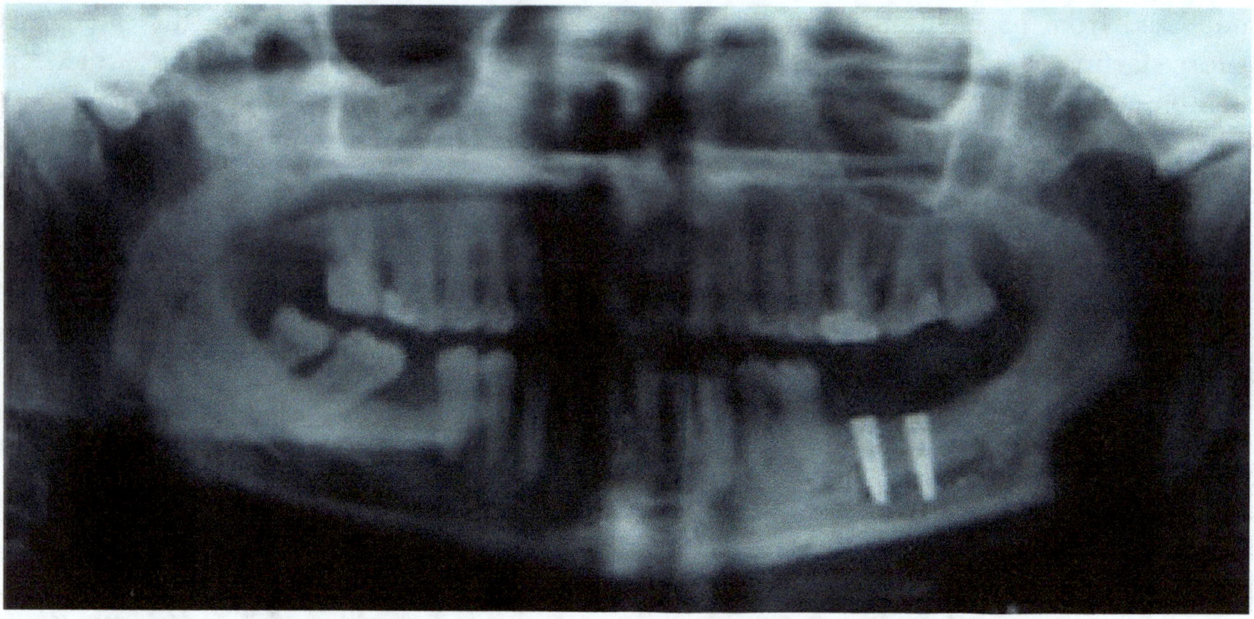

Fig. 5. The ends of the implants are positioned inferior to the canal.

We didn't examine any neurologic disturbance at postoperative controls. The present study investigated neurosensorial disturbances related to IAN lateralization for up to 6 month follow-up. Subjective criteria, sensory function of the IAN returned to normal 6 weeks after surgery. IAN lateralization is a precise technique requiring high clinical competence, which should only be carried out by specialists. IAN lateralization is a useful method for managing the atrophic posterior mandible with dental implants. The risk of permanent damage of the IAN appears to be small.

5. References

Ardekian, L., Salnea, J., Abu el-Naaj, I., Gutmacher, T., & Peled, M. (2001). "Inferior alveolar nerve repositioning in implant surgery." *Refuat Hapeh Vehashinaym* 18(2): 39-41, 62.

Aldskogius, H., Arvidsson, J. & Grant, G. (1985). "The reaction of primary sensory neurons to peripheral nerve injury with particular emphasis on transganglionic changes." *Brain Res* 357(1): 27-46.

Anderson, LC., Kosinski, TF., & Mentag, PJ. (1991). "A review of the intraosseous course of the nerves of the mandible." *J Oral Implantol* 17(4): 394-403.

April, EW. (1990). Clinical anatomy. *The National Medical Series for Independent Study*. 2nd ed. Harwal Publishing Company, USA.

Babbush, CA. (1998). "Transpositioning and repositioning the inferior alveolar and mental nerves in conjunction with endosteal implant reconstruction." *Periodontology 2000* 17: 183-90.

Becerra, L., Morris, S., Bazes, S., Gostic R., Sherman, S., Gostic J., Pendse G., Moulton, E., Scrivani, S., Keith D., Chizh B., & Borsook D. (2006). "Trigeminal neuropathic pain alters responses in CNS circuits to mechanical (brush) and thermal (cold and heat) stimuli." *J Neurosci* 26: 10646–57.

Bodner, L., Oberman, M., & Shteyer, A. (1989). "Mental nerve neuropathy associated with compound odontoma." *Oral Surg Oral Med Oral Pathol* 63(6): 658-60.

Bovi M. (2005) "Mobilization of the inferior alveolar nerve with simultaneous implant insertion: a new technique. Case report." *Int J Periodontics Restorative Dent* 25(4): 375-83.

Chand, V., Sweeney, C., & Agger, WA. (1997). "Mental neuropathy in patients with AIDS-associated malignant lymphoma." *Clin Infect Dis* 24(3): 521-2.

Chrcanovic, BR., & Custodio, AL. (2009). "Inferior alveolar nerve lateral transposition." *Oral Maxillofac Surg* 13(4): 213-9.

Cummings, CW., Fredrickson, JM., Harker, LA., Krause, CJ., & Schuller, DE. (1993). *Otolaryngology-Head and Neck Surgery*. 2nd ed. Vol I, Mosby Year Book, , pp312.

Deeb, GR., Dierks, E., So, YT. (2000). "Sensory nerve conduction study of the mental nerve." *Muscle Nerve* 23(7):1121-4.

Di Lenarda, R., Cadenaro, M., & Stacchi, C. (2000). "Paresthesia of the mental nerve induced by periapical infection: A case report." *Oral Surg Oral Med Oral Pathol Oral Radiol Endod* 90(6):746-9.

Essick, G. (2004). "Psychophysical assessment of patients with post- traumatic neuropathic trigeminal pain." *J Orofac Pain* 18: 345–54.

Ferrera, PC., & Chandler, R. (1994). Anesthesia in the emergency setting: Part II. Head and neck, eye and rib injuries. *Am Fam Physician* 15;50(4):797-800.

Gary, G., & Dennis, T. (2006). "The mental foramen and nerve: clinical and anatomical factors related to dental implant placement: a literature review." *J Periodontol* 77(12): 1933-43.

Gilbert, BO., & Dickerson, AW 2nd. (1981). "Paresthesia of the mental nerve after an acute exacerbation of chronic apical periodontitis." *J Am Dent Assoc* 103(4):588-90.

Greenstein, G., & Tarnow, D. (2006). "The mental foramen and nerve: clinical and anatomical factors related to dental implant placement: a literature review." *J Periodontol* 77(12): 1933-43.

Gregg, JM. (2000). Neuropathic complications of mandibular implant surgery: review and case presentations. *Ann R Australas Coll Dent Surg* 15:176-80.

Grover, PS., & Lorton, L. (1983). "Bifid mandibular nerve as a possible cause of inadequate anesthesia in the mandible." *J Oral Maxillofac Surg* 41(3): 177-9.

Jensen, O. & Nock, D. (1987). "Inferior alveolar nerve repositioning in conjunction with placement of osseointegrated implants: a case report." *Oral Surg Oral Med Oral Pathol* 63(3): 263–8.

Johansson AS, Isberg A, & Isacsson G. (1990). "A radiographic and histologic study of the topographic relations in the temporomandibular joint region: Implications for a nerve entrapment mechanism." *J Oral Maxillofac Surg* 48: 953–61.

Haghighat, K. (2007). "Bone augmentation techniques." *J Periodontol* 78(3): 377-96.

Hashemi, HM. (2010). "Neurosensory function following mandibular nerve lateralization for placement of implants." *Int J Oral Maxillofac Surg* 39(5): 452–6.

Hilu, RE., & Zmener, O. (1999). "Mental nerve paresthesia associated with an amalgam filling: A case report." *Endod Dent Traumatol* 15(6): 291-3.

Hu, KS., Yun, HS., Hur, MS., Kwon, HJ., Abe, S., & Kim, HJ. (2007). "Branching patterns and intraosseous course of the mental nerve." *J Oral Maxillofac Surg* 65(11): 2288-94.

Kieser, J., Kuzmanovic, D., Payne A, Dennison J., & Herbison P. (2002). "Patterns of emergence of the human mental nerve." *Arch Oral Biol* 47(10): 743-7.

Khan, MM., Darwish, HH., & Zaher, WA. (2010). "Perforation of the inferior alveolar nerve by the maxillary artery: An anatomical study." *Br J Oral Maxillofac Surg* 48(8): 645-7.

Kim, ST., Hu, KS., Song, WC., Kang, MK., Park HD. & Kim HJ. (2009). "Location of the mandibular canal and the tomography of its neurovascular structures." *J Craniofac Surg* 20(3):936-9.

Klokkevold PR, Miller DA, & Friedlander AH. (1989). "Mental nerve neuropathy: A symptom of Waldenström's acroglobulinemia." *Oral Surg Oral Med Oral Pathol* 67(6):689-93.

Krmpotic-Nemanic, J., Vinter, I., & Jalsovec, D. (2001). "Accessory oval foramen." *Ann Anat* 183:293–5.

Krogstad O, & Omland G. (1997). "Temporary paresthesia of the lower lip: A complication of orthodontic treatment. A case report." *Br J Orthod* 24(1): 13-5.

LaBanc JP. (1992). "Reconstructive microneurosurgery of the trigeminal nerve." In: Bell WH. editors. *Modern practice in orthognathic and reconstructive surgery*. Philadelphia: W. B. Saunders Cop. p: 1083–89.

Labanc, JP. (1988). "Diagnostic evaluation and management of inferior alveolar and lingual nerve injuries." *Fla Dent J* 59(4): 50-4.

Langlais, RP., Broadus, R., & Glass BJ. (1985). "Bifid mandibular canals in panoramic radiographs." *J Am Dent Assoc* 110(6): 923-6.

Levine, MH., Goddard, AL., & Dodson, TB. (2007). "Inferior alveolar nerve canal position: a clinical and radiographic study." *J Oral Maxillofac Surg* 65(3): 470-4.

Loughner, BA., Larkin, LH., & Mahan, PE. (1990). "Nerve entrapment in the lateral pterygoid muscle." *Oral Surg Oral Med Oral Pathol* 69(3):299–306.

Lundborg, G. (1988). "Intraneural microcirculation." *Orthop Clin North Am* 19(1): 1-12.

Manikandhan, R., Mathew, PC., Naveenkumar, J., Anantanarayanan, P. (2010). "A rare variation in the course of the inferior alveolar nerve." *Int J Oral Maxillofac Surg* 39(2): 185-7.

Mardinger O, Chaushu G, Arensburg B, Taicher S, & Kaffe I. (2000). "Anterior loop of the mental canal: An anatomical-radiologic study." *Implant Dentistry* 9(2):120-5.

Metzger, MC., Bormann, KH., Schoen, R., Gellrich, NC., & Schmelzeisen, R. (2006). "Inferior alveolar nerve transposition an in vitro comparison between piezosurgery and conventional bur use." *J Oral Implantol* 32(1): 19-25.

Meyer, RA., Bagheri, SC. (2011) "Nerve injuries from mandibular third molar removal." *Atlas Oral Maxillofac Surg Clin North Am* 19(1):63-78.

Misch, CE., & Resnik, R. (2010). "Mandibular nerve neurosensory impairment after dental implant surgery: management and protocol." *Implant Den*t 19(5): 378-86.

Mizbah, K., Gerlach, N., Maal, TJ., Bergé, SJ., & Meijer GJ. (2010). "Bifid and trifid mandibular canal. A coincidental finding." *Ned Tijdschr Tandheelkd* 117(12): 616-8.

Morrison, A, Chiarot, M, & Kirby, S. (2002). "Mental nerve function after inferior alveolar nerve transposition for placement of dental implants." *J Can Dent Assoc* 68:46-50.

Moore, KL. (1983). *Clinically orianted anatomy*. The Williams and Wilkind Company USA.

Nortjé, CJ., Farman, AG., & de V Joubert JJ. (1977). "The radiographic appearance of the inferior dental canal: an additional variation." *Br J Oral Surg* 15(2): 171-2.

Oktem H., Oktem F., Sanli E., Menevse GT., & Tellioğlu AT. (2008). "An anatomic variation of mental nerve." *J Plast Reconstr Aesthet Surg* 61(11):1408-9;

Ordás, CM., Cuadrado, ML., Simal, P., Barahona, R., Casas, J., Matías-Guiu Antem, J., & Porta-Etessam, J. (2011). "Wallenberg's syndrome and symptomatic trigeminal neuralgia." *J Headache Pain* Feb 10. [Epub ahead of print].

Paparella, MM., Shumrick, DA., Gluckman, JL., & Meyerhoff, WL. (1991). *Otolaryngology, Vol I,II,III*. 3rd ed. WB. Saunders Company, pp123, 2958,2050;

Piagkou, M., Demesticha, T., Skandalakis, P., & Johnson, EO. (2011). "Functional anatomy of the mandibular nerve: Consequences of nerve injury and entrapment." *Clin Anat* 24(2):143-50.

Polland, KE., Munro, S., Reford, G., Lockhart, A., Logan, G., Brocklebank, L., & McDonald SW. (2001). "The mandibular canal of the edentulous jaw." *Clin Anat* 14(6): 445-52.

Prado, FB., Groppo, FC., Volpato, MC., & Caria, PH. (2010). "Morphological changes in the position of the mandibular foramen in dentate and edentate Brazilian subjects." *Clin Anat* 23(4):394-8;

Ramadhan, A., Messo, E., & Hirsch, JM. (2010). "Anatomical variation of mental foramen. A case report." *Stomatologija* 12(3):93-6.

Scarano, A., Carinci, F., Assenza, B., Piattelli, M., Murmura, G., & Piatelli, A., (2011). "Vertical ridge augmentation of atrophic posterior mandible using an inlay technique with a xenograft without miniscrews and miniplates: case series." *Clin Oral Implants Res*

Seddon, HJ. (1943). "Three types of nerve injuries." *Brain* 66: 237–43.

Seo, K., Tanaka, Y., Terumitsu, M., & Someya, G. (2005). "Characterization of different paresthesias following orthognathic surgery of the mandible." *J Oral Maxillofac Surg* 63(3):298-303.

Siéssere, S., Hallak Regalo, SC., Semprini, M., Honorato De Oliveira, R., Vitti, M., Mizusaki Iyomasa, M., Mardegan Issa, JP., & De Sousa, LG. (2009). "Anatomical variations of the mandibular nerve and its branches correlated to clinical situations." *Minerva Stomatol* 58(5):209-15;

Smiler, DG. (1993). "Repositioning the inferior alveolar nerve for placement of endosseous implants: Technical note." *Int J Oral Maxillofac Implants* 8(2): 145-50.

Snell, RS. (2011). Clinical Anatomy. Williams and Wilkins 8th ed.Walters Kluwer, USA.

Standring, S., Ellis, H., Healy, JC., Johnson, D., Williams, A. & Collins, P. (2005). *Gray's Anatomy* (ed 39). London, Churchill Livingstone, p 513;

Sunderland, S., (1951) "A Classification of Peripheral Nerve Injuries Producing Loss of Function." *Brain* 74(4): 491-516.

Takazakura, D., Ueki, K., Nakagawa, K., Maruka, K., Shimada, M., Shamiul, A., & Yamamoto, E. (2007). "A comparison of postoperative hypoesthesia between two types of sagittal split ramus osteotomy and intraoral vertical ramus osteotomy, using the trigeminal somatosensory-evoked potential method." *Int J Oral Maxilofac Surg* 36: 11–4.

Van de, Graaff. (1998). *Human Anatomy 5th ed.* WBC McGraw-Hill Companies, USA, pp395

Westermark, A., Bystedt, H., & von Konow, L. (1998). "Inferior alveolar nerve function after mandibular osteotomies." *Br J Oral Maxillofac Surg* 36(6):425-8.

Wismeijer, D., van Waas, MA., Vermeeren, JI., & Kalk W. (1997). "Patients' perception of sensory disturbances of the mental nerve before and after implant surgery: A prospective study of 110 patients." *Br J Oral Maxillofac Surg* 35:254-9

Woodburne, RT, & Burkel, WE. *Essentials of Human Anatomy* (ed 9). New York, Oxford University Press, 1994, p 268.

4

Clinical Complications of Dental Implants

Su-Gwan Kim
Dept. of Oral and Maxillofacial Surgery, School of Dentistry, Chosun University
Republic of Korea

1. Introduction

Dental implant surgery has become routine treatment in dentistry and is generally considered to be a safe surgical procedure with a high success rate. However, complications should be taken into consideration because they can follow dental implant surgery as with any other surgical procedure. Many of the complications can be resolved without severe problems; however, in some cases, they can cause dental implant failure or even life-threatening circumstances. Avoiding complications begins with careful treatment planning based on accurate preoperative anatomic evaluations and an understanding of all potential problems. This chapter contains surgical complications associated with dental implant surgery and management.

2. Complications associated with implant surgery

2.1 Hemorrhage

The submental artery (2mm in average diameter) (Greenstein et al., 2008 as cited in Hofschneider et al., 1999) is a branch of the facial artery. The sublingual artery (2 mm in average diameter) arises from the lingual artery and is found coronal to the mylohyoid muscle (Greenstein et al., 2008 as cited in Martin et al., 1993). The arterial blood supply of the floor of the mouth is formed by an anastomosis of the sublingual and submental arteries. In the canine area, the vessels are located closer to the lingual plate and alveolar crest than they are in more posterior areas (Dubois et al., 2010). Intraosseous hemorrhage is not a serious event, and control of the hemorrhage can be ensured by compressing the area with a directional indicator, an abutment, or the implant (Annibali et al., 2009). However, severe bleeding and the formation of massive hematomas in the floor of the mouth are the result of an arterial trauma. A vascular wound may occur after detrimental surgical manipulations or tearing of the lingual periosteum, but in most cases, it is attributed to perforations of the lingual cortical plate. Mechanical pressure exerted by the expanding hematomas displaces the tongue and floor of the mouth both superiorly and posteriorly (Kalpidis & Setayesh, 2004). This occurrence may lead to extensive bleeding into the submandibular space, resulting in a life-threatening acute airway obstruction within the first few hours after surgery (Goodacre et al., 1999). The hemorrhage can easily spread in the loose tissues of the floor of the mouth (Fig. 1.), the sublingual area, and the space between the lingual muscles, which may require intubation or an emergency tracheostomy (Dubois et al., 2010). The surgeons also should consider other sources of potential hemorrhage and subsequent hematoma formation, including injuries to muscles or other soft tissues (Isaacson, 2004) (Fig.

2.). The escalating symptomatology of massive bleeding and progressive respiratory distress strongly resemble the clinical development of Ludwig's angina. Most important is the immediate bimanual compression at the suspected site of perforation and transport of the patient to the nearest hospital to secure the airway without delay (Dubois et al., 2010).

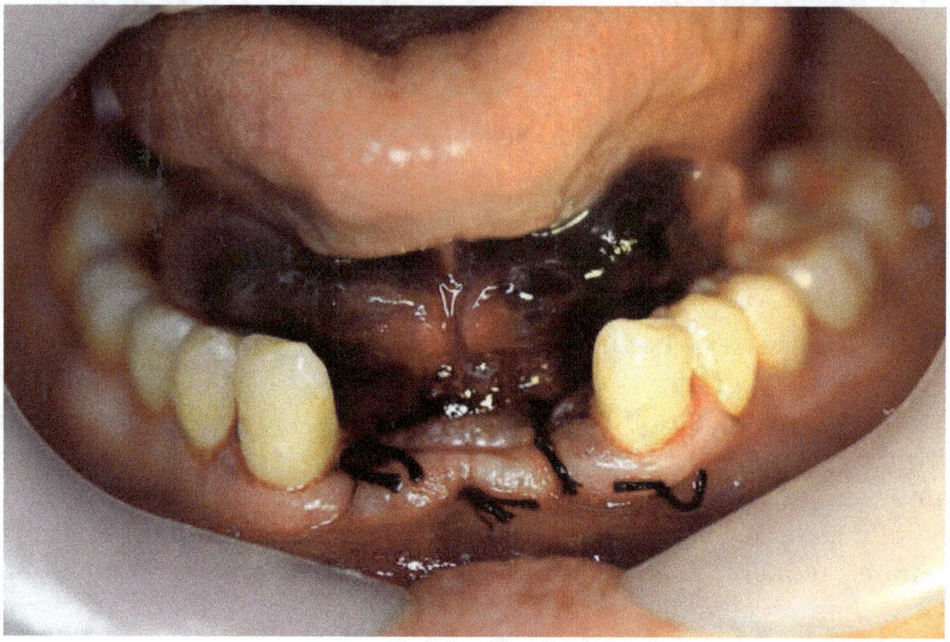

Fig. 1. A severe hematoma on the anterior floor of the mouth after implant placement in the anterior mandible.

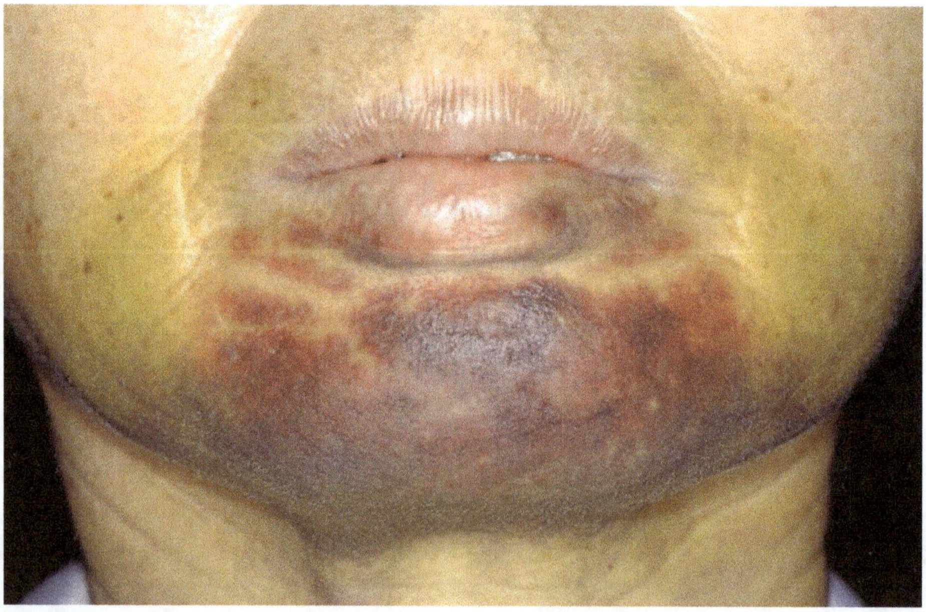

Fig. 2. Ecchymosis on the chin after implant placement in the anterior mandible.

Once the airway is controlled, efforts are undertaken for the definitive resolution of the hemorrhage (Kalpidis & Setayesh, 2004 as cited in Givol, 2000). Hemorrhages can be controlled by gauze tamponage, application of hemostatic agents, cauterization, or digital compression. If a hemorrhage cannot be controlled by these methods, ligation of the bleeding vessel should be performed. An endovascular angiography is an alternative diagnostic tool that can overcome unsuccessful attempts to define and isolate the bleeding source (Fig. 3.) (Kalpidis & Setayesh, 2004). Incisions in the mucosa to relieve the hematoma should be avoided because they may promote further bleeding. The removal of an already inserted implant would also be ineffective (Fig. 4.) (Kalpidis & Setayesh, 2004) (Table 1).

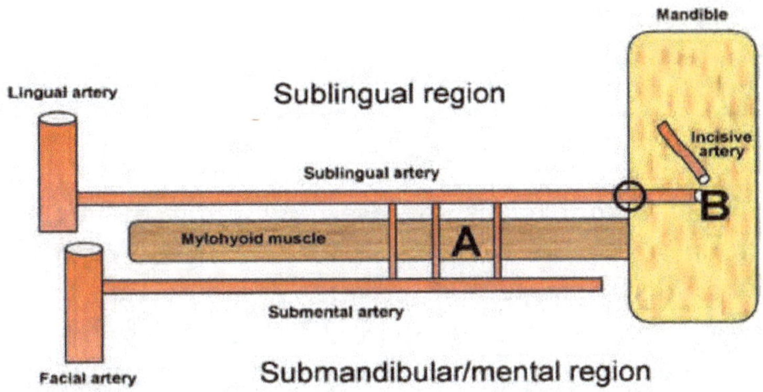

Fig. 3. A schematic representation of the arterial anatomy in the floor of the mouth (Kalpidis & Setayesh, 2004).

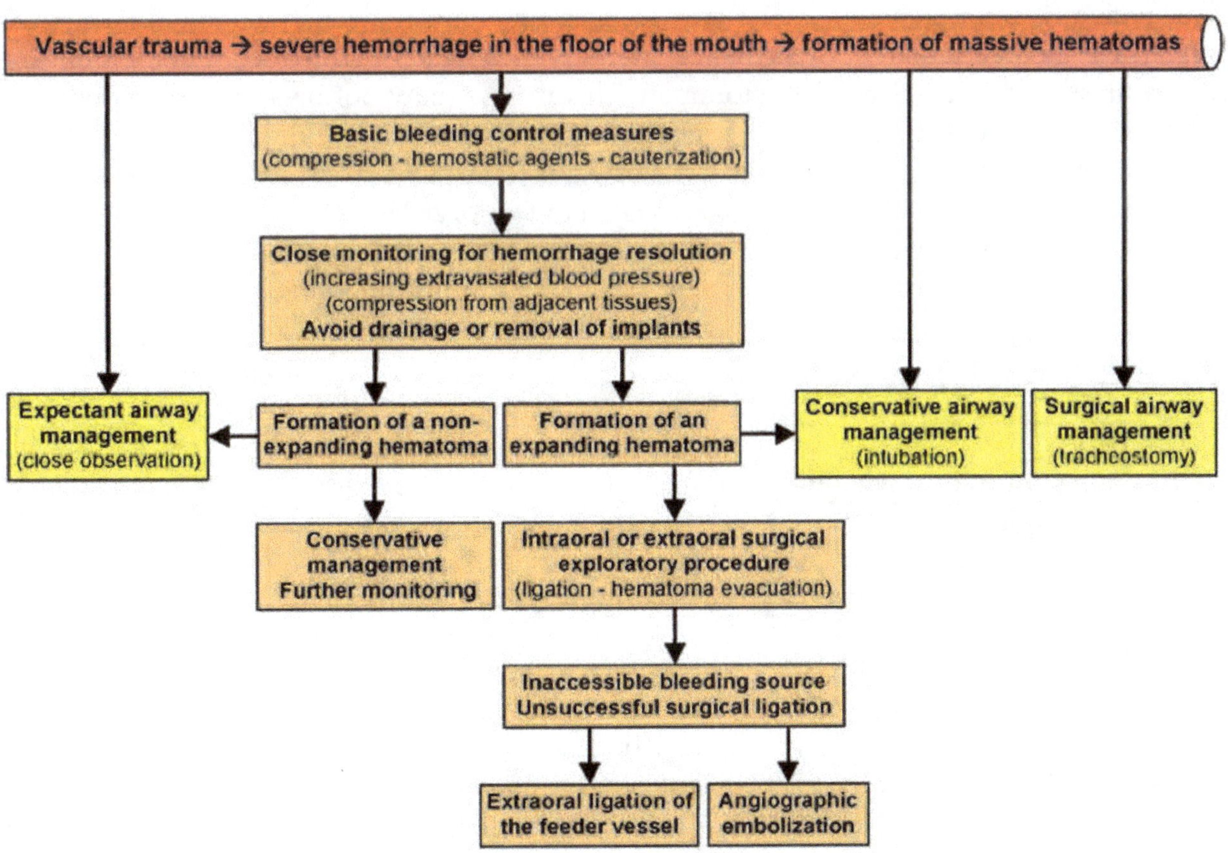

Fig. 4. A flow diagram of airway management and control of massive hemorrhage in the floor of mouth associated with implant placement in the anterior mandibular region (Kalpidis & Setayesh, 2004).

Bleeding site during implant osteotomy	Arteries	Treatments
Posterior mandible	Mylohyoid	Finger pressure at the site
Middle lingual of mandible	Submental	Surgical ligation of facial and lingual arteries
Anterior lingual of mandible	Terminal branch of sublingual or submental	Compression, vasoconstriction, cauterization, or ligation
Invading the mandibular canal	Inferior alveolar artery	Bone graft

Table 1. Treatment of a hemorrhage at an implant osteotomy site (Park & Wang, 2005)

To prevent unintentional hemorrhages in cases involving the immediate placement of implants or recent tooth extractions, the practitioner should be careful not to use the extraction socket as a guide for angulation because this may lead to the perforation of the lingual cortex (Isaacson, 2004 as cited in Givol, 2000). Soft-tissue management during the procedure is essential, and clinicians should make every attempt to avoid subperiosteal tears (Isaacson, 2004).

2.2 Neurosensory disturbances

The inferior alveolar nerve is midway between the buccal and lingual cortical plates in the first molar region (Tammisalo et al., 1992). In about 1% of patients, however, the mandibular canal bifurcates in the inferior superior or medial lateral planes. Thus, a bifurcated mandibular canal will manifest more than one mental foramen. This may or may not be seen on panoramic or periapical films. Accordingly, Dario suggested that clinicians should consider obtaining a preoperative tomogram to avoid nerve injuries prior to implant placement above the inferior alveolar canal (Greenstein & Tarnow, 2006 as cited in Dario, 2002).

A mean incidence of neurosensory disturbance incidence after implant surgery was 6.1% (Goodacre et al., 1999) to 7% (Goodacre et al., 2003), with a range between 0.6% and 39%. Nerve damage can have results ranging from mild paresthesia to complete anesthesia or even disabling dysesthesia (Table 2).

Neurapraxia	There is no loss of continuity of the nerve; it has been stretched or has undergone blunt trauma. The parasthesia will subside, and feeling will return in days to weeks.
Axonotmesis	Nerve is damaged but not severed; feeling returns within 2 to 6 months.
Neurotmesis	Severed nerve; poor prognosis for resolution of parasthesia.

Table 2. Classification of nerve injuries (Greenstein & Tarnow, 2006 as cited in Jalbout & Tabourian, 2004)

Possible causes of nerve injury include poor flap design, traumatic flap reflection, accidental intraneural injection, traction on the mental nerve in an elevated flap, penetration of the osteotomy preparation and compression of the implant body into the canal (Fig. 5.)(Misch & Wang, 2008). Nerve injuries may be caused indirectly by postsurgical intra-alveolar edema or hematomas that produce a temporary pressure increase, especially inside the mandibular canal. Direct traumas are the most frequent causes of nerve injury, and they may occur through five mechanisms: compression, stretch, cut, overheating, and accidental puncture

(Annibali et al., 2009). Finally, prolonged pressure from neuritis may lead to the permanent degeneration of the affected nerve (Park & Wang, 2005).

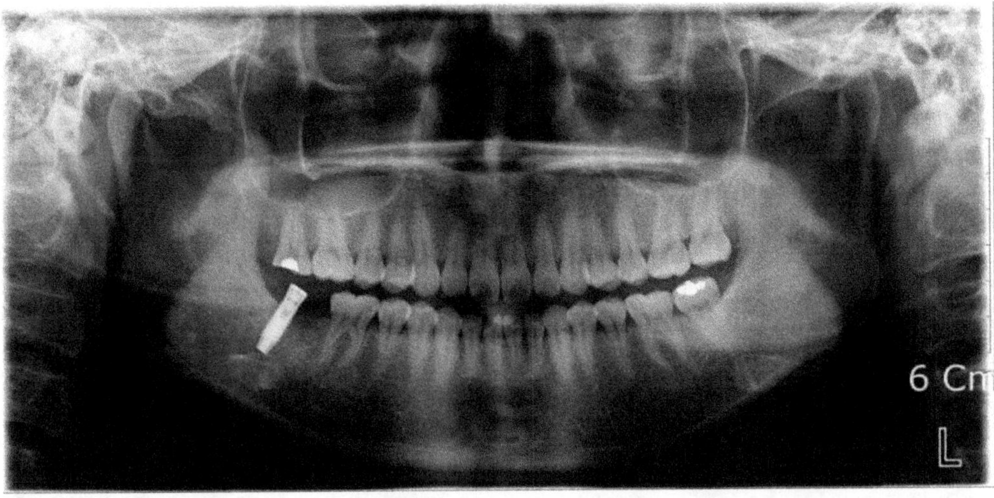

Fig. 5. An inferior alveolar nerve injury after implant placement of #47.

The mental nerve is at particular risk of iatrogenic injury because it arises from asymmetric foramina and forms a concave loop anteriorly. In edentulous patients, it may be very close to the bone surface or the top of the crest.

The nerve injury may cause one of the following conditions: parasthesia (numb feeling), hypoesthesia (reduced feeling), hyperesthesia (increased sensitivity), dysthesia (painful sensation), or anesthesia (complete loss of feeling) of the teeth, the lower lip, or the surrounding skin and mucosa (Greenstein & Tarnow, 2006 as cited in Sharawy & Misch, 1999).

Overpenetration occurs when the cortical portion of the alveolar crest places resistance on the drill. However, as it enters the marrow spaces, a drill may drop into the neurovascular bundle unless the surgeon has excellent control (Misch & Wang, 2008).

For implants placed in the atrophic posterior mandible, the routine use of intraoperative periapical radiographs during the drilling sequence can help avoid the risk of injury to the inferior alveolar nerve. Periapical radiographs used intraoperatively to obtain working length measurements are similar in concept to techniques used in root canal therapy. This method can reliably determine safe distances between the implant and the inferior alveolar canal, thus avoiding the risk of injury to the nerve altogether (Burstein et al., 2008).

The appropriate magnification correction factor should be used, and drill guards can be placed on burs to avoid the unintentional overpenetration of the drill. A safety margin of 2 mm between the entire implant body and any nerve canal should be maintained (Greenstein et al., 2008, as cited in Greenstein & Tarnow, 2006; Worthington, 2004). Additionally, surgical placements of implants should be at least 3 mm in front of the mental foramen (Greenstein & Tarnow, 2006). When placing implants in proximity to the mental foramen, the clinician must take into consideration the anterior loop of the nerve and the available bone above the mental foramen, because the inferior alveolar nerve often rises as it approaches the mental foramen (Kraut & Chahal, 2002). Finally, although the depths of the implant bur are variable, the drill bur may be longer than the implant according to the manufacturers (Table 3).

Be sure to include nerve injury as an item in the informed consent document. Measure the radiograph with care. Apply the correct magnification factor. Consider the bony crestal anatomy: If the ridge is thin buccolingually, is this useless bone or should an augmentation procedure be done? Is the buccolingual position of the crestal peak of bone influencing the measurement of available bone? Consider the buccolingual position of the nerve canal.	Use coronal true-size tomograms where needed. Allow a 1 to 2 mm safety zone. Use a drill guard. Take care with countersinking not to lose support of the crestal cortical bone. Use the aforementioned formula to calculate implant length. Keep the radiograph and the calculation in the patient's chart as powerful evidence of meticulous patient care.

Table 3. Recommendations to avoid nerve injuries during implant placement (Worthington, 2004)

The mental foramen may be located at or near the crest of an atrophic mandible. To avoid damage to the mental nerve in patients with atrophic mandibles, the clinician may need to make incisions in the area of the mental foramen that are lingual to the crest of the mandible (Kraut & Chahal, 2002).

If an implant is in danger of violating the canal, its depth should be decreased in the bone (i.e., by unscrewing it a few turns) and left short of the canal or removed. Because the altered sensation may be due to an inflammatory reaction, a course of steroid treatment or a high dose of nonsteroidal anti-inflammatory medication (e.g., ibuprofen [800 milligrams] three times per day) should be prescribed for three weeks (Kraut & Chahal, 2002). Adjunct drugs such as clonazepam, carbamazepine, or vitamin B-complex might alleviate neuritis via their known neuronal anti-inflammatory actions.

If improvement is noted at three weeks on the basis of a repeated neurosensory examination, the clinician can prescribe an additional three weeks of anti-inflammatory drug treatment. If the improvement is seen, however, the patient should be referred to a microneurosurgeon (Kraut & Chahal, 2002).

The patient should be referred for microsurgery if total anesthesia persists, or if after 16 weeks, dysesthesia is ongoing (Misch & Wang, 2008, as cited in Day, 1994; Nazarian et al., 2003).

Many studies have reported favorable patient responses to inferior alveolar nerve repairs. All have emphasized the need for repair before Wallerian degeneration of the distal portion of the inferior alveolar nerve has occurred; because this degeneration is a slow process, repair is possible four to six months after the injury has occurred (Kraut & Chahal, 2002).

2.3 Injury to adjacent teeth

Damage to teeth adjacent to the implant site may occur subsequent to the insertion of implants along an improper axis or after placement of excessively large implants (Figs. 6, 7.). This problem arises more frequently with single implants (Annibali et al., 2009). Adjacent teeth should be evaluated before implant placement. Pulpal and periradicular conditions such as small periapical radiolucencies, root resorption and large restorations in/near the vital pulp are often misdiagnosed. Dilacerated roots and excessive tilting in the mesiodistal direction that invades the implant space often prevent ideal placement (Misch & Wang, 2008). The tilt of adjacent teeth should be assessed before drilling. The damage of an adjacent tooth by implant placement may cause the tooth to become non-vital, and the tooth may require subsequent endodontic treatment. This will not only result in damage to an adjacent tooth but also implant failure (Sussman, 1998). Use of a surgical guide, radiographic analysis and CT scan can help locate the implant placement, thereby avoiding damage to adjacent teeth. The angulation of adjacent teeth and dilacerations of roots must be radiographically assessed prior to implant placement. Ideally, 1.5 to 2 mm of bone should be present between an implant and the adjacent tooth. Furthermore, inspection of a radiograph with a guide pin at a depth of 5 mm will facilitate osteotomy angulation corrections (Greenstein et al., 2008). To prevent a latent infection of the implant from the potential endodontic lesion, endodontic treatment should be performed (Sussman, 1998). Discrepancies between the apical and crestal interdental spaces as a result of mesial or distal tipping of the roots can be corrected orthodontically (Annibali et al., 2009).

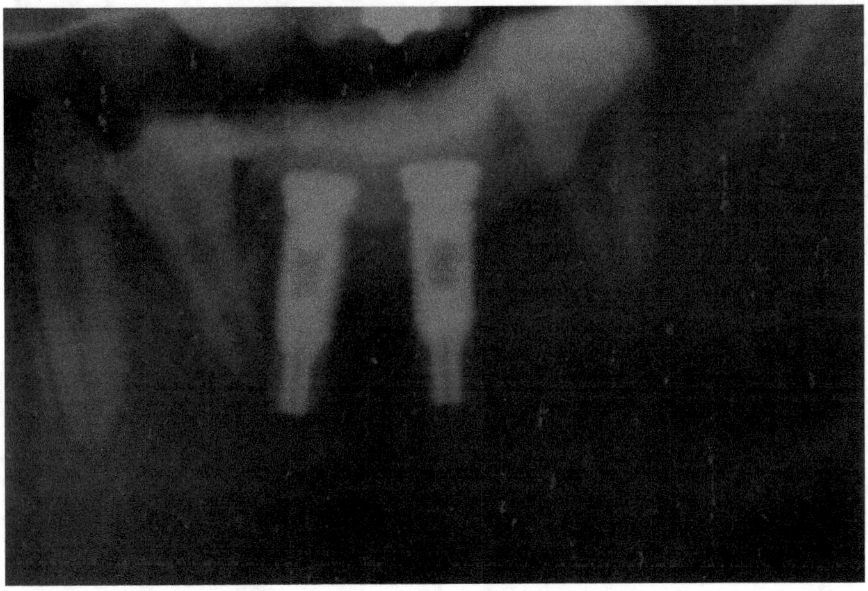

Fig. 6. Injury of an adjacent tooth by a malpositioned implant.

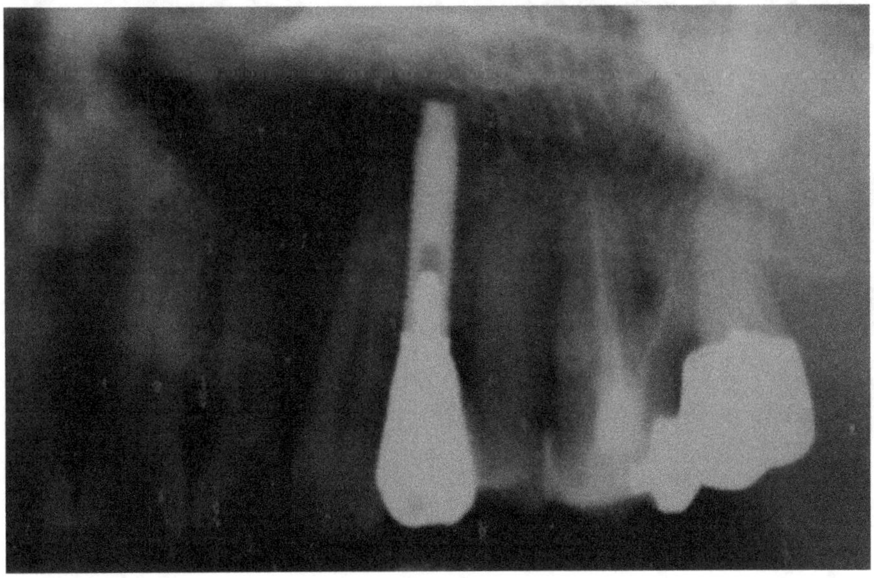

Fig. 7. A malpositioned implant hitting an adjacent tooth.

2.4 Flap dehiscence and exposure of graft material or barrier membrane

The most common postoperative complication is wound dehiscence, which sometimes occurs during the first 10 days (Greenstein et al., 2008). Contributing factors of dehiscence and exposure of the graft material or barrier membrane include flap tension, continuous mechanical trauma or irritation associated with the loosening of the cover screw, incorrect incisions and formation of sequestration of bone debris (Park & Wang, 2005). Premature exposure of barrier membranes may also cause contamination of the graft and its eventual loss (Figs. 8, 9.).

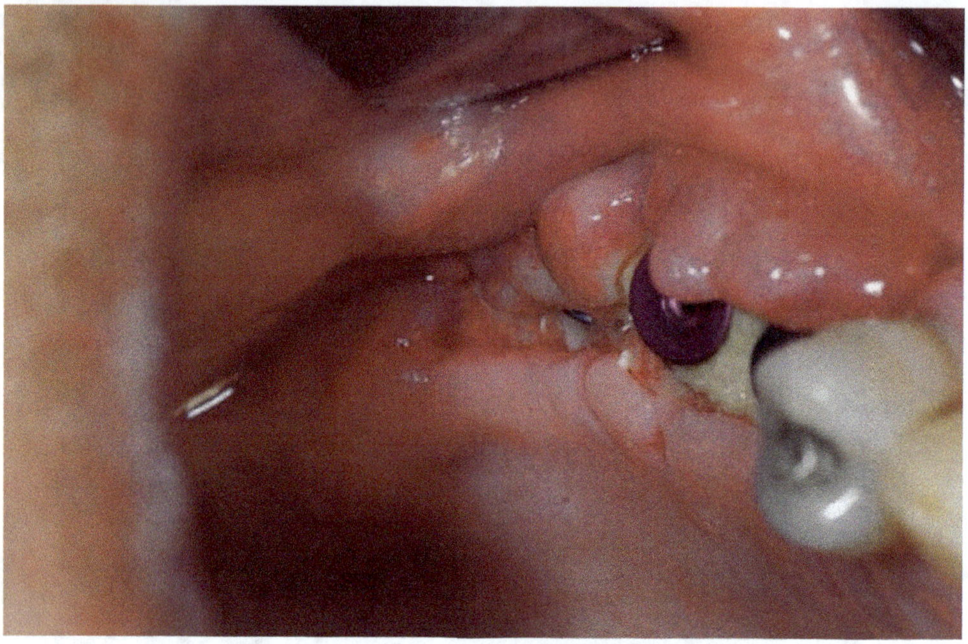

Fig. 8. A dehiscence after guided bone regeneration and implant placement using a non-resorbable membrane.

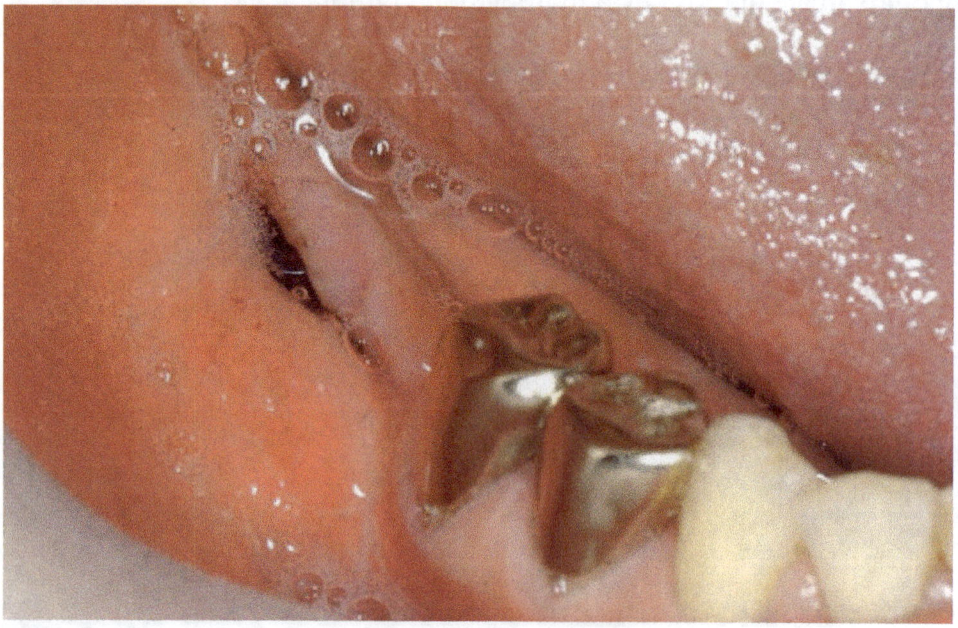

Fig. 9. A dehiscence after implant placement.

To avoid wound dehiscence, tension-free closure using a buccal releasing incision is most important. Dentures should be relieved with a tissue conditioner. Mattress sutures combined with interrupted sutures are also useful. When the dehiscence is small and occurs within 24 to 48 hours, the clinician can immediately resuture the dehiscence. Once the diameter of the wound is large (2 to 3 cm) or the time elapsed is > 2 days, it is suggested that the margins of the wound be excised and resutured (Fig. 10.) (Greenstein et al., 2008 as cited in Sadig & Almas, 2004). If the suture is not possible, chlorhexidine rinses twice a day and/or systemic antibiotics should be considered.

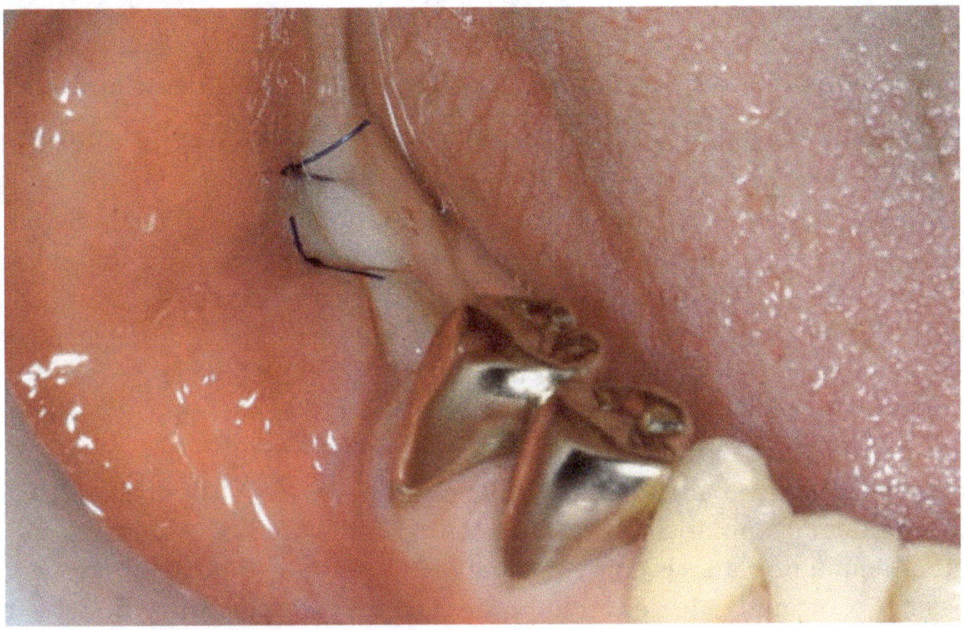

Fig. 10. Resuturing was performed to achieve closure of the dehiscence.

2.5 Bisphosphonate-related osteonecrosis

Bisphosphonates are drugs that inhibit bone resorption; they are widely used for the treatment of osteoporosis, multiple myeloma and skeletal complications of bone metastases (Table 4). The American Association of Oral and Maxillofacial Surgeons (AAOMS) states that patients are considered to have bisphosphonate-related osteonecrosis of the jaw (BRONJ) if they have the following three characteristics: current or previous treatment with a bisphosphonate, exposed or necrotic bone in the maxillofacial regin that has persisted for more than 8 weeks, and no history of localized radiotherapy to the jaws (Advisory Task Force on Bisphosphonate-Related Ostenonecrosis of the Jaws, 2007). The risk of BRONJ associated with oral bisphosphonates appears to increase when the duration of therapy more than 3 years. This time may be shortened in the presence of certain comorbidities. Type 2 diabetes mellitus (Abu-Id et al., 2008), prolonged steroid therapy (Advisory Task Force on Bisphosphonate-Related Ostenonecrosis of the Jaws, 2007), and health-threatening habits such as smoking (Wessel et al., 2008; Yarom et al., 2007) were suggested as predisposing conditions for the development of BRONJ.

If systemic conditions permit, discontinuation of oral bisphosphonates for a period of 3 months prior to and 3 months after elective invasive dental surgery may lower the risk of BRONJ. The risk reduction may vary depending on the duration of bisphosphonate exposure (Advisory Task Force on Bisphosphonate-Related Ostenonecrosis of the Jaws, 2007).

Active ingredient	Trade name	Administered
Alendronate	Fosamax®,Fosavance®	Orally
Etidronate	Osteum®, Difosfen®	Orally
Resedronate	Actonel®, Acrel®	Orally
Tiludronate	Skelid®	Orally
Zoledronate	Zometa®, Aclasta®	Intravenously
Pamidronate	Aredia®, Linoten®, Pamifos®, Xinsidona®	Intravenously
Ibandronate	Bondronat®	Orally, Intravenously
Clodronate	Bonefos®	Orally, Intravenously

Table 4. Different types of bisphosphonates in current usage (Montoya-Carralero et al., 2010)

Currently, there are no reliable or widely available tests for the risk of BRONJ. Marx et al. recommend a blood test, specifically involving a serum C-terminal telopeptide test (CTX) to assess a surrogate marker of bone turnover in patients taking oral bisphosphonates. Categorization of <100 pg/mL as high risk, 100 pg/mL to 150 pg/mL as moderate risk, and >150 pg/mL as minimal risk provides the clinician (Marx et al., 2007).

Many articles have confirmed that implant surgery in patients receiving oral bisphosphonate therapy does not result in BRONJ. (Bell &Bell, 2008; Fugazzotto et al., 2007; Grant et al.,2008; Jeffcoat, 2006) Nevertheless, patients taking bisphosphonates who either had implants that failed to integrate or had integrated implants that subsequently failed have been reported (Goss & Backhous, 2007; Stark & Epker, 1995; Wang et al., 2007).

The prognosis of dental implants that have been placed remains uncertain, and the use of osseointegrated dental implants is controversial.

AAOMS does not contraindicate dental implant placement in patients who have been taking bisphosphonates orally for less than three years prior to surgery, provided that they do not present other risk factors such as medications with corticosteroids or advanced age (e.g., older than seventy years). It has been reported that oral bisphosphonates had a lower risk because they took longer to develop bisphosphonate-induced osteonecrosis given their slower accumulation rates in bone (Ruggiero et al., 2004). Moreover, a drug holiday is recommended 3 to 6 months in duration before dental implant placement in patients with a history of oral bisphosphonate use for longer than 3 years (Ruggiero et al., 2009). Finally, current guidelines contraindicate the placement of dental implants in cancer patients treated with intravenous bisphosphonates (Ruggiero et al., 2009; Khan et al., 2008).

Although bisphosphonates tend to accumulate in sites of active bone remodeling like the jaws, surgical trauma to the alveolar bone during implant surgery could further stimulate the postoperative accumulation of the drug in the implanted site. The localized interference of bisphosphonates on areas of bone turnover may reduce the peri-implant bone resistance to oral bacteria in the long term, thus increasing the risk of peri-implantitis. The potential role of infection on implant failure and BRONJ occurrence is still debated. However, at least one study has reported a reduced incidence of BRONJ in patients who were given prophylactic antibiotics (Montefusco et al., 2008). In addition, the use of perioperative antibiotics and a chlorhexidene mouth wash have been suggested. Great attention should be paid to the oral hygiene and plaque control of implant-prosthetic restorations (Bedogni et al., 2010). Patients treated with bisphosphonates who receive implants should be followed for long periods of time. All patients treated with

oral bisphosphonates must be informed of the potential complications of implant failure and BRONJ development in both the short and long term before the placement of dental implants (Bedogni et al., 2010).
AAOMS has proposed the use of the following staging categories and treatment guidelines regarding BRONJ (Table 5).

BRONJ Staging	Treatment Strategies
At risk category: No apparent exposed/ necrotic bone in patients who have been treated with either oral or IV bisphosphonates	No treatment indicated Patient education
Stage 1: Exposed/necrotic bone in patients who are asymptomatic and have no evidence of infection	Antibacterial mouth rinse Clinical follow-up on a quarterly basis Patient education and review of indications for continued bisphosphonate therapy
Stage 2: Exposed/necrotic bone associated with infection as evidenced by pain and erythema in the region of the exposed bone with or without purulent drainage	Symptomatic treatment with broad-spectrum oral antibiotics, e.g., penicillin, cephalexin, clindamycin, or first generation fluoroquinolone Oral antibacterial mouth rinse Pain control Only superficial debridements to relieve soft tissue irritation
Stage 3: Exposed/necrotic bone in patients with pain, infection, and one or more of the following: pathologic fracture, extraoral fistula, or osteolysis extending to the inferior border	Antibacterial mouth rinse Antibiotic therapy and pain control Surgical debridement/resection for longer term palliation of infection and pain

Table 5. Staging and treatment strategies (Advisory Task Force on Bisphosphonate-Related Ostenonecrosis of the Jaws, 2007)

3. Complications associated with maxillary sinus lift

3.1 Schneiderian membrane perforation

The Schneiderian membrane, which is characterized by periosteum overlaid with a thin layer of pseudociliated stratified respiratory epithelium, constitutes an important barrier for the protection and defense of the sinus cavity. The integrity of the sinus membrane is essential in maintaining the healthy and normal function of the maxillary sinus (Ardekian et al., 2006).
The mucociliary apparatus protects the sinus against infection while the membrane also acts as a biologic barrier. If a perforation occurs, the membrane perforation could represent a window for bacterial penetration and invasion into the grafted area (Zijderveld et al., 2008). Failure to atraumatically elevate the Schneiderian membrane may result in graft migration or loss, exposure of the graft or the implant to the sinus, and postoperative site infection. In addition to contaminating the recipient site, disruption of the mucosa may alter the normal

mucociliary flow patterns, causing retention of secretions and infections around the foreign body (Ward et al., 2008).

The most common intraoperative complication seems to be Schneiderian membrane perforation, which occurs in 10% to 60% of all procedures (Ardekian et al., 2006; Pikos, 1999; Proussaefs et al., 2004). The risk of membrane perforation increases when anatomical variations such as a maxillary sinus septum, spine, or sharp edge are present (Chanavaz, 1990; van den Bergh et al., 2000). Very thin or thick maxillary sinus walls create higher risks of perforating the Schneiderian membrane. The angulation between the medial and lateral walls of the maxillary sinus seemed to exert an especially large influence on the incidence of membrane perforation. For example, sharper angles observed at the inner walls of the sinus in the vicinity of the second upper bicuspid presents a higher risk of perforation (Zijderveld et al., 2008).

The occurrence of iatrogenic sinus membrane perforations during surgery does not seem to be related to sinusitis in healthy people (Ardekian et al., 2006). However, large tears can cause sinusitis, graft infection, or graft displacement into the sinus, which could compromise new bone formation and implant survival (Reiser et al., 2001).

To minimize Schneiderian membrane perforations, surgeons must evaluate the maxillary sinus anatomy while considering the lateral thickness of the lateral wall, slope of the sinus wall, location of septa, membrane thickness through the radiography and CT analysis before maxillary sinus augmentation. Piezoelectric surgery is usually more time-consuming than other techniques, though the frequency and number of Schneiderian membrane perforations or lacerations are generally lower. If the bony lateral wall is thick, a reduction of the thickness of the wall before formation of the lateral window is recommended. In cases involving a very thin maxillary sinus wall, careful reflection of the mucoperiosteum is recommended while the Schneiderian membrane already shines a dark grayish-bluish color through the sinus wall. It is advised that clinicians not begin the lateral door preparation with a round stainless-steel burr; they should use a round diamond bur directly, thereby reducing the risk of a membrane perforation (Zijderveld et al., 2008). To prevent a perforation, some additional small holes in the suction device are recommended to diminish the suction power and to avoid the direct contact of the suction device with the Schneiderian membrane (Zijderveld et al., 2008).

If a tear in the membrane occurs along the periphery of the osteotomy and it is difficult to reengage the membrane, this situation can be managed by extending the outline of the osteotomy several millimeters past the original window and reestablishing contact with the membrane (Greenstein et al., 2008). In general, small tears (<5 to 8 mm) are mitigated simply by folding the membrane up against itself as the membrane is elevated (Chanavaz, 1990). Larger tears do not lend themselves to closure by infolding, and they would need additional methods to contain the graft in its desired position. It has been reported that large sinus membrane perforations should be repaired with collagen or a fibrin adhesive. In severe perforations, some investigators have even suggested abandoning the procedure for 6 to 9 months while the membrane regenerates (Karabuda et al., 2006).

3.2 Hemorrhage

The blood supply of the maxillary sinus is derived from the infraorbital artery, the greater palatine artery and the posterior superior alveolar artery (Chanavaz, 1990; Uchida et al., 1998a). Bleeding during sinus augmentation is rare because the main arteries are not within the surgical area. Although accidental laceration of the vessel is not life-threatening because of the small size of the artery, an impaired visualisation may compromise the elevation of the Schneiderian membrane and interfere with the placement of the graft material (Elian et al., 2005; Testori et al., 2010).

The blood supply to the buccal antral portions relevant to sinus floor elevation surgery occurs via two arteries: the posterior superior alveolar artery and the infraorbital artery, as well as their intraosseous branches and anastomoses (Solar et al., 1999). Anatomically, anastamosis between the posterior superior alveolar artery and infraorbital artery is always found at the lateral antral wall (Traxler et al, 1999); bleeding via damage to these arteries may occur during the formation of the lateral window. The average distance from the artery to the alveolar crest was 16.4 mm (Elian N et al., 2005) to 18.9 mm (± 2.82 mm) (Solar et al., 1999).

The height of the residual bony ridge appears to play a significant role in the location of the vessel. In classes A, B and C (Lekholm & Zarb classification (Lekholm & Zarb, 1985)), the vessel was found >15 mm from the alveolar crest, but in classes D and E, the value was >7 mm (mean 10.4 mm). It is recommended, therefore, to place the superior border of the osteotomy up to 15 mm from the alveolar crest in classes A, B and C, which is sufficient for sinus exposure and placement of long dental implants. In severely atrophic ridges, or classes D and E, where the surgeon has a tendency to place the osteotomy of the sinus wall too far cranially, there is a high probability of transecting the vessel (Mardinger et al., 2007b). Such bleeding can usually be controlled by pressure with a moist gauze pad (Fig. 11.)(Elian et al., 2005).

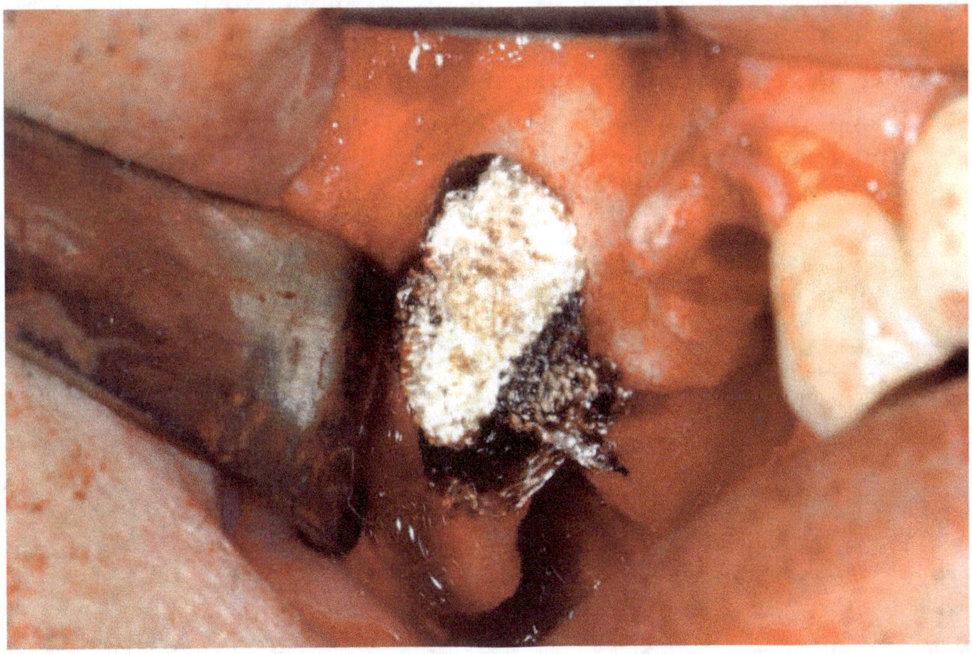

Fig. 11. Hemostasis was achieved using Surgicel during maxillary sinus augmentation.

A preoperative CT examination is essential to detect the location of the intraosseous anastomoses. In addition, piezoelectric surgical inserts may be beneficial in minimizing lacerations of vessels and membrane (Testori et al., 2010). A vestibular extraosseous anastomosis runs below the zygomatic process (Solar et al., 1999). This anastaomosis is located in the area of the periosteum overlying the lateral wall at a higher level than the intraosseous anastamosis. The vascular compromise would be the result of an inappropriate anterior releasing incision or vertical incision (Elian et al., 2005). To avoid damage to the extraosseous anastomosis, vertical mucosal incisions should extend superiorly as little as possible, and the periosteum should be prepared carefully (Solar et al., 1999).

3.3 Loss of the implant or graft materials into the maxillary sinus

The displacement of implants or graft materials into the maxillary sinus can result in a foreign-body reaction and cause serious complications. Migration of a dental implant into the maxillary sinus may present a risk for the development of maxillary sinusitis. Immediate implant insertion should be performed only if the residual bone is stable and high enough to ascertain high primary stability (Becker et al., 2008).

An implant can easily migrate into the sinus without apparent force in the posterior maxilla, clearly showing a lack of osseointegration (Fig. 12.). Various mechanisms have been proposed to explain the migration of an implant into the maxillary sinus, which fall under three main categories: changes in intrasinal and nasal pressures; autoimmune reaction to the implant, causing peri-implant bone destruction and compromising osseointegration; and resorption produced by an incorrect distribution of occlusal forces (Galindo et al., 2005). The changes in intrasinal and nasal air pressures produce a suction effect because of the negative pressure exerted by these cavities. A portion of the bone grafting material can become dislodged in the maxillary sinus at either the initial ridge augmentation or during the implant placement surgery. The natural ciliary movement in the maxillary sinus will transport foreign material toward the ostium (Hunter et al., 2009). In cases with less than 5 mm of bone, mastication can cause the implants to move during the graft maturation timeframe (Peleg et al., 2006). The implants must be immediately retrieved surgically via an intraoral approach or endoscopically via the transnasal route to avoid inflammatory complications (Ueda & Kaneda, 1992). To avoid complications when bone volume is inadequate to support an implant with sufficient length, a bone reconstruction procedure of the maxilla should be performed.

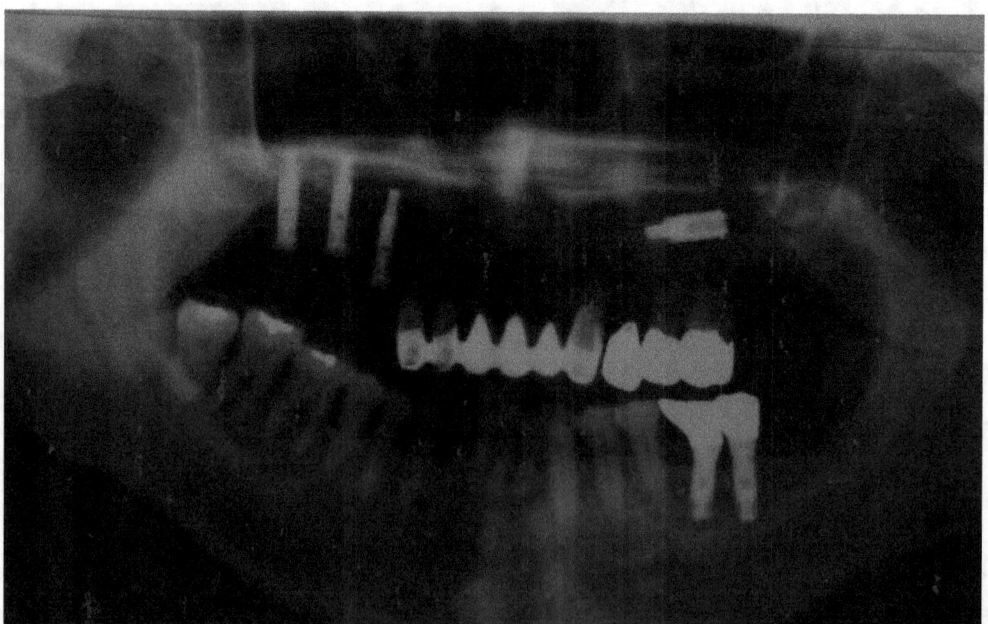

Fig. 12. Displacement of an implant into the maxillary sinus.

3.4 Postoperative maxillary sinusitis

The mean height of the maxillary sinus is 36 to 45 mm, the mean width mesiodistally is 25 to 35 mm, and the mean depth is 38 to 45 mm (laterally–medially). The average total maxillary sinus volume is 13.6±6.4 cc. The minimum maxillary sinus volume is 3.5 cc, while the maximum is 31.8 cc (Uchida, 1998b). The ostium is located on the superior aspect of the medial wall of the maxillary sinus above the first molar (van den Bergh et al., 2000). The normal drainage pattern of the maxillary sinus is into the middle nasal meatus by way of a naturally occurring ostium.

The ostium is usually 35 mm superior to the floor of the maxillary sinus (Zinner et al., 2008). This information can be used to prevent maxillary sinus complications such as sinusitis by the obstruction of the ostium. Radiographic imaging of the osteo-meatal complex is crucial in fully evaluating the physiologic health of the maxillary sinus and the likelihood of avoiding infections following maxillary bone grafting (Zinner et al., 2008).

Maxillary sinusitis can occur as a result of contamination of the maxillary sinus with oral or nasal pathogens or via ostial obstruction caused by postoperative swelling of the maxillary mucosa, hematoma and seroma. Mucosal swelling may lead to the reduction of the patency of the ostio-meatal unit (Figs. 13, 14.). This unit plays a key role in the development of sinusitis, through impairment of the mucociliar cleansing system (Bertrand & Eloy, 1992). Maxillary sinusitis can also occur because of non-vital bony fragments floating freely in the maxillary sinus. Another cause is the lack of asepsis during sinus augmentation (Timmenga et al., 2001). Maintenance of normal maxillary sinus physiology should be a major goal while ostium patency must be preserved. Therefore, the use of a systemic decongestant, such as pseudoephedrine, and a nasal spray containing a vasoconstrictor, such as phenylephrine, is recommended after implant surgery (Regev et al., 1995).

The development of sinusitis following sinus augmentation can be directly related to drainage disturbances, mainly as a result of septal deviation and allergies combined with oversized inferior and middle turbinates (Mardinger, 2007a). In the event of an inadvertent laceration or puncture of the Schneiderian membrane and inoculation of the maxillary sinus

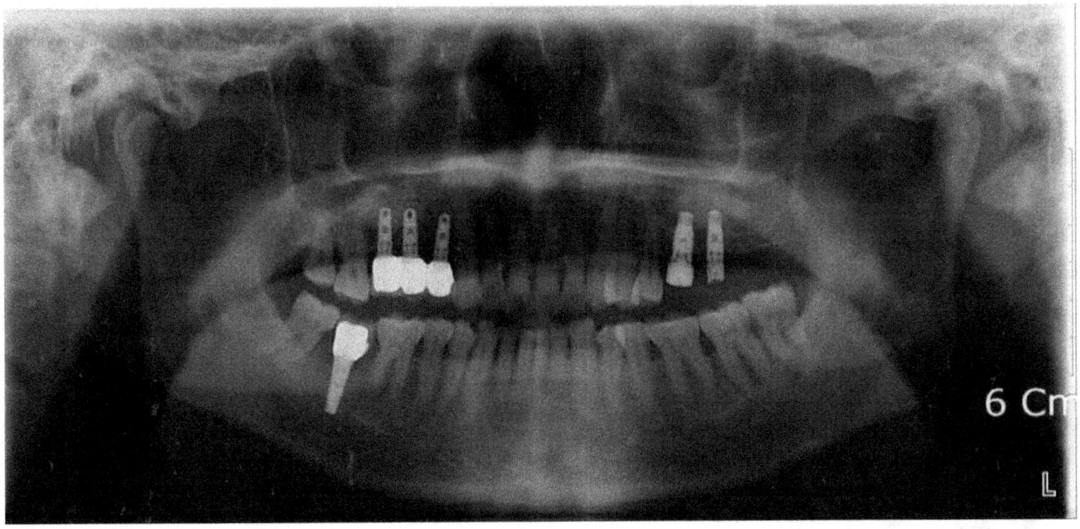

Fig. 13. Panoramic view showing an area of opacification on the left maxillary sinus.

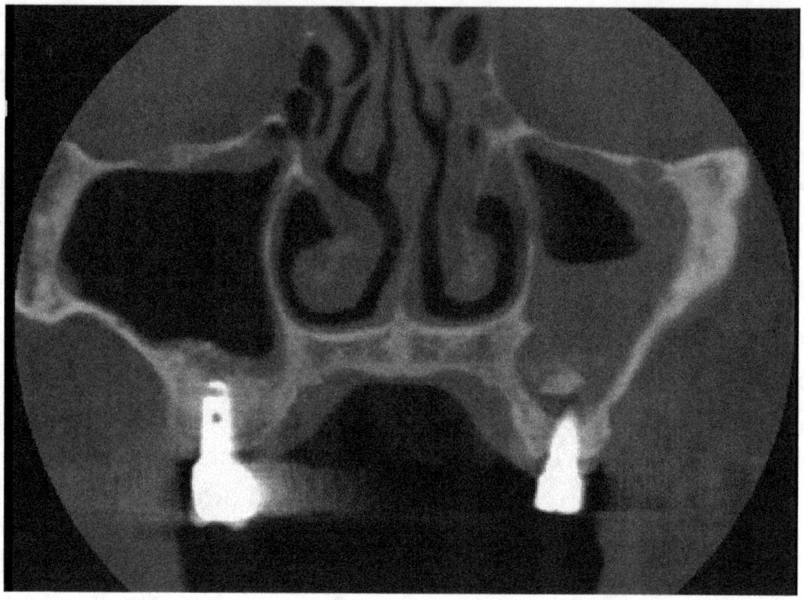

Fig. 14. Computed tomography scan clearly shows significant mucosal thickening along the entire lining of the sinus.

with oral bacteria, a healthy sinus with a patent osteo-meatal complex will usually remove the offending bacteria and remain healthy (Zinner et al., 2008). With no patent drainage pathway, the maxillary sinus quickly became obstructed, inflamed, and then infected (Hunter et al., 2009).

Timmenga et al. reported that the occurrence of postoperative sinusitis after bone grafting of the sinus floor is limited to patients with a predisposition for sinusitis (Timmenga et al., 1997). To minimize the occurrence of a postoperative infection, possible causes should be removed prior to sinus augmentation.

A history of excessive yellow or green nasal discharge, particularly with worsening nasal obstruction, is a relatively strong predictor of possible chronic bacterial sinusitis and may warrant further assessment for chronic sinusitis (Ward et al., 2008). A nasoendoscopic evaluation should be considered for patients with a history of frequent sinusitis to rule out the presence of an obstructive phenomenon as a risk factor before undergoing sinus augmentation (Manor et al., 2010).

Most implant failures occur 3 to 6 months after surgery, and they are usually not associated with an infection of the maxillary sinus (Becker et al., 2008). The clinical diagnosis of sinusitis is characterized by a triad of symptoms: nasal congestion, secretion or obstruction, and headache (Manor et al., 2010). If an infection develops (e.g., pain, redness, and tenderness) without fluctuance, antibiotics are administered. Once there is fluctuance, incision and drainage are performed in conjunction with systemic antibiotics (Barone et al., 2006; Regev et al., 1995).

Pathogens found have included *β-hemolytic Strepococcus, Enterococcus, Peptostreptococcus, Pneumococcus, Staphylococcus* (Doud Galli et al., 2001) and *Actinomycosis* (Roth & Montone, 1996). The antibiotics most effective in alleviating sinus infections are amoxicillin, trimethoprim sulfamethoxazole, and cefaclor. Amoxicillin with clavulanic acid and clindamycin also are commonly used (Regev et al., 1995). General guidelines for treatment of sinusitis was represented in Tables 6, 7.

Transient sinusitis	Chronic sinusitis
1. Use of decongestants and antibiotics 2. Follow-up after 2 weeks 3. If no recovery, transient sinusitis has possibly evolved into subacute sinusitis needing further treatment: a. Continuation of decongestants and antibiotics b. Maxillary drains for sinus irrigation c. CT scanning and consideration of functional endoscopic sinus surgery if no recovery within 3 weeks	1. Use of decongestants and antibiotics 2. CT scanning and functional endoscopic sinus surgery

Table 6. General guidelines for the treatment of transient and chronic maxillary sinusitis after maxillary sinus augmentation (Timmenga et al., 2001)

1. Preoperative evaluation of sinus clearance-related factors 2. Postsurgery: a nasal decongestant (xylomethazoline 0.05%) and topical corticosteroid (dexamethasone 0.01%) to prevent postsurgery obstruction of the ostium 3. Perioperative antibiotic prophylaxis (cephradine 1 g 3 times daily, starting 1 hour before surgery and continued for 48 hours after surgery)

Table 7. General guidelines for the prevention of transient and chronic maxillary sinusitis after maxillary sinus augmentation (Timmenga et al., 2001)

4. Conclusions

Although serious complications are uncommon, dental implant placement is not free of complications, as complications may occur at any stage (Table 8). Therefore, careful analysis via imaging, precise surgical techniques and an understanding of the anatomy of the surgical area are essential in preventing complications. One should be aware of the possible complications related to implant placement so that the patient can be properly informed. Prompt recognition of a developing problem and proper management are needed to minimize postoperative complications.

Problems	Possible causes	Solutions
Nerve injury	Mechanical injury by stretching, compression, and partial or total trans-section	Remove implant Wait for a period Rivotril®, Tegretol®, Vitamin B6
Hemorrhage during drilling	Injury of an artery	Extraoral pressure from the submental against the body of mandible Implant placement will stop bleeding

Fracture of mandible	Atrophic mandible	Immediate implant retrieval Bone graft Monocortical miniplates
Penetration of nasal/sinus floor	Type IV bone	Primary closure Antibiotic, decongestant, chlorhexidine
Lack of primary stability	Type IV bone, grafted bone, imprecise preparation, excessive countersinking	Remove implant, replace with larger diameter or longer implant
Maxillary sinus lift	Preexisting condition, surgical handling	Seal by folding the excess membrane, collagen membrane, bone graft, primary closure Antibiotics, decongestant, chlorhexidine
Significant bleeding	Subclinical bleeding diathesis, surgical handling	Atraumatic surgical technique, compression for >10min
Devitalization of adjacent teeth	Not enough space in between implant and adjacent tooth	Endodontic treatment

Table 8. Intraoperative surgical-related complications (Park & Wang, 2005)

5. References

Abu-Id, MH.; Warnke, PH. & Gottschalk J. (2008). "Bis-phossy jaws"- High and low risk factors for bisphosphonate-induced osteonecrosis of the jaw. *J Craniomaxillofac Surg,* Vol. 36, No. 2, (January 2008), pp. 95-103, ISSN 1010-5182, Edinburgh, Scotland

American Association of Oral and Maxillofacial Surgeons. (2007). Advisory Task Force on Bisphosphonate-Related Osteonecrosis of the Jaws, American Association of Oral and Maxillofacial Surgeons position paper on bisphosphonate-related osteonecrosis of the jaws. *J Oral Maxillofac Surg,* Vol. 65, No. 3, (March 2007), pp. 369-76, ISSN 0278-2391, Philadelphia, Pennsylvania, USA

Annibali, S.; Ripari, M., La Monaca, G., Tonoli, F. & Cristalli MP. (2009). Local accidents in dental implant surgery: prevention and treatment. *Int J Periodontics Restorative Dent* Vol. 29, No. 3, (June 2009), pp. 325-31, ISSN 0278-2391, Philadelphia, Pennsylvania, USA

Ardekian, L.; Oved-Peleg, E., Mactei, E. & Peled, M. (2006). The clinical significance of sinus membrane perforation during augmentation of the maxillary sinus. *J Oral Maxillofac Surg,* Vol. 64, No. 2, (February 2006), pp. 277-82, ISSN 0278-2391, Philadelphia, Pennsylvania, USA

Barone, A.; Santini, S., Sbordone, L., Crespi, R. & Covani, U. (2006). A clinical study of the outcomes and complications associated with maxillary sinus augmentation. *Int J*

Oral Maxillofac Implants, Vol. 21, No. 1, (Jan-Fab 2006), pp. 81-5, ISSN 0882-2786, Illinois, USA

Becker , ST.; Terheyden, H., Steinriede, A., Behrens, E., Springer, I. & Wiltfang, J. (2008). Prospective observation of 41 perforations of the Schneiderian membrane during sinus floor elevation. *Clin Oral Implants Res*, Vol. 19, No. 12, pp. 1285-9, ISSN 0905-7161, Oxford, England

Bedogni, A.; Bettini, G., Totola, A., Saia, G. & Nocini, PF. (2010). Oral bisphosphonate-associated osteonecrosis of the jaw after implant surgery: a case report and literature review. *J Oral Maxillofac Surg*, Vol. 68, No. 7, pp. 1662-6, ISSN 0278-2391, Philadelphia, Pennsylvania, USA

Bell, BM.; Bell R. (2008). Oral bisphosphonates and dental implants: A retrospective study. *J Oral Maxillofac Surg*, Vol. 66, Vol. 5, pp. 1022-4, ISSN 0278-2391, Philadelphia, Pennsylvania, USA

Bertrand, B.; Eloy, P. (1992). Relationship of chronic ethmoidal sinusitis, maxillary sinusitis, and ostial permeability controlled by sinusomanometry: statistical study. *Laryngoscope*, Vol. 102, No. 11, (Nov 1992), pp. 1281-4, ISSN 0023-852X, Philadelphia, Pennsylvania, USA

Burstein, J.; Mastin, C. & Le, B. (2008). Avoiding injury to the inferior alveolar nerve by routine use of intraoperative radiographs during implant placement. *J Oral Implantol*, Vol. 34, No. 1, pp. 34-8, ISSN 0160-6972, Kansas, USA

Chanavaz, M. (1990). Maxillary sinus: Anatomy, physiology, surgery, and bone grafting related to implantology—Eleven years of surgical experience. *J Oral Implantol*, Vol. 16, No. 3, pp. 199-209, ISSN 0160-6972, Kansas, USA

Dario, LJ. (2002). Implant placement above a bifurcated mandibular canal: a case report. *Implant Dent*, Vol. 11, No. 3, pp. 258-61, ISSN 1056-6163, Philadelphia, Pennsylvania, USA

Day, RH. (1994). Microneurosurgery of the injured trigeminal nerve. *Oral Maxillofac Surg Knowledge Update*, Vol. 1, pp. 91-116

Doud Galli, SK.; Lebowitz, RA., Giacchi, RJ., Glickman, R. & Jacobs, JB. (2001). Chronic sinusitis complicating sinus lift surgery. *Am J Rhinol*, Vol. 15, No. 3, (May-Jun 2001), pp. 181-6, ISSN 1050-6586, Rhode Island, USA

Dubois, L.; de Lange, J., Baas. E. & Van Ingen, J. (2010). Excessive bleeding in the floor of the mouth after endosseus implant placement: a report of two cases. *Int J Oral Maxillofac Surg*, Vol. 39, No. 4, (Apr 2010), pp. 412-5, ISSN 0901-5027, Edinburgh, Scotland

Elian, N.; Wallace, S., Cho, SC., Jalbout, ZN. & Froum, S. (2005). Distribution of the maxillary artery as it relates to sinus floor augmentation. *Int J Oral Maxillofac Implants*, Vol. 20, No. 5, (Sep-Oct), pp. 784-7, ISSN 0882-2786, Illinois, USA

Fugazzotto, PA.; Lightfoot, WS., Jaffin, R. & Kumar, A. (2007). Implant placement with or without simultaneous tooth extraction in patients taking oral bisphosphonates: Postoperative healing, early follow-up, and the incidence of complications in two private practices. *J Periodontol*, Vol. 78, No. 9, (Sep 2007), pp. 1664-9, ISSN 0022-3492, Chicago, Illinois, USA

Galindo, P.; Sánchez-Fernández, E., Avila, G., Cutando, A. & Fernandez, JE. (2005). Migration of implants into the maxillary sinus: two clinical cases. *Int J Oral Maxillofac Implants*, Vol.20, No. 2, (Mar-Apr 2005), pp. 291-5, ISSN 0882-2786 Illinois, USA

Givol, N.; Chaushu, G., Halamish-Shani, T. & Taicher, S. (2000). Emergency tracheostomy following life-threatening hemorrhage in the floor of the mouth during immediate implant placement in the mandibular canine region. *J Periodontol*, Vol. 71, No. 12, (Dec 2000), pp. 1893-5, ISSN 0022-3492, Chicago, Illinois, USA

Goodacre, CJ.; Kan, JY. & Rungcharassaeng, K. (1999). Clinical complications of osseointegrated implants. *J Prosthet Dent*, Vol. 81, No. 5, (May 1999), pp. 537-52, ISSN 0022-3913, New York, USA

Goodacre, CJ.; Bernal, G., Rungcharassaeng, K. & Kan, JY. (2003). Clinical complications with implants and implant prostheses. *J Prosthet Dent*, Vol. 90, No. 2, (Aug 2003), pp. 121-32, ISSN 0022-3913, New York, USA

Goss, AN.; Backhouse, P. (2007). Bisphosphonates and osteonecrosis of the jaws. *Aust Prescriber*, Vol. 30, pp. 96-7, ISSN 0312-8008, Deakin, Australia

Grant, BT.; Amenedo, C., Freeman, K. & Kraut, RA. (2008). Outcomes of placing dental implants in patients taking oral bisphosphonates: A review of 115 cases. *J Oral Maxillofac Surg*, Vol. 66, No. 2, (Feb 2008), pp. 223-30, ISSN 0278-2391, Philadelphia, Pennsylvania, USA

Greenstein, G.; Tarnow, D. (2006). The mental foramen and nerve: clinical and anatomical factors related to dental implant placement: a literature review. *J Periodontol*, Vol. 77, No. 12, (Dec 2006), pp. 1933-43, ISSN 0022-3492, Chicago, Illinois, USA

Greenstein, G.; Cavallaro, J., Romanos, G. & Tarnow, D. (2008). Clinical recommendations for avoiding and managing surgical complications associated with implant dentistry: a review. *J Periodontol*, Vol. 79, No. 8, pp.1317-29, ISSN 0022-3492, Chicago, Illinois, USA

Hofschneider, U.; Tepper, G., Gahleitner, A. & Ulm, C. (1999). Assessment of the blood supply to the mental region for reduction of bleeding complications during implant surgery in the interforaminal region. *Int J Oral Maxillofac Implants*, Vol. 14, No. 3, (May-Jun 1999), pp. 379-83, ISSN 0882-2786, Illinois, USA

Hunter, WL 4th.; Bradrick, JP., Houser, SM., Patel, JB. & Sawady, J. (2009). Maxillary sinusitis resulting from ostium plugging by dislodged bone graft: case report. *J Oral Maxillofac Surg*, Vol. 67, No. 7, pp. 1495-8, ISSN 0278-2391, Philadelphia, Pennsylvania, USA

Isaacson, TJ. (2004). Sublingual hematoma formation during immediate placement of mandibular endosseous implants. *J Am Dent Assoc*, Vol. 135, No. 2, (Feb 2004), pp. 168-72, ISSN 0002-8177, Chicago, Illinois, USA

Jalbout, Z.; Tabourian, G. (2004). Glossary of Implant Dentistry, *Proceedings of International Congress of Oral Implantologists*, Upper Montclair, New Jerjey 2004

Jeffcoat, MK. (2006). Safety of oral bisphosphonates: Controlled studies on alveolar bone. *Int J Oral Maxillofac Implants*, Vol. 21, No. 3, (May-Jun 2006), pp. 349-53, ISSN 0882-2786, Illinois, USA

Kalpidis, CD.; Setayesh, RM. (2004). Hemorrhaging associated with endosseous implant placement in the anterior mandible: a review of the literature. *J Periodontol* , Vol. 75, No. 5, (May 2004), pp. 631-45, ISSN 0022-3492, Chicago, Illinois, USA

Karabuda, C.; Arisan, V. & Ozyuvaci, H. (2006). Effects of sinus membrane perforations on the success of dental implants placed in the augmented sinus. *J Periodontol* , Vol. 77, No. 12, (Dec 2006), pp. 1991-7, ISSN 0022-3492, Chicago, Illinois, USA

Khan, AA.; Sándor, GK., Dore, E., Morrison, AD., Alsahli, M., Amin, F., Peters, E., Hanley, DA., Chaudry, SR., Dempster, DW., Glorieux, FH., Neville, AJ., Talwar, RM., Clokie, CM., Al Mardini, M., Paul, T., Khosla, S., Josse, RG., Sutherland, S., Lam, DK., Carmichael, RP., Blanas, N., Kendler, D., Petak, S., St-Marie, LG., Brown, J., Evans, AW., Rios, L. & Compston, JE. (2008). Canadian consensus practice guidelines for bisphosphonate associated osteonecrosis of the jaw. *J Rheumatol* Vol. 35, No. 7, pp. 1391-7, ISSN 0315-162X, Toronto, Ontario, Canada

Kraut, RA.; Chahal, O. (2002). Management of patients with trigeminal nerve injuries after mandibular implant placement. *J Am Dent Assoc*, Vol. 133, No. 10, (Oct 2002), pp. 1351-4, ISSN 0002-8177, Chicago, Illinois, USA

Lekholm, U.; Zarb, GA. (1985). Patient selection and preparation, In: *Tissue- Integrated Prostheses: Osseointegration in Clinical Dentistry*, Bra°nemark, PI., Zarb, GA. & Albrektsson, T., pp. 199-209, Quintessence, ISBN: 0-86715-129-3, Illinois, USA

Manor, Y.; Mardinger, O., Bietlitum, I., Nashef, A., Nissan, J. & Chaushu, G. (2010). Late signs and symptoms of maxillary sinusitis after sinus augmentation. *Oral Surg Oral Med Oral Pathol Oral Radiol Endod*, Vol. 110, No. 1, (Jul 2010), pp. e1-4, ISSN 1079-2104, New York, USA

Mardinger, O.; Manor, I., Mijiritsky, E. & Hirshberg, A. (2007). Maxillary sinus augmentation in the presence of antral pseudocyst: a clinical approach. *Oral Surg Oral Med Oral Pathol Oral Radiol Endod*, Vol. 103, No. 2, (Feb 2007), pp. 180-4, ISSN 1079-2104, New York, USA

Mardinger, O.; Abba, M., Hirshberg, A. & Schwartz-Arad, D. (2007). Prevalence, diameter and course of the maxillary intraosseous vascular canal with relation to sinus augmentation procedure: a radiographic study. *Int J Oral Maxillofac Surg*, Vol. 36, No. 8, (Aug 2007), pp. 735-8, ISSN 0901-5027, Edinburgh, Scotland

Martin, D.; Pascal, JF., Baudet, J., Mondie, JM., Farhat, JB., Athoum, A., Le Gaillard, P. & Peri, G. (1993). The submental island flap: a new donor site. Anatomy and clinical applications as a free or pedicled flap. *Plast Reconstr Surg*, Vol. 92, No. 5, (Oct 1993), pp. 867-73, ISSN 0032-1052, Philadelphia, Pennsylvania, USA

Marx, RE. ; Cillo, JE. Jr. & Ulloa, JJ. (2007). Oral bisphosphonate-induced osteonecrosis: risk factors, prediction of risk using serum CTX testing, prevention, and treatment. *J Oral Maxillofac Surg*, Vol. 65, No. 12, (Dec 2007), pp. 2397-410, ISSN 0278-2391, Philadelphia, Pennsylvania, USA

Misch, K.; Wang, HL. (2008). Implant surgery complications: etiology and treatment. *Implant Dent*, Vol. 17, No. 2, (Jun 2008), pp. 159-68, ISSN 1056-6163, Philadelphia, Pennsylvania, USA

Montefusco, V.; Gay, F., Spina, F., Miceli, R., Maniezzo, M., Teresa Ambrosini, M., Farina, L., Piva, S., Palumbo, A., Boccadoro, M. & Corradini, P. (2008). Antibiotic prophylaxis before dental procedures may reduce the incidence of osteonecrosis of the jaw in patients with multiple myeloma treated with bisphosphonates. *Leuk Lymphoma* Vol. 49, No. 11, (Nov 2008), pp. 2156-62, ISSN 1042-8194, Ebingdon, England

Montoya-Carralero, JM.; Parra-Mino, P., Ramírez-Fernández, P., Morata-Murcia, IM., Mompeán-Gambín Mdel, C. & Calvo-Guirado, JL. (2010). Dental implants in patients treated with oral bisphosphonates: a bibliographic review. *Med Oral Patol Oral Cir Bucal*, Vol. 15, No. 1, (Jan 2010), pp. e65-9, ISSN 1698-4447, Valencia, Spain

Nazarian, Y.; Eliav, E. & Nahlieli, O. (2003). Nerve injury following implant placement: Prevention, diagnosis and treatment modalities. *Refuat Hapeh Vehashinayim*, Vol. 20, No. 3, (Jul 2003), pp. 44-50, ISSN 0792-9935, Israel

Park, SH.; Wang, HL. (2005). Implant reversible complications: classification and treatments. *Implant Dent*, Vol. 14, No. 3, pp. 211-20, ISSN 1056-6163, Philadelphia, Pennsylvania, USA

Peleg, M.; Garg, AK. & Mazor, Z. (2006). Predictability of simultaneous implant placement in the severely atrophic posterior maxilla: A 9-year longitudinal experience study of 2132 implants placed into 731 human sinus grafts. *Int J Oral Maxillofac Implants*, Vol. 21, No. 1, pp. 94-102, ISSN 0882-2786, Illinois, USA

Pikos, M. (1999). Maxillary sinus membrane repair. Report of a technique for large perforations. *Implant Dent*, Vol. 8, No. 1, pp. 29- 34, ISSN 1056-6163, Philadelphia, Pennsylvania, USA

Proussaefs, P. ; Lozada, J., Kim, J. & Rohrer, MD. (2004). Repair of the perforated sinus membrane with a resorbable collagen membrane: A human study. *Int J Oral Maxillofac Impl*, Vol. 19, No. 3, (May-Jun 2004) pp. 413-420, ISSN 0882-2786, Illinois, USA

Regev, E.; Smith, RA., Perrott, DH. & Pogrel, MA. (1995). Maxillary sinus complications related to endosseous implants. *Int J Oral Maxillofac Implants*, Vol. 10, No. 4, (Jul-Aug 1995), pp. 451-61, ISSN 0882-2786, Illinois, USA

Reiser, GM.; Rabinovitz, Z., Bruno, J., Damoulis, PD. & Griffin, TJ. (2001). Evaluation of maxillary sinus membrane response following elevation with the crestal osteotome technique in human cadavers. *Int J Oral Maxillofac Implants*, Vol. 16, No. 6, (Nov-Dec 2001), pp. 833-40, ISSN 0882-2786, Illinois, USA

Roth, M.; Montone, KT. (1996). Actinomycosis of the paranasal sinuses: a case report and review. *Otolaryngol Head Neck Surg*, Vol. 114, No. 6, pp. 818-21, ISSN 0194-5998, New York, USA

Ruggiero, SL.; Mehrotra, B., Rosenberg, TJ. & Engroff, SL. (2004). Osteonecrosis of the jaws associated with the use of bisphosphonates: a review of 63 cases. *J Oral Maxillofac Surg*, Vol. 62, No. 5, (May 2004), pp. 527-34, ISSN 0278-2391, Philadelphia, Pennsylvania, USA

Ruggiero, SL.; Dodson, TB., Assael, LA., Landesberg, R., Marx, RE. & Mehrotra, B. (2009). American Association of Oral and Maxillofacial Surgeons: Position paper on bisphosphonate-related osteonecrosis of the jaws—2009 update. *J Oral Maxillofac Surg*, Vol. 67, No. 5 suppl, pp. 2-12, ISSN 0278-2391, Philadelphia, Pennsylvania, USA

Sadig, W.; Almas, K. (2004). Risk factors and management of dehiscent wounds in implant dentistry. *Implant Dent*, Vol. 13, No. 2, pp. 140-147, ISSN 1056-6163, Philadelphia, Pennsylvania, USA

Schwartz-Arad, D.; Herzberg, R. & Dolev, E. (2004). The prevalence of surgical complications of the sinus graft procedure and their impact on implant survival. *Journal of Periodontology*, Vol. 75, No. 4, (Apr 2004), pp. 511-516, ISSN 0022-3492, Chicago, Illinois, USA

Sharawy, M.; Misch, CE. (1999). Anatomy for dental implants. In: *Contemporary Implant Dentistry, 2nd ed,* Misch, CE. pp. 217-224, The CV Mosby Company, ISBN 0815170599, St. Louis, USA

Shlomi, B.; Horowiz, I., Kahn, A., Dobriyan, A. & Chaushu, G. (2004). The effect of sinus membrane perforation and repair with Lambone sheet on the outcome of maxillary sinus floor augmentation: A radiographic assessment. *Int J Oral Maxillofac Implants*, Vol. 19, No. 4, (Jul-Aug 2004), pp. 559-62, ISSN 0882-2786, Illinois, USA

Solar, P.; Geyerhofer, U., Traxler, H., Windisch, A., Ulm, C. & Watzek, G. (1999). Blood supply to the maxillary sinus relevant to sinus floor elevation procedures. *Clin Oral Implants Res*, Vol. 10, No. 1, (Feb 1999), pp. 34-44, ISSN 0905-7161, Oxford, England

Stark, WJ.; Epker, BN. (1995). Failure of osseointegrated dental implants after bisphosphonate therapy for osteoporosis. A case report. *Int J Oral Maxillofac Implants*, Vol. 10, No. 1, (Jan-Feb), pp. 74-8, ISSN 0882-2786, Illinois, USA

Sussman, HI. (1998). Tooth devitalization via implant placement: a case report. *Periodontal Clin Investig*, Vol. 20, No. 1, pp. 22-4, ISSN 1065-2418, USA

Tammisalo, T.; Happonen, RP. & Tammisalo, EH. (1992). Stereographic assessment of mandibular canal in relation to the roots of impacted lower third molar using multiprojection narrow beam radiography. *Int J Oral Maxillofac Surg*. Vol. 21, No. 2, (Apr 1992), pp. 85-9, ISSN 0901-5027, Edinburgh, Scotland

Testori, T.; Rosano, G., Taschieri, S. & Del Fabbro, M. (2010). Ligation of an unusually large vessel during maxillary sinus floor augmentation. A case report. *Eur J Oral Implantol*, Vol. 3, No. 3, (Autumn 2010), pp. 255-8, ISSN 1756-2406

Timmenga, NM.; Raghoebar, GM., Boering, G. & Weissenbruch, R. (1997). Maxillary sinus function after sinus lifts for the insertion of dental implants. *J Oral Maxillofac Surg*, Vol. 55, No. 9, pp. 936-9, ISSN 0278-2391, Philadelphia, Pennsylvania, USA

Timmenga, NM.; Raghoebar, GM., van Weissenbruch, R. & Vissink, A. (2001). Maxillary sinusitis after augmentation of the maxillary sinus floor: a report of 2 cases. *J Oral Maxillofac Surg*, Vol. 59, No. 2, Feb 2001), pp. 200-4, ISSN 0278-2391, Philadelphia, Pennsylvania, USA

Traxler, H.; Windisch, A., Geyerhofer, U., Surd, R., Solar, P. & Firbas, W. (1999). Arterial blood supply of the maxillary sinus. *Clin Anat*, Vol. 12, No. 6, pp. 417-421, ISSN 0897-3806, New Jersey, USA

Uchida, Y.; Goto, M., Katsuki, T. & Akiyoshi, T. (1998) A cadaveric study of maxillary sinus size and aid in bone grafting of the maxillary sinus floor. *Journal of Oral and Maxilofacial Surgery*, Vol. 56, No. 10, (Oct 1998), pp. 1158-1163, ISSN 0278-2391, Philadelphia, Pennsylvania, USA

Uchida, Y.; Goto, M., Katsuki, T. & Soejima, Y. (1998). Measurement of maxillary sinus volume using computerized tomographic images. *Int J Oral Maxillofac Implants*, Vol. 13, No. 6, (Nov-Dec 1998), pp. 811-8, ISSN 0882-2786, Illinois, USA

Ueda, M.; Kaneda, T. (1992). Maxillary sinusitis caused by dental implants: report of two cases. *J Oral Maxillofac Surg*, Vol. 50, No. 3, (Mar 1992), pp. 285-7, ISSN 0278-2391, Philadelphia, Pennsylvania, USA

van den Bergh, JP.; ten Bruggenkate, CM., Disch, FJ. & Tuinzing, DB. (2000). Anatomical aspects of sinus floor elevations. *Clin Oral Implants Res*, Vol. 11, No. 3, (Jun 2000), pp. 256-265, ISSN 0905-7161, Oxford, England

Wang, HL.; Weber, D. & McCauley, LK. (2007). Effect of long-term oral bisphosphonates on implant wound healing: Literature review and a case report. *J Periodontol*, Vol. 78, No. 3, (Mar 2007), pp. 584-94, ISSN 0022-3492, Chicago, Illinois, USA

Ward, BB.; Terrell, JE. & Collins, JK. (2008). Methicillin-resistant Staphylococcus aureus sinusitis associated with sinus lift bone grafting and dental implants: a case report. *J Oral Maxillofac Surg*, Vol. 66, No. 2, (Feb 2008), pp. 231-4, ISSN 0278-2391, Philadelphia, Pennsylvania, USA

Wessel, JH.; Dodson, TB. & Zavras, AI. (2008). Zoledronate, smoking, and obesity are strong risk factors for osteonecrosis of the jaw: A case-control study. *J Oral Maxillofac Surg*, Vol. 66, No. 4, pp. 625-31, ISSN 0278-2391, Philadelphia, Pennsylvania, USA

Worthington, P. (2004). Injury to the inferior alveolar nerve during implant placement: a formula for protection of the patient and clinician. *Int J Oral Maxillofac Implants*, Vol. 19, No. 5, (Sep-Oct 2004), pp. 731-4, ISSN 0882-2786, Illinois, USA

Yarom, N.; Yahalom, R., Shoshani, Y., Hamed, W., Regev, E. & Elad, S. (2007). Osteonecrosis of the jaw induced by orally administered bisphosphonates: Incidence, clinical features, predisposing factors and treatment outcome. *Osteoporos Int*, Vol. 18, No. 10, (Oct 2007), pp. 1363-70, ISSN 0937-941X, Godalming, England

Zijderveld, SA.; van den Bergh, JP., Schulten, EA. & ten Bruggenkate, CM. (2008). Anatomical and surgical findings and complications in 100 consecutive maxillary sinus floor elevation procedures. *J Oral Maxillofac Surg*, Vol. 66, No. 7, (Jul 2008), pp. 1426-38, ISSN 0278-2391, Philadelphia, Pennsylvania, USA

Zinner, ID.; Shapiro, HJ., Gold, SD. (2008). Sinus graft complications. Problem solving. *N Y State Dent J*, Vol. 74, No. 4, (Jun-Jul 2008), pp. 40-3, ISSN 0028-7571, New York, USA

5

An Overview Regarding Contemporary Biomechanical Aspects on Immediate Loading Dental Implants

José Mauricio dos Santos Nunes Reis, Lígia Antunes Pereira Pinelli, Nicolau Conte Neto, Marcelo Silva Monnazzi and José Cláudio Martins Segalla
UNESP - Univ Estadual Paulista / Araraquara Dental School
Brazil

1. Introduction

The use of dental implants for the treatment of partially or completely edentulous patients has become an effective therapy in the last years (Romeo et al., 2004). Therefore, the development of dental implants represents a remarkable advance in trends of Dentistry allowing to oral edentulous patients rehabilitation characterized by a high and long-term success.

Despite the great use of dental implants, many factors regarding its biomechanical aspects remain incompletely understood. According to Gross (2008), a preliminary consideration of the natural anatomy of the dentition, occlusion and alveolar support mechanisms would be helpful to provide a perspective for planning of implant supported restorations. Criteria as primary stabilization, bone quality, number, distribution, width, length and design of the dental implants, surface treatments, implant-abutment connection, and occlusion aspects must be also considered for the success of immediate, early or delayed loading dental implants (Casap et al., 2011).

In the delayed loading period, the implants are kept load free during the osseointegration period (varying from 3 to 6 months according to the insertion anatomic place and implant system requirements) and are rehabilitated afterward. In the early loading period, the rehabilitation of the implant is done during the first 3 months after the implantation, and according to Esposito et al. (2009), it is now recognized to generate harmful mechanical loading forces on the implants just at the time as the healing bone process has started and has not been finished yet.

In the immediate loading period, the waiting between implantation and loading is limited at a maximum of 48 hours, and the loading is only performed when good primary stability has been achieved. This procedure reduces the number of clinical steps and appears to allow a more comfortable and acceptable condition for the patients (Al-Omiri et al., 2005). Among the reasons for the immediate loading dental implants is the surgical trauma, which is minimized, in a one-step surgical procedure (Misch et al., 2004a). According to Misch et al. (2004a), the reduction of the surgical trauma in immediate loading procedures can be obtained by reducing heat during the surgical steps and reducing the stress on the bone-implant interface. The great advantage, besides avoiding a second surgical procedure, is the

possibility to carry the dental implants (provisionalization) immediately after the surgery or some brief period after it (Misch et al., 2004a, 2004b). Several *in vitro* and *in vivo* studies have observed similar success between immediate and/or delayed loading implants (Attard & Zarb, 2005; Becker et al., 1997; Brånemark et al., 1999; Chiapasco et al., 2001; Chow et al., 2001; Degidi & Piattelli, 2003; Degidi & Piattelli, 2005; Ericsson et al., 1994; Gatti et al., 2000; Misch & Wang, 2003; Misch et al., 2004a, 2004b; Morton et al., 2004; Nkenke et al., 2005; Schnitman et al., 1997). However, in order to achieve success in immediate loading techniques its required a proper planning prior to implantation and considerable coordination among the oral surgeon, the prosthodontist and the laboratory. And it's thus required the exactly intraoperative transfer of the previously planned. Furthermore, the patient is very often required to wait many hours after the implant surgery for the completion of the immediate prosthetic work in the laboratory and it´s installation.
Based on the above information, the aim of this Chapter was to accomplish an overview regarding contemporary biomechanical aspects on immediate loading dental implants.

2. Primary stabilization

Primary stabilization is influenced by the surgical procedures, implants design and bone quality and quantity. After dental implant insertion, bone responds to the local stimulus, thus propitiating its repair through properties of bone plasticity, resorption and apposition. A bone remodelation begins on the bone-implant interface, accelerated by the low intensity loads, which induce the bone cells stimulation (Kenney & Richards, 1998). The patient's diet has a major importance during the bone apposition and remodelation after the immediate loading procedures. Consequently, soft diet should be indicated during the initial period (3 to 4 months) of the healing process and bone deposition (Misch et al., 2004a, 2004b). Most of the immature bone tissues formed is substituted by lamellar bone 3 to 6 months after the surgical placement of the implants in the delayed loading procedures (Duyck et al., 2001). Therefore, the immediate loading dental implants not only can reduce the risks of development of fibrous tissues, but also can minimize the development of immature bone, promoting a faster maturation of the immature bone to lamellar bone (Duyck et al., 2001; Zubery et al., 1999). Load transfer depends on successful osseointegration, which is characterized as a direct structural and functional connection between the bone and the implant surface (Adell et al., 1981; Brånemark et al., 1977). Thus, increasing the bone-implant contact surface area, directly related to implant diameter and length, can improve the osseointegration of implant to bone and establish implant stability. According to Misch et al. (2004a, 2004b), the smaller the applied stress to the bone, the smaller will be its micro-deformation and an increased surface area on the bone-implant interface will be expected. Short and long-term histological studies have demonstrated that immediate loading implants do not necessarily result in excessive stress on the bone-implant interface (Piattelli et al., 1993).

3. Bone quality and quantity

The close relationship between the bone and the implant is the core of osseointegration. Occlusal overloading on poor-quality bone can be a crucial factor in implant success and longevity. Different bone density may be observed for each region of the jaws. The posterior regions of the jaws usually have less dense bone than the anterior regions (Misch et al.,

1999). Generally, the mandible has a denser and thicker cortical layer than the maxilla, with the cortical layer becoming thinner and more porous posteriorly. According to Morris et al. (2001), poor quality and quantity of surrounding bone was ranked as the most influential factor for reducing the success rate of dental implant treatments. Misch et al. (1999) stated that the density of the bone is directly proportional to the strength of the bone, with less density demonstrating strength reduction of 50% to 80% compared to higher density bone tissues. In addition, Goodacre et al. (2003) reported that dental implants loaded in lower density bone averaged 16% higher failure rates compared to more ideal bone quality. In a multicenter study by Weng et al. (2003), the posterior maxilla produced a 25% failure rate when short implants were used to support the prosthesis, and the implant failure occurred during the first 18 months of loading. Consequently, researchers have been unanimous for the indication of a larger number of implants for the rehabilitations of partially or completely edentulous maxillae. Therefore, the greater the number, the smaller will be the biomechanical risk. The design of the implants is more associated to the area of functional surface than to its size. Cylindrical implants without threads and with larger diameter possess smaller surface area in comparison to a screw implant of smaller diameter (Misch et al., 2004b). Consequently, implants with threads should be the most appropriate for the immediate loading procedures. This aspect will be focused in another section of this Chapter. Finally, following the recommendations of Attard & Zarb (2005), the posterior region of the jaws should be carefully evaluated for the indication of immediate loading implants. The cantilever elimination and the accomplishment of bilateral ferulization seem to be advantageous in order to reduce the stress concentrations on peri-implant bone.

4. Implant design

Several efforts have been focused to the knowledge and control of all factors that could enhance the osseointegration process, which includes those related to the implant design. The implant design refers to three-dimensional architecture of an implant system (Sykaras et al., 2000; Triplet et al., 2003), that is closely related to biological and biomechanical issues, especially those associated to the force transfer characteristics of implants (Geng et al., 2004; Siegele & Soltesz, 1989; Strong et al., 1998; Sykaras et al., 2000). Several aspects can be addressed in trends of implant design, but features related to the fixation shape, type of prosthetic interface and surface characteristics (surface topography and chemical composition) have been considerate the most important aspects within this context (Sykaras et al., 2000).

4.1 Dental implant shape

The Implant shape determines the surface area available for stress transfer and governs the initial stability of the fixation (Steigenga et al., 2003). Different kinds of implant shape designs have been described in the literature; however the root form implants have been dominating the implant market since it was developed. These dental implants are characterized by a body that works as a vertical bone column (Misch, 2008) and it can be presented as one or two-pieces implants (Jones & Cochran, 2006), solid or hollow, with a parallel, tapered/conical, or stepped shape/outline and a flat, round, or pointed apical end (Sykaras et al., 2000; Triplet et al., 2003).

4.1.1 Cylindrical vs tapered dental implants

Finite Element Analysis (FEA) and *in vivo* studies have demonstrated that taper implants are associated with advantages over cylindrical implants, including a greater initial stability (Lee et al., 2010) and the avoidance of "punching" stresses (Rieger et al., 1990). However, from a biomechanical perspective, studies have shown that cylindrical implants produced a more desirable stress profile than the conical shaped counterparts (Holmgren et al., 1998; Mailath et al., 1989; Siegele & Soltesz, 1989).

Within this context, recent studies have shown that in order to induce controlled compressive forces in the cortical bone layer during the implant insertion, a new hybrid self-tapping implant has been specifically designed for the use in critical quality bone, which combines the advantages of a conical implant with those of a cylindrical shape (Toyoshima et al., 2011).

4.1.2 One-piece vs two-pieces dental implants

Another category of implant design classify theses fixations as one-piece implant (non-submerged placement) which comprises the implant body and the soft tissue healing abutment manufactured as one piece, or two-pieces implants (submerged placement) that consist of an implant body and a separate abutment (Jones & Cochran, 2006). Regarding biomechanical issue, it was demonstrated that one and two-pieces implants have similar low force transmission characteristics under vertical loading (M.C. Cehreli et al., 2004) and since these stresses are extremely low, they do not seem to have any clinical relevance on the mechanical as well as the biomechanical outcomes (Pilliar et al., 1986; Szmukler-Moncler et al., 1998).

5. Dental implant prosthetic interface

The prosthetic interface represents the level in which the superstructure or the abutment connects to the implant body (Sykaras et al., 2000; Triplet et al., 2003). It is considered an important aspect of implant design since it can influence the force transmission mechanism by implant-prosthesis system (Bozkaya & Muftu, 2003; Geng et al., 2001) and the amount of bacterial invasion of the implant internal part (Tesmer et al., 2009). To date, both these factors are markedly implicated with the pathological bone loss around dental implants (Misch, 2008), which can compromise the maintenance of peri-implant aesthetic harmony or implant system stability.

The implant-abutment connection can be classified as external, which includes hexagonal, octagonal, and spline, with its interdigitating projections and slots, or internal that includes the morse-taper interface, the internal hexagon, and the internal octagon (Sykaras et al., 2000; Triplet et al., 2003). In general, morse-taper connections are associated with better outcomes regarding the maintenance of the peri-implant bone, since they have been associated with a lesser bacterial infiltration (Mangano et al., 2009) and a better force transmission mechanism by implant-prosthesis system (Merz et al., 2000), although other studies have found similar marginal bone levels and biological outcomes of different implant designs (Engquist et al., 2002; Heydenrijk et al., 2002).

As described previously, one limitation with the implant-suport rehabilitation relates to the marginal bone loss that still is seen in some implant systems. The probable factors are: a possible bacterial colonization located between implant and abutment (Goodacre et al., 2003) and/or a stress concentration at the neck of implants resulting from prosthesis overloading leading to bone microfractures. In an attempt to reduce this stress concentration in the bone-implant interface, the companies put on the market different types of connections attached to the prosthetic abutment. From a biomechanical perspective, the major distinction among implant systems is the implant-abutment connection. Mechanical failures, such as loosening and/or fracture of occlusal screws, abutment screws or abutments, are related to the type of implant-abutment connection (Akca et al., 2003). When it comes to biomechanics, an internal conical joint design is mechanically more stable than an external hexagonal or butt-joint implant-abutment connection, which improves the clinical outcome (Merz et al., 2000).

In another words, the type of connection is important because it directly interfere in the prosthetic restoration, and the restoration must receive and transmit the masticatory loads to the implants in a controlled manner to avoid mechanical and biological failure after the osseointegration. When inadequate tensions occur in the bone-implant interface, bone resorption may occur in incompatible levels with the maintenance of osseointegration. There are already some experimental, numerical, and clinical studies evaluating the influence of implant-abutment connection on osseointegrated implants (Pessoa et al., 2010). For Hebel & Gajjar (1997), the success of implant-supported restoration and the health of surrounding tissues are related to the accuracy and fit between the components, stability at implant-abutment interface, and the resistance of this interface submitted to masticatory loads (Hebel & Gajjar, 1997). The stability at implant-abutment interface may be influenced by several factors, such as, connection type (M. Cehreli et al., 2004) and retention system (Pellizzer et al., 2010).

5.1 External hexagon

The initial purpose of external hexagon implants was to transmit torque during surgical placement. Afterwards, the external hexagon was also shown to work as an antirotational mechanism and to orient the abutment in single tooth prostheses (Davi et al., 2008). The biomechanical complications reported are loosening or fracturing of the abutment and prostheses screws (Merz et al., 2000). Therefore, the external hexagon connection continues to be comprehensively used (Figures 1, 2 and 3) and studied with the aim of improving the dimensional machining tolerances of the components (Schulte, 1994), and making this screwed junction more stable.

The external hexagon system has advantages such as (a) suitable for the two stage method, (b) an anti-rotation mechanism and retrievability and (c) compatibility among different systems. Possible disadvantages of the external hex are: (a) micro-movements because of the size of the hex, (b) higher centre of rotation that leads to lower resistance for rotational and lateral movements and (c) a micro gap leading to bone resorption. However, the weak-link to the fixture of the external hexagon configuration, is often referred as a fail-self mechanism for over-loading situations (Maeda et al., 2006).

Davi et al. (2008) evaluated the integrity of the external hexagon of an implant system with internal and external hexagons but with prosthetic connection through the external hexagon (internal torque) in comparison with that of an implant system with external hexagon with mount (external hexagon). They concluded that the internal torque implant system may be preferable in clinical situations where implant placement within a certain bone density could generate torques higher than 60 N.cm. After application of an 80 N.cm torque, the external hexagon did not support the torque, suffering deformation of its external hexagon. According to the authors, the fragility of the external hexagon of some systems can compromise the future dental prosthesis if deformation of the hexagon vertices occurs due to the torque applied in the implant mount when the implant is placed. Greater rotation at the interface implant-abutment transfers stress to the implant components and to the bone, which could lead to screw loosening or fracturing, microfractures of bone, and loss of osseointegration.

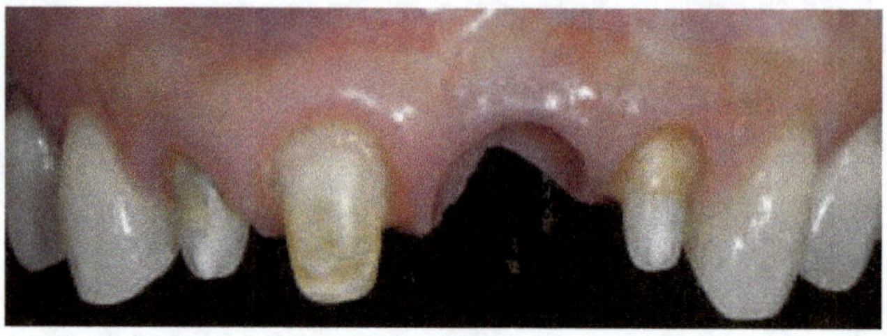

Fig. 1. Buccal view of a 3i external hexagon dental implant after provisionalization and soft tissue conditioning

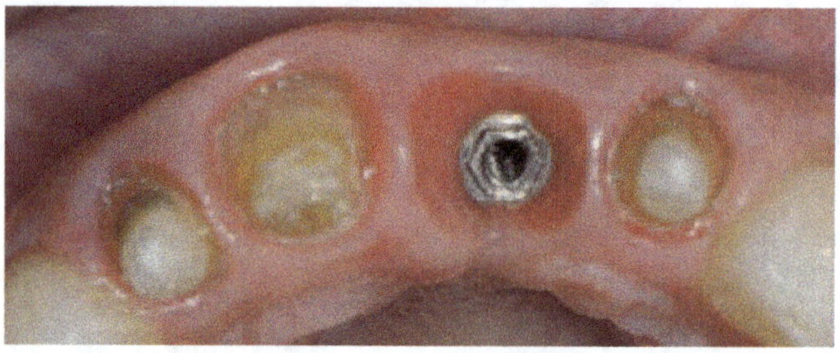

Fig. 2. Occlusal view of the 3i external hexagon dental implant

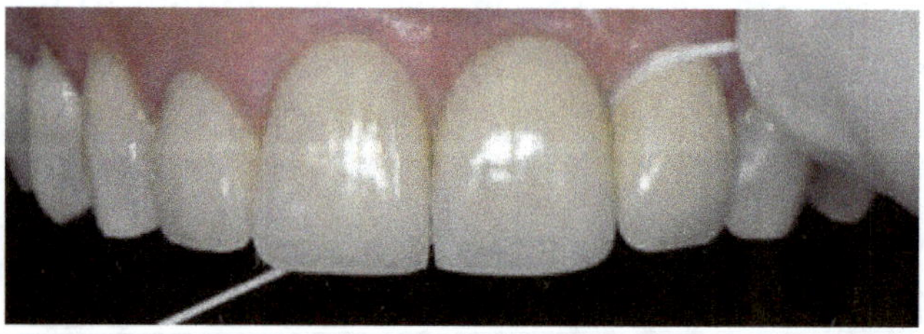

Fig. 3. Zirconia-based ceramic crowns after installation

5.2 Internal hexagon

One of the most important advances in the Implantology was the development of internal prosthetic connections, such as internal hexagon and morse-taper, in which excellent mechanical stability has been demonstrated *in vitro* (Merz et al., 2000). To ensure stability of the implants in long-term, science has turned its attention to improving the accuracy and passivity of prosthetic components, since it is unclear the level of mismatch between components that can affect the treatment success. Recently, some internal implant connections have appeared on the market, which are able to receive higher torques during surgical placement, with effective screw joint stability.

The internal hexagon system has advantages such as (a) ease in abutment connection, (b) suited for one stage implant installation, (c) higher stability and antirotation because of a wider area of connection and suited for single tooth restoration, (d) higher resistance to lateral loads because of the lower centre of rotation and (e) better force distribution; while its disadvantages are (a) thinner lateral fixture wall at the connecting part and (b) difficulty in adjusting divergences in angles between fixtures (Maeda et al., 2006).

From a biomechanical point of view, the design of the internal hexagon implant establishes a greater hexagon retention depth and the more precise and safer antirotational components of the internal hexagon system reducing the stress at the neck of the implant and retention screw (Hunt et al., 2005; Krennmair et al., 2002). In a study conduced by da Silva et al. (2010) evaluating the influence of connector and implant design on implant-tooth-connected prostheses, when the internal hexagon implant was assessed in the three types of connection (rigid connection, semirigid connection and rigid connection with oclusal screw), it was observed that the stresses on it occurred more in the apical region in comparison with the external hexagon, probably because of the greater depth of union of the denture to implant, and that the internal hexagon presented better stress dissipation characteristics than the external hexagon design. According to Krennmair et al. (2002), transferring the fulcrum point from the neck of the implant (external hexagon) to close to the middle third of the implant (internal hexagon), as well as the greater denture retention depth in the internal hexagon implant, reduced the power arm in the face of biomechanical behavior, making the implant more stable, with less tendency to screw loosening of fracturing, and improving the dissipations of tensions.

Bone resorption around the implant neck or cervical area may be explained by many other factors, however, smaller stress at cervical area of the internal hexagon system might contribute to the bone preservation, while larger stress at tip area might be one of the risk factors for bone resorption or fixture fracture (Maeda et al., 2006). Maeda et al. (2006), in an attempt to clarify the difference in the stress distribution patterns between implants with external or internal-hexagon connection systems using *in vitro* models, suggested that fixtures with internal-hexagon showed widely spread force distribution down to the fixture tip compared with external hexagon ones.

Pellizzer et al. (2010) evaluated the stress distribution of different retention systems (screwed or cemented) associated to different prosthetic connections (external hexagon, internal hexagon and morse-taper) in 3-unit implant-supported fixed partial prostheses through photoelasticity, and concluded that the internal hexagon implant was more favorable according to the biomechanical standpoint and also that the oblique load increased stress in all systems and connections tested. They believed that the stability at the implant-abutment interface, with internal connections, exhibits better contacts between the surfaces of abutment and implant, which decreases the micromovements during loading. In their study, among the internal connections, the morse-taper indicated better stress distribution.

5.2.1 Morse-taper

While high incidences of mechanical complications were reported for external-hexagon implants (Binon, 1996; Merz et al., 2000), insignificant episodes of abutment loosening were reported for solid-screw morse-taper implants (Levine et al., 1999). A different type of internal connection, known as morse-taper, was developed in an attempt to solve some biomechanical problems that still occur with internal hexagons implants. The implants have a conical union between implant and abutment, and this bond strength is proportional to the force used to insert. Tapered interference fits provide a reliable connection method between the abutment and the implant (Bozkaya & Muftu, 2003) and can also withstand prolonged lateral force applications (Merz et al., 2000). In the most common mechanical attachment method, a retaining-screw (abutment screw) is used to fix the abutment with respect to the implant. Another approach is to use a screw with a relatively large tapered end; the term taper integrated screwed-in (TIS) abutment is used to indicate an abutment, which uses simultaneously a screw and a tapered fit. A tapered interference fit (TIF) between the abutment and the implant is also used in some implant systems to provide the connection (Bozkaya & Muftu, 2005). For the systems using a screw, the connection between the implant and the abutment depends on the screw-preload, which is generated by applying a predetermined amount of torque during installation (Bozkaya & Muftu 2003). Designs in which the screw has a large tapered end essentially work like a tapered interference fit, and the screw threads do not appear to contribute to the connection; this mechanism relies on the large contact pressure and resulting frictional resistance, in the mating region of the implant–abutment interface, to provide a secure connection. In the morse-taper connection the bitting force acts in the direction of the abutment insertion, hence aids to secure the connection. This situation is in direct contrast to implants using screws where the biting force lowers the pretension in the screw (Bozkaya & Muftu, 2003).

Based on the previously information, it is clear that the morse-taper implant-abutment connection possesses higher mechanical behaviour than the external-hexagon (butt-joint) designs. In the external-hexagon implant design, the abutment screw alone is primarily responsible for maintaining the implant-abutment complex assembly under functional loads (Akca et al., 2003). Therefore, the axial preload of the abutment screw is a determining factor for the stability of the connection (Burguete et al., 1994). However, in the morse-taper connection, lateral loading is resisted mainly by the tapered design, which prevents the abutment from tilting (Akca et al., 2003). Because of the tapered design, a high normal pressure is maintained in the contact area, allowing stable retention of position by frictional forces (Merz et al., 2000). Taper joint connections with a conical seal, or Morse's taper, have advantages of better sealing capabilities in closing the micro-gap on top of those in an internal hexagon system (Maeda et al., 2006).

Regarding immediately loading implants, it was demonstrated that the implant-abutment connection design did not significantly influence the bone strain and the implant displacement. On the other hand, the Morse-taper connection presented superior abutment stability and the least stress concentration in the abutment screw, and the internal hexagon and external hexagon implants presented the lowest strain levels (Pessoa et al., 2010). Pieri et al. (2011) compared the clinical and radiographic outcomes of single implants immediately placed and restored with two different implant-abutment connections, prosthetic abutments with a Morse-taper connection and a platform switch (test group), and conventional abutments with an internal connection and a matching diameter (control group). No statistical significant differences were found between the two groups for periodontal parameters, marginal soft tissue level change, or papilla height, but greater marginal bone loss was observed at the control sites compared to the test sites. Although the control group demonstrated a slight increase in marginal bone loss compared to the test group, the peri-implant soft tissues were very stable with both types of implant-abutment connection after 12 months of loading.

5.3 Platform switching

According to Serrano-Sánchez et al. (2011), the platform switching effect was accidentally established in the 1980s and early 1990s when different dental implant manufacturers introduced implants of larger diameter before producing the corresponding abutments of the same measures. Thus, it involves reducing the abutment diameter in comparison with the diameter of the dental implant. Sánchez reported that it is possible to use abutments with a diameter smaller than the implant body width, or alternatively an implant design can be used in which the neck diameter is increased with respect to the implant body width, like suggested by Calvo-Guirado et al. (2009). The contemporary literature is unanimous in affirm that the use of platform switching dental implants improves bone crest preservation, contributes to biological space reposition, and, therefore, is directly related to excellent aesthetic outcomes. Conversely, Sabet et al. (2009) reported that the platform switching should be not used in mandibular implant-mucosal support prostheses, since reduction of the diameter of the junction lessens the abutment resistance in response to occlusal loading applied in the posterior area of the overdentures.

6. Surface characteristics

The surface characteristics have been considerate by Albrektsson et al. (1981) as relevant factors that could influence the establishment of a reliable osseointegration. In fact, it was demonstrated that the surface properties could influence the healing dynamics around bone-interfacing implants (Lee et al., 2008). Within this context, topographic and chemical properties have been considerate the most relevant features related to surface characteristics since they play a major role in the biological events that follow implantation (Le Guéhennec et al., 2007).

6.1 Topographic properties

According to Stanford (2008) the evaluation of an implant surface refers to macroscopic and microscopic features that, when combined, are used to describe the surface topography, being considered a relevant issue, since it can produce orientation and guide locomotion of specific cell types and has the ability to directly affect cell shape and cell function (Brunette & Chehroudi, 1999; Chou et al., 1998; Qu et al., 1996).

6.1.1 Macroarchitecture

The main characteristics regarding the macroarchitecture include the presence or absence of threads as well its design which are considered important factors that could affects the osseointegration process (Vidyasagar & Apse, 2004), because they play an important role in load transfer from dental implant to the surrounding bone (Schenk & Buser, 1998), affecting the stress distribution and marginal bone resorption (Chun et al., 2002). Furthermore, threads are used to maximize the initial contact, improve stability (Sykaras et al., 2000; Triplet et al., 2003) and enlarge the implant surface area (Kong et al., 2008). According to Misch et al. (2006), the greater the number of threads, the greater will be the surface area, if all other factors are equal. On the other hand, the thread number may be more significant for the shorter implant in the posterior regions of the mouth with reduced bone density.

Regarding thread design, a sort of varying geometric pattern that determine the functional thread surface can be found relating to thread depth, thread pitch, thread helix angle, thread thickness and thread face angle (Misch, 2008). These two last geometric aspects determine the shape of the thread, which can be V-shape, reverse buttress or a square thread (Strong et al., 1998; Thakur, 1997) and this last one is associated to the highest contact area (Lee et al., 2008).

6.1.2 Microarchitecture

The surface microarchitecture of dental implants refers to the classification of the implant design based on the average surface roughness (Sa). According to Triplet et al. (2003) most of the papers have described the dental implants surface as smooth (Sa ≤ 1.0 µm) or rough (Sa > 1.0 µm), although other terms, such as porous, minimally rough (0.5-1.0 µm), intermediately rough (1-2.0 µm), and rough (2-3.0 µm) have also been proposed (Wennerberg et al., 1995).

a. **Smooth surfaces**

The original Brånemark implant (Nobel Biocare, Göteborg, Sweden) is a turned screw of minimal surface roughness (Sa between 0.5 and 1.0 µm) that represents the main example for smooth surfaces. Nowadays, these surfaces have not been indicated yet, since they are associated with several disadvantages, including: slower biological processes at the bone-implant interface (BIC) (Elias et al., 2008), poor mechanical integration with bone, since these surfaces provide no resistance to mechanical forces at the BIC, allowing epithelial down growth and are associated with deeper peri-implant pockets (Puleo, 2006).

b. **Rough surfaces**

The development of rough implant surfaces represents a great advance to solve the problems of smooth surfaces. In fact, rough surfaces typically result in better clinical outcomes, probably due to the advantages offered by these superficies, such as lesser crestal bone loss (Wiskott & Belser, 1999), faster rate and higher degree of bone formation (Abrahamsson et al., 2004), higher percentage of contact at the BIC (Suzuki et al., 1997), increased surface energy, improves matrix protein adsorption, bone cell migration and proliferation, and finally osseointegration (Dohan Ehrenfest et al., 2009).

On the other hand, surface roughness may lead to negative consequences due to the changes on surface microcomposition (M. Cehreli et al., 2004), such as increased risk of peri-implantitis, especially in high surface roughness (Albrektsson & Wennerberg, 2004), since rough surfaces acts in favor to plaque accumulation (van Steenberghe et al., 1999) and increased risk of ionic leakage, since greater surface roughness gives greater tissue-implant contact and hence ionic leakage (Albrektsson & Wennerberg, 2004).

The main clinical indication for using an implant with a rough surface includes areas with poor quality or volume of the host bone, since in these unfavorable clinical situations early and high bone-to-implant contact would be beneficial for allowing high levels of loading (Conner et al., 2003; Testori et al., 2001).

c. **Porous surfaces**

Some papers have described the Porous surface, which represents those with an extremely high Sa. These surfaces are characterized by pore size, pore shape, pore volume, pore depth and different from the rough surfaces due to the lack of sharp edges (Sykaras et al., 2000). It is evident that bone ingrowth into porous implant surfaces may result in improved osseointegration and mechanical stability by interlocking the surrounding bone tissue with the implant (Götz et al., 2004). These surfaces are produced when spherical powders of metallic or ceramic material become a coherent mass with the metallic core of the implant body (Sykaras et al., 2000, Triplet et al., 2003), being affected by the size of spherical particles, temperature and pressure conditions of the sintering chamber (Esposito et al., 1998).

6.2 Physicochemical properties

These properties usually refer to factors such as surface energy, charge and composition of the titanium implants (Albrektsson & Wennerberg, 2004; Puleo, 2006). These characteristics differ, depending on their bulk composition and surface treatments; affecting biological process including the protein adsorption and cell attachment (Le Guéhennec et al., 2007), as well largely determines the chemical stability/reactivity (Kasemo & Lausma, 1988).

The surface energy is a relevant issue, since affects directly the hydrophilicity of the surface. It is well know that highly hydrophilic surfaces (higher surface energy) seem more desirable than hydrophobic ones in view of their interactions with biological fluids, cells and tissues (Buser et al., 2004; Zhao et al., 2005).

7. Methods of surface modification

In order to improve the osseointegration of titanium dental implants, clinical efforts have been done to develop methods to provide an enhanced osseous stability through microsurface mediated events (Stanford, 2008) by the micro and nanoscale modifications of dental implant surface roughness and chemistry.

With surface treatment, it is possible to change the surface features of the titanium dental implant, such as chemical composition, energy level, morphology, topography and roughness (Upp et al., 2006). To date, several methods used to increase roughness, frequently tend to change the surface chemistry as well as texture (Puleo, 2006), such as Alkali and heat treatments (Lee et al., 2002).

For didactic reasons, only the main methods usually employed to modify surface properties will be discussed in detail in this Chapter and they can be classified as ablative (remove material from the surface) or additive (deposit material on implant surfaces) (M. Cehreli et al., 2004; Puleo, 2006).

7.1 Ablative methods

a. Grit blasting

This method consists in blasting the implants with hard ceramic particles, resulting in different surface roughnesses according to the ceramic particles sizes, time of blasting, pressure and distance from the source of particles to the implant surface (Sykaras et al., 2000; Triplet et al., 2003). Several ceramic particles have been used, such as alumina, titanium oxide and calcium phosphate particles (Le Guéhennec et al., 2007).

b. Acid etching

In this method the metallic implant is immersed into an acidic solution such as HCl, H_2SO_4, HNO_3 and HF (Le Guéhennec et al., 2007) which erodes the implant surface, creating pits of specific dimensions and shape that vary according to the concentration of the acidic solution, time, and temperature (Sykaras et al., 2000). Through acid etching it is possible to control the roughness, number, size and porous distribution on micrometer and nanometer scales (Elias et al., 2008).

c. Grit blasting followed by acid etching

This surface was produced by blasting implants with 250 to 500 mm corundum grit followed by acid etching in a hot solution of hydrochloric acid and sulfuric acid (Puleo, 2006) that have been developed by Institute Straumann (Basel, Switzerland) (Buser et al.,

1998). Sandblasting produces macro-roughness onto which acid etching superimposes micro-roughness (Cochran et al., 1998).

7.2 Additive methods

a. Plasma-spraying

Plasma spray coating is one of the most common methods for surface modification. This method consists in injecting both Ti or HA powders into plasma torch at high temperature (Le Guéhennec et al., 2007). Thickness depends on particle size, speed and time of impact, temperature, and distance from the nozzle tip to the implant surface area (Sykaras et al., 2000, Triplet et al., 2003).

It is relevant to state that by coating implants with hydroxyapatite (HA) both the roughness and surface chemistry are altered, resulting in an increased roughness with a dramatically change in surface chemistry from TiO_2 to a bone-like ceramic with the potential to chemically bonding to bone (Puleo, 2006). Furthermore, beyond plasma spray coating, other methods have been developed to coat metal implants, such as sputter-deposition, sol-gel coating, electrophoretic deposition or biomimetic precipitation (Le Guéhennec et al., 2007).

b. Anodization

This method produces modifications in the microstructure and the crystallinity of the titanium oxide layer (Sul et al., 2002) (Figures 4 to 9). It consists of preparing a porous oxide surface by potentiostatic or galvanostatic anodization of titanium in strong acids (H_2SO_4, H_3PO_4, HNO_3, HF) at high current density (200 A/m^2) or potential (100 V) (Le Guéhennec et al., 2007). The properties (thickness, microstructure, composition) of the oxide will depend on different process parameters such as electrolyte composition, anodic potential, current, temperature, and electrode geometry (Triplet et al., 2003).

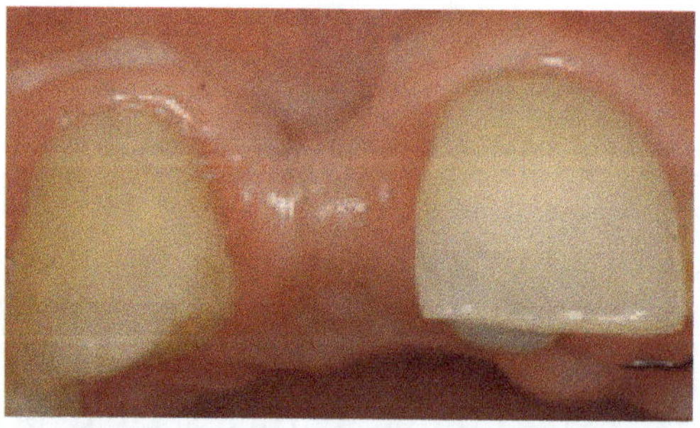

Fig. 4. Preoperative clinical aspect of the edentulous space

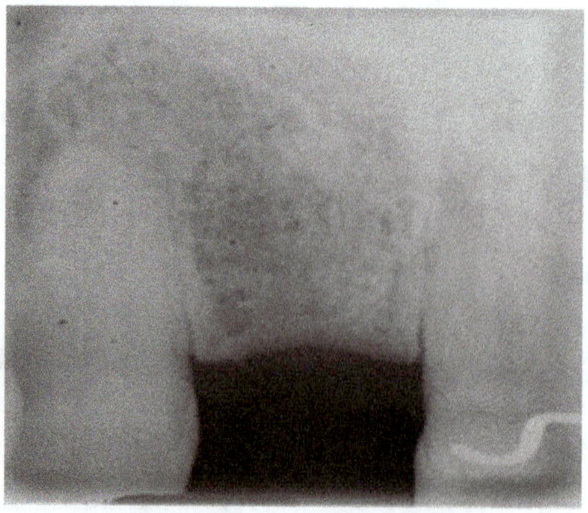

Fig. 5. Preoperative periapical radiographic

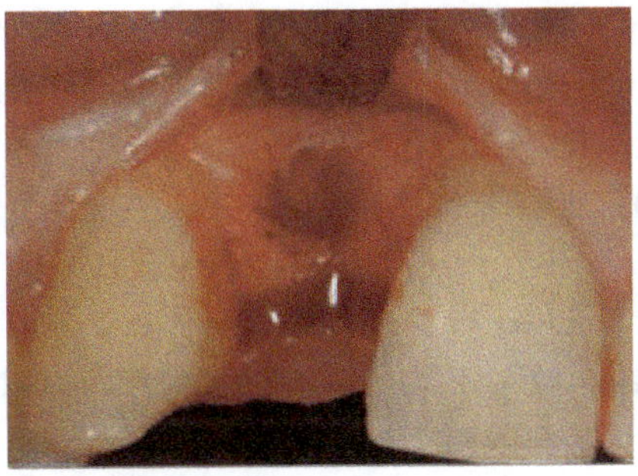

Fig. 6. Surgical approach to the alveolar bone

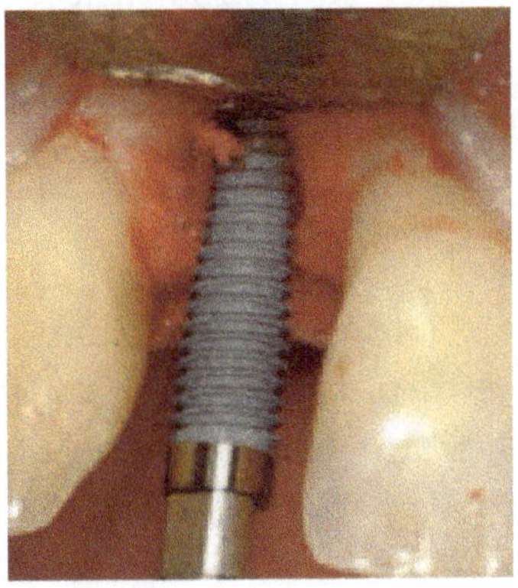

Fig. 7. Nobel Replace Select dental implant being positioned

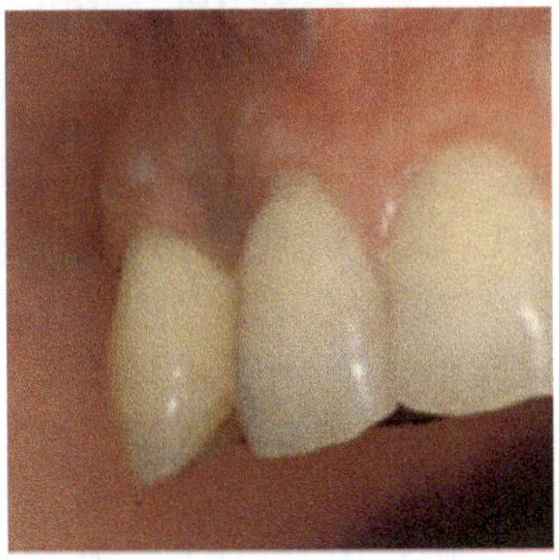

Fig. 8. Postoperative clinical aspect of the final prosthesis

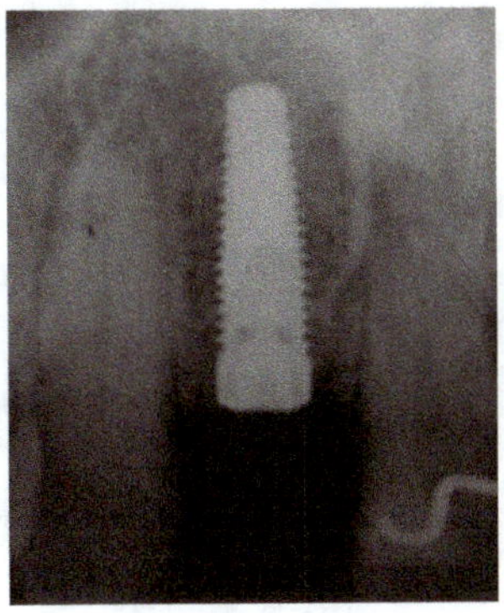

Fig. 9. Postoperative radiographic aspect of the dental implant

7.3 Incorporation of biologically active drugs into titanium dental implants

Modern trends associated with dental surface modification include the incorporation of several growth and differentiation factors either alone or combined as biocoatings of conventional implants. These factors include the bone morphogenetic proteins (BMPs), in particular BMP-2 and BMP-7 or osteogenic protein-1 (OP-1), and growth factors such as platelet-derived growth factor (PDGF), insulin-like growth factor (IGF), and transforming growth factor-beta 1 (TGF,-1) alone or combined with IGF-1, and TGF (Mavrogenis et al., 2009).

Other biological coatings that have been used to improve osseointegration of titanium implants include collagen and other extracellular matrix proteins such as fibronectin and vitronectin (Ku et al., 2005), and systemic administration of pharmacological agents such as ibandronate and human parathyroid hormone (Dayer et al., 2010).

8. Short implants

In a multicenter retrospective 6-year case series study, Misch et al. (2006) stated that there are three risk factors that increase stress and may explain why posterior short implants may have a higher failure rate compared to longer implants in the literature: 1) an increased crown height, 2) higher bite forces, and 3) bone density in the region. An increased crown height results in a vertical cantilever (Figure 10), in which the load transfer to the implant may be increased by 100% (Bidez et al., 1992). In order to reduce the stress at bone-implant interface the authors included 1) no cantilevers on the prostheses, 2) no angled forces to the posterior restorations, and 3) splinting multiple implants together. Splinted implants increase functional surface area of support whenever a load is applied to the prosthesis (Bidez et al., 1992). In addition, eliminating lateral contacts in mandibular excursions and cantilevers on the prosthesis helps to reduce forces on the implants. Increasing the implant number and splinting multiple implants in the prosthesis result in more functional area, in which the forces are applied and transferred. According to Gross (2008) studies after 1997 taking into account bone density and surface finish with microtexture versus machined co-variables, report comparable survival rates for short and standard length implants. These observations are corroborated by the study of Misch et al. (2006), in which, through employing properties of biomechanical stress reduction, high implant success rates in short implants of 7.0 and 9.0 mm can be predictably attained as reported in this and other studies.

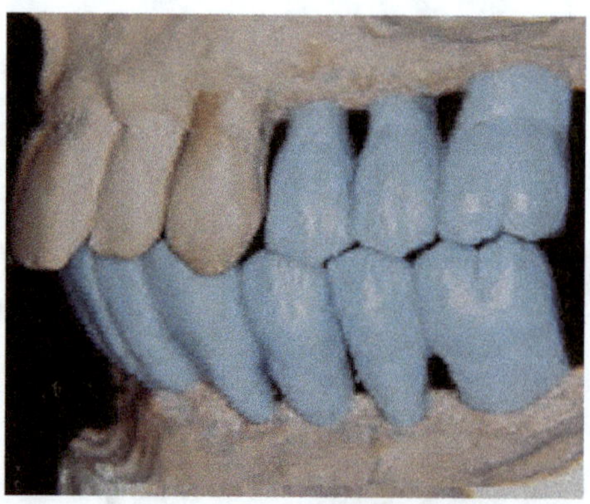

Fig. 10. Set-up wax of increased crowns height resulting in a vertical cantilever. Splinting must be considered

9. Guided dental implant surgery

Many methods to speed up the prosthetic stage have been devised in which devices could guide the surgeon on the implants placement, such as the Ohio State University Framework (Turkyilmaz et al., 2009) or the Novum System (Nobel Biocare, Göteborg, Sweden). However, these methods have not completely succeed because they solve a limited number of immediate planned loading cases because the failure in to feet individual anatomic variation.

The previous planning includes the patient complete anamnesis, the extra and intraoral examination in order to verify all anatomic and aesthetics components that are missing or should be improved. During the planning period conventional two-dimensional radiographs are necessary to evaluated available bone and the relationship between the implant insertion area and relevant anatomic structures, such as the inferior alveolar nerve and the maxillary sinus, and some templates representing the prosthetic setup could be made over these radiographs. However, this kind of preoperative planning neglects information about the third dimension of the patient´s anatomy.

Computer tomography has been providing medicine with some kind of three-dimensional anatomic information for at least thirty years, although for dentistry it was restricted to selected cases. At the last years the increasing availability, reduced radiation and lower costs of 3-D (three dimensional) imaging exams thanks to cone bean computer tomography development the 3-D implant planning is becoming more often used in dentistry and maxillo-facial surgery (Schneider et al., 2009). In conjunction with the 3-D tomography several manufactures developed computer software allowing virtual implant placement using the acquired digital data from the computed tomography (CT) scan (Mandelaris et al., 2010).

The transfer of the previously planned at the computer software according to the 3-D anatomic data scanned of the patients face, can be done by the use of stereolithographicsurgical guides created by computer-aided design and computer-aided manufacturing (CAD-CAM) technology or by "navigation" systems that use intra-operative optical tracking of the hand-piece position and guide the surgeon in real-time during the surgery providing visual feedback on a screen. The first one described is the more often used due to the inferior costs and because the high technology development required to use "navigations" systems are not available everywhere. Computer-aided implantation minimizes the error in implant positioning compared to conventional surgical guide implant placement and allows the provisory restoration to be manufactured prior to surgery (Yamada et al., 2011). Thereafter even the CAD-CAM technology provide the surgeon very precise information about the anatomy and the correct placement of the implants, so precise that allows the surgeon to perform flapless surgeries (Barnea et al., 2010; Patel, 2010).

The flapless surgery for placement of dental implants has some advantages such as the maintenance of the periosteum attachment and blood supply to the bone, avoids gingival profile modification following the contour of the surgical incision, reduces the postoperative edema, bleeding, pain and discomfort for the patients and clearly make the surgical time shorter (Abad-Gallegos et al., 2010; Azari & Nikzad, 2008). These advantages seem to increase the success rates of immediate loading, probably due to the blood supply preservation (Fortin et al., 2003; Malo et al., 2007). The flapless surgery is only possible with the use of surgical guides that should be precisely made; with this methodology it is always possible to avoid inadequate positioning of the implant and the unintentionally anatomic structures contact with the implant surface. Remembering always that in this kind of surgery both the safety and success of treatment depend on the surgeon and prosthodontist accuracy. But despite many benefits described about the flapless implantation, this type of procedure could be perceived as a blind procedure due to the difficulty in evaluation alveolar bone contours and fenestrations or different angulations, setbacks that increases the chances of cortical plates perforation or fenestration when performed unassociated to the guided planning, however, the new 3-D computer guided planning technology made the implant insertion so precise that the setbacks of the flapless surgery were almost all vanished.

Some protocols for rehabilitation of completely edentulous jaws with flapless surgery and the placement of immediate fixed prostheses through computer guided surgery seems to be effective and predictable according to Puig (2010), besides with high potential for the patients acceptance, however, the author states that this techniques, for example the "all-on-four" and "all-on-six" protocols, could be sensitive to the experience of the surgeon and like all other surgical techniques its requires a learning curve from the surgeons who intend to perform they.

However, complications may occur during computer-guided surgery and the superstructure, sometimes, cannot be inserted immediately. Complications like insufficient primary implant stability or misfit of the restoration due to transfer mistakes, mistakes that can be justified due the mucosa anatomic alterations in flapless surgeries, unstable fixation of the surgical guide, imprecise impressions and incorrect pouring of the casts. Also the incorrect acquisition of tomographic image and processing could lead to errors (Almeida et al., 2010). Because of this some potentially complications, some author do recommend the application of guided surgery with flapless approach in cases with adequate bone volume and states that the guided technique can also be used in sites with insufficient bone volume, but a mucoperiosteal flap procedure is recommended (Fitzgerald et al., 2010).

The guided surgery has been indicated for complete and partial edentulism, for booth maxilla and mandibular bones. Thus many authors agree that the mainly advantage of this method is the use in the maxilla because of its anatomic peculiarities (Meloni et al., 2010; Vasak et al., 2011). Jung et al. (2009) revealed, after a systematic review including 29 different image guidance systems, a high mean implant survival rate of 96.6% after only 12 months of observation in different clinical indications.

There is no doubt that the computer guided surgery is a very advanced treatment and it's belong to the future of the implant treatment, although it seems to be a safe and predictable treatment, future long-term clinical data are necessary to identify the right clinical indications and to justify additional radiation doses, efforts and costs associated with this technique; because until now, despite all described advantages there is no evidence to suggest that computer guided surgery is superior to conventional procedures in terms of safety, outcomes, morbidity or yet success rates.

9.1 Surgical and prosthetic sequence

The virtual planning was first executed over the images acquired with the computerized tomography of the patient (Figures 11, 12 and 13), planning the implants position according to the desired teeth future positioning and to the existing bone support.

Afterwards the implant´s company makes the surgical guide based on the previous virtual planning done by the surgeon using the specific software that this company supplies for the surgeons (Figure 14).

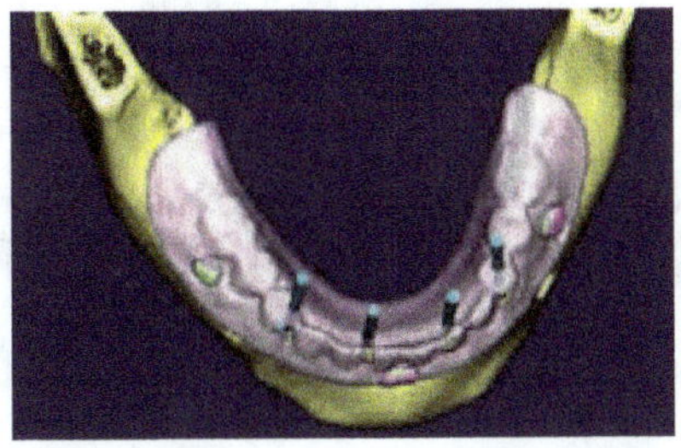

Fig. 11. Virtual planning occlusal view

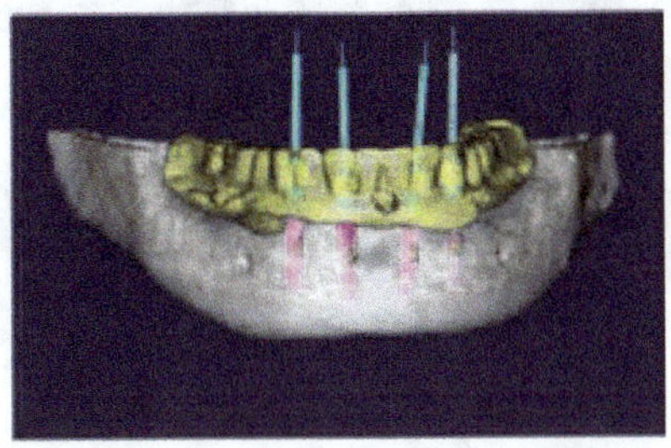

Fig. 12. Virtual planning frontal view

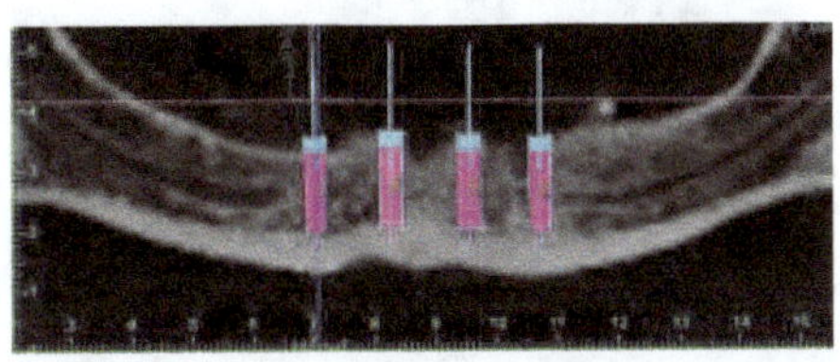

Fig. 13. Virtual planning on the panoramic view of the computerized tomography

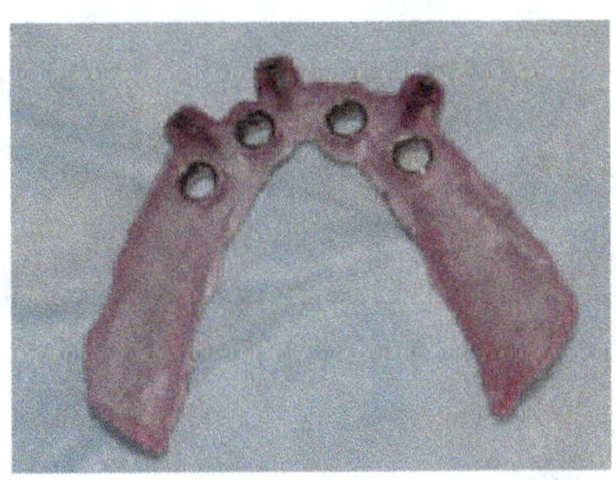

Fig. 14. Surgical guide made by the implant system company

The preoperative frontal view of the patient's mouth can be seen in Figure 15. With the surgical guide in hands the surgeons shall performs the surgery, after the anesthetization the surgeons most secure the surgical guide by drilling three or four holes at the exactly spots and locking the guide with the proper devices (Figure 16).

After locking the surgical guide starts the drilling steps, following the exactly drill sequence designed by the implant company in order to make the implant insertion with the same inclinations that previously virtually planned (Figure 17). The implants were inserted by flapless surgery guided through the surgical guide (Figure 18). After the complete insertion, the prothetical abutments are locked over the implants (Figure 19) and the total prosthesis was installed (Figure 20).

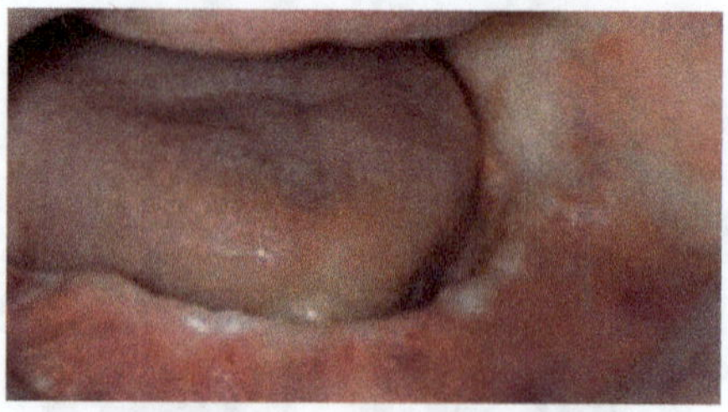

Fig. 15. Preoperative patient´s mouth view

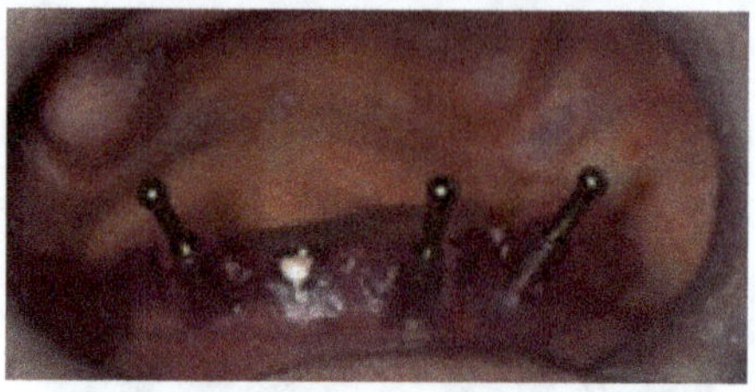

Fig. 16. Surgical guide in place and locked

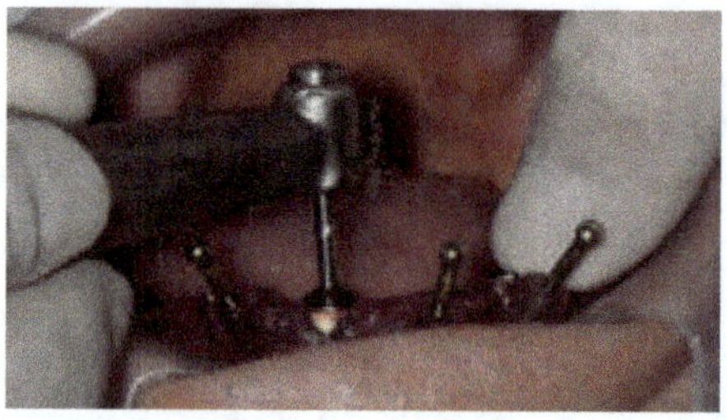

Fig. 17. Drilling steps according to the manufacturer´s orientation

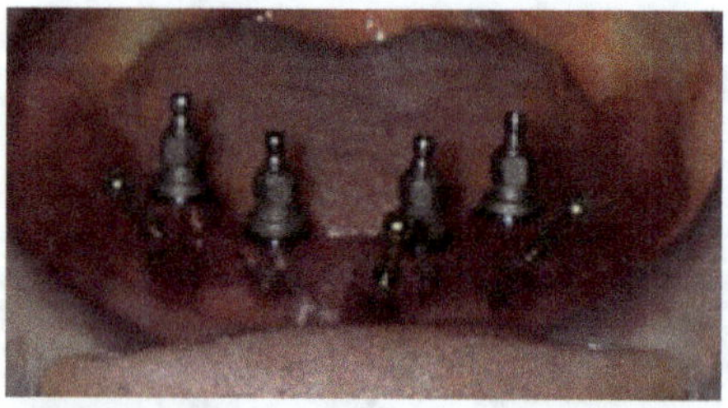

Fig. 18. Implants insertion completed

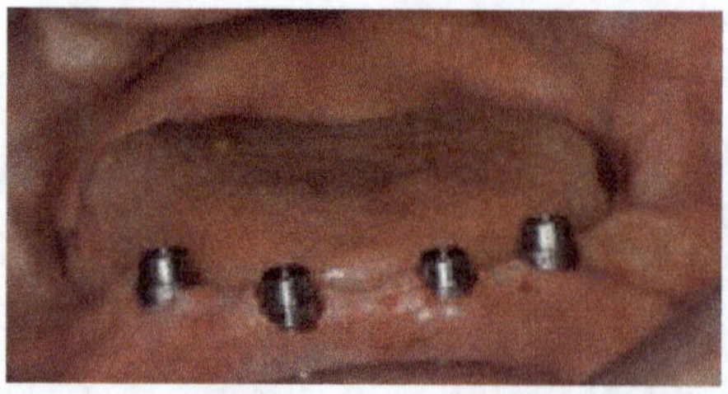

Fig. 19. Removal of the surgical guide and abutment insertion

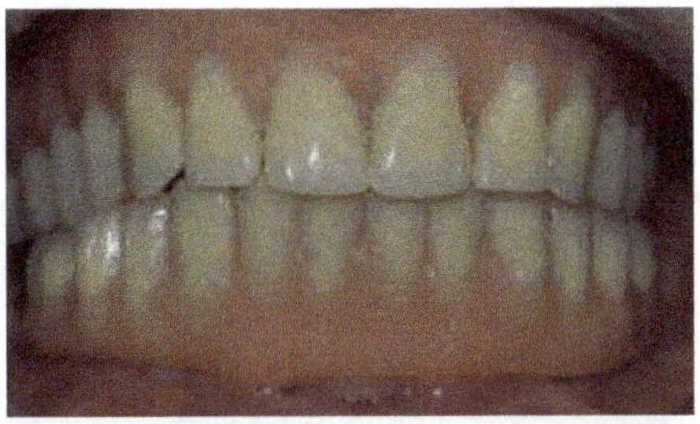

Fig. 20. Clinical case completed with the total inferior prosthesis installation in less than 24 hours (Courtesy of Prof. Dr. Valfrido Pereira Antonio Filho)

10. Occlusion aspects

Although the etiological factors underlying bone loss have not been fully established (Prosper et al., 2009), Canay & Akça (2009) stated that the main contributory factors of bone loss are occlusal overload and peri-implantitis. Current concepts are mixed regarding the peri-implant response to occlusal overload. Gross (2008) reported that a phenomenon of fatigue microtrauma has been proposed as the process of cervical and progressive bone loss as bone "modeling" due to excessive occlusal load. When the rate of fatigue microdamage exceeds the reparative rate, cervical bone is irreversibly lost. According to Kozlovsky et al. (2007), the overloading aggravated plaque-induced bone resorption, and increased bone loss of the dental implants. The decreasing of the functional surface of the dental crowns, the loads being directed to the long axis of the implants, the provisionalization and an adequate occlusal adjustment seem to favor the immediate loading implants result. In addition to poor bone quality, unfavorable force direction and concentration may increase failure rates of implants (Becktor et al., 2002; Chen et al., 2008). The question of splinting is also relevant to a discussion of occlusion as previously described. Some authors (Nokar et al., 2010; Zarone et al., 2003) advocated separation of mandibular superstructures in the midline (Figures 21 to 24) and cite mandibular flexure as a potential source of distal implant morbidity in full-arch restorations. However, additional studies about bone loss and prosthesis failure are necessary to confirm these findings.

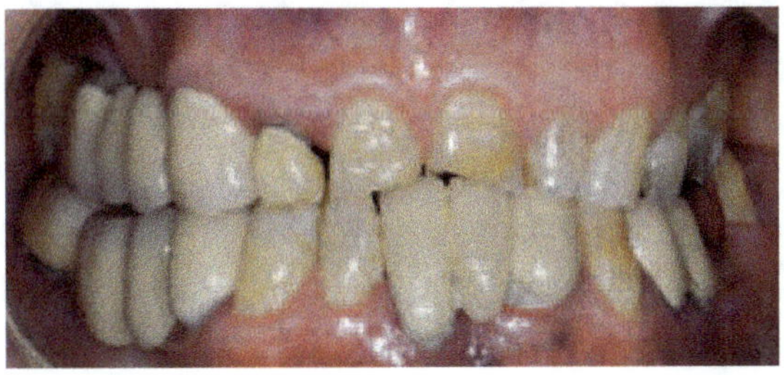

Fig. 21. Initial clinical aspect

Gross (2008) suggested that the occlusion should be viewed as consisting of three basic elements: posterior support, occlusal vertical dimension (Figure 25) and eccentric or anterior guidance. The degree of vertical and horizontal overlap determines whether the anterior teeth disclude the posterior teeth in protrusion and whether the working side discludes the non-working side in latero-protrusive movements (anterior disclusion). Mutual protection is directly dependent on posterior support, in which the molars protect the anterior teeth during occlusion and the anterior teeth protect the posteriors in excursive movements. Gross also recommends to avoid creation of excursive guidance on single implant

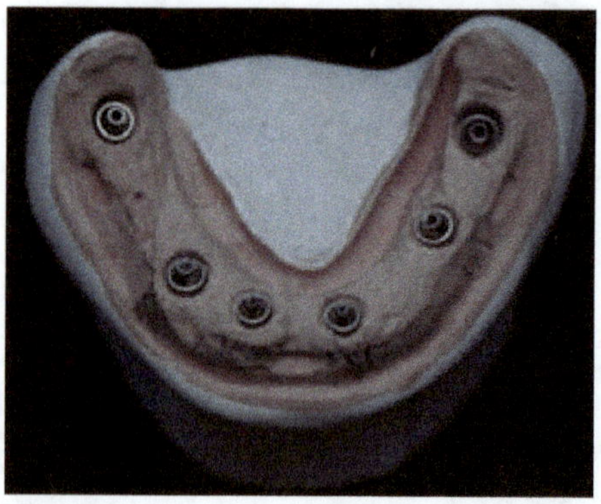

Fig. 22. Cast after the impression of immediate placed dental implants

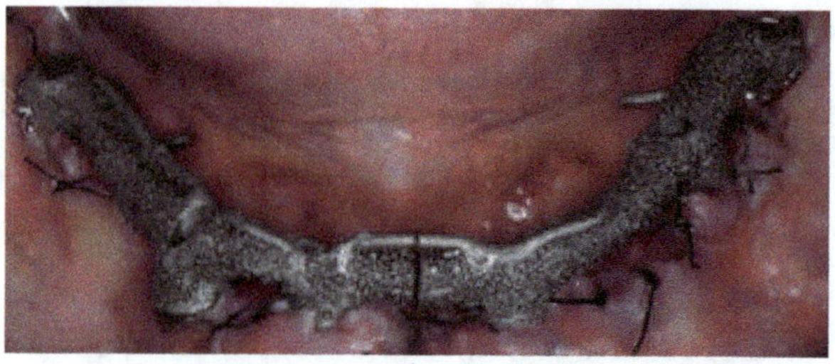

Fig. 23. Bar casted in two rigid segments, with a minimum separation in the anterior region

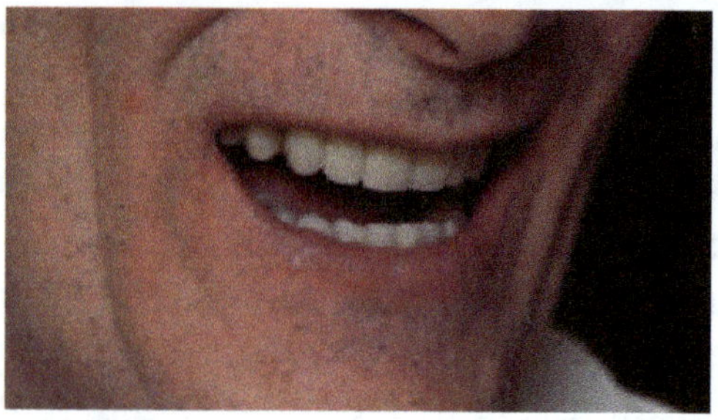

Fig. 24. Final aspect of the oral rehabilitation

restorations in order to prevent overloading to the prosthesis, abutment, implant and, therefore, to bone-implant interface. Cantilevers must be also avoided (Figure 26) or decreased (Figure 27) when possible. It must be remembered that the greater the bucco-lingual (Figure 28), mesial, distal or vertical cantilever, the greater will be the biomechanical failure risk. Finally, the decreasing of the functional surface of the crowns, the loads being directed to the long axis of the implants, the absence of cantilevers during the provisionalization and an adequate occlusal adjustment seem to favor the immediate loading implants results (Misch & Bidez, 1995).

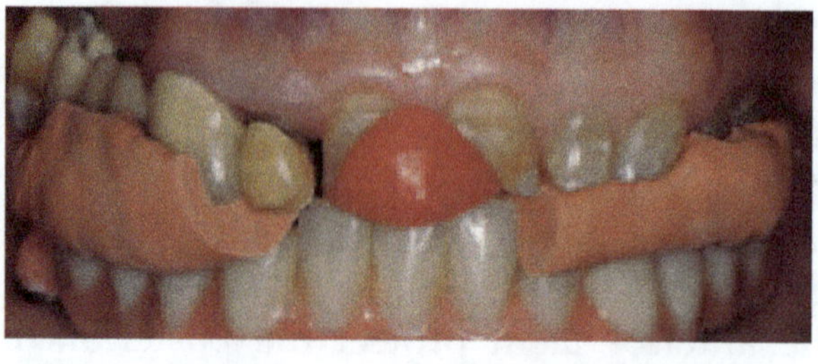

Fig. 25. Occlusion vertical dimension determined by a Lucia's Jaw Interference Guide (JIG)

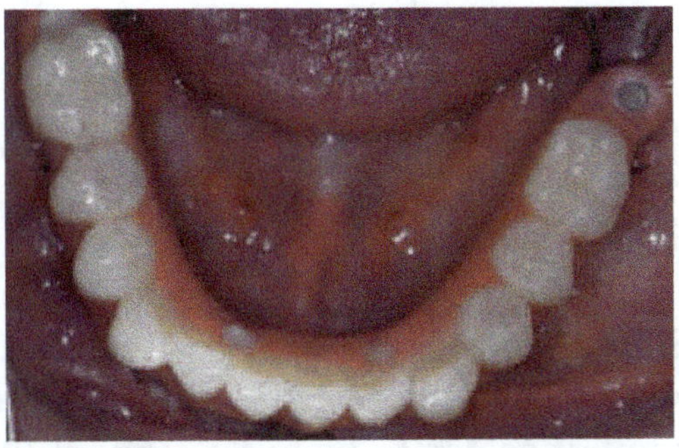

Fig. 26. Total implant-supported prosthesis with no cantilever

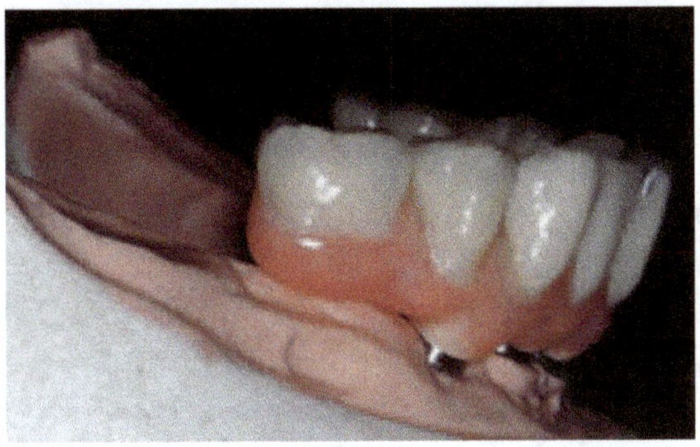

Fig. 27. Shortened dental arch concept reducing the length of the cantilever by using one premolar for each quadrant

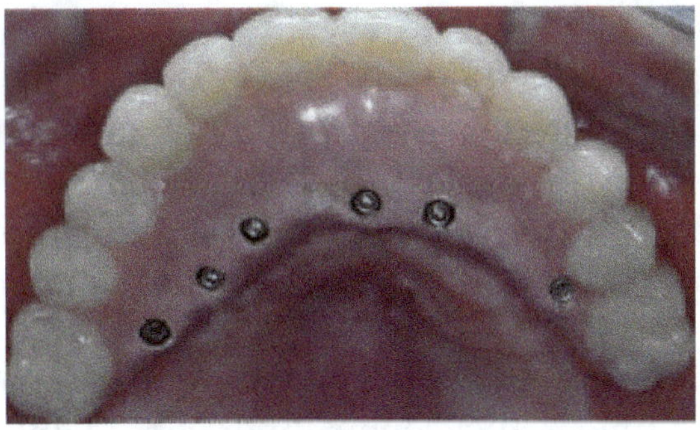

Fig. 28. Unsatisfactory implant-supported prosthesis. See the great bucco-lingual cantilever and the inadequate orientation of the teeth

11. Ferulization

A key factor for success or failure of dental implants is the manner in which stresses are transferred to bone-implant interface (Geng et al., 2001). Finite Element Analysis (FEA) is a useful tool for the determination of stresses and displacements in mechanical objects and materials, but is also frequently used in biological systems like in dentistry. Bevilacqua et al. (2008) reported that stress at the bone-implant interface increased with increasing single implant inclinations. Therefore, these authors demonstrated that vertical implants remain the first choice for single implants, given that stress transmitted to the bone-implant interface increases with increasing implant inclinations. On the other hand, different results were found in another study made by Bevilacqua et al. (2011), regarding the stress distribution in maxillary implant-supported fixed dentures, in which tilted implants were used in fixed denture designs. In this study, tilted distal implants, rigidly splinted, decreased peri-implant bone stresses as compared to a vertical implant model with cantilevered segments. From the results of this investigation the authors concluded that the use of distal tilted implants results in a reduction in stresses in the peri-implant bone and in metal frameworks secondary to cantilever length reduction and implant length increase. Therefore, the concept of splinted arch seems to be very pertinent when immediate loading procedures are indicated for patients with extensive implant-supported prostheses and for edentulous patients. In addition, it seems to be quite evident the use of a larger number of implants and their splinting (if possible) when one-step surgical procedures are indicated (Attard & Zarb, 2005).

12. Parafunctional habits

Another relevant aspect that must be taken into account is the presence of parafunctional habits. Parafunctional habits may generate overloading and may contribute with up to 75% of the immediate loading implants failure. These non-functional habits may increase the looseness or fracture risk of the abutments and of the restorations (Mish et al., 2004b). According to Gross (2008), eccentric occlusal parafunction may generate extremely high and potentially destructive loads, sufficient to wear down the teeth, fracture crowns and roots, decement or break fixed partial dentures, dislodge or break abutment screws, fracture porcelain or superstructures, traumatize supporting bone and break implants. Thus, bruxism should be diagnosed and addressed as a complicating and additional risk factor. In agreement with some authors (Colomina, 2001; Misch et al., 2004a), when the parafunctional habits are not normalized, its presence may be an exclusion criterion for the immediate loading dental implants. Regardless the procedure (immediate, early or delayed) for the dental implants and prosthesis insertion, the use of a full-arch night splint may be beneficial in reducing potential overload from nocturnal parafunction. Despite the fact that some reviews show that bruxism has not been causally linked to supporting bone morbidity, its potential for creating complication in the superstructure and implant stack are very real (Gross, 2008).

Parafunction is a significant factor in the planning of excursive guidance and the creation of an occlusal scheme with abutment and bone support optimally designed to minimize the potentially destructive forces of bruxism (Gross, 2008). Therefore, flattening guiding inclines, increasing implant numbers and bone support, splinting multiple implants together, reducing occlusal vertical dimension to decrease crown-root ratio and minimizing functional occlusal surfaces and cupids without excessively compromising tooth shape should be also considered.

13. Conclusions

Physical and biomechanical procedures, such as splinting and appropriate occlusal adjustment, must be always followed in order to avoid the overloading risks and the stress on bone-implant interface.

Short implants, cantilevered segments and external hexagon connections may be associated with increased problems such as screw loosening, as well as screw, denture teeth, denture base, and framework fractures.

The treated surface dental implants and morse-taper implant-abutment connection possesses higher biomechanical behavior than the non-treated dental implants, and the conventional external and internal hexagon designs, respectively

Restorations should be planned on an articulator with a diagnostic wax set-up, and radiographic and surgical guides used when possible and necessary.

Computerized guidance systems may improve the accuracy of surgical procedures, especially in clinical situations in which the bone ridge and the anatomical relations are unfavorable.

14. Acknowledgments

We would like to thanks Prof. Dr. João Gustavo Rabelo Ribeiro, Prof. Dr. Marcelo Antonialli Del'Acqua, Prof. Dr. Valfrido Antonio Pereira Filho, Prof. Dr. Leandro Eduardo Kluppel and Ricardo Pasquini Filho for the courtesy of some clinical Figures.

15. References

Abad-Gallegos, M.; Gómez-Santos, L.; Sánchez-Garcés, M.A.; Piñera-Penalva, M.; Freixes-Gil, J.; Castro-García, A. & Gay-Escoda, C. (2010). Complications of guided surgery and immediate loading in oral implantology: a report of 12 cases. *Medicina Oral Patologia Oral y Cirurgia Bucal,* Vol.15, (August 2010), (Epub ahead of print), ISSN 1698-6946

Abrahamsson, I.; Berglundh, T.; Linder, E.; Lang, N.P. & Lindhe, J. (2004). Early bone formation adjacent to rough and turned endosseous implant surfaces. An experimental study in the dog. *Clinical Oral Implants Research,* Vol.15, No.4, (August 2004), pp. 381–392, ISSN 0905-7161

Adell, U.; Lekholm, U.; Rockler, B. & Brånemark, P.I. (1981). A 15-year study of osseointegrated implants in the treatment of endentulous jaw. *International Journal of Oral Surgery,* Vol.10, No.6, (December 1981), pp. 387-416, ISSN 0300-9785

Akca, K.; Cehreli, M.C. & Iplikcioglu, H. (2003). Evaluation of the mechanical characteristics of the implant-abutment complex of a reduced-diameter morse-taper implant. A nonlinear finite element stress analysis. *Clinical Oral Implants Research,* Vol.14, No.4, pp. 444-454. ISSN 0905-7161

Albrektsson, T.; Brånemark, P.I.; Hansson, H.A. & Lindstrom, J. (1981). Osseointegrated titanium implant. Requirements for long lasting, direct bone-to-implant anchorage in man. *Acta Orthopaedica Scandinavica,* Vol.52, No.2, pp. 155–170, ISSN 0001-6470

Albrektsson, T. & Wennerberg, A. (2004). Oral Implant Surfaces: Part 1—Review Focusing on Topographic and Chemical Properties of Different Surfaces and In Vivo Responses to them. *The International Journal of Prosthodontics,* Vol.17, No.5, (September-October 2004), pp. 536–543, ISSN 0893-2174

Almeida, E.O.; Pellizer, E.P.; Goiatto, M.C.; Margonar, R.; Rocha, E.P.; Freitas-Jr, A.C. & Anchieta, R.B. (2010). Computer-guided surgery in implantology: Review of basic concepts. *The Journal of Craniofacial Surgery,* Vol.21, No. 6, (November 2010), pp. 1917-1921, ISSN 1049-2275

Al-Omiri M.; Hantash R.A. & Al-Wahadni A. (2005). Satisfaction with dental implants: a literature review. *Implant Dentistry,* Vol.14, No.4, (December 2005), pp. 399-406, ISSN 1056-6163

Attard N.J. & Zarb G.A. (2005). Immediate and early implant loading protocols: a literature review of clinical studies. *The Journal of Prosthetic Dentistry,* Vol.94, No.3, (September 2005), pp. 242-58, ISSN 0022-3913

Azari, A. & Nikzad, S. (2008). Flapless implant surgery: review of the literature and report of 2 cases with computer-guided surgical approach. *Journal of Oral and Maxillofacial Surgery,* Vol.66, No.5, (May 2008), pp. 1015-1021, ISSN 0278-2391

Barnea, E.; Alt, I.; Kolerman, R. & Nissan, J. (2010). Accuracy of a laboratory-based computer implant guiding system. *Oral Surgery Oral Medicine Oral Pathology Oral Radiology Endodonty,* Vol.109, No.5, (May 2010), pp. e6-e10, ISSN 1079-2104

Becker, W.; Becker, B.E.; Israelson, H.; Lucchini, J.P.; Handelsman, M.; Ammons, W.; Rosenberg, E.; Rose, L.; Tucker, L.M. & Lekholm, U. (1997). One-step surgical placement of Brånemark implants: a prospective multicenter clinical study. *The International Journal of Oral & Maxillofacial Implants.* Vol.12, No.4, (July-August 1997), pp. 454-62, ISSN 0882-2786

Becktor, J.P.; Eckert, S.E.; Isaksson, S. & Keller, E.E. (2002). The influence of mandibular dentition on implant failures in bone-grafted edentulous maxillae. *The International Journal of Oral & Maxillofacial Implants,* Vol. 17, No.1, (January-February 2002), pp. 69-77, ISSN 0882-2786

Bevilacqua, M.; Tealdo, T.; Menini, M.; Pera, F.; Mossolov, A.; Drago, C. & Pera, P. (2008). Three-dimensional finite element analysis of load transmission using different implant inclinations and cantilever lengths. *The International Journal of Prosthodontics,* Vol.21, No.6, (November-December 2008), pp. 539-42, ISSN 0893-2174

Bevilacqua, M.; Tealdo, T.; Menini, M.; Pera, F.; Mossolov, A.; Drago, C. & Pera P. (2011). The influence of cantilever length and implant inclination on stress distribution in maxillary implant-supported fixed dentures. *The Journal of Prosthetic* Dentistry, Vol.105, No.1, (January 2011), pp. 5-13, ISSN 1097-6841

Bidez, M.W. & Misch, C.E. (1992). Force transfer in implant dentistry: Basic concepts and principles. *Journal of Oral Implantology,* Vol.18, No.3, pp. 264-274. ISSN 0160-6972

Binon, P.P. (1996) The effect of implant/abutment hexagonal misfit on screw joint stability. *The International Journal of Prosthodontics,* Vol.9, No.2, (March-April 1996), pp. 149-160, ISSN 0893-2174

Bozkaya, D. & Muftu, S. (2003). Mechanics of the tapered interference fit in dental implants. *Journal of Biomechanics,* Vol.36, No.11 (November 2003), pp. 1649–1658, ISSN 0021-9290

Bozkaya, D. & Muftu, S. (2005) Mechanics of the taper integrated screwed-in (tis) abutments used in dental implants. *Journal of Biomechanics,* Vol.38, No.1 (January 2005), pp. 87-97, ISSN 0021-9290

Brånemark, P.I.; Hansson, B.O.; Adell, R.; Breine, U.; Lindström, J.; Hallén, O. & Ohman A. (1977). Osseointegrated implants in the treatment of the endentulous jaw. Experience from a 10-year period. *Scandinavian Journal of Plastic and Reconstructive Surgery,* Vol.16, pp. 1-132, ISSN 0581-9474

Brånemark, P.I.; Engstrand, P.; Ohrnell, L.O.; Grondahl, K.; Nilsson, P.; Hagberg, K.; Darle, C. & Lekholm, U. (1999). Brånemark Novum: a new treatment concept for rehabilitation of the edentulous mandible. Preliminary results from a prospective clinical follow-up study. *Clinical Implant Dentistry and Related Research*, Vol.1, No.1, pp. 2-16, ISSN 1523-0899

Brunette, D.M. & Chehroudi, B. (1999). The effects of the surface topography of micromachined titanium substrata on cell behavior in vitro and in vivo. *Journal of Biomechanical Engineering*, Vol.121, No.1, (February 1999), pp. 49–57 ISSN 0148-0731

Burguete, R.L.; Johns, R.B.; King, T. & Patterson, E.A. (1994) Tightening characteristics for screwed joints in osseointegrated dental implants. *The Journal of Prosthetic Dentistry*, Vol.71, No.6, (June 1994), pp. 592-599 ISSN 0022-3913

Buser, D.; Broggini, N.; Wieland, M.; Schenk, R.K.; Denzer, A.J.; Cochran, D.L.; Hoffmann, B.; Lussi, A. & Steinemann, S.G. (2004). Enhanced bone apposition to a chemically modified SLA titanium surface. *Journal of Dental Research*, Vol.83, No.7, (July 2004), pp. 529–533, ISSN 0022-0345

Buser, D.; Nydegger, T.; Hirt, H.P.; Cochran, D.L. & Nolte, L.P. (1998). Removal torque values of titanium implants in the maxilla of miniature pigs. *The International Journal of Oral & Maxillofacial Implants*, Vol.13, No.5, (September-October 1998), pp. 611–619, ISSN 0882-2786

Calvo-Guirado, J.L.; Ortiz-Ruiz, A.J.; López-Marí, L.; Delgado-Ruiz, R.; Maté-Sánchez, J. & Bravo Gonzalez, L.A. (2009). Immediate maxillary restoration of single-tooth implants using platform switching for crestal bone preservation: a 12-month study. *The International Journal of Oral & Maxillofacial Implants*, Vol.24, No.2 (March-April 2009), pp. 275-281, ISSN 0882-2786

Canay, S. & Akça, K. (2009). Biomechanical aspects of bone-level diameter shifting at implant-abutment interface. *Implant Dentistry*, Vol.18, No.3, (June 2009), pp. 239-248, ISSN 1538-2982

Casap, N.; Laviv, A. & Wexler, A. (2011). Computerized navigation for immediate loading of dental implants with a prefabricated metal frame: a feasibility study. *Journal of Oral and Maxillofacial Surgery*, Vol.69, No.2, (February 2011), pp. 512-519, ISSN 0278-2391

Cehreli, M.; Sahin, S. & Akca, K. (2004). Role of mechanical environment and implant design on bone tissue differentiation: current knowledge and future contexts. *Journal of Dentistry*, Vol.31, No.4, (February 2004), pp. 123–132, ISSN 0300-5712

Cehreli, M.C.; Akça, K. & Iplikçioğlu, H. (2004). Force transmission of one- and two-piece morse-taper oral implants: a nonlinear finite element analysis. *Clinical Oral Implants Research*, Vol.15, No.4, (August 2004), pp. 481-489, ISSN 0905-7161

Chen, Y.Y.; Kuan, C.L. & Wang, Y.I. (2008). Implant occlusion: biomechanical considerations for implant-supported prostheses. *Journal of Dental Sciences*, Vol.3, No. 2, pp. 65-74, ISSN 1991-7902

Chiapasco, M.; Abati, S.; Romeo, E. & Vogel, G. (2001). Implant-retained mandibular overdentures with Brånemark System MKII implants: a prospective comparative study between delayed and immediate loading. *The International Journal of Oral & Maxillofacial Implants*, Vol. 16, No.4, (July-August 2001), pp. 537-546, ISSN 0882-2786

Chou, L.; Firth, J.D.; Uitto, V.J. & Brunette, D.M. (1998). Effects of titanium substratum and grooved surface topography on metalloproteinase- 2 expression in human fibroblasts. *Journal of Biomedical Materials Research*, Vol.39, No.3, (March 1998), pp. 437–445, ISSN 1549-3296

Chow, J.; Hui, E.; Liu, J.; Li, D.; Wat, P.; Li, W.; Yau, Y.K. & Law, H. (2001). The Hong Kong Bridge Protocol. Immediate loading of mandibular Brånemark fixtures using a fixed provisional prosthesis: preliminary results. *Clinical Implant Dentistry and Related Research*, Vol. 3, No.3, pp. 166-174, ISSN 1523-0899

Chun, H.J.; Cheong, S.Y.; Han, J.H.; Heo, S.J.; Chung, J.P.; Rhyu, I.C.; Choi, Y.C.; Baik, H.K.; Ku, Y. & Kim M.H. (2002). Evaluation of design parameters of osseointegrated dental implants using finite element analysis. *The Journal of Oral Rehabilitation*, Vol.29, No.6, (June 2002), pp. 565–574, ISSN 0305-182X

Cochran, D.L.; Schenk, R.K.; Lussi, A.; Higginbottom, F.L. & Buser, D. (1998). Bone response to unloaded and loaded titanium implants with a sandblasted and acid-etched surface: a histometric study in the canine mandible. *Journal of Biomedical Materials Research,* Vol. 40, No.1, (April 1998), pp. 1–11, ISSN 1549-3296

Colomina, L.E. (2001). Immediate loading of implant-fixed mandibular prostheses: a prospective 18-month follow-up clinical study-preliminary report. *Implant Dentistry*, Vol.10, No.1, pp. 23-29, ISSN 1056-6163

Conner, K.; Sabatini, R.; Mealey, B.; Takacks, V.; Mill, M. & Cochran, D. (2003). Guided bone regeneration around titanium plasma-sprayed, acid-etched and hydroxyapatite-coated implants in the canine model. *Journal of Periodontology,* Vol.74, No.5, (May 2003), pp. 658–668, ISSN 0022-3492

Da Silva, E.F.; Pellizzer, E.P.; Quinelli Mazaro, J.V. & Garcia Júnior, I.R. (2010). Influence of the connector and implant design on the implant-tooth-connected prostheses. *Clinical Implant Dentistry and Related Research*, Vol.12, No.3, (May 2010), pp. 254-262. ISSN 1523-0899

Davi, L.R.; Golin, A.L.; Bernardes, S.R.; Araujo, C.A. & Neves, F.D. (2008). In vitro integrity of implant external hexagon after application of surgical placement torque simulating implant locking. *Brazilian Oral Research,* Vol.22, No. 2, (April-June 2010), pp. 125-131, ISSN 1807-3107

Dayer, R.; Brennan, T.C.; Rizzoli, R. & Ammann, P. (2010). PTH improves titanium implant fixation more than pamidronate or renutrition in osteopenic rats chronically fed a low protein diet. *Osteoporosis International*, Vol.21, No. 6, (June 2010), pp. 957-967, ISSN 0937-941X

Degidi, M. & Piattelli, A. (2003). Immediate functional and non-functional loading of dental implants: a 2- to 60-month follow-up study of 646 titanium implants. *Journal of Periodontology*, Vol.74, No.2, (February 2003), pp. 225-241, ISSN 0022-3492

Degidi, M. & Piattelli A. (2005). Comparative analysis study of 702 dental implants subjected to immediate functional loading and immediate nonfunctional loading to traditional healing periods with a follow-up of up to 24 months. *The International Journal of Oral & Maxillofacial Implants*, Vol.20, No.1, (January-February 2005), pp. 99-107, ISSN 0882-2786

Dohan Ehrenfest D.M.; Coelho, P.G.; Kang, B.S.; Sul1, Y.T. & Albrektsson, T. (2009). Classification of osseointegrated implant surfaces: materials, chemistry and topography. *Trends in Biotechnology*, Vol.28, No.4, (April 2009), pp. 198-206, ISSN 0167-9430

Duyck, J.; Ronold, H.J.; Van Oosterwyck, H.; Naert, I.; Vander Sloten, J. & Ellingsen, J.E. (2001). The influence of static and dynamic loading on marginal bone reactions around osseointegrated implants: an animal experimental study. *Clinical Oral Implants Research*, Vol.12, No.3, (June 2001), pp. 207-218, ISSN 0905-7161

Elias, C.N.; Oshida, Y.; Lima, J.H. & Muller, C.A. (2008). Relationship between surface properties (roughness, wettability and morphology) of titanium and dental implant removal torque. *Journal of the Mechanical Behavior of Biomedical Materials*, Vol.1, No.3, (July 2008), pp. 234-242, ISSN 1751-6161

Engquist, B.A.; Strand, P.; Dahlgren, S.; Engquist, E.; Feldmann, H. & Grondahl, K. (2002). Marginal bone reaction to oral implants: a prospective comparative study of Astra Tech and Brånemark system implants. *Clinical Oral Implants Research*, Vol.13, No.1, (February 2002), pp. 30–37, ISSN 0905-7161

Ericsson, I.; Randow, K.; Glantz, P.O.; Lindhe, J. & Nilner, K. (1994). Clinical and radiographical features of submerged and nonsubmerged titanium implants. *Clinical Oral Implants Research*, Vol.5, No.3, (September 1994), pp. 185-189, ISSN 0905-7161

Esposito, M.; Hirsch, J.M.; Lekholm, U. & Thomsen, P. (1998). Biological factors contributing to failures of osseointegrated oral implants. (I) Success criteria and epidemiology. *European Journal of Oral Sciences*, Vol.106, No.1 (February 1998), pp. 527–551, ISSN 0909-8836

Esposito, M.; Grusovin, M.G.; Achille, H.; Coulthard, P. & Worthington, H.V. (2009). Interventions for replacing missing teeth: different times for loading dental implants. *Cochrane Database Systematic Review*, Vol.21, CD 003878, DOI 10.1002/14651858

Fitzgerald, M.; O´Sullivan, M.; O´Connell.B. & Houston, F. (2010). Accuracy of bone mapping and guided flapless implant placement in human cadavers using a model-based planning procedure.*The International Journal of Oral & Maxillofacial Implants*, Vol.25, No.5, (September-October 2010), pp. 999-1006, ISSN 0882-2786

Fortin, T.; Bosson, J.L.; Coudert, J.L. & Isidori, M. (2003). Reliability of preperative planning of an image-guided system for oral implant placement based on 3-dimensional images: An in vivo study. *The International Journal of Oral Maxillofacial Implants*, Vol. 18, No.6, (November-December 2003), pp. 886-893, ISSN 0882-2786

Gatti, C.; Haefliger, W. & Chiapasco, M. (2000). Implant-retained mandibular overdentures with immediate loading: A prospective study of ITI implants. *The International Journal of Oral Maxillofacial Implants*, Vol.15, No.3, (May-June 2000), pp. 383-388, ISSN 0882-2786

Geng, J.; Tan, K.B.C. & Liu, G. (2001). Application of finite element analysis in implant dentistry: a review of the literature. *The Journal of Prosthetic Dentistry*, Vol.85, No.6 (June 2001), pp. 585–598, ISSN 0022-3913

Geng, J.P.; Ma, Q.S.; Xu, W.; Tan, K.B. & Liu, G.R. (2004). Finite element analysis of four thread form configurations in a stepped screw implant. *The Journal of Oral Rehabilitation*, Vol.31, No.3 (March 2004), pp. 233–239, ISSN 0305-182X

Goodacre, C.J.; Bernal, G.; Runcharassaeng, K. & Kan, J.Y.K. (2003). Clinical complications with implants and implant prostheses. *The Journal of Prosthetic Dentistry*, Vol. 90, No.2, (August 2003), pp. 121-132, ISSN 0022-3913.

Götz, H.E.; Müller, M.; Emmel, A.; Holzwarth, U.; Erben, R.G. & Stangl, R. (2004). Effect of surface finish on the osseointegration of laser-treated titanium alloy implants. *Biomaterials*, Vol.25, No.18, (August 2004), pp. 4057-4064, ISSN 0142-9612

Gross, M.D. (2008). Occlusion in implant dentistry. A review of the literature of prosthetic determinants and current concepts. *Australian Dental Journal,* Vol.53, No.1, (June 2008), pp. S60-S68, ISSN 1834-7819

Hebel, K.S. & Gajjar, R.C. (1997). Cement-retained versus screw-retained implant restorations: Achieving optimal occlusion and esthetics in implant dentistry. *The Journal of Prosthetic Dentistry,* Vol.77, No., (January 1997), pp. 28-35, ISSN 0022-3913

Heydenrijk, K.; Raghoebar, G.M.; Meijer, H.J.A.; van der Reijden, W.A.; van Winkelhoff, A.J. & Stegenga, B. (2002). Two-stage IMZ implants and ITI implants inserted in a single stage procedure. A prospective comparative study. *Clinical Oral Implants Research,* Vol.13, No.4, (August 2002), pp. 371–380, ISSN 1523-0899

Holmgren, E.P.; Seckinger, R.J.; Kilgren, L.M. & Mante, F. (1998). Evaluating parameters of osseointegrated dental implants using finite element analysis—a two-dimensional comparative study examining the effects of implant diameter, implant shape, and load direction. *Journal of Oral Implantology,* Vol. 24, No.2, pp. 80–88, ISSN 0160-6972

Hunt, P.R.; Gartner, J.L. & Norkin, F.J. (2005). Choice of a dental implant system. *Compendium of Continuing Education in Dentistry,* Vol.26, No.4, (April 2005), pp. 239-240, 242,245-248 passim, quiz 251, 271, ISSN 1548-8578

Jones, A.A. & Cochran, D.L. (2006). Consequences of implant design. *Dental Clinics of North America,* Vol.50, No.3, (July 2006), pp. 339-360, ISSN 0011-8532.

Jung, R.E.; Schneider, D.; Ganeles, J.; Wismeijer, D.; Zwahlen, M.; Hämmerle, C.H.F. &Tahmaseb, A. (2009). Computer technology applications in surgical implant dentistry: A systematic review. *The International Journal of Oral & Maxillofacial Implants,* Vol.24, (Suppl 2009), pp. 92-109, ISSN 0882-2786

Kasemo, B. & Lausma, J. (1998). Biomaterial and implant surfaces: a surface science approach. *The International Journal of Oral & Maxillofacial Implants,* Vol.3, No.4, (Winter 1988), pp. 247-259, ISSN 0882-2786

Kenney, R. & Richards, M.W. (1998). Photoelastic stress patterns produced by implant-retained overdentures. *The Journal of Prosthetic Dentistry,* Vol.80, No.5, (November 1998), pp. 559-564, ISSN 0022-3913

Kong, L.; Sun, Y.; Hu, K.; Liu, Y.; Li, D.; Qiu, Z. & Liu, B. (2008). Selections of the cylinder implant neck taper and implant end fillet for optimal biomechanical properties: a three-dimensional finite element analysis. *Journal of Biomechanical,* Vol.41, No. 5, (February 2008), pp. 1124-1130, ISSN 0021-9290

Kozlovsky, A.; Tal, H.; Laufer, B.Z.; Leshem, R.; Rohrer, M.D.; Weinreb, M. & Artzi, Z. (2007). Impact of implant overloading on the peri-implant bone in inflamed and non-inflamed peri-implant mucosa. *Clinical Oral Implants Research,* Vol. 18, No.5, (October 2007), pp. 601- 610, ISSN 0905-7161

Krennmair, G.; Schmidinger, S. & Waldenberger, O. (2002). Single-tooth replacement with the frialit-2 system: A retrospective clinical analysis of 146 implants. *The International Journal of Oral & Maxillofacial Implants,* Vol.17, No.1, (January-February 2002), pp. 78-85, ISSN 0882-2786

Ku, Y.; Chung, C.P. & Jang, J.H. (2005). The effect of the surface modification of titanium using a recombinant fragment of fibronectin and vitronectin on cell behaviour. *Biomaterials,* Vol.26, No.25, (September 2005), pp. 5153-5157, ISSN 0142-9612

Le Guéhennec, L.; Soueidan, A.; Layrolle, P. & Amouriq, Y. (2007). Surface treatments of titanium dental implants for rapid osseointegration. *Dental Materials*, Vol.23, No.7, (July 2007), pp. 844-854, ISSN 0109-5641

Lee, B.H.; Do Kim, Y.; Shin, J.H. & Hwan Lee, K. (2002). Surface modification by alkali and heat treatments in titanium alloys. *Journal of Biomedical Materials Research*, Vol.61, No.5, (September 2002), pp. 466-473, ISSN 1549-3296

Lee, B.H.; Lee, C.; Kim, D.G.; Kuiwon, C.; Lee, K.H. & Young, D.K. (2008). Effect of surface structure on biomechanical properties and osseointegration. *Materials Science and Engineering. C*, Vol.28, No.8, (December 2008), pp. 1448-1461, ISSN 0928-4931

Lee, C.C.; Lina, S.C.; Kanga, M.J.; Wua, S.W. & Fu, P.Y. (2010). Effects of implant threads on the contact area and stress distribution of marginal bone. *Journal of Dental Sciences*, Vol.5, No.3, (September 2010), pp. 156-165, ISSN 1343-4934

Levine, R.A.; Clem, D.S.; Wilson, T.G.; Higginbottom, F. & Solnit, G. (1999). Multicenter retrospective analysis of the ITI implant system used for single-tooth replacements: Results of loading for 2 or more years. *The International Journal of Oral and Maxillofacial Implants*, Vol.14, No.4, (July-August 1999), pp. 516-520, ISSN 0882-2786

Maeda, Y.; Satoh, T. & Sogo, M. (2006). In vitro differences of stress concentrations for internal and external hex implant-abutment connections: A short communication. *The Journal of Oral Rehabilitation*, Vol.33, No.1, (January 2006), pp. 75–78, ISSN 0305-182X

Mailath, G.; Stoiber, B.; Watzek, G. & Matejka, M. (1989). Bone resorption at the entry of osseointegrated implant - a biomechanical phenomenon. Finite element study. *Z Stomatol*, Vol.86, No.4, (June 1989), pp. 207–216, ISSN 0175-7784

Malo, P.; Araujo-Nobre, M. & Lopes, A. (2007). The use of computer-guided flapless implant surgery and four implants placed in immediate function to support a fixed denture: Preliminary results after a mean follow-up period of thirteen months. *The Journal of Prosthetic Dentistry*, Vol.97, No.6, (Suppl 2007), pp. 26-34, ISSN 0022-3913

Mandelaris, G.A.; Rosenfeld, A.L.; King, S.D. & Nevins, M.L. (2010). Computer-guided implant dentistry for precise implant placement: combining specialized stereolithographically generated drilling guides and surgical implant instrumentation. *The International Journal of Periodontics and Restorative Dentistry*, Vol.301, No.3, (June 2010), pp.275-281, ISSN 0198-7569

Mangano, C.; Mangano, F.; Piattelli, A.; Iezzi, G.; Mangano, A. & La Colla L. (2009). Prospective clinical evaluation of 1920 Morse taper connection implants: results after 4 years of functional loading. *Clinical Oral Implants Research*, Vol.20, No.3, (March 2009), pp. 254-261, ISSN 1523-0899

Mavrogenis, A.F.; Dimitriou, R.; Parvizi, J. & Babis, G.C. (2009). Biology of implant osseointegration. *Journal of Musculoskeletal and Neuronal Interactions*, Vol.9, No.2, (April-June 2009), pp. 61-71, ISSN 1108-7161

Meloni, S.M.; De Riu, G.; Pisano, M.; Cattina, G. & Tullio, A. (2010). Implant treatment software planning and guided flapless surgery with immediate provisional prosthesis delivery in the fully edentulous maxilla. A retrospective analysis of 15 consecutively treated patients. *European Journal of Oral Implantology*, Vol.3, No.3, (Autumn 2010), pp. 245-251, ISSN 1756-2406

Merz, B.R.; Hunenbart, S. & Belser, U.C. (2000). Mechanics of the implant abutment connection: an 8-degree taper compared to a butt joint connection. *International*

Journal of Oral and Maxillofacial Implants, Vol.15, No.4, (July-August 2000), pp. 519-526, ISSN 0882-2786

Misch, C.E. & Bidez, M.W. (1995). Implant-protected occlusion. *Practical Periodontics and Aesthetic Dentistry*, Vol.7, No.5, (June-July 1995), pp. 25-29, ISSN 1042-2722

Misch, C.E.; Qu, Z. & Bidez, M.W. (1999). Mechanical properties of trabecular bone in the human mandible: Implications for dental implant treatment planning and surgical placement. *Journal of Oral Maxillofacial Surgery*, Vol.57, No.6, (June 1999), pp. 700-706, ISSN 0278-2391

Misch, C.E. & Wang, H.L. (2003). Immediate occlusal loading for fixed prostheses in implant dentistry. *Dentistry Today*, Vol. 22, No.8, (August 2003), pp. 50-56, ISSN 8750-2186

Misch, C.E.; Wang, H.L.; Misch, C.M.; Sharawy, M.; Lemons, J.; Judy, K.W. (2004a). Rationale for the application of immediate load in implant dentistry: Part I. *Implant Dentistry*, Vol.13, No.3, (September 2004), pp. 207-217, ISSN 1056-6163

Misch, C.E.; Wang, H.L.; Misch, C.M.; Sharawy, M.; Lemons, J. & Judy, K.W. (2004b). Rationale for the application of immediate load in implant dentistry: part II. *Implant Dentistry*, Vol.13, No.4, (December 2004), pp. 310-321, ISSN 1056-6163

Misch, C.E.; Steignga, J.; Barboza, E.; Misch-Dietsh, F.; Cianciola, L.J. & Kazor, C. (2006). Short dental implants in posterior partial edentulism: a multicenter retrospective 6-year case series study. *Journal of Periodontology*, Vol.77, No.8, (August 2006), pp. 1340-1347, ISSN 0022-3492

Misch, C.E. (2008). Contemporary Implant Dentistry (3rd ed), Mosby, ISBN 0323043739, St Louis, USA

Morris, H.F.; Winkler, S.; Ochi, S. & Kanaan, A. (2001). A new implant designed to maximize contact with trabecular bone: survival to 18 months. *Journal of Oral Implantology*, Vol.27, No.4, pp. 164-173, ISSN 0160-6972

Morton, D.; Jaffin, R. & Weber, H.P. (2004). Immediate restoration and loading of dental implants: Clinical considerations and protocols. *The International Journal of Oral Maxillofacial Implants*, Vol.19, (Suppl 2004), pp. 103-108, ISSN 0882-2786

Nkenke, E.; Lehner, B.; Fenner, M.; Roman, F.S.; Thams, U.; Neukam, F.W. & Radespiel-Tröger M. (2005). Immediate versus delayed loading of dental implants in the maxillae of minipigs: follow-up of implant stability and implant failures. *The International Journal of Oral & Maxillofacial Implants*, Vol.20, No.1, (January-February 2005), pp. 39-47, ISSN 0882-2786

Nokar, S. & Baghai Naini, R. (2010). The effect of superstructure design on stress distribution in peri-implant bone during mandibular flexure. *The International Journal of Oral & Maxillofacial Implants*, Vol.25, No.1, (January-February 2010), pp. 31-37, ISSN 0882-2786

Patel, N. (2010). Integrating three-dimensional digital technologies for comprehensive implant dentistry. *The Journal of the American Dental Association*, Vol.141, (Suppl 2), pp. 20S-24S, ISSN 0002-8177

Pellizzer, E.; Tonella, B.; Ferraco, R.; Falcon-Antenucci, R.M.; de Carvalho, P.S. & Goiato, M. (2010). Photoelastic analysis of cemented or screwed implant-supported prostheses with different prosthetic connections. *The Journal of Oral Implantology*,. Vol.16 (August 2010), pp. 1-19, ISSN 0160-6972

Pessoa, R.S.; Muraru, L.; Junior, E.M.; Vaz, L.G.; Sloten, J.V.; Duyck, J. & Jaecques, S.V. (2010). Influence of implant connection type on the biomechanical environment of immediately placed implants - ct-based nonlinear, three-dimensional finite element analysis. *Clinical Implant Dentistry and Related Research,* Vol.12, No.3, (September 2010), pp. 219-234, ISSN 1708-8208

Piattelli, A.; Ruggeri, A.; Franchi, M.; Romasco, N. & Trisi, P.A. (1993). An histologic and histomorphometric study of bone reactions to unloaded and loaded non-submerged single implants in monkeys: a pilot study. *Journal of Oral Implantology,* Vol.19, No.4, pp. 314-320, ISSN 0160-6972

Pieri, F., Aldini, N.N., Marchetti, C. & Corinaldesi, G. (2011). Influence of implant-abutment interface design on bone and soft tissue levels around immediately placed and restored single-tooth implants: A randomized controlled clinical trial. *The International Journal of Oral & Maxillofacial Implants,* Vol.26, No.1, (January-February 2011), pp. 169-178, ISSN 0882-2786.

Pilliar, R.M.; Lee, J.M. & Maniatopoulos, C. (1986) Observation of the effect of movement on the bone ingrowth into porous surfaced implants. *Clinical Orthopaedics and Related Research,* Vol.208 (July 1986), pp. 108–113, ISSN 0009-921X

Prosper, L.; Redaelli, S.; Pasi, M.; Zarone, F.; Radaelli, G. & Gherlone, E.F. (2009). A randomized prospective multicenter trial evaluating the platform- switching technique for the prevention of postrestorative crestal bone loss. *The International Journal of Oral & Maxillofacial Implants,* Vol.24, No.2, 9 (March-April 2009), pp. 299-308, ISSN 0882-2786

Puig, C.P. (2010). A retrospective study of edentulous patients rehabilitated according to the "all-on-four" or the "all-on-six" immediate function concept using flapless computer-guided implant surgery. *European Journal of Oral Implantology,* Vol.3, No.2, (Summer 2010), pp. 155-163, ISSN 1756-2406

Puleo, D.A. (2006). Thomas MV. Implant surfaces. *Dental Clinics of North America,* Vol.50, No.3, (July 2006), pp. 323-338, ISSN 0011-8532

Qu, J.; Chehroudi, B.; Brunette, D.M. (1996). The use of micromachined surfaces to investigate the cell behavioral factors essential to osseointegration. *Oral Disease,* Vol.2, No.1, (March 1996), pp. 102–115, ISSN 1354-523X

Rieger, M.R.; Adams, W.K. & Kinzel, G.L. (1990). A finite element survey of eleven endosseous implants. *The Journal of Prosthetic Dentistry,* Vol.63, No.4, (April 1990), pp. 457-465. ISSN 0022-3913

Romeo, E.; Lops, D.; Margutti, E.; Ghisolfi, M.; Chiapasco, M. & Vogel, G. (2004). Long-term survival and success of oral implants in the treatment of full and partial arches: a 7-year prospective study with the ITI dental implant system. *The International Journal of Oral & Maxillofacial Implants,* Vol.19, No.2, (March-April 2004), pp. 247-259, ISSN 0882-2786

Sabet, M.E.; El-Korashy, D.I. & El-Mahrouky, N.A. (2009). Effect of platform switching on strain developed around implants supporting mandibular overdenture. *Implant Dentistry,* Vol.18, No.4, (August 2009), pp. 362-370, ISSN 1538-2982

Schenk, R. K. & Buser, D. (1998). Osseointegration: a reality. *Periodontology 2000,* Vol.17, No.1, (June 1998), pp. 22-35, ISSN 0906-6713

Schneider, D.; Marquardt, P.; Zwahlen, M. & Jung, R.E. (2009). A systematic review on the accuracy and the clinical outcome of computer-guided template-based implant dentistry. *Clinical Oral Implants Research,* Vol.20, (Suppl 4 2009), pp. 73-86, ISSN 0905-7161

Schnitman, P.A.; Wöhrle, P.S.; Rubenstein, J.E.; DaSilva, J.D. & Wang, N.H. (1997). Ten-years results for Brånemark implants immediately loaded with fixed prostheses at implant placement. *The International Journal of Oral & Maxillofacial Implants*, Vol.12, No.4, (July-August 1997), pp. 495-503, ISSN 0882-2786

Schulte, J.K. (1994) External hex manufacturing tolerances of six implant systems: A pilot study. *Implant Dentistry*, Vol.3, No.1, (Spring 1994), pp. 51-53, ISSN 1056-6163

Serrano-Sánchez, P.; Manzanera-Pastor, E.; Lorrio-Castro, C.; Bretones-López, P.; Garcia-Serrano, A. & Calvo-Guirado, J.L. (2011). Influence of platform switching in dental implants. A literature review. *Medicina Oral Patologia Oral y cirurgia Bucal* , Jan 3. [Epub ahead of print]. ISSN 1698-6946

Siegele, D. & Soltesz, U. (1989). Numerical investigations of the influence of implant shape on stress distribution in the jaw bone. *The International Journal of Oral & Maxillofacial Implants*, Vol.4, No.4 (Winter 1989), pp. 333-340, ISSN 0882-2786

Stanford C.M. (2008). Surface modifications of dental implants. *Australian Dental Journal*, Vol.53, (Suppl S1 June 2008), pp. S26-S33, ISSN 0045-0421

Steigenga J.T.; al-Shammari, K.F.; Nociti, F.H.; Misch, C.E. & Wang, H.L. (2003). Dental implant design and its relationship to long-term implant success. *Implant Dentistry*, Vol.12, No.4, pp. 306-317, ISSN 1056-6163

Strong, J.T.; Misch, C.E.; Bidez, M.W. & Nalluri, P. (1998). Functional surface area: thread-form parameter optimization for implant body design. *Compendium of Continuing Education in Dentistry*, Vol.19, No.3, (supplement 2 1998), pp. 4-9, ISSN 1548-8578

Sul, Y.T.; Johansson, C.B.; Roser, K. & Albrektsson, T. (2002). Qualitative and quantitative observations of bone tissue reactions to anodized implants. *Biomaterials*, Vol.23, No.8, (April 2002), pp. 1809-1817, ISSN 0142-9612

Suzuki, K.; Aoki, K. & Ohya, K. (1997). Effects of surface roughness of titanium implants on bone remodeling activity of femur in rabbits. *Bone*, Vol.21, No.6, (December 1997), pp. 507-514, ISSN 8756-3282

Sykaras, N.; Iacopino, A.M.; Marker, V.A., Triplett, R.G. & Woody, R.D. (2000). Implant materials, designs, and surface topographies: their effect on osseointegration. A literature review. *The International Journal of Oral & Maxillofacial Implants*, Vol.15, No.5, (September-October 2000), pp. 675-690. ISSN 0882-2786

Szmukler-Moncler, S.; Salama, H.; Reingewirtz, Y. & Dubruille, J.H. (1998). Timing of loading and effect of micromotion on bone-dental implant interface: review of experimental literature. *Journal of Biomedical Materials Research*, Vol.43, No.2, (Summer 1998), pp. 192–203, ISSN 1549-3296

Tesmer, M.; Wallet, S.; Koutouzis, T. & Lundgren, T. (2009). Bacterial colonization of the dental implant fixture-abutment interface: an in vitro study. *Journal of Periodontology*, Vol.80, No.12, (December 2009), pp. 1991-1997, ISSN 1566-0702

Testori, T.; Wiseman, L.; Woolfe, S. & Porter, S. (2001). A prospective multicenter clinical study of the Osseotite implant: four-year interim report. *The International Journal of Oral & Maxillofacial Implants*, Vol.16, No.2, (March-April 2001), pp. 193–200. ISSN 0882-2786

Thakur, A.J. (1997). *The Elements of Fracture Fixation* (1st ed), Churchill Livingstone, ISBN 0443055475, New York, USA

Toyoshima, T.; Wagner, W.; Klein, M.O.; Stender, E.; Wieland, M. & Al-Nawas, B. (2011). Primary stability of a hybrid self-tapping implant compared to a cylindrical nonself-tapping implant with respect to drilling protocols in an ex vivo model. *Clinical Implant Dentistry and Related Research*, Vol.13, No.1, (March 2011), pp. 71-78, ISSN 0905-7161

Triplett, R.G.; Frohberg, U.; Sykaras, N. & Woody, R.D. (2003). Implant materials, design, and surface topographies: their influence on osseointegration of dental implants. *Journal of Long-Term Effects of Medical Implants*, Vol.13, No.6, pp. 485-501, ISSN 1050-6934

Turkyilmaz, I.; Suarez, J.C.; Company, A.M. & McGlumphy EA. (2009). Early load mandibular hybrid prosthesis using the OSU acrylic frame requiring no final impression. *Australian Dental Journal*, Vol.54, No.3, (September 2009), pp. 255-261, ISSN 1834-7819.

Upp, F.; Scheideler, L.; Olshanska, N.; de Wld, M.; Wieland, M. & GeisGesttorfer, J. (2006). Enhancing surface free energy and hydrophilicity through modification of microstructured titanium implant surface. *Journal of Biomedical Materials Research*, Vol.76, No.2, (February 2006), pp. 323-324, ISSN 1552-4965

van Steenberghe, D.; Naert, I.; Jacobs, R. & Quirynen, M. (1999). Influence of inflammatory reactions vs. occlusal loading on peri-implant marginal bone level. *Advances in Dental Research,* Vol.13, (June 1999), pp. 130-135, ISSN 0895-9374

Vasak, C.; Watzak, G.; Gahleitner, A.; Strbac, G.; Schemper, M. & Zechner, W. (2011). Computed tomography-based evaluation of template (NobelGuide)-guided implant positions: a prospective radiological study. *Clinical Oral Implants Research,* doi: 10.1111/j.1600-0501.2010.02070, ISSN 0905-7161

Vidyasagar, L. & Apse, P. (2004). Dental implant design and biological effects on bone-implant interface. *Baltic Dental and Maxillofacial Journal*, Vol.6, No.2, (June 2004), pp. 51-54, ISSN 1392-8589

Weng, D.; Jacobson, Z.; Tarnow, D.; Hürzeler, M.B.; Faehn, O.; Sanavi, F.; Barkvoll, P. & Stach, R.M. (2003). A prospective multicenter clinical trial of 3i machined-surface implants: Results after 6 years of follow-up. *The International Journal of Oral & Maxillofacial Implants*, Vol.18, No.3, (May-June 2003), pp. 417-423, ISSN 0882-2786

Wennerberg, A.; Albrektsson, T. & Andersson, B. (1995). An animal study of cp titanium screws with different surface topographies. *Journal of Materials Science: Materials in Medicine,* Vol.6, No.5, pp. 302–309, ISSN 0957-4530

Wiskott, H.W. & Belser, U.C. (1999). Lack of integration of smooth titaniumsurfaces: A working hypothesis based on strains generated in the surrounding bone [review]. *Clinical Oral Implants Research*, Vol.1, No.6, (December 1999), pp. 429–444. ISSN 0905-7161

Yamada, K.; Hoshina, H.; Arashiyama, T.; Arasawa, M.; Arai, Y.; Uoshima, K.; Tanaka, M. & Nomura, S. (2011). Immediate implant loading following computer-guided surgery. *Journal of Prosthodontic Research,* doi:10.1016/j.por.2010.11.002, ISSN 1883-1958

Zarone, F.; Apicella, A.; Nicolais, L.; Aversa, R. & Sorrentino, R. (2003). Mandibular flexure and stress build-up in mandibular full-arch fixed prostheses supported by osseointegrated implants. *Clinical Oral Implants Research*, Vol.14, No.1, (February 2003), pp. 103-114, ISSN 0905-7161

Zhao, G.; Schwartz, Z.; Wieland, M.; Rupp, F.; Geis-Gerstorfer, J.; Cochran, D.L. & Boyan, B.D. (2005). High surface energy enhances cell response to titanium substrate microstructure. *Journal of Biomedical Materials Research Part A,* Vo.74, No.1, (July 2005), pp. 49-58. ISSN 1552-4965

Zubery, Y.; Bichacho, N.; Moses, O. & Tal, H. (1999). Immediate loading of modular transitional implants: a histologic and histomorphometric study in dogs. *International Journal of Periodontics & Restorative Dentistry,* Vol.19, No.4, (August 1999), pp. 343-353, ISSN 0198-7569

6

Load Transfer Along the Bone-Implant Interface and its Effects on Bone Maintenance

Samira Faegh, Hsuan-Yu Chou and Sinan Müftü
Northeastern University, Department of Mechanical Engineering
Boston, Massachusetts
USA

1. Introduction

The long term success of dental implant treatment relies on the proper stability of the implant within the host bone. This condition is achieved through osseointegration, which is characterized as a direct functional and structural connection between ingrown bone tissue and implant surface (Brånemark et al., 1977; Simmons et al., 2001). Osseointegration begins with rapid growth of random and unorganized woven bone around the implant, while a biomechanically favorable environment at the bone-implant interface develops (Leucht et al., 2007; Schenk & Buser, 1998). This initial bony structure is maintained by bone remodeling and bone adaptation, where woven bone is slowly replaced by more organized lamellar bone. Adaptation of bone morphology in response to functional loads continues throughout life (Schenk & Buser, 1998).

The load transfer from the implant to the host bone depends on the amount of bone surrounding the implant and in turn affects the success of treatment, by the load transfer from the implant to the host bone. X-ray imaging, computerized tomography (CT), and histomorphometric evaluation of the extracted implants provide insightful information about the quality and quantity of peri-implant bone. However, systematic evaluation of the mechanism of load transfer and its effect on peri-implant bone remodeling is difficult via aforementioned techniques, due to the cost and effort involved and due to the associated ethical concerns. Reliable computational models can be useful to predict the long term outcome of a dental implant treatment, and thus help with the decisions related to implant treatments and design. In this paper, a state of the art review of the computational models used in evaluating the biomechanics of dental implant systems is provided. The literature shows that load transfer along the bone-implant interface is not well understood, despite the fact that the bone loading starts along this interface.

Recently a systematic investigation of the effects of various parameters related to a dental implant's contour including the implant's diameter, body-length, collar length and slope, and the morphology of the external threads was carried out by Faegh and Müftü (2010). The variation of normal and shear stresses along the bone dental-implant interface was investigated. Here, in order to generalize the bone morphology an elliptical contour is used. The results are compared to a similar recent study in which the bone contour was drawn from a CT image of the incisor region (Faegh & Müftü, 2010).

1.1 Factors that influence the load transfer from implant systems to bone

Load transfer from the implant to the bone has been identified as one of the critical factors that determine the long term success of dental implant treatment (Duyck et al., 1997; Morris et al. 2001). Load transfer is influenced by several factors including: (i) the loading type, (ii) the length and diameter of implant, (iii) the implant shape, (iv) the structure of the implant surface, and (v) the bone quality (Duyck et al., 1997). A simple, analytical solution of the stress/strain distribution in the bone for an implant treatment scenario is not feasible, due to the complex geometry of the bone and the dental implant system. Photoelesticity (Farah et al., 1979; Kinni et al., 1987; Munir et al., 1975) and finite element analyses have been increasingly used in this field (Cook et al., 1980, 1982a, 1982b; Geng et al., 2001;) to analyze the stress distribution for different root form implant designs (Bozkaya et al., 2004; Hansson, 1999; Holmgren et al, 1998; Rieger, 1988; Rieger et al., 1989a, 1989b, 1990a, 1990b; Siegele & Soletz, 1989) prosthesis designs (Papavasiliou, et al. 1996a, 1996b; Stegaroiu et al. 1998a, 1998b) and for various clinical scenarios (Akça & İplikçioğlu, 2001; Canay et al., 1996; Gross & Laufer, 1997; İplikçioğlu & Akça, 2002; Meijer et al., 1994; Pierrisnard et al., 2002; Tuncelli et al., 1997; van Oosterwyck et al, 2002).

Over the years, numerous implant designs and clinical protocols emerged, sometimes dictated by market demands (Brunski, 1999). Currently, there are more than 50 implant designs available in the market. Research and development in the dental implant field led to significant progress in areas and applications that were previously limited. For example, implants can be successfully inserted in areas of reduced bone height and high functional load, such as the posterior segments of mandible and the maxilla. Moreover, advances in our understanding of the mechanobiology led to design of implant systems that can function immediately after insertion (Balshi & Wolfinger, 1997a; Brånemark et al., 1999; Brunski, 1999; Chow et al., 2001; Ericsson et al., 2000; Jaffin et al., 2000; Salama et al., 1995; Tarnow et al., 1997).

1.1.1 Bone-implant connection

One of the main drivers for different implant designs is to improve bone-to-implant connection. Osseointegeration, first described by Brånemark et al. (1977, 1985), defines the direct connection of bone and implant. Osseointegration involves chemical bonding of the tissue to the implant, as well as micro- and macro-level mechanical interlocking of the bone with the features on the implant surface. Chemical and morphological modifications of the outside surface of the implant material have been shown to enhance connection strength and reduce the healing time. To this end, bioactive ceramics such as hydroxyapatite have been used as coatings on the implant surface. Such coatings have been shown to improve bone-implant fixation through chemical bonding between the implant and the surrounding tissues. Surface morphology of implants can be modified in macro-level through the designs of external threads, undercuts and layers of wires, and in micro-level by increasing surface roughness.

Shape and chemistry of the bone-implant interface influence the stress distribution in the bone for different implant designs (Bidez et al., 1988; Hipp et al., 1985). Siegele and Soltesz (1989) modeled different bone-to-implant connection types by using frictional contact. Their work showed that high levels of bone stresses occur in the apex region of the implant if perfect osseointegration is assumed, whereas the high stress region occurs in the alveolar crest for frictional sliding contact condition. Similar results for the perfectly bonded interface have been reported by Weinstein et al. (1976).

Strength of bone fixation depends in part on the mechanical properties of the bone surrounding the implant. One common metric of bone quality is the bone density levels (Lekholm and Zarb, 1985). Whether the implant is surrounded by cortical bone or trabecular bone makes a significant difference in interfacial stresses (Borchers & Reichart, 1983; Lavernia et al., 1982). Lavernia et al. (1981) reported significant change in stress magnitude when bone properties are switched between trabecular and cortical. Kitoh et al. (1978) and Bozkaya et al. (2004) showed that the occlusal force applied to the implant is supported primarily by the cortical bone.

1.1.2 Implant-contour

The long term outcome of the implant treatment is influenced by the loading experienced by the bone, in several different respects. In general, excessive micro-motion of the bone-implant interface should be avoided, while providing adequate stimulation to promote healing and remodeling response (Brunski, 1999). The shape of the implant contour, and its local features have a considerable influence on bone healing and maintenance. Siegele and Soltesz (1989) compared the load transfer characteristics of five different implant shapes. Considered contours were cylindrical, conical, stepped, internally hollow cylindrical and externally threaded. They showed that under vertical load, lower stresses are induced in the bone with smoother implant shapes such as cylindrical, rather than implants with small radii of curvature such as the conical shape and implants with geometric discontinuities such as stepped implant contours. Under lateral loading, large stresses were observed in the apex area of the hollow cylindrical implant, and below the uppermost thread of the externally threaded implants. Holmgren et al. (1998) reported that the stepped implant design levels out the stress distribution better than a cylindrical design. Rieger et al. (1989a, 1990a, 1990b) investigated the effect of implant geometry and the elastic modulus of the implant materials on the stress distribution for different implant designs. A tapered design made of a material with high elastic modulus was concluded to be the most suitable design in their study. Weinstein et al. (1976) investigated a porous rooted dental implant and concluded that high bone-level stresses are induced near the apex of the implant in a model with continuously bonded interface. In their comparative evaluation of five commercially available implant systems, Bozkaya et al. (2004) showed that implant systems with internally sloping crestal modules are better at reducing the bone overload in the cortical bone, whereas systems with widening crestal-modules cause bone overload in compression. Kong et al. (2008) suggested that neck taper (collar slope) ranging from 64° to 70°and end (apex) fillet exceeding 0.8 mm result in the optimal stability of implant.

Siegele and Soltesz (1989) reported a high failure rate in the hollow cylindrical implants due to low primary stability. Moreover, the conical or shoulder-type implants distributed high stress level at the bone interface. Rounding off the corners of the implant was found to have a significant effect on reducing the stress (Siegele & Soltesz, 1989). Faegh and Müftü (2010) showed that cylindrical implants with no external threads induce low stresses along the bone-implant interface in the trabecular region, and indicated that this might lead to inadequate bone stimulation. Cylindrical implants are no longer recommended due to problems with osseointegration and high failure rates (Schenk & Buser, 1998).

Vaillancourt et al. (1995) investigated the possible causes of bone loss in the crestal bone surrounding both porous-coated implant and non-porous-coated regions of a partially coated implant designs. They reported that lower stress level was transferred to the crestal bone region in the case of partially-porous implant, where crestal bone loss was mostly observed. They attributed this to disuse atrophy. A sufficient stress level of 1.6 MPa was reported to avoid bone loss resulting from disuse atrophy by histological studies.

1.1.2.1 Externally threaded implants

There are several advantages associated with externally threaded implants. Threads improve primary implant stability during the implant insertion (Misch, 1999b) and thus reduce micro-motion during the post insertion healing period until the stable osseointegration is established. This characteristic is of more importance in the regions of low bone density and in the submerged implant placement modality (Frandsen et al, 1984). In addition, applied (mastication) forces are diverted in normal and tangential directions to the faces of the thread and amplified in certain thread locations. This is beneficial in providing adequate loading for long term bone maintenance (Faegh & Müftü, 2010). Finally, bone growth between the threads provides the macro-level interlocking. There are different types of externally threaded implants available in the market, which vary in thread pitch, shape and depth. Since the morphology of screw threads plays an important role in the load transfer from dental implant to the surrounding bone (Frandsen et al, 1984), usage of different thread configurations for different bone qualities have been suggested (Misch, 1999a, 1999b; Misch et al., 1998, 1999, 2001).

In a finite element study carried out by Moser and Nentwig (1989), it was observed that using screw threads with an apically increasing screw thread depth reduces tension in the cervical area when implant was apically loaded. Similarly, Huang et al. (2010) suggested that external threads reduce the stress and sliding at the interface. Chun et al. (2002) reported that maximum effective stress in the cortical bone is higher in the plateau design as compared to the triangular or square thread designs. In another study carried out by Patra et al. (1998), tapered thread design implants were found to distribute higher stress levels in bone as compared to the parallel profile thread. Use of external threads on the implant body with some micro-scale roughness was reported to enhance osseointegration (Skalak, 1988). It was observed that inclined faces of threads allow for normal stress to be carried perpendicular to the interface. Transmission of shear stress can benefit from microasperities on the interface which work along each of the faces of a screw in a similar way that the screw threads work (Skalak, 1988). Faegh & Müftü (2010) carried out a systematic analysis of various implant designs with and without external threads. They showed that threads increase the interfacial stresses locally and could help in stimulating bone remodeling.

1.1.2.2 Implant diameter

Wider diameter implants provide increased implant-bone contact area, enable the engagement of the implant to the buccal and lingual (BL) faces of the bone, and have the ability to occupy the tooth socket especially in the posterior regions. These inherent characteristics of wide diameter implants significantly improve initial implant stability, which leads to the increase in likelihood of osseointegration (Langer et al., 1993; Renouard et al., 1999; Trauhlar et al., 1997). Wide diameter implants also provide higher mechanical strength to avoid implant fractures (Jarvis, 1996). Wide and short implants provide the advantage of avoiding sinus elevations and extensive bone augmentation procedures in regions of limited bone height due to the existence of alveolar nerve in the mandible and maxillary sinus in the maxilla, and potentially prevent the costs associated with bone grafting procedures (Blatz et al., 1998; Graves et al., 1994; Jarvis, 1996; Langer et al., 1993). Overall advantages of wide diameter implants include improved prosthetic stability, reduced screw loosening, reduced incidents of implant fracture, and more optimal force distribution in qualitatively and quantitatively poor bone (Mahon et al., 2000).

Griffin et al. (2004) conducted a clinical study investigating the application of 6×8 mm hydroxyapatite coated screw retained implants in the mandibular and maxillary molar regions and reported a 100% success rate. They observed that significant stress concentration distributed to the crestal cortical bone, at the level of the first few threads and concluded that the use of long implants to provide a larger surface area for stress distribution is not necessary. Instead larger surface area provided by wide diameter implants was deemed to be better. On the other hand in a retrospective study conducted by Aparicio & Orozco (1998) the success rates of 5 mm- and 3.75 mm-diameter implants were reported to be similar in the maxilla, while higher success rate was observed for 3.75 implants in the mandible. They attributed the high failure rate in the mandible to the overheating during surgical bone drilling, excessive tightening force during implant placement, and variations of the remodeling response of the cortical bone caused by extensive drilling.

Geramy & Morgano (2004) conducted a finite element analysis comparing displacement of a standard diameter and a wide diameter implant under an occlusal load applied at the distobuccal cusp tip, and concluded that increasing the diameter of the implant will reduce both mesiodistal and buccolingual displacement of the implant system by approximately 50%.

Davarpanah et al. (2001) evaluated the resistance to fracture and depth of insertion of wide diameter implants versus standard diameter implants. They found that wider diameter implants demonstrate more resistance to fracture than standard implants, which is attributed to increased surface area. Jarvis (1997) compared the 3.7 mm and 4.7 mm diameter implants and concluded that wider diameter implants decrease the induced load on the abutment screw which results in reducing implant fracture, and also the vibration of the implant that leads to loosening. Mahon et al. (2000) evaluated the stress distribution using implants with diameters 3.25, 3.75, 4, 5, and 6 mm under a load of 176 N applied 5 mm off axis. They observed that the mean stress level was highest for the 3.25 mm-diameter implant, and lowest for the 6 mm-diameter implant. High stress levels were located at the necks of the 3.25 mm implant which was consistent with the high deformation which occurred in these regions. They observed that stress level for 3.75, 4, and 5 mm diameter implants did not demonstrate large differences, however, 6 mm diameter implants showed the most reduction in the stress level. Due to this observation, they concluded that the implant diameter must be greater than a certain value in order to reduce the stress significantly. Li et al. (2011) suggested that implant with diameter greater than 4.0 mm and length longer than 12.0 mm is the optimal selection to treat tooth loss at the at locations with poor bone quality (ie. posterior mandible). Huang and Tsai (2003) reported that increasing the implant diameter and consequently the bone-implant contact area reduces stress concentration and results in improving implant stability. Chou et al. (2010) showed that the insertion depth and implant diameter affect the biomechanical response of bone, particularly between the plateaus of an implant. They indicated that the strain distribution can be optimized for long-term bone maintenance by adjusting the insertion depth for different levels of bone quality in the alveolar ridge.

1.1.2.3 Multiple implants

Using two narrow implants to support prosthesis in posterior regions has been an alternative solution to the wide diameter implant (Langer et al., 1993; Lazzara, 1994; Moscovitch, 2001). Balshi & Wolfinger, (1997b) stated that two implants maintain a more natural replacement of the missing tooth in position and direction, and allow for the preservation of the crestal bone. Mahon et al. (2000) and Trauhlar et al., (1997) stated that use of two implants also provides a more appropriate support against buccolingual and mesiodistal bending, decreases the rotating forces around the implant axis, offers greater surface area and better biomechanical properties, and maintains prosthesis retrievability. However, there are some restrictions on using two narrow implants in the posterior regions. One of these is the cone space availability buccolingually and mesiodistally (Graves et al., 1994).

Geramy et al. (2004) compared the use of a wide diameter implant with the use of two implants and reported that use of two implants to support the restoration reduces the buccolingual displacement to the same level as the 5 mm-diameter implant. Stress distribution for both wide diameter implants and two implant design systems were compared by Balshi and Wolfinger (1997b), who concluded that the percentage of stress reduction was almost identical for both designs. In a study conducted by Bahat and Handelsman (1996), the failure rate of the 5 mm-diameter implants was 2.3% compared to the 1.6% failure rate of the double implants. They suggested using double implants to support restorations rather than a single implant in the molar regions, even though there were some disadvantages associated with using double implants, such as greater bone loss and higher prosthesis mobility. On the other hand, Sato et al. (2000) concluded that using double implants in molar areas does not always reduce loads on the implants however eliminates torque. They observed higher stress levels near the marginal ridge of the superstructure compared to stress field on the wide diameter implants.

1.2 Bone remodeling (cell interactions)

Unlike the bone growth or bone modeling which mostly occurs in the early age of skeletal development, bone remodeling is a process of continuous cellular activities to replace aged, injured and dead bone. Bone remodeling is a process that is composed of two consecutive, and interrelated physiological activities, namely bone resorption and bone formation. Remodeling is carried out by basic multicellular/bone metabolic units (BMUs). Normally, osteoclasts, which are responsible for resorption, are inhibited by osteoprotegerin (OPG), which is a protein secreted by osteoblasts as inhibitory signal (Carda et al., 2005). The osteoclastic resorption is signaled by the circulating parathyroid hormone and locally secreted receptor activator nuclear kappa-b ligand (RANKL), which binds to RANK receptors on the membrane of osteoclasts (Marx, 2007). In addition to OPG, osteoblasts also secrete RANKL so that the activation of osteoclasts and the amount of resorption are regulated.

When remodeling is activated, osteoclasts are first recruited to bone surface and start to excavate the bone by releasing hydrochloric acid to dissolve the inorganic matrix, and collagenases to break down the organic matrix (Marx, 2007). A tunnel with approximately 200 μm in diameter and 300 μm long is dug at the rate of 40 μm/day (Martin et al., 1998). Following the resorption, there is reversal phase before the initiation of formation. A cylindrical space in the tunnel can be observed and the length of this region varies with the lag between the resorption and formation.

During bone resorption, some bone morphogenic proteins and insulin-like growth factors are released as active cytokines (growth and differentiation factors), which induce the differentiation of stem cells into osteoblasts (Marx, 2007). Bone formation is conducted by the osteoblasts, which refill the space with unmineralized bone matrix, osteoid, at a rate of about 1-2 μm/day (Martin et al., 1998). As the osteoblastic activity continues, a tunnel with 40-50 μm in diameter called Haversian canal is left for the transportation of the nutrients to bone cells. Finally, the bone matrix deposited by osteoblasts is mineralized and turns into Haversian system, osteon. Osteoclastic activity restores to quiescent condition under the influence of osteoblasts, and bone is maintained until the aging or diseased bone triggers the secretion of RANKL by osteoblasts (Marx, 2007).

1.2.1 Theoretical models of bone remodeling

Wolff (1892, 1986) observed that internal structure and density of bone depends on the load that it carries. It is generally well established that this functional adaptation is the result of the BMU activity as described above, which is triggered by some mechanical stimulus that BMUs can sense. Several theoretical models were formulated in order to quantitatively describe the functional adaptation of the bone (Hart, 2001). These models assume that a mechanical control signal (remodeling stimulus) governs the bone density regulation, and the BMU has the capability to respond to the changes in this signal. A biomechanical equilibrium or homeostatic state is assumed, so that bone remodeling is only triggered when the control signal deviates from this equilibrium state. Remodeling activity continues until the biomechanical equilibrium is restored and new bone morphology is established. This approach neglects the effects of hormonal, genetic and metabolic factors on bone regulation.

1.2.1.1 Mechanostat hypothesis

Frost proposed the mechanostat, which is a non-linear switch, to explain his experimental observations of bone remodeling (Frost, 1987, 2003). He used strain as the mechanical control signal, and divided the remodeling response to four different regimes. Each regime, which he called "window," is separated by threshold strains levels. These minimum strain levels were called minimum effective strain (MES). The disuse window (DW) is the lowest strain regime. If the bone is exposed to strain levels in DW for a prolonged duration, Frost's hypothesis states that decrease in bone mass will occur. Adapted window (AW) is where bone strength is naturally accepted to sustain the strain level caused by normal daily activities. Increased strain level to the mild overload window (MOW) promotes increase of bone mass. However, further increase of strain will lead to the pathologic overload window (POW) and generate internal micro damage that cannot be repaired by normal cell activities. The following relation gives a compact representation of the mechanostat hypothesis in terms of the MES:

$$\text{Bone tissue response} = \begin{cases} \text{DW: reduced bone mass;} & \text{strain} < \text{MESr} \\ \text{AW: constant bone mass;} & \text{MESr} < \text{strain} < \text{MESm} \\ \text{MOW: increased bone mass;} & \text{MESm} < \text{strain} < \text{MESp} \\ \text{POW: bone damage;} & \text{MESp} < \text{strain} \end{cases} \quad (1)$$

where MESr is the threshold of disuse remodeling; MESm is the modeling threshold; and MESp is the pathologic threshold. Note that what type of strain measure to be used in this theory was not precisely stated.

1.2.1.2 Bone remodeling base on strain energy density

Huiskes et al. (1987) suggested strain energy density U as the remodeling stimulus, and they proposed that the change of bone's elastic modulus (E) can be described as,

$$\frac{dE}{dt} = \begin{cases} C_e\left(U-(1+s)U_n\right); & U > (1+s)U_n \\ 0; & (1-s)U_n \le U \le (1+s)U_n \\ C_e\left(U-(1-s)U_n\right); & U < (1-s)U_n \end{cases} \quad (2)$$

where C_e is a remodeling constant, U is the strain energy density of bone due to loading, U_n is the homeostatic equilibrium strain energy density, and s is the fraction of U_n indicating the width of lazy zone, where no net change of elastic modulus takes place. The lazy zone and the AW appear to describe the same phenomena where the bone's elastic modulus does not depend on the remodeling stimulus, in other words it is in equilibrium.
Weinans et al. (1992) proposed a remodeling stimulus (S) that depends on, not only the strain energy density, but, but also on the bone density ρ, and on different types of loadings as follows,

$$S = \frac{1}{n}\sum_{i=1}^{n}\left(\frac{U_i}{\rho}\right) \tag{3}$$

where n is the total number of load types (i) that induce strain energy density (U_i). The density change was expresses as,

$$\frac{d\rho}{dt} = \begin{cases} A_1\left(S-(1+s)K\right)^2; & S > (1+s)K \\ 0; & (1-s)K \le S \le (1+s)K \\ A_2\left(S-(1-s)K\right)^3; & S < (1-s)K \end{cases} \tag{4}$$

where A_1 and A_2 are remodeling constant, s is the width of lazy zone, K is the homeostatic stimulus for remodeling equilibrium. The exponents of bone formation and bone resorption are set to be 2 and 3, respectively, to simulate that resorption is a faster process than formation.

1.2.1.3 Bone remodeling based on daily effective stress

Carter et al. (1987) stated that a minimum amount of daily remodeling stimulus is required for bone maintenance (Carter et al., 1987; Beaupré et al., 1990). This daily remodeling stimulus (Ψ_b) characterizing the magnitude and cycles of loads is defined as,

$$\Psi_b = \left(\sum_{day} n_i \bar{\sigma}_i^{\,m}\right)^{1/m} \tag{5}$$

where n_i is the number of cycles of load type i, and m is an empirical constant to weight the relative importance of stress magnitude and number of load cycles, and $\bar{\sigma}_i$ is the continuum level effective stress, which is defined as,

$$\bar{\sigma}_i = \sqrt{2EU} \tag{6}$$

where E is the continuum average elastic modulus and U is the strain energy density. The velocity of surface remodeling in response to the daily remodeling stimulus was formulated as follows,

$$\dot{r} = \begin{cases} C_1\left(\Psi_b - \Psi_{bAS}\right) + \left(C_1 - C_2\right)w_1; & \Psi_b - \Psi_{bAS} < -w_1 \\ C_2\left(\Psi_b - \Psi_{bAS}\right); & -w_1 \le \Psi_b - \Psi_{bAS} < 0 \\ C_3\left(\Psi_b - \Psi_{bAS}\right); & 0 \le \Psi_b - \Psi_{bAS} \le w_2 \\ C_4\left(\Psi_b - \Psi_{bAS}\right) + \left(C_3 - C_4\right)w_2; & \Psi_b - \Psi_{bAS} > w_2 \end{cases} \tag{7}$$

where Ψ_{bAS} is the attractor stimulus for remodeling equilibrium, C_1 - C_4 are rate constants, and w_1 and w_2 are the boundaries of the normal activity region. Biologically, bone remodeling only occurs at the bone surface so the remodeling potential depends on the amount of available bone surface. Bone specific surface is used to quantify available bone surface for remodeling in bulk bone. The relation between the rate of density change and the rate of surface change can be expressed as,

$$\dot{\rho} = kS_v\rho_t\dot{r} \tag{8}$$

where k is the fraction of local area, which is actively remodeling, S_v is the bone-specific surface, which is determined according to apparent bone density (Martin, 1984), and ρ_t is the density of the fully mineralized tissue.

1.2.2 Modeling dental implant induced bone remodeling

Numerous clinical and histologic studies have been carried out to understand osseointegration in order to improve dental implant designs, surfaces and surgical protocols. Developing mathematical models of dental bone remodeling can help uncover biomechanical factors controlling short and long term survivability of implant treatments. Mathematical models mentioned previously were originally developed to study the phenomenon of bone adaptation to functional loads in long bone. However, simulations of bone remodeling in other bone regions such as acetabulum, proximal tibia, metacarpal, calcaneus and mandible (Carter & Beaupré, 2001; Pérez et al., 2010; Reina et al., 2007) have been reported. These long bone remodeling theories were used to study the bone remodeling, as a result of biomechanical alteration of the equilibrium state in the jaw bone due to use of dental implants (Lin et al., 2009a). Long term bone maintenance following fixed partial denture treatment was simulated by Field et al. (2010). A qualitative validation was reported by comparing the prediction of dental implant induced mandibular bone remodeling to clinical follow-up x-ray images over 48 months (Lin D. et al. 2010). Marginal bone loss is a common problem following dental implantation. Crupi et al. (2004), Li et al. (2007) and Lin C.-L. et al (2010) investigated the biomechanical causes of marginal bone loss by adding an overload bone loss criteria to remodeling equations. Lian et al. (2010) examined the effect of initial bone implant contact percentage on long term peri-implant bone remodeling and showed that 58-60% bone implant contact state develops at the equilibrium state no matter what initial contact percentage was assumed. Chou et al. (2011), investigated the effects of bone grafts in peri-implant bone remodeling in fresh extraction sockets and predicted that graft materials that are relatively stiff and that have high equilibrium stimulus values are likely to result in increased bone loss in the long term. In addition to studying clinical scenarios, factors influencing peri-implant bone remodeling is also of great interest to implant designers. A functionally graded dental implant, where the material composition varies from hydroxyapatite at the implant apex to titanium at the implant collar, was suggested. Lin et al. (2009b) predicted that the bone density can increase for implants made of functionally graded materials, but the initial stability of implant can be compromised due to the excessive vertical displacement due to the overall reduction in implant stiffness.

In Section 3, the strain energy density based remodeling theory (Section 1.2.1.2) is adopted to investigate the effects of various dental implant designs on bone remodeling. Equation (4) is first solved by the forward Euler time integration method, which gives,

$$\rho^{j+1} = \begin{cases} \rho^j + A_1\left(S^j - (1+s)K\right)^2 \Delta t; & S^j > (1+s)K \\ 0; & (1-s)K \le S^j \le (1+s)K \\ \rho^j + A_2\left(S^j - (1-s)K\right)^3 \Delta t; & S^j < (1-s)K \end{cases} \tag{9}$$

where j is the integration time step. Parameters A_1, A_2 and Δt can be treated as a single constant. To implement these formulations into finite element analysis, bone density must be related to material properties. The general relation of density and linear isotropic elasticity is,

$$E = C\rho^d \tag{10}$$

(Carter & Hayes, 1977), where E is the elastic modulus of bone. Empirical parameters C and d are set to be 3.79 and 3, respectively. The minimum modulus is 1 kPa. The maximum modulus is taken as 13 GPa, which corresponded to a density of 1.508 g/cm³.

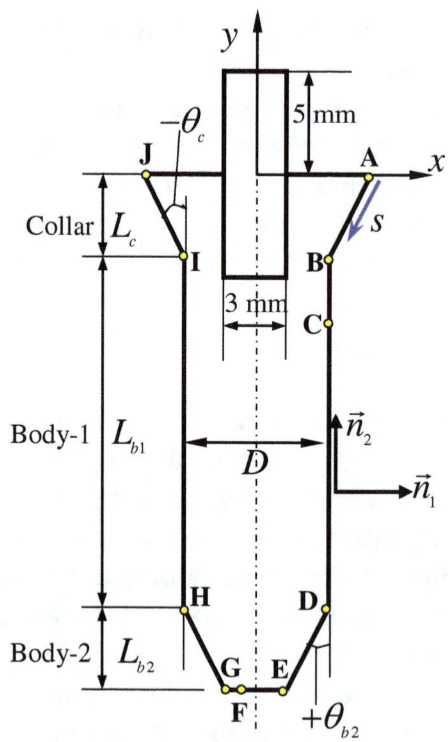

Fig. 1. The definitions of the parameters used to identify the contour of a generic dental implant.

2. Load transfer along the bone-implant interface

In order to investigate the nature of load transfer along the bone implant interface, a comprehensive parametric study of different implant designs was carried out. A generic implant with adjustable contour features, much like Faegh and Müftü (2010), was used. The normal and shear stress components, σ_{11} and σ_{12} acting normal and parallel to the implant surface, respectively, (Figure 1) were computed and plotted along the s-coordinate axis placed on the bone implant interface. Note that $s = 0$ represents the buccal-side and it is also marked as point-A, whereas point-J is the end of the interface path.

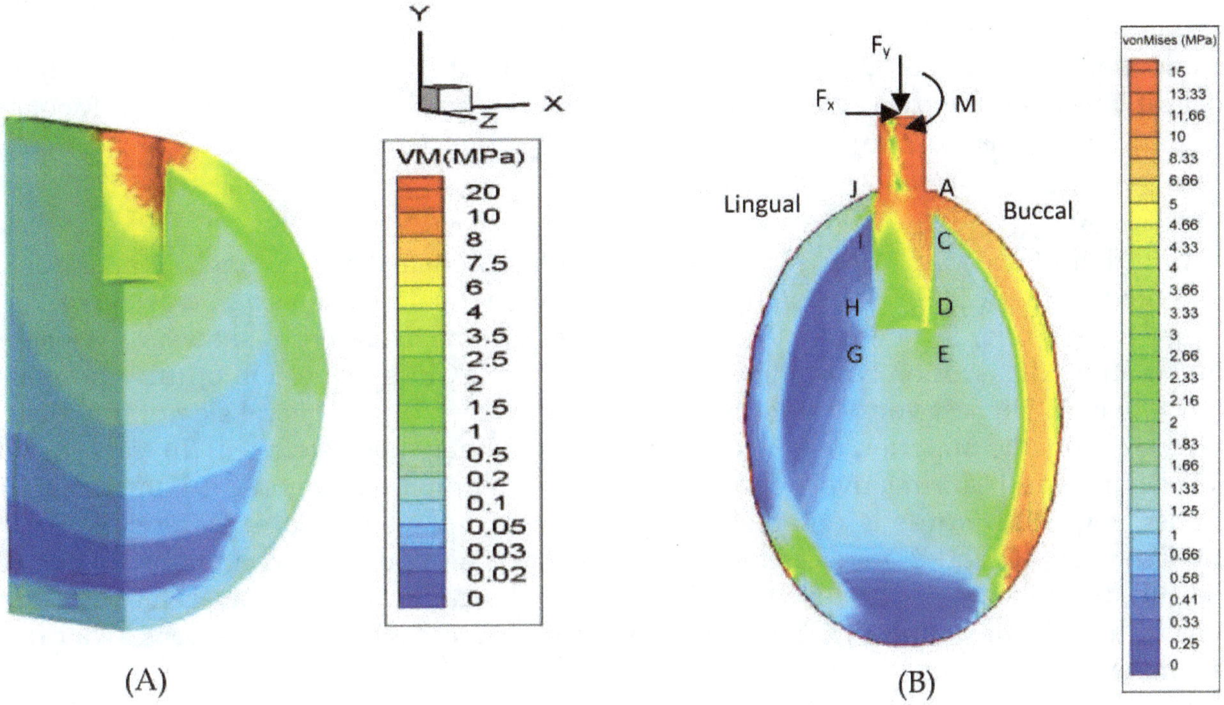

Fig. 2. von Mises stress distribtution in (A) the 3D model, (B) the 2D model.

2.1 Methods

Four main regions were designated to define implant geometry as the *collar*, *body*-1, *body*-2, and *apex* regions. The effects of the length, L_c, and slope, θ_c, of the collar region, the length, L_{b1}, and the diameter, D, of the body-1 region and the length, L_{b2}, and the slope, θ_{b2}, of the body-2 region were investigated. The apex was modeled to be flat. Faegh and Müftü (2010) investigated the effects of four common external thread shapes. The values they used were chosen according to the commercially available dental implants. Here we only report on the effect of a triangular thread shape, as the results and conclusions are similar. The thread geometry is defined by using three parameters. These are the *thread pitch*, p_t, the *thread depth* h_t, and the *thread slope* θ_t. The thread depth was $h_t = 0.32$ mm and the thread pitch was $p_t = L_{b1}/7$ in this study.

The implant-abutment connection was assumed to be monolithic; and, all of the components, (implant, abutment, cortical bone, and trabecular bone) were assumed to be perfectly bonded along their individual interfaces. The (x, y) coordinate system was placed at the center of the superior surface of the implant, as shown in Figure1 and the locations of the key points (A – J) on implant geometry, were programmed to be variable. In order to eliminate effects of bone morphology, which vary in individual jaws, the external geometry of bone was simplified as an ellipse. The major and minor axes of the bone model were idealized as 30 and 18 mm respectively, and a cortical layer of 2 mm was assumed.

Finite Element Method (FEM) was used and the system was modeled in ANSYS ver. 11 (Canonsburg, PA, USA). The analysis was carried out in 2D plane-strain. However, a 3D analysis was conducted to verify the level of validity of the 2D analysis. In 3D, the bone was modeled as an elliptical cylinder. The model was gradually meshed by creating extra regions around the implant with very high mesh density as in Faegh and Müftü (2010). 3D and 2D models were meshed with the structural solid elements, SOLID 185 and PLANE 42 of ANSYS respectively. An occlusal load of 113 N was applied at the center of abutment with the direction of 11 degrees with respect to the main axis, and a moment of 90 N.mm to mimic the biting force on the prosthesis. The elastic moduli of the implant system (Ti), the cortical bone, and the trabecular bone were set to 113, 13 and 1 GPa, respectively (Rieger et al., 1989a; Steinemann, 1996).

2.2 Results

Distribution of the von Mises stress in the bone, as predicted by 2D and 3D analyses, is presented in Figure 2, for a smooth faced implant with the dimensions θ_c = -10 degrees, L_c = 1 mm, L_{b1} = 5 mm, L_{b2} = 3 mm, θ_{b2} = 5 mm, D = 3.3 mm. This figure shows a reasonably similar stress distribution both in magnitude and trend. Close inspection of this figure also shows that: (i) Highest von Mises stress levels are observed on the buccal side of the cortical bone, and on the superior region of implant and abutment system; (ii) In general, the trabecular bone bears relatively low levels of stress compared to cortical bone; and, (iii) Higher von Mises stress is observed near the bone implant interface. Differences in the details of the 2D and 3D stress contours are due to the boundary conditions. In the 3D analysis, the bone was restricted at the distal ends, whereas in the 2D analysis the restriction is near the inferior periphery. This results in some distinct variations in regions away from the implant, as shown in the figure.

The effect of external thread shape on the von Mises stress distribution is presented for a smooth faced-implant and an externally threaded implant in Figure 3. The general contour parameters of these two cases are described above. This figure shows the load transfer along the bone-implant interface, via the normal σ_{11} and shear σ_{12} stresses. For the smooth (threadless) implant the normal stress σ_{11} is primarily compressive along the collar region and the apex of the implant, but it is small and tensile along the smooth faces of the body-1 and -2 regions. Jumps and stress concentrations are observed at the locations with abrupt changes in geometry and material properties. The collar region on the lingual side is seen to experience roughly 1/10th of the compressive stress experienced on the buccal side. Variation of the normal σ_{11} and shear σ_{12} stresses along the bone-implant interface for the externally threaded implant is presented in Figure 3B. It is observed that the interfacial normal and shear stresses increase around the external threads. In particular, on the first thread of the buccal side, where the thread is engaged with the cortical bone, a significant σ_{11} stress peak is observed. On the other hand, the general behavior of σ_{11} and σ_{12}, between the two implant types shows that the overall load transfer characteristics in the bone-implant interface are similar. It appears that at a local level the externally threaded implant is able to transfer higher loads to the tarbecular region. This can have significant effects on long term bone maintenance. Effects of different thread shapes are presented by Faegh & Müftü (2010).

The effects of different implant contours are investigated by changing the implant design parameters (θ_c, L_c, L_{b1}, L_{b2}, θ_{b2}, D) systematically (Table 1). Analysis of the interfacial stresses showed that the parameters that have the highest impact on the stress magnitude are the implant diameter D, the collar parameters θ_c and L_c, and the length of the body-1 region L_{b1}. The effects of these four parameters are summarized in Figure 4. Note that this analysis was carried out for smooth (threadless) implants. Figure 4 gives the maximum normal and shear stress values transferred to the bone. Incidentally all of the maximum values are found in the collar region of the buccal side. The results presented in Figure 4 are summarized as follows:

- For implants with larger diameter D the largest normal σ_{11} and shear stress σ_{12} transferred to the bone is reduced (Figures 4A-C).
- Increasingly negative collar slope (θ_c) causes the maximum normal stress transferred to the bone to increase, but it causes the maximum shear stress to decrease (Figure 4A).
- Increasing the length (L_c) of the collar and length (L_{b1}) of the body-1 regions cause the maximum normal stress and the maximum shear stress transferred to the bone to decrease (Figures 4B,C).

Parameter	Values
Length of Collar, L_c (mm)	1, 2
Angle of Collar, θ_c (degrees)	-10, -5, 0, 5, 10
Length of body-1, L_{b1} (mm)	4, 5, 6
Diameter of body-1, D (mm)	3.3, 3.5, 4
Length of body-2, L_{b2} (mm)	3, 4
Angle of body-2, θ_{b2} (degrees)	5, 10

Table 1. Implant dimensions that were varied in this work. See Figure 1 for the definitions of these variables. Note that θ_c as drawn in this figure is defined to be a negative angle, whereas θ_{b2} is defined to be positive.

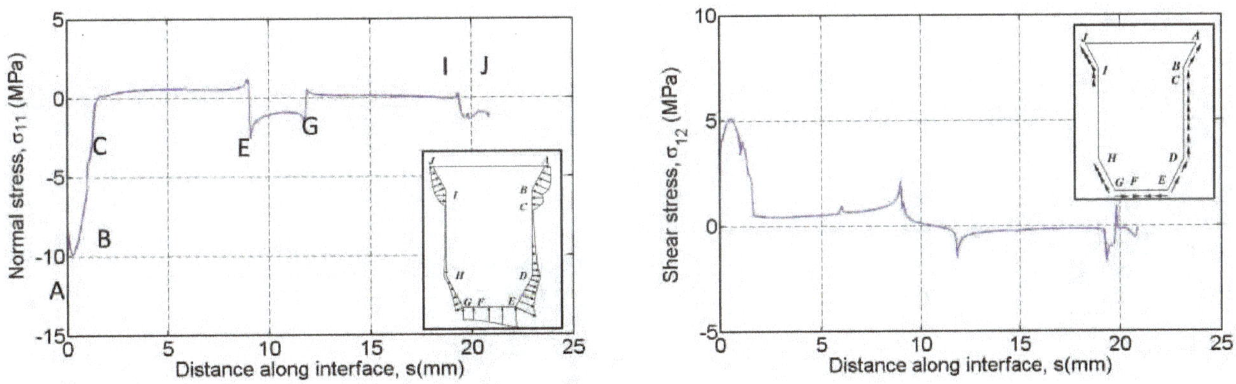

(A) σ_{11} and σ_{12} for smooth faced implant

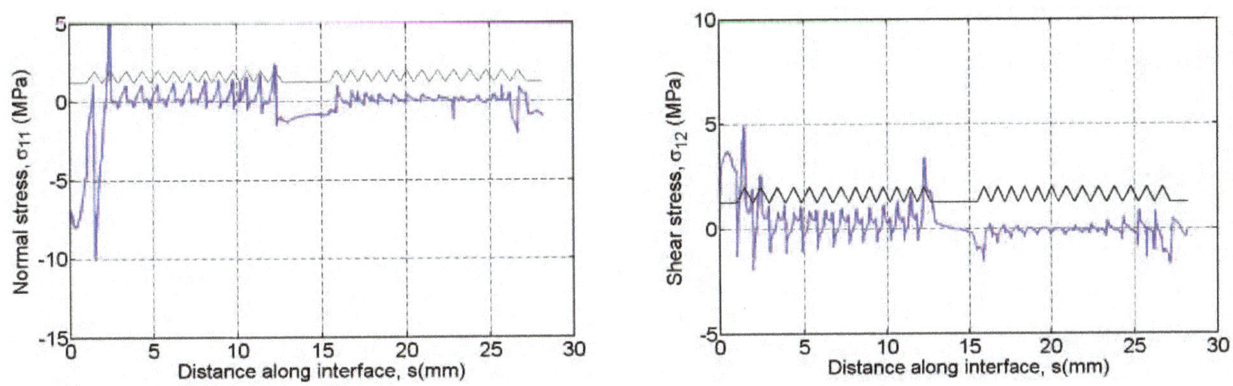

(B) σ_{11} and σ_{12} for externally threaded implant

Fig. 3. Normal and shear stresses along the interface for an implant with (A) no-external thread, and (B) triangular external thread. The other parameters of the implants are as follows: θ_c = -10 degrees, L_c = 1 mm and L_{b1} = 5 mm, L_{b2} = 3 mm, θ_{b2} = 5 degrees, D = 3.3 mm.

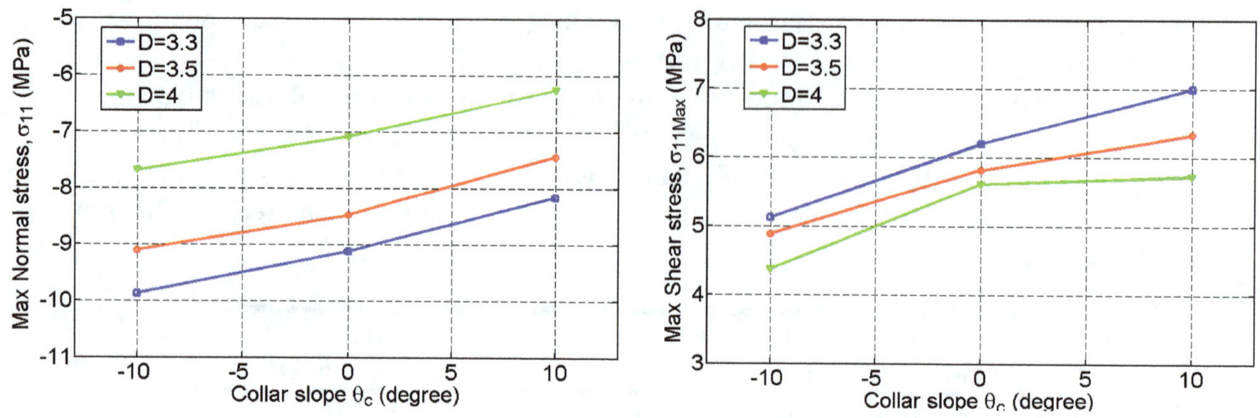

(A) Effect of θ_c

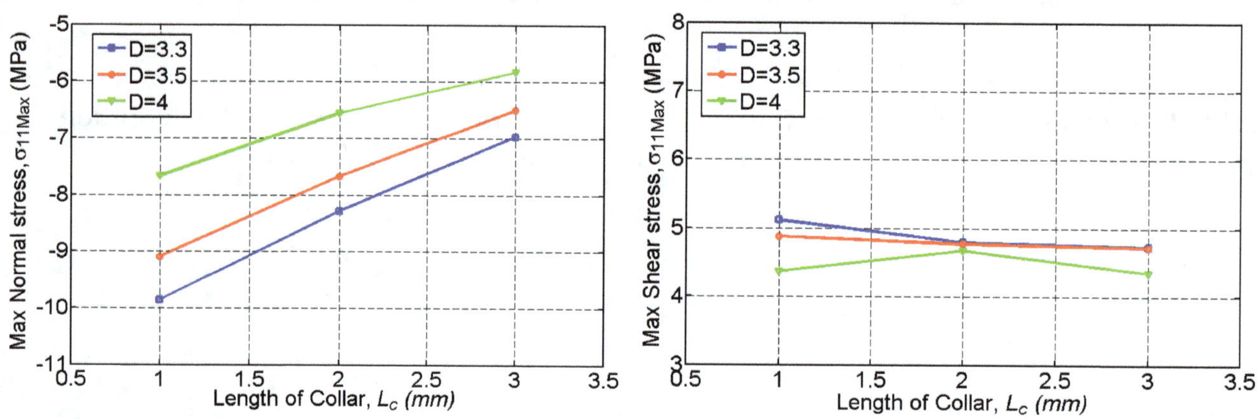

(B) Effect of L_c

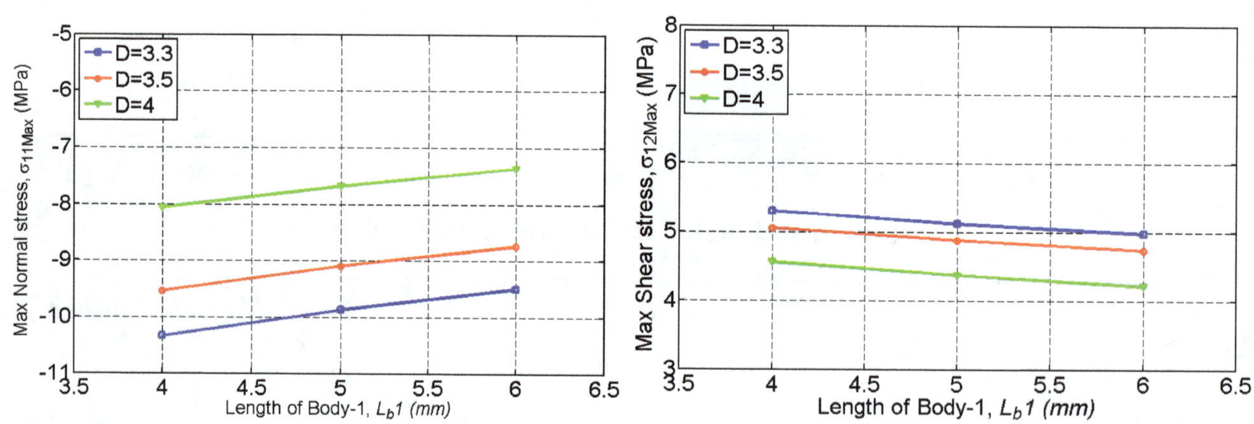

(C) Effect of L_{b1}

Fig. 4. Maximum normal and shear stress components σ_{11}, σ_{12} along the bone-implant interface with respect to contour parameter (A) collar slope, θ_c, (B) length of collar, L_c, (C) length of body-1, L_{b1}.

3. Simulation of dental implant induced bone remodeling

3.1 Methods

Bone remodeling around implant systems was modeled by using the remodeling theory presented by Huiskes and co-workers. Finite element method was used to assess the strain energy density in loading. Equations (9) and (10) were programmed into ANSYS. Two separate analyses are presented. The first one is a 2D plane strain analysis of bone remodeling originally presented by Chou et al. (2008), and the second one is a 3D analysis of bone remodeling by Chou et al. (2011). In the 2D analysis, the external bone contour of the mandible was obtained from a slice of CT scans at the premolar region in the buccal-lingual plane. A layer of cortical bone with a thickness of 1 mm was assigned. Elastic modulus and Poisson's ratio of this cortical layer are 13 GPa and 0.3, respectively. Dental implant systems considered were assumed to be made of titanium alloy (Ti-6Al-4V). Elastic modulus and Poisson's ratio are 113.8 GPa and 0.3 (Misch & Bidez, 1999), respectively. Quadrilateral elements were used to mesh the implant bone complex, and the bottom of mandible was constrained as shown in Figure 5. Occlusion was modeled as a concentrated force, F_o = 100 N, applied on the abutment in the buccal-lingual plane at 11° with respect to vertical axis (Chou et al., 2008). In addition, a uniform pressure (P_{mf} = 500 kPa) was assumed on the outer periphery of cortical bone to simulate the effect of mandibular flexure during jaw movement. Remodeling algorithm was applied only to the trabecular region, which was initially assumed to have a uniform density of 0.808 g/cm^3 corresponding to an elastic modulus of 2 GPa. Poisson's ratio was taken as 0.3. Remodeling parameters in Equation (9) were K = 25 J/kg, s = 0.65 and $A_i\Delta t$ = 5×10^{-3} for i = 1, 2.

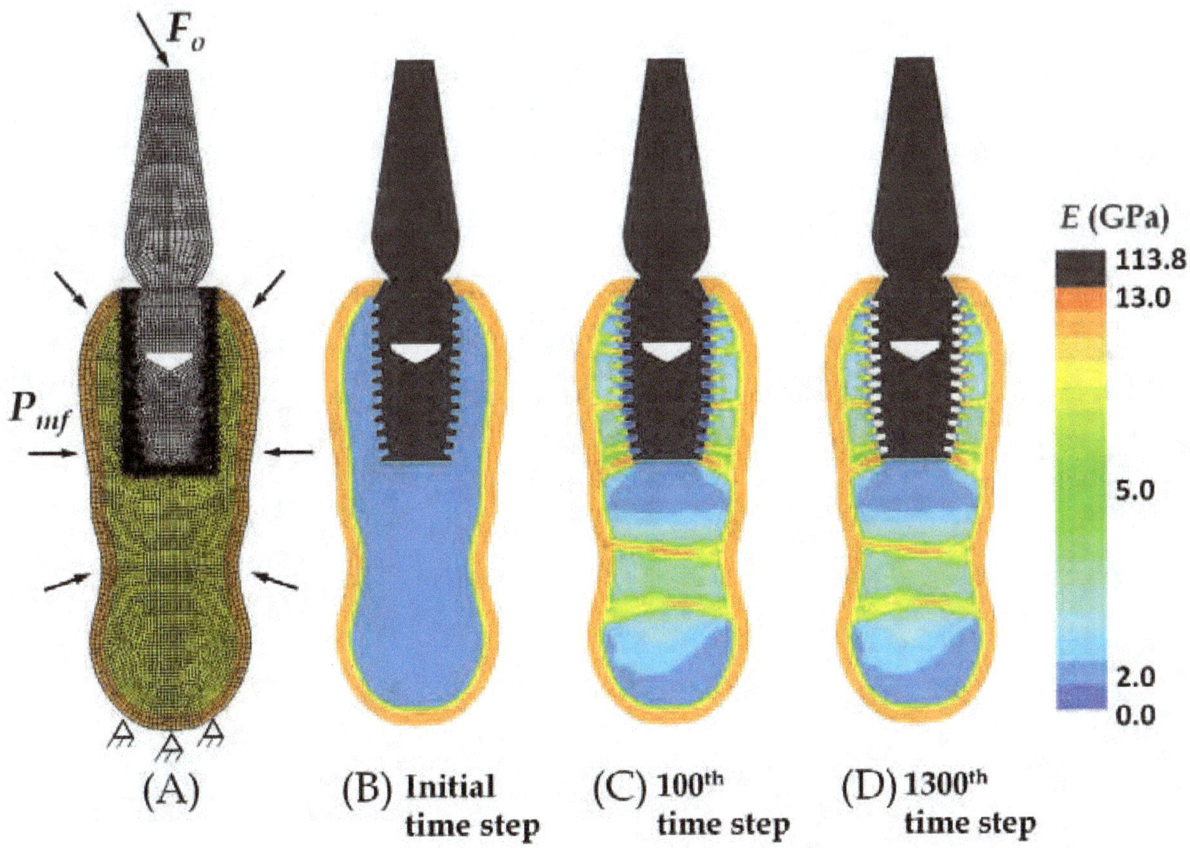

Fig. 5. (A) Two dimensional finite element mesh and loading conditions. Fine mesh is assigned at the bone implant interface. Elastic modulus distribution at (B) initial time step, (C) 100th time step, and (D) 1300th time step (Chou et al, 2008). (Printed with permission from Elsevier Limited).

3.2 Results and discussion

The transient change in the bone's elastic modulus at time steps 1, 100 and 1,300 is presented in Figure 5. This figure shows that the bone density, and hence the elastic modulus, changes gradually form a uniform initial state to a non-uniform state that is reflective of the local loading conditions. It is seen that high modulus bone is developed in the first 100 time steps, and no significant update takes place afterward. It is also observed that the tips of the external threads promote high density bone (high elastic modulus) but the area between the threads experience some bone resorption in the later stages of remodeling. As the Huiskes' model of bone remodeling doesn't have an effective means to handle actual time and loading rates, the time steps in this figure have arbitrary units. Nevertheless, one can see that bone density redistribution takes place quickly, but stays stable for prolonged loading.

Effects of four different implant contours on trabecular bone remodeling are presented in Figure 6. Three smooth faced implants systems and one externally threaded implant system are considered. Details of the geometrical differences are given in the figure. Cylindrical implant with the flat apex (Figure 6A) results in the largest amount of bone loss. The cylindrical implant with the rounded apex (Figure 6B) causes a similar response, albeit with less bone loss. The root form implant (Figure 6C) further reduces this bone loss region with the narrow apex design. For these three smooth faced implants, high density trabecular bone develops near the apical corners, and some high density struts emerging from the implant body are found in Figures 6A-6C. The main bodies of these implants fail to stimulate the bone sufficiently to induce significant bone remodeling. A study carried out by Watzak et al. (2005) in baboons investigates the effects of surface features such as threads and chemical modifications to the surface also show similar results. Note the lack of tarbecular bone under the flat apex of the implant in Figure 6A. Watzak et al. (2005) also indicate that signs of bone remodeling at the surface of cylindrical implant were absent.

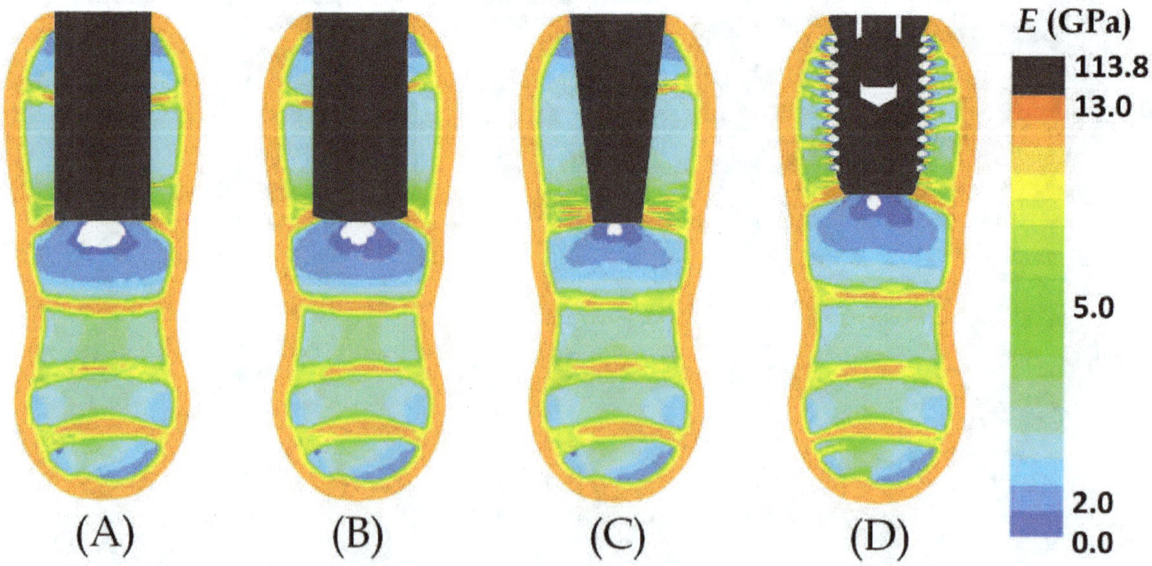

Fig. 6. Elastic modulus distribution predicted around a (A) cylindrical implant, a (B) cylindrical implant with rounded apex, a (C) root from implant and a (D) threaded implant. (Chou et al., 2008). (Printed with permission from Elsevier Limited).

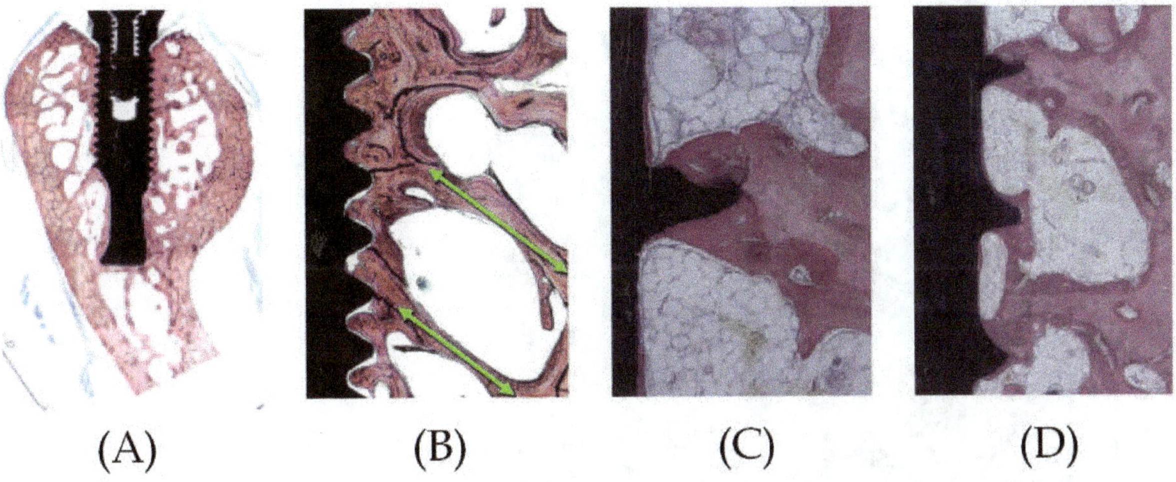

Fig. 7. Histologic studies show (A) bone remodeling around dental implant (Watzak et al., 2005), (B) trabeculae like dense struts at implant surface (Watzak et al., 2005), (C) and (D) bone growth around implant threads (Schenk & Buser, 1998). (Printed with permission from John Wiley and Sons.)

The predictions for the externally threaded implants (Figures 5D and 6D) are significantly different from smooth faced implants. In the case of threaded design, development of high density bone around the threads is evident. Similar remodeling patterns were reported in the histologic observations of Watzak et al. (2005) in Figures 7A and 7B, and those of Schenk & Buser (1998) in Figures 7C and 7D. Note that while Figures 7B-7D show bone density increase around the threads some resorption is also observed between the threads in Figures 7C and 7D similar to our simulations.

In the study presented above, the homeostatic stimulus, *K*, was assumed to be constant. Although satisfying results were predicted by this simplification, it implies that bone remodels toward a spatially homogenous biomechanical field, despite the fact that the biological environment (i.e. the cells and the nutrients) varies among bone sites. In order to address this issue, we used a site dependant homeostatic stimulus, $K(x,y,z)$ in a 3D analysis of bone remodeling around a dental implant. This approach was also used by Huiskes et al. (1992) and Weinans, et al. (1993) to simulate bone remodeling around hip prostheses. In addition, we hypothesize that the site specific homeostatic stimulus must be similar to that induced by a natural tooth in its supporting bone. Therefore, the site-specific *K* value was computed, first for a model with a natural tooth that is shown in Figure 8A. These *K* values were subsequently used for predicting the bone remodeling around a dental implant system. Details are presented by Chou et al. (2011).

A three-dimensional mandibular segment was constructed from the CT-scan of the premolar region of the mandible. Same material properties and occlusal load, as above, were applied to the finite element models of bone tooth and bone implant prosthesis complexes shown in Figure 8. The elastic modulus of the tooth and the prosthesis were taken as 20 GPa and 80 GPa, respectively; and the Poisson's ratios were assumed to be 0.3. Similar to clinical practice, the interstitial gap created by the incongruence of dental implant with extraction socket is filled with a (virtual) bone graft in the finite element model. The elastic modulus of the graft was set to be the same as trabecular bone. The mandible segment was constrained in all directions on the distal buccal-lingual plane, and symmetry boundary condition was applied to the mesial buccal-lingual plane shown in Figure 8.

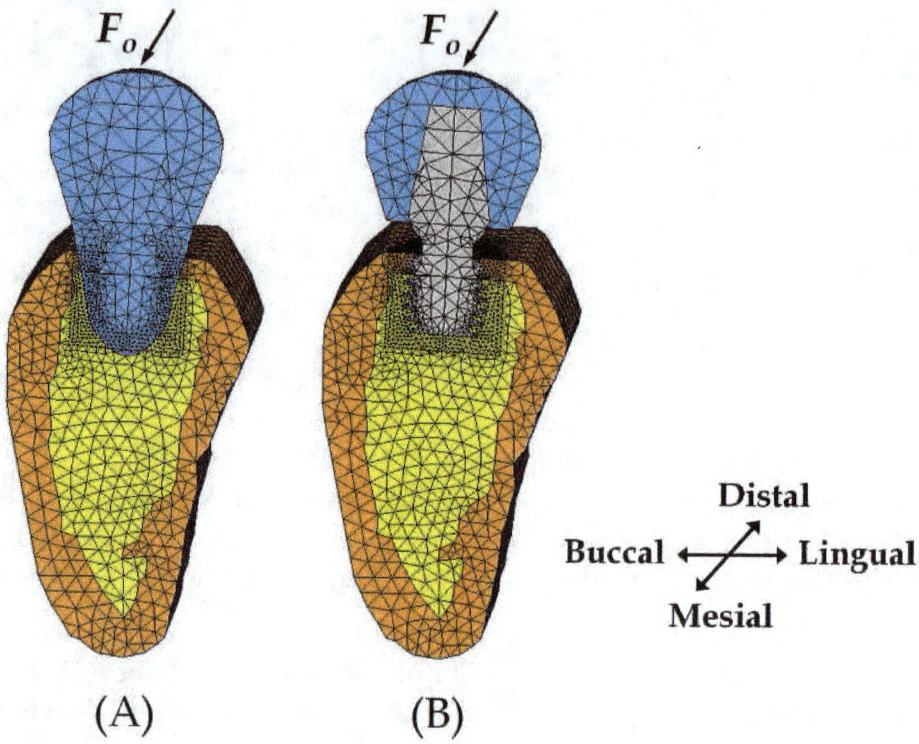

Fig. 8. Finite element models of (A) bone tooth and (B) bone implant prosthesis complexes. A concentrated force F_o is used to simulate occlusion.

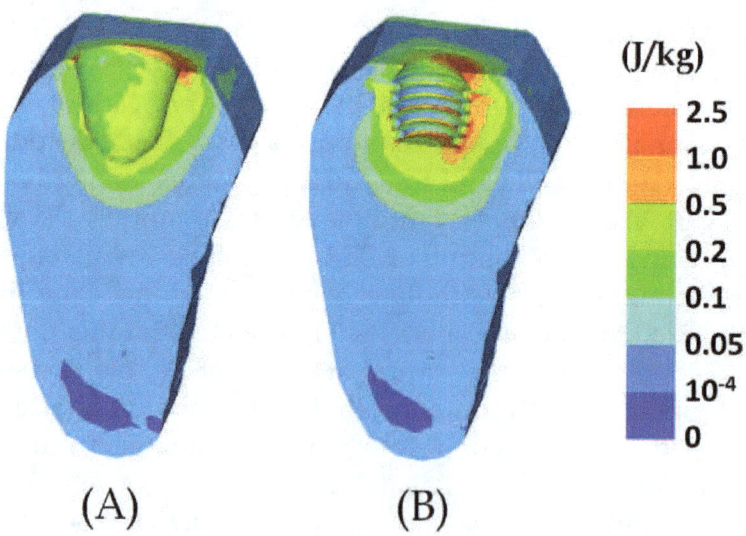

Fig. 9. (A) Homeostatic stimuli distribution in bone induced by tooth. (B) Remodeling stimuli distribution in bone induced by dental implant prior to bone remodeling (Initial time step).

The site dependant homeostatic stimuli K was based on the strain energy per unit bone mass, induced by the occlusal force acting on the natural tooth. Next, homeostatic stimuli in the graft region had to be assumed. This assumption was based on the stimulus levels near the tooth. Therefore, a constant value K_g = 0.25 J/kg was used to represent the homeostatic stimulus of the bone graft. This parameter is treated as the potential of bone graft to induce

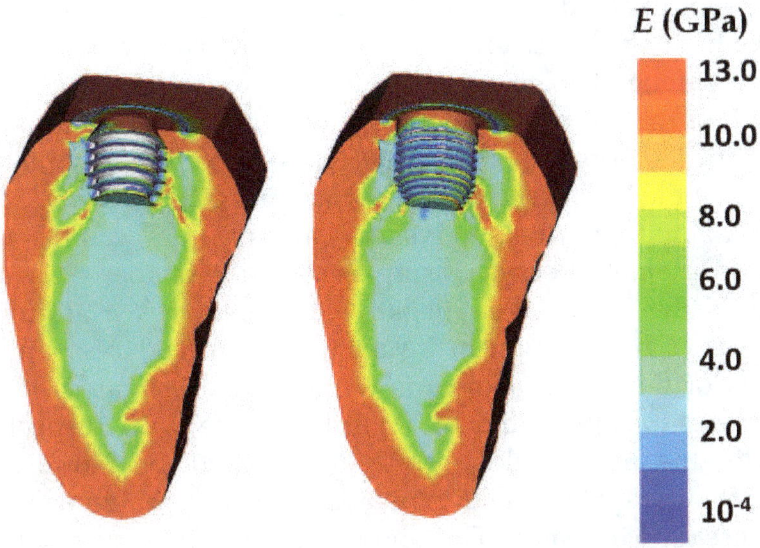

Fig. 10. Elastic modulus distribution predicted around two different implant designs at remodeling equilibrium.

bone remodeling (Chou et al., 2011). Figure 9A shows the computed site specific *K* distribution, and Figure 9B shows the initial remodeling stimuli *S* distribution around the implant It is seen that the variations of the homeostatic stimuli *K*. It is seen that the homeostatic stimuli *K* and the remodeling stimulus *S* are localized around the tooth and the dental implant. In fact, it can be stated that a certain degree of biomimetic match has been obtained in this case. For implants with longer body-1 and body-2 regions, the remodeling stimulus is markedly different than that of the tooth (Chou et al., 2011).

Figure 10 shows the elastic modulus distribution at remodeling equilibrium for two wide-diameter, short implants with different thread profiles. Trabeculae like dense bone struts develop at the implant surface and extend toward cortical layer. Implant threads show same characteristics as in 2D analysis; bone apposition occurs at the thread tips, and the regions between the implant threads are prone to bone resorption. The predicted results also demonstrate that bone remodeling is a localized event, and it decays with increasing distance away from implant surface. A histologic study by Coelho et al. (2009) reported high levels of osteoactivity taking place near the implant surface. This can be observed in the predictions in Figure 10.

4. Summary and conclusions

Dental implants provide an attractive alternative to classical prosthodontic techniques in the treatment of edentulism. It has been shown clinically that the bone loss after tooth extraction is reversed by the placement of dental implant, since the first human study reported by Brånemark et al. (1977). The mechanical loads exerted by occlusion are transferred into jawbone through the dental implant, and can potentially affect the bone remodeling according to Wolff's law (Wolff, 1892). Therefore, it is critical to develop a sound understanding of the load transfer mechanism from the implant to the bone. It is equally important, to supply a dental implant with critical chemical and contour features on its surface. If the ideal load transfer characteristics can be identified, it may be possible to improve the osseointegration.

A systematic analysis of the load transfer along the bone-implant interface was carried out by using finite element analysis. Various implant systems were designed by changing their contour parameters. Among all design parameters, the diameter, the collar slope, the collar length and the length of the implant were found to be the most influential parameters to the interfacial variations of the normal and shear stresses. Maximum normal and shear stresses were found to occur on the buccal side of the cortical bone, as in many other studies. It was shown that both maximum normal and shear stress values can be reduced by either widening the implant diameter, or increasing the lengths of the collar and body regions. Varying the slope of the collar from negative to positive was found to increase the maximum normal stress, but to reduce the maximum shear stress transferred along the interface. The effects of the external threads were also investigated. It was seen that the general interfacial load transfer behavior doesn't change with respect to smooth faced implants, but locally the interfacial stresses are elevated around the threads. A bone remodeling algorithm was implemented to analyze the bone maintenance characteristics of smooth faced and threaded implants. This showed poor bone maintenance around smooth faced implants. On the other hand, significant remodeling and densification was predicted around threaded implants. It was shown that the thread tips promote the development of dense bone. Total bone resorption was predicted in the areas between the threads. Similar remodeling phenomenon around implant threads was reported in histologic studies by Schenk & Buser (1998) and Watzak et al. (2005). It appears that adequately high interfacial stresses are introduced by using externally threaded implants.

This study contributes to our understanding of the complex problem of load transfer mechanism in the bone-dental implant interface and the subsequent peri-implant bone remodeling. Despite the interesting conclusions drawn from the results, the computational predictions are still limited by the assumptions and simplifications of loading, geometry and material properties made in this study.

5. References

Akça, K., Iplikçioğlu, H. (2001). Finite element stress analysis of the influence of staggered versus straight placement of dental implants. *The International Journal of Oral & Maxillofacial Implants*, Vol.16, No.5, (Sep-Oct 2001 Sep-Oct), pp. 722-30

Aparicio, C., Orozco, P. (1998). Use of 5 mm diameter implants: Periotest values related to a clinical and radiographic evaluation. *Clinical Oral Implants Research*, Vol.9, No.6, (Dec 1998), pp. 398-406

Bahat, O., Handelsman, M. (1996). Use of wide implants and double implants in the posterior jaw: a clinical report. *The International Journal of Oral & Maxillofacial Implants*,Vol.11, No.3, (May-Jun 1996), pp. 379-86

Balshi, T.J., Wolfinger, G.J. (1997a). Immediate loading of branemark implants in edenulous mandibles: a preliminary report. *Implant Dentistry [Implant Dent]*, Vol.6, No.2, (Summer 1997), pp. 83-8, ISSN: 1056-6163

Balshi, T.J., Wolfinger, G.J. (1997b). Two implant supported single molar replacement: interdental space requirements and comparison to alternative options. *The International Journal of Periodontics & Restorative Dentistry*, Vol.17, No.5, (Oct 1997), pp. 426-35

Beaupre, G.S., Orr, T.E. & Carter, D.R. (1990). An approach for time-dependent bone modeling and remodeling-theoretical development. *Journal of Orthopaedic Research*, Vol. 8, No. 5, (September 1990), pp. 651-661, ISSN 1554-527X

Bidez, M.W., Stephens, B.J., Lemons, J.E. (1988). A comparison of interfacial assumptions in a three dimensional stress analysis of a CP-Ti dental implant system, *Transactions Third World Biomaterials Congress*, 117, Kyoto, Japan, 1988

Blatz, M.B., Strub, J.R., Glaser, R., Beghart, W. (1998). Use of wide-diameter and standard diameter implants to replace single molars: Two case presentations. *Int J Proshodont*, Vol. 11, pp. 356-363

Borchers, L., Reichart, P. (1983). Three-dimensional stress distribution around a dental implant at different stages of interface development. *J. Dent. Res.*, Vol.62, No.2, pp. 155-9

Bozkaya, D., Müftü, S., Müftü, A. (2004). Evaluation of Load Transfer Characteristics of Five Different Implants in Compact Bone at Different Load Levels by Finite Element Analysis, *Journal of Prosthetic Dentistry*, Vol. 92, No. 6 pp. 523-530

Brånemark, P.I., Hansson, B.O., Adell, R., Breine, U., Lindström, J., Hallén, O. & Ohman, A. (1977). Osseointegrated implants in the treatment of endentulous jaw. Experience from a 10-year period. *Scandinavian Journal of Plastic and Reconstructive Surgery Supplementum*, Vol. 16, pp. 1-132, ISSN 0581-9474

Brånemark, P.I., Engstrand, P., Ohrnell, L.O., Gröndahl, K., Nilsson, P., Hagberg, K., Darle, C., Lekholm, U. (1999) Branemark Novum: a new treatment concept for rehabilitation of the edenrulous mandible. Preliminary results from a prospective clinical follow-up study. *Clinical Implant Dentistry And Related Research*, Vol.1, No.1, pp. 2-16

Brånemark, P.I., Zarb, G., Alberktsson, T. (1985). Tissue Integrated Prostheses, Quintessence, Chicago

Brunski, J.B. (1999). In vivo bone response to biomechanical loading at the bone/dental-implant interface. *Adv Dent Res 1999*. Vol.13, pp. 99-119

Canay, S., Hersek, N., Akpinar, I., Aşik, Z. (1996). Comparison of stress distribution around vertical and angled implants with finite element analysis. *Quintessence International (Berlin, Germany: 1985)*, Vol.27, No.9, 591-8

Carda, C., Silvestrini, G., Gomez de Ferraris, M.E., Peydró, A. & Bonucci, E. (2005). Osteoprotegerin (OPG) and RANKL expression and distribution in developing human craniomandibular joint. Tissue and Cell, Vol. 37, No. 3, (Jun 2005), pp. 247-255, ISSN 0040-8166

Carter, D.R., Fyhrie, D.P. & Whalen, R.T. (1987). Trabecular bone dnsity and loading history: regulation of connective tissue biology by mechanical energy. *Journal of Biomechanics*, Vol. 20, No. 8, pp. 785-794

Carter, D.R. & Beaupré, G.S. (2001). *Skeletal Function and Form: Mechanobiology of Skeletal Development, Aging, and Regeneration*. Cambridge University Press, ISBN 052179000X, New York

Carter D.R., Hayes W.C. (1977).The behavior of bone as a two-phase porous structure. *J. Bone Joint Surg*. Vol. 59A, pp. 954-962

Chou, H.-Y., Jagodnik, J. & Müftü, S. (2008). Predictions of bone remodeling around dental implant systems. *Journal of Biomechanics*, Vol. 41, No. 6, (April 2008), pp. 1365-1373, ISSN 0021-9290

Chou, H.-Y., Müftü, S. & Bozkaya, D. (2010). Combined effects of implant insertion depth and alveolar bone quality on periimplant bone strain induced by a wide-diameter, short implant and a narrow-diameter, long implant. *The Journal of Prosthetic Dentistry*, Vol. 104, No. 5, (November 2010), pp. 293-300, ISSN 0022-3913

Chou, H.-Y., Romanos, G., Müftü, A. & Müftü, A. (2011). Peri-Implant Bone Remodeling Around a Fresh Extraction Socket: Predictions of Bone Maintenance by Finite Element Method, *International Journal of Oral and Maxilliofacial Implants*, in review.

Coelho, P.G., Cardaropoli, G., Suzuki, M. & Lemons, J.E. Histomorphometric evaluation of a nanothickness bioceramic deposition on endosseous implants: a study in dogs. (2009). Clinical Implant Dentistry Res, Vol. 11, No. 4, (December 2009), pp. 292-302 ISSN 1708-8208

Chow, J., Hui, E., Liu, J., Li, D., Wat, P., Li, W., Yau, Y.K., Law, H. (2001). The Hong Kong Bridge Protocol. Immediate loading of mandibular branemark fixures using a fixed provisional prosthesis: preliminary results. *Clin Implant Dent Relat Res*, Vol.3, No.3, pp. 166-74

Chun, H.J., Cheong, S.Y., Han, J.H., Heo, S.J., Chung, J.P., Rhyu, I.C., Choi, Y.C., Baik, H.K., Ku, Y., Kim, M.H. (2002). Evaluation of design parameters of osseointegrated dental implants using finite element analysis. *J Oral Rehabil*, Vol.29, No.6, pp. 565-574

Cook, S.D., Klawitter, J.J., Weinstein, A.M. Lavernia, C.J. (1980). The design and evaluation of dental implants with finite element analysis, In: *Finite Elements in Biomechanics.*, R.A. Gallagher, (Ed.), 159-168, University of Arizona Press, Tuscon, AZ

Cook, S.D., Klawitter, J.J., Weinstein, A.M. (1982a). The influence of implant geometry on the stress distribution around dental implants. *J. Biomed. Mater. Res.*, Vol.16, No.4, pp. 369-79

Cook, S.D., Weinstein, A.M., Klawitter, J.J. (1982b). Parameters affecting the stress distribution around LTI carbon and aluminum oxide dental implants. *J. Biomed. Mater. Res.*, Vol.16, No.6, pp. 875-85

Crupi, V., Guglielmino, E., La Rosa, G., Vander Sloten, J. & Van Oosterwyck, H. (2004). Numerical analysis of bone adaptation around an oral implant due to overload stress. *Proceedings of the Institution of Mechcanical Engineers. Part H: Journal of Engineering in Medicine*. Vol. 218, No. 6, pp. 407-415, ISSN 0954-4119

Davarpanah, M., Martinez, H., Kebir, M., Etienne, D., Tecucianu, J.F. (2001). Wide diameter implants: new concepts. The *International Journal of Periodontics & Restorative Dentistry*, Vol. 21. No.2, (Apr 2001), pp. 149-59, ISSN 0198-7569

Duyck, J., Naert, I.E., Van Oosterwyck, H., Van der Sloten, J., De Cooman, M., Lievens, S., Puers, B. (1997). Biomechanics of dental implant: a review of the literature. *Technology and Health care 1997*, Vol.5, pp. 253-273

Ericsson, I., Nilson, H., Lindh, T., Nilner, K., Randow, K. (2000). Immediate functional loading of branemark single tooth implants. An 18 months' clinical pilot follow-up study. *Clinical Oral Implants Research*, Vol.11, No.1 (February 2000), pp. 26-33

Faegh, S., Müftü, S. (2010). Load transfer along the bone-dental implant interface. *Journal of Biomechanics*, Vol. 43, pp. 1761-1770

Farah, J.W., Craig, R.G., Yapp, R.A. (1979-80). Stress distribution caused by blade type implant. *Implantologist*, 1979-80; Vol.1, No.4, pp. 77-86

Field, C., Li, Q., Li, W., Thompson, M. & Swain, M. (2010). Prediction of mandibular bone remodelling induced by fixed partial dentures. *Journal of Biomechanics*, Vol. 43, No. 9, (March 2010), pp. 1771-1779, ISSN 0021-9290

Frandsen, P.A., Christoffersen, H., Madsen, T. (1984). Holding power of different screws in the femoral head. A study in hyman cadaver hips. *Acta Orthopaedica Scandinavica*, Vol.55, No.3, (Jun 1984), pp. 349-51

Frost, H.M. (1987). Bone "mass" and the "mechanostat": a proposal. *The Anatomical Record*, Vol. 219, No. 1, (September 1987), pp. 1-9, ISSN 1932-8486

Frost, H.M. (2003). Bone's mechanostat: a 2003 update. *The Anatomical Record*, Vol. 275A, No. 2, (December 2003), pp. 1043-1121, ISSN 1932-8486

Geng, J.P., Tan, K.B., Liu, G.R. (2001). Application of finite element analysis in implant dentistry: a review of the literature. *J Prosthet Dent*, Vol.85, No.6, pp. 585-598

Geramy, A., Morgano, S.M. (2004). Finite element analysis of three designs of an implant-supported molar crown. *The Journal of Prosthetic Dentistry*, Vol.92, No.5, pp. 434-40

Graves, S.L., Siddiqui, A.A., Jansen, C.E., Beaty, K.D. (1994). Wide diameter implants: Indications, considerations and preliminary results over a two-year period. *Australian prosthodontic Journal*, Vol.8, pp. 31-37

Griffin, T.J., Cheung, W.S. (2004). The use of short, wide implants in posterior area with reduced bone height: a retrospective investigation. *The Journal of Prosthetic Dentistry*, Vol.92, No.2, (Aug 2004), pp. 139-44

Gross, M., Laufer, B.Z. (1997). Splinting osseointegrated implants and natural teeth in rehabilitation of partially edentulous patients. Part I: laboratory and clinical studies. *Journal Of Oral Rehabilitation*, Vol.24, No.11, (Nov 1997), pp. 863-70

Hansson, S. (1999). The implant neck: smooth or provided with retention elements: A biomechanical approach. *Clinical Oral Implants Research*, Vol.10, No.5, pp. 394-405

Hart, R..T. (2001). Bone modeling and remodeling: theories and computation, In: *Bone Mechanics Handbook* (2nd edition), Cowin, S.C., (Ed.), 31_1-31_42, CRC Press, ISBN 0849391172, Boca Rotan, FL

Holmgren, E.P., Seckinger, R.J., Kilgren, L.M., Mante, F. (1998). Evaluating parameters of osseointegrated dental implants using finite element analysis-a two dimensional comparative study examining the effects of implant diameter, implant shape, and load direction. *The Journal of Oral Implantology*, Vol.24, No.2, pp. 80-8

Hipp, J.A., Brunski, J.B., Shephard, M.S., Cochran, G.V.B. (1985). Finite element models for implants in bone: interfacial assumptions, In: *Biomechanics, Current Interdisciplinary Research,* 447-452, E. Schneider and S.A. Perren. M. Nijhoff, (Ed.), Dordrecht, The Netherlands

Huang, H.-L, Hsu, J.-T., Fuh L.-J., Lin, D.-J. & Chen, M.Y.-C., (2010). Biomechanical simulation of various surface roughnesses and geometric designs on an immediately loaded dental implant. *Computers in Biology and Medicine*, Vol.40, No.5, pp. 525-532

Huang, S.-C. & Tsai, C.-F. (2003). Finite element analysis of a dental implant. *Biomedical Engineering: Applications, Basis and Communications*, Vol. 15, No. 2, pp. 82-85

Huiskes, R., Weinans, H., Grootenboer, H.J., Dalstra, M., Fudala, B. & Sloof, T.J. (1987). Adaptive bone remodeling theory applied to prosthetic-design analysis. *Journal of Biomechanics*, Vol. 20, No. 11-12, pp. 1135-1150, ISSN 0021-9290

Huiskes, R., Weinans, H. & van Rietbergen, B. (1992). The relationship between stress shielding and bone resorption around total hip stems and the effects of flexible materials. *Clinical Orthopaedics and Related Research*, Vol. 274, (January 1992), pp. 124-134, ISSN 0009-921X

Iplikcioglu, H., Akca, K. (2002). Comparative evaluation of the effect of diameter, length and number of implants supporting three-unit fixed partial prostheses on stress distribution in the bone. *J Dent*, Vol.30, No.1, pp. 41-46

Jaffin, R.A., Kumar, A., Berman, C.L. (2000). Immediate loading of implants in partially and fully edentulous jaws; a series of 27 case reports. *Journal of Periodontology*, Vol.71, No.5, (May 2000), pp. 833-8

Jarvis, W.C. (1996). Know when to use wide bodied implants to limit bone stress. *Dental Implantology Update*, Vol.7, No.12, (Dec 1996) pp. 89-92

Jarvis, W.C. (1997). Biomechanical advantage of wide diameter implants. *Compendium of Continuing Education In Dentistry (Jamesburg, N.J.: 1995)*, Vol.18, No.7, (Jul 1997), pp. 687-92

Kinni, M., E., Hokama, S. N., Caputo, A.A. (1987). Force transfer by osseointegration implant devices. *Int. J. Oral Maxillofac. Implants*, Vol.2, No.1, pp. 11-14

Kitoh M., Suetsugu T., Murakami Y., Tabata T. (1978). A biomathematical study on implant desing and stress distribution. *The Bulletin Of Tokyo Medical And Dental University*, Vol.25, No.4, pp. 269-76

Kong, L., Sun, Y., Hu, K., Liu, Y., Li D., & Liu, B. (2008). Selections of the cylinder implant neck taper and implant end fillet for optimal biomechanical properties: A three-dimensional finite element analysis. *Journal of Biomechanics*, Vol. 41, No. 5, pp. 1124-1130

Langer, B., Langer, L., Herrmann, I., Jorneus, L. (1993). The wide fixture: a solution for special bone situation and a rescue for the compromised implant. *The International Journal of Oral & Maxillofacial Implants*, Vol.8, No.4, pp. 400-8

Lavernia, C.J., Cook, S.D., Weinstein, A.M., Llawitter, J.J. (1981). An analysis of stresses in a dental implant system. *J. Biomech.*, Vol.14, No.8, pp. 555-60

Lavernia, C.J., Cook, S.D., Weinstein, A.M., Klawitter, J.J. (1982). The influence of the bone-implant interface on stress profiles surrounding Al_2O_3 and carbon implants. *Ann. Biomed. Engng*, Vol.10, No.3, pp. 129-38

Lazzara, R.J. (1994). Criteria for implant selection: Surgical and prosthetic considerations. *Pract Peno & Aest Dent* Vol.6, No.9, pp, 62

Lekholm U., Zarb G.A. (1985) Patient selection and preparation. In: *Tissue-integrated prostheses: osseointegration in clinical dentistry*, Brånemark P.I., Zarb G.A., Albrektsson T., (Ed.), Quintessence, Chicago, pp. 199-209

Leucht, P., Kim, J.B., Wazen, R., Currey, J.A., Nanci, A., Brunski, J.B. & Helms, J.A. (2007). Effect of mechanical stimuli on skeletal regeneration around implants. *Bone*, Vol. 40, No. 4, (April 2007), pp. 919-930, ISSN 8756-2382

Li, J., Li, H., Shi, L., Fok, A.S.L., Ucer, C., Devlin, H., Horner, K. & Silikas, N. (2007). A mathematical model for simulating the bone remodeling process under mechanical stimulus. *Dental Materials*, Vol. 23, No. 9, (November, 2006), pp. 1073-1078, ISSN 0109-5641

Li, T., Hu, K., Cheng, L., Ding, Y., Ding, Y., Shao, J. & Kong, L., (2011). Optimum selection of the dental implant diameter and length in the posterior mandible with poor bone quality - A 3D finite element analysis. *Applied Mathematical Modelling*, Vol. 35, No.1, pp. 446-456

Lian, Z., Guan, H., Ivanovski, S., Loo, Y.-C., Johnson, N.W. & Zhang, H. (2010). Effect of bone to implant contact percentage on bone to implant contact percentage on bone remodelling surrounding a dental implant. *International Journal of Oral and Maxillofacial Surgery*, Vol. 39, No. 7, (July 2010), pp. 690-698, ISSN 0901-5027

Lin, D., Li, Q., Li, W. & Swain , M. (2009a). Dental implant induced bone remodeling and associated algorithms. *Journal of the Mechanical Behavior of Biomedical Materials*, Vol. 2, No. 5, (December 2008), pp. 410-432, ISSN 1751-6161

Lin, D., Li, Q., Li, W., Zhou, S. & Swain, M.V. (2009b). Design optimization of functionally graded dental implant for bone remodeling. Composites Part B: Engineering, Vol. 40, No. 7, (October 2009), pp. 668-675, ISSN 1359-8368

Lin, D., Li, Q., Li, W., Duckmanton, N. & Swain, M. (2010). Mandibular bone remodeling induced by dental implant. *Journal of Biomechanics*, Vol. 43, No. 2, (January 2010), pp. 287-293, ISSN 0021-9290

Lin, C.-L., Lin, Y.-H. & Chang, S.-H. (2010). Multi-factorial analysis of variables influencing the bone loss of an implant placed in the maxilla: prediction using FEA and SED bone remodeling algorithm. *Journal of Biomechanics*, Vol. 43, No. 4, (November 2009), pp. 644-651, ISSN 0021-9290

Mahon, J.M., Norling, B.K., Phoenix, R.D. (2000). Effects of varying fixture width on stress and strain distribution associated with an implant stack system. *Implant Dentistry*, Vol.9, No.4, pp. 310-20

Martin, R.B. (1984). Porosity and specific surface in bone. *Critical Reviews in Biomedical Engineering*, Vol. 10, No. 3, pp. 179-222, ISSN 0278-940X

Martin, R.B., Burr, D.B. & Sharkey, N.A. (1998). *Skeletal Tissue Mechanics*. Springer, ISBN 0387984747, New York

Marx, R.E. (2007). Bone and bone graft healing. *Oral and Maxillofacial Surgery Clinics of North America*, Vol. 19, No. 4, (November 2007), pp. 455-466, ISSN 1042-3699

Meijer, H.J., Starmans, F.J., Steen, W.H., Bosman, F. (1994). A three-dimensional finite element study on two versus four implants in an edentulous mandible. *The International Journal of Prosthodontics*, Vol.7, No.3, (May-Jun 1994), pp. 217-9

Misch, C.E., Hoar, J., Beck, G., Hazen, R., Misch, C.M. (1998). A bone quality based implant system: a preliminary report of stage I & stage II. *Implant Dentistry*, Vol.7, No.1, pp. 35-42

Misch, C.E., Dietsh-Misch, F., Hoar, J., Beck, G., Hazen, R., Misch, C.M. (1999). A bone quality based implant system: first year of prosthetic loading. *The Journal of Oral Implantology*, Vol.25, No.3, pp. 185-97

Misch, C.E. (1999a). Implant design considerations for the posterior regions of the mouth. *Implant Dentistry*, Vol.8, No.4, pp. 376-86

Misch, C.E. (1999b). *Contemporary Implant Dentistry*, Mosby, St. Louis

Misch, C.E. & Bidez, M.W. (1999). A scientific rationale for dental implant design, In: *Contemporary Implant Dentistry* (2nd edition), Misch, C.E., (Ed.), 329-343, Mosby, ISBN 0815170599, St. Louis, MO

Misch, C.E., Bidez, M.W., Sharawy, M. (2001). A bioengineered implant for a predentermined bone cellular response to loading forces. *Journal of Periodontology*, Vol.72, No.9, (Sep 2001), pp. 1276-86

Morris, H.F., Winkler, S., Ochi, S., Kanaan, A. (2001). A new implant designed to maximize contact with trabecular bone: Survival to 18 months. *Journal of Oral Implantology*, Vol.27, No.4, pp. 164-173

Moscovitch, M. (2001). Molar restorations supported by 2 implants: An alternative to wide implants. J *can Dent assoc*, Vol.67, pp. 535-539

Moser, W. Nentwig, G.H. (1989). Finite Element Studien zur Optimierung von Implantat-gewindeformen. *Z Zhanarztl Implantol*, Vol.5, pp. 29-32

Munir, Z.A., Richards, L.W., Prado, M.E. (1975). Photoelastic studies of the stress distributions on blade-type endosteal dental implants. *J. Oral Implantol.*, Vol.5, No.3, pp. 296-332

Papavasiliou, G., Kamposiora, P., Bayne S.C., Felton D.A. (1996a). Three-dimensional finite element analysis of stress distribution around single tooth implants as a function of bony support, prosthesis type, and loading during function. *The Journal of Prosthetic Dentistry*, Vol.76, No.6, pp. 633-40

Papavasiliou, G., Tripodakis, A.P., Kamposiora, P., Strub, J.R., Bayne S.C. (1996b). Finite element analysis of ceramic abutment-restoration combinations for osseointegrated implants. *The International Journal of Prosthodontics*, Vol.9, No.3, (May-Jun 1996), pp. 254-60

Patra, A.K., DePaolo, J.M., D'Souza, K.S., DeTolla, D., Meenaghan, M.A. (1998). Guidelines for analysis and redesign of dental implants. *Implant Dentistry*, Vol.7, No.4, pp. 355-68

Pérez, M.A., Fornells, P., Doblaré, M. & García-Aznar, J.M. (2010). Comparative analysis of bone remdelling models with respect to computerised tomography-based finite element models of bone. Computer Methods in Biomechanics and Biomedical Engineering, Vol. 13, No. 1, (February 2010), pp. 71-80, ISSN 1476-8259

Pierrisnard, L., Hure, G., Barquins, M., Chappard, D. (2002). Two dental implants designed for immediate loading: a finite element analysis. *Int J Oral Maxillofac Implants*, Vol.17, No.3, pp. 353-362

Renouard, F., Arnous, J.P., Sarment, D.P. (1999). Five-mm-diameter implants without a smooth surface collar: Report on 98 consecutive placements. *Int J Oral Maxillofac Implants*. Vol 14:101-107

Rieger, M.R. (1988). Finite element stress analysis of root-form implants. *The Journal Of Oral Implantology*, Vol.14, No.4, pp. 472-84

Rieger, M.R., Fareed, K., Adams, W.K., Tanquist, R.A. (1989a). Bone stress distribution for three endosseous implants. *The Journal of Prosthetic Dentistry*, Vol.61, No.2, (Feb 1989), pp. 223-8

Rieger, M.R., Adams, W.K., Kinzel, G.L., Brose, M.O. (1989b). Finite element analysis of bone-adapted and bone-bonded endosseous implants, *J. Prosth. Dent*, Vol.64, No.5, pp. 436-40

Rieger, M.R., Adams, W.K., Kinzel G.L. (1990a). A finite element survey of eleven endosseous implants. *The Journal Of Prosthetic Dentistry*, Vol.63, No.4, pp. 457-65

Rieger, M.R., Mayberry, M., Brose, M.O. (1990b). Finite element analysis of six endosseous implants. *The Journal of Prosthetic Dentistry*, Vol.63, No.6, pp. 671-6

Reina, J.M., García-Aznar, J.M., Dominguez, J. & Doblaré, M. (2007). Numerical estimation of bone density and elastic constants distribution in a human mandible. *Journal of Biomechanics*, Vol. 40, No. 4, (May 2006), pp. 828-836, ISSN 0021-9290

Salama, H., Rose, L.F., Salama, M., Betts, N.J. (1995). Immediate loading of bilaterally splinted titanium root-form implants in fixed prosthodontics-a technique reexamined: two case reports. *The International Journal of Periodontics & Restorative Dentistry*, Vol.15, No.4, (August 1995), pp. 344-61

Sato, Y., Shindoi, N., Hosokawa, R., Tsuga, K., Akagawa, Y. (2000). Biomechanical effects of double or wide implants for single molar replacement in the posterior mandibular region. *Journal of Oral Rehabilitation*, Vol.27, No.10, pp. 842-5

Schenk, R.K. & Buser, D. (1998). Osseointegration: a reality. *Periodontology 2000*, Vol. 17, (Jun 1988), pp. 22-35, ISSN 1600-0757

Siegele, D., Soltesz, U. (1989). Numerical investigations of the influence of implant shape on stress distribution in the jaw bone. *The International Journal Of Oral & Maxillofacial Implants*, Vol.4, No.4, (Winter 1989), pp. 333-40

Simmons, C.A., Meguid, S.A. & Pilliar, R.M. (2001). Differences in osseointegration rate due to implant surface geometry can be explained by local tissue strains. *Journal of Orthopaedic Research*, Vol. 19, No. 2, (March 2001), pp. 187-194, ISSN 1554-527X

Skalak, R. (1988). Stress transfer at the implant interface. *J Oral Implantol*. Vol.13, pp. 531-593

Stegaroiu, R., Kusakari, H., Nishiyama, S., Miyakawa, O. (1998a). Influence of prosthesis material on stress distribution in bone and implant: a 3-dimensional finite element analysis. *The International Journal of Oral & Maxillofacial Implants*, Vol.13, No.6, (Nov-Dec 1998), pp. 781-90

Stegaroiu, R., Sato, T., Kusakari, H., Miyakawa, O. (1998b). Influence of restoration type on stress distribution in bone around implants: a three-dimensional finite element analysis. *The International Journal of Oral & Maxillofacial Implants*, Vol.13, No.1, (Jan-Feb 1998), pp. 82-90

Steinemann, S. (1996). The properties of titanium, In: *Oral implantology. Basics. ITI Dental Implant system.* A. Schroeder, F. Sutter, D. Biser, G. Drekeler, (Ed.) 37-59, Thieme Medical Publishers, New York

Tarnow, D.P., Emtiaz, S., Classi, A. (1997). Immediate loading of threaded implants at stage 1 surgery in edentulous arches: ten consecutive case reports with 1- to 5- year data.

The International Journal of Oral & Maxillofacial Implants, Vol.12, No.3, (May-June 1997), pp. 319-24

Trauhlar, R.S., Farish, S.E., Scheitler,L.E., Morris, H.F., Ochi, S. (1997). Bone quality and implant design-related outcomes through stage II surgical uncovering of spectra-system root form implants. *J Oral Maxillofac Surg*. Vp;/ 55, pp. 46-54

Tuncelli, B., Poyrazoglu, E., Köylüoglu, A.M., Tezcan, S. (1997). Comparison of load transfer by angulated, standard and inclined implant abutments. *The European Journal Of Prosthodontics And Restorative Dentistry*, Vol.5, No.2, (Jun 1997), pp. 85-8

Vaillancourt, H., Pilliar, R.M., McCammond, D. (1995). Finite element analysis of crestal bone loss around porous coated dental implants. *Journal of Applied Biomaterials*. Vol.6, No.4, pp. 267-282

Van Oosterwyck, H., Duyck, J., Vander Sloten, J., Van Der Perre, G., Naert, I. (2002). Peri-implant bone tissue strains in cases of dehiscence: a finite element study. *Clin oral Implants Res 2002*, Vol.13, No.3, pp. 327-333

Watzak, G., Zechner, W., Ulm, C., Tangl, S., Tepper, G. & Watzek, G. (2005). Histologic and histomorphometric analysis of three types of dental implants following 18 months of occlusal loading: a preliminary study in baboons. *Clinical Oral Implants Research*, Vol. 16, No. 4, (August 2005), pp. 408-416, ISSN 1600-0501

Weinans, H., Huiskes, R., & Grootenboer, H.J. (1992). Effects of material properties of femoral hip components on bone remodeling, *Journal of Orthopaedic Research*, Vol. 10, No. 6, (November 1992), pp. 845-853, ISSN 1554-527X

Weinans, H., Huiskes, R., van Rietbergen, B., Sumner, D.R., Turner, T.M. & Galante, J.O. (1993). Adaptive bone remodeling around bonded noncemented total hip arthroplasty: a comparison between animal experiments and computer simulation. *Journal of Orthopaedic Research*, Vol. 11, No. 4, (July 1993), pp. 500-513, ISSN 1554-527X

Weinstein A.M., Klawitter J.J., Anand S.C., Schuessler R. (1976). Stress analysis of porous rooted dental implants. *Journal Of Dental Research*, Vol.55, No.5, (Sep-Oct 1976), pp. 772-7

Wolff, J. (1892). *Das Gesetz der Transformation der Knochen*, Hirschwald, Berlin

Wolff, J. (1986). *The Law of Bone Remodelling*, Springer, ISBN 354016281X, Berlin

7

Titanium: A New Allergen

Laurence Evrard
Stomatology and Maxillo-facial Surgery Department
Hopital Erasme – ULB Brussels
Belgium

1. Introduction

Buccal allergies represent a growing problem and often go undiagnosed by health professionals. There is an increase in the prevalence of oral allergies to dental materials, and especially to metals used in dental materials.

Titanium, used in orthopaedic devices and oral implants, although considered an inert material, can actually induce toxicity or allergic type I or IV reactions.

Cases of an allergy to titanium described in the literature reflect the difficulty in the diagnosis of this allergy. In case of a suspected contact allergy, epicutaneous patch tests can be done, which consist of applying the allergens which are to be tested to the patient's back. These tests are known to have a diagnostic efficiency of 75% for metal allergy, and can therefore underdiagnose a titanium sensitization or allergy. Blood tests which can be used for the diagnosis of allergies are based on lymphoblastic transformation. They are more sensitive than patch tests, but sometimes lack specificity.

The occurrence of an allergy to titanium could be responsible for successive unexplained cases of failure of dental implants in some patients (known as "cluster patients"). It has been reported that the risk of an allergy to titanium is increased in patients who are allergic to other metals.

In these patients, an allergy evaluation is recommended, in order to exclude any problem with titanium dental implants.

1.1 Types of allergies

The term "allergy" is used to define a specific immune reaction to one or more exogenic substances (allergens).

Four types of allergies have been described. For a review see Gell and Coombs, 1963.

Type I allergy, known as immediate sensitivity, is characterized by interactions between an allergen and IgE present on the surface of mastocytes inducing histamine and other vasopeptide leakage. This is sometimes associated with atopy. This type of allergy may manifest clinically by acute reaction of anaphylaxis, which can represent a life-threatening condition. Type I allergy also causes urticarial reactions on the skin, in the form of erythematous plaques or papules, accompanied by pruritus or tingling sensations.

Type II allergy, known as cytotoxic, or antibody-dependent hypersensitivity, consists of an autoimmune cytotoxic reaction involving IgG and IgM and is encountered, for example, in acute transplant rejection or autoimmune haemolytic anaemia.

Type III allergy, or immune complex disease, is due to precipitation of immune complex formed by antigen-IgG in the blood vessel walls and can induce vasculitic lesions, manifesting in the form of the Arthus reaction, glomerulonephritis associated with streptococcal throat infection or systemic lupus erythematosus.

Type IV allergy, known as delayed-type hypersensitivity, or cell-mediated immune memory response, antibody-independent or contact allergy, is by far the most frequent type of allergy. It is defined as a cell-mediated delayed sensitization reaction (mediated by Langerhans cells and T-lymphocytes), and occurs after exposure to allergens for between ten days and several years. Type IV sensitization is induced by repeated contact of an allergen with skin or mucosa, and follows several steps (Figure 1). In the first step, a hapten penetrates through the skin or through the epithelium of the mucosa, and combines with endogenous proteins to form an antigenic molecule: the allergen. This allergen is captured by the Langerhans cells, which present it to the T-lymphocytes, which become sensitized and thereafter carry on their surface a specific receptor to the allergen. These lymphocytes are known as "memory lymphocytes", and are able to recognize the allergen. Following another contact, the allergen binds to the specific receptor of the memory lymphocytes, which multiply and produce a set of cytokines. An allergic cellular inflammatory reaction takes place within 48 to 72 hours, and is responsible for the clinical manifestations of type IV allergy (Axell, 2001, Grevers and Röcken, 2002, Gawrodger, 2005). Type IV allergy is more frequently encountered in the skin than in the oral mucosa. This has been explained by the fact that Langerhans cells are about ten times more numerous in the layers underlying the skin than in those underlying the oral mucosa. Another reason is the rich network of capillary vessels which characterizes oral mucosa vascularization and which, in turn, eliminates the allergens more quickly from the area (Forte et al, 2008). Clinically, it may manifest as chronic transplant rejection, or more often as chronic dermatitis (eczema).

Allergy types I, III and IV may manifest in the orofacial region (Axell, 2001, Grevers, 2002, Gawkrodger, 2005).

A hapten penetrates skin or mucosa and combines with endogenous proteins to form an allergen. Langerhans cells capture the allergen, and present it to the T-lymphocytes, which become sensitized and thereafter carry on their surface a specific receptor to the allergen. These lymphocytes are known as "memory lymphocytes".

1.2 Clinical manifestations of an allergy in the orofacial region

Patients with an oral allergy complain of various symptoms such as burning or tingling sensations, with or without swelling, oral dryness or loss of taste (Garhammer et al, 2001, Lygre et al, 2003, Gawrodger 2005), or sometimes more general symptoms such as headache, dyspepsia, asthenia, arthralgia, myalgia (Lygre et al, 2003, Vamnes et al, 2004).

The signs of an oral allergy include erythema of the oral mucosa, labial oedema or purpuric patches on the palate, mouth ulcers, hyperplastic gingivitis, areas of depapillation on the tongue, angular cheilitis, perioral eczematous eruption, or lichenoid reactions localized on the oral mucosa (Alanko et al, 1996, Leigh et al, 2001, Vamnes et al, 2004).

Type I allergy may manifest clinically in the orofacial region, in the acute form by Quincke's oedema, characterized by swelling, which, if it involves the upper respiratory tract, can become life-threatening for the patient. In serious forms, it gives rise to urticarial reactions and/or tingling sensations or pruritus, localized in the oral or pharyngeal cavity (Axell, 2001, Grevers and Röcken, 2002, Gawrodger, 2005).

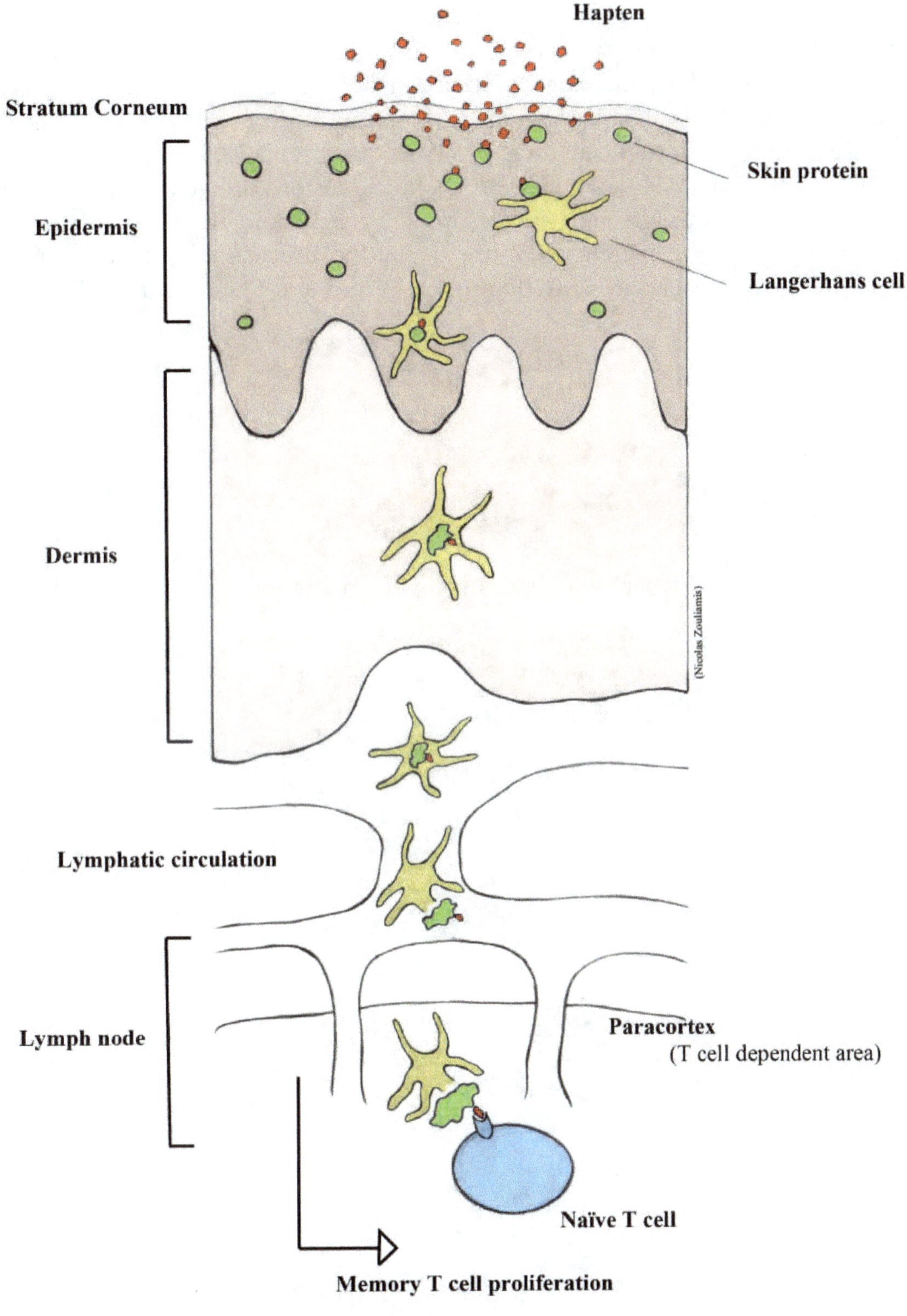

Fig. 1. Development of type IV sensitivity.

Type III allergy in the buccal area can take the form of aphthous ulcerations of the oral mucosa or, in more serious cases, the form of erythema multiforme, with large ulcerations of the oral mucosa found in association with typical skin lesions "en cocarde" (Axell, 2001, Grevers and Röcken, 2002, Gawrodger, 2005).

Type IV allergy is by far the most frequent allergy encountered in the orofacial region (Gawkrodger, 2005). This type IV allergy may manifest clinically by eczema, angular cheilitis, cheilitis (Figure 2), erythema of the oral mucosa, hyperplastic gingivitis (Figure 3), lichenoid reactions of the oral mucosa (Figure 4), perioral dermatitis or a loss of lingual papillae that can mimic "geographical tongue" (Waroquier et al, 2009) (Figure 5) (Vamnes et al., 2004, Leigh et al., 2001, Alanko et al., 1996). Clinical lesions are generally localized next to structures containing the allergen, as illustrated by lichenoid reactions just in front of amalgam fillings containing mercury (Figure 6), or the mucosa of the palate next to a prosthesis containing methacrylate resin (Figure 7) (Evrard and Parent, 2010).

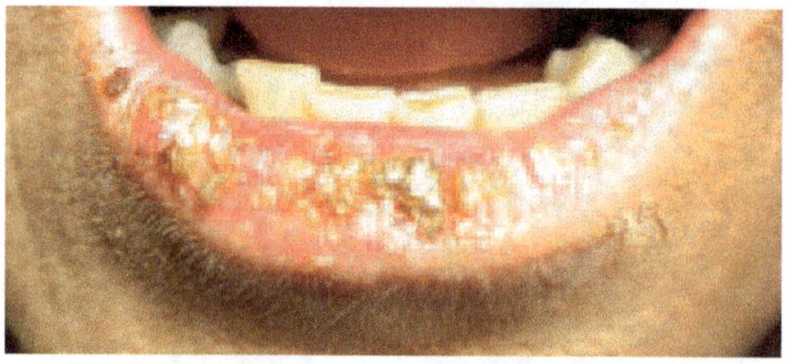

Fig. 2. Contact cheilitis in a patient who has developed an allergy to a component of her lipstick.

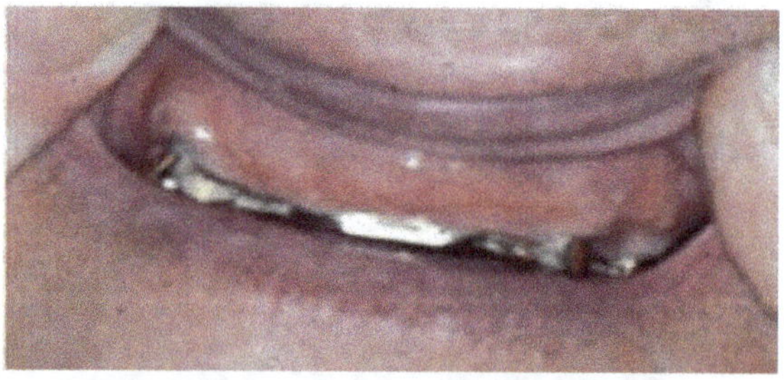

Fig. 3. Hyperplastic gingivitis associated with a contact allergy to gold. There is a prosthetic gold bar in the upper jaw.

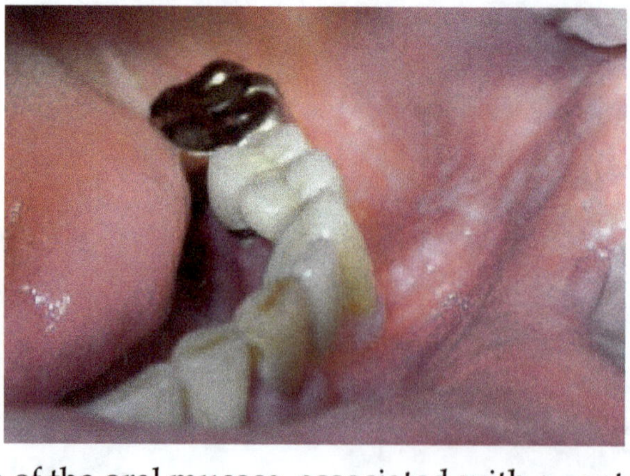

Fig. 4. Lichenoid reaction of the oral mucosa, associated with a contact allergy to gold. The patient has a gold crown on tooth 36.

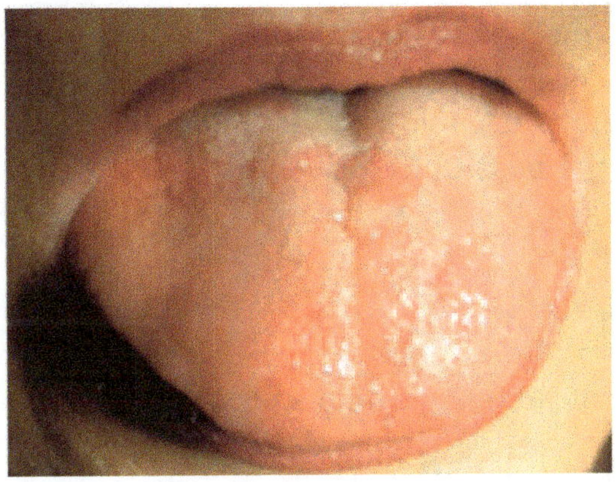

Fig. 5. Depapillation of the tongue, mimicking a geographical tongue, associated with a contact allergy to mercury and gold.

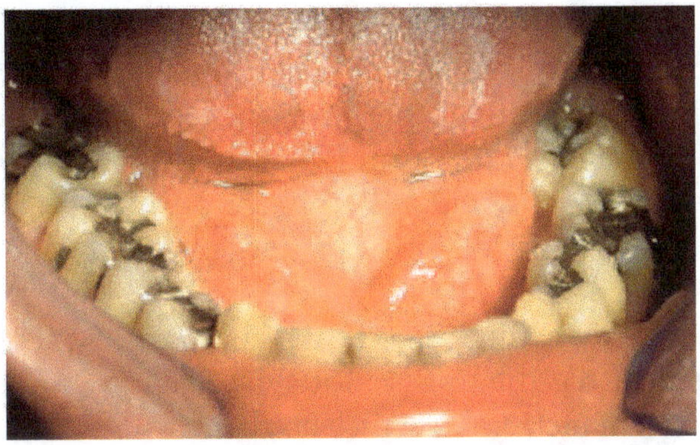

Fig. 6. Lichenoid reactions on the mucosa of the tongue, associated with a contact allergy to mercury. The patient has amalgam filling in his teeth.

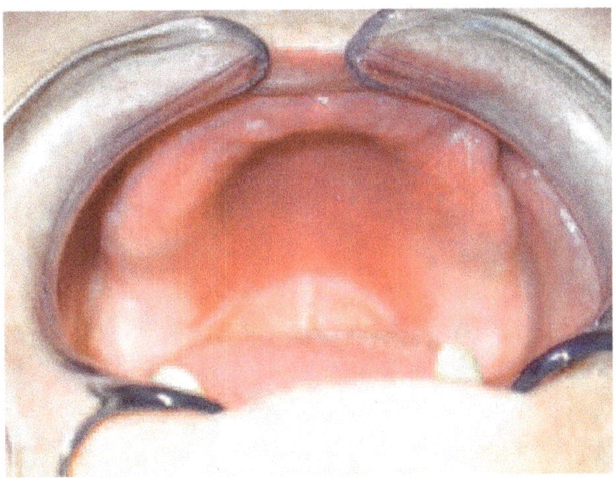

Fig. 7. Erythema of the palate in the area in contact with a resin prosthesis, in association with a contact allergy to methyl methacrylate.

In type IV allergy, patients complain of burning or tingling sensations of the oral mucosa, sometimes of dryness of the mouth, or a metallic taste (Lygre et al., 2003, Gawkrodger, 2005). Burning sensations ("burning mouth") can reach a frequency of 72% in patients with a contact allergy to dental materials (Garhammer et al, 2001, Waroquier et al, 2007). Other causes can give rise to the same signs and symptoms as those found in allergy; in such cases it is necessary, when faced with burning sensations and/or erythematous patches on the oral mucosa, to exclude metabolic causes such as iron, B12 or folate deficiency by doing a blood test, and to rule out the possibility of a fungal infection, taking a swab of the lesion and culturing it, before going on to allergy testing.

1.3 Diagnostic tests for allergy

The diagnosis of a contact/type IV allergy is typically based on the patient's medical record, clinical findings and the results of epicutaneous tests.

Epicutaneous tests are known as "patch tests". The principle is to apply different allergens which are to be tested on the patient's back. The results are read after 48 and 72 hours for most allergens, and also after 10 days for gold testing (because gold can give rise to late reactions). If the test is positive for an allergen, the area of skin corresponding to the tested allergen will show an eczematous reaction: erythema and/or vesicles and pruritus (Alanko et al, 1996, Grevers and Röcken, 2002, Gawrodger, 2005). There is a limit to the utility of patch tests, given their poor sensitivity, which has been shown to be about 75% for type IV metal allergy (Forte et al, 2008). Some authors report a lack of standardization in the patch tests, especially for allergens such as titanium (Fischer, 2008, Forte et al, 2008). According to these authors, patch tests have been validated only for dermal sensitization to allergens, and their relevance for systemic sensitization to allergens such as titanium (mucosal and internal) is limited.

Thus, patch test may underestimate the real prevalence of a metal allergy.

Skin tests (prick tests) help in the diagnosis of a type I allergy. They consist of intradermal inoculation of the antigen (Yamauci et al, 2000). The results are read within 15 to 30 minutes. If the test is positive, there will be a red, papular and/or vesicular reaction of the skin. Prick tests are not routinely done for the diagnosis of an oral allergy to a dental material, because most of the reactions to dental material are Type IV. Nevertheless, prick tests are used in the diagnosis of a food allergy, which may manifest by aphthous lesions of the oral mucosa (Scully, 2004).

A blood test can help in the diagnosis of a type IV allergy. *In vitro* testing with the lymphocyte transformation test (LTT) can detect both dermally and non-dermally (mucosal) sensitizing allergens. It has been used to detect hypersensitivity leading to both local and systemic effects resulting from dental allergies, in particular in the optimized version of LTT known as MELISA (Stjekstal et al, 1994, Muller and Valentine-Thon, 2006). The patient's lymphocytes are exposed to the allergen to be tested. If they have previously been sensitized to the allergen, they will undergo proliferation, which is measured using incorporation of radioactive nucleotides (tritiated thymidine). Some authors have reported that non-relevant proliferation of lymphocytes could happen in non-sensitized patients (Fisher's, 2008), leading to some false-positive results.

It would be valuable in the future to have a test that would respond with good sensitivity and good specificity, thus providing a better diagnostic tool.

2. Allergy to dental materials

There are various dental materials that have been shown to be capable of triggering an allergic reaction in the oral cavity, and contain metals (nickel, cobalt, chromium, gold, palladium, mercury), fragrances (balsam of Peru, fragrance mix, eugenol, cinnamic aldehyde, essential oils), topical medicines (including some synthetic steroids), preservatives, resins, colourings and other products contained in toothpastes (Lesueur and Lannias, 2003, Evrard and Parent 2010).

It has been shown that dental materials can give rise to type I, type III or type IV hypersensitivity. In type IV allergy, which is by far the most frequent type encountered in the oral cavity, signs and symptoms can appear between a few days and several years after the beginning of contact with the allergen (Gawrodger 2005, Vamnes et al, 2004, Garhammer et al, 2001, Lesueur and Yiannias, 2003, Evrard and Parent, 2010).

2.1 Dental metals involved in oral allergy

In the field of dentistry, dental metals are used in precious and non-precious alloys, for producing removable or fixed prostheses, or dental fillings. Titanium is used for its excellent biocompatibility in implantology and maxillo-facial surgery and will be the subject of Chapter 3.

Metals contained in dental alloys may corrode in an electrolytic solution such as saliva. Corrosion will be greater in the case of multiple metals, given the electric potential difference induced following contact between different metals (Messer and Wahata, 2002) (Figure 6).

It has been described that the mercury contained in amalgam dental fillings and gold used in alloys for fixed prostheses can give rise to allergic reactions, in the form of lichenoid reactions of the oral mucosa (Koch and Bahmer, 1999, Yiannias et al, 2000, Laine et al, 1997, Evrard and Parent 2010). In a study on 19 patients with lichenoid reactions of the oral mucosa in the vicinity of amalgam fillings (Koch and Bahmer, 1999), it has been shown that 78.9% of patients proved to be sensitized to mercury and that the removal of dental amalgams allowed healing of the mucosal lesions in 86% of cases. In another study on 46 patients with an oral lichen planus (Yiannias et al, 2000), 14 patients had an epicutaneous test positive to gold. In this study, after removal of gold from the mouth, the oral lichen planus disappeared in 10 patients out of 14. Another study on 118 patients with lichenoid lesions in the mouth (Laine et al, 1997), shows that 80 of them had a contact allergy (type IV allergy) to one or more metals: 78 to mercury, 11 to gold, 17 to nickel, 4 to cobalt, 3 to tin, 2 to palladium and 1 to chromium.

All the authors point out that healing of the lesions takes place in a large number of cases after removal of amalgam dental fillings or prostheses containing gold, in the case of a diagnosed contact allergy to mercury or gold (Lygre et al, 2003, Koch and Bahmer, 1999, Yiannias et al, 2000, Laine et al, 1997, Evrard and Parent 2010).

Cobalt is a metal used in alloys in removable or fixed prostheses, and represents a known allergen giving rise to oral manifestations in the case of an allergy (Forte et al, 2008). In a recent study (Waroquier et al, 2009), it has been shown that the burning sensations and intense pruritus on a geographical tongue were due to the cobalt contained in the hook of a removable resin prosthesis replacing a tooth 51 lost through trauma in a 7-year-old child. In this case, type IV allergy had been diagnosed by a positive patch test to cobalt. After removal of the hook containing cobalt, all the patient's signs and symptoms had disappeared.

Burning sensations represent a frequent complaint in patients allergic to one or more dental metals (Alanko et al, 1996). Our team conducted a pilot study to try and establish the prevalence of oral allergies to dental materials in patients complaining of burning sensations of the oral mucosa (Warroquier et al, 2007). In this study, other causes of burning sensations were excluded by a blood test (in order to rule out a metabolic disturbance such as iron, B12 or folate deficiency), and by swabbing and culture, in order to rule out a fungal infection. Allergy testing revealed that, among that population of 26 "burning mouth" patients, 34.6% were allergic to nickel, 19% to chromium, 11.5% to gold, 11.5% to cobalt and 7.7% to mercury. Only 11.5% of the patients did not display a positive result for an allergy to any of the metals tested. These results are about three times higher than the known percentages of allergies to metals in the general European population, which have been reported to be 20% for nickel, 5.4% for chromium, 6% for gold, 6.5% for cobalt and 2.9% for mercury (Forte et al, 2008).

In a study on 294 patients complaining of both general and local signs (including burning sensations of the oral mucosa), epicutaneous tests have shown an allergy to nickel in 28% of the patients, to gold in 23%, to cobalt in 14%, to palladium in 9% and to mercury in 6% of cases.

All these studies show that the prevalence of allergies to metals in patients presenting signs or symptoms of an oral allergy is higher than the prevalence of allergies in a general European population.

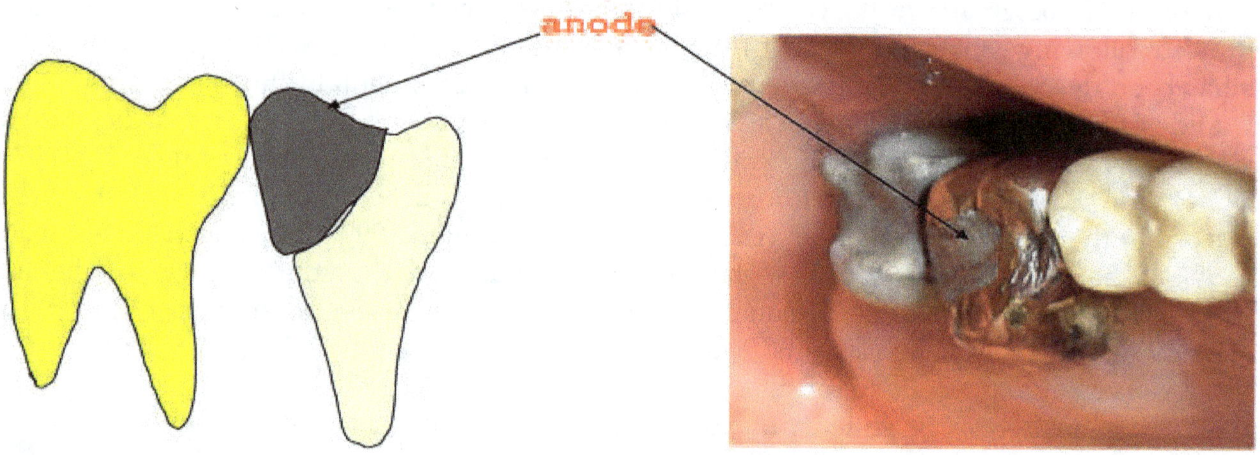

Fig. 6. Multiple metals in contact with each other.

Gold alloy in contact with silver amalgam restoration. The silver amalgam represents the anode pole, and gold alloy the cathode pole. There is an electric potential difference, and electrolytic corrosion within the electrolytic saliva solution may occur.

3. Titanium: a metal allergen of growing significance

Titanium is a metal used in medical and dental fields, because of its properties of strength, corrosion resistance behaviour and excellent biocompatibility due to the formation of an oxide layer on its surface (Steinemann, 2000). In oral and maxillofacial surgery, titanium alloys are used for ostheosynthesis plates used in traumatology or maxillofacial surgery, and for dental implants. In implantology, titanium is used most often in the form of "commercially pure" titanium (cpTi: grade I to IV alloys). CpTi contains trace elements (N, C, H, Fe, O, Al, V), that can represent 1% of its volume, and can enhance its mechanical properties and resistance to fracture (Steinemann, 2000, Messer and Wahata, 2002, Geetha et al, 2009). In implantology, titanium is used also in the form of an alloy (grade V titanium): Ti-6Al-4V, Nitinol (Ti-Ni), Ti-Co (Geetha et al, 2009) or titanium-zirconium, especially in cases where narrow implants are recommended (Evrard and Atash, 2009).

The insertion of titanium dental implants can cause internal exposure, and it has been proved that concentrations of 100-300 ppm titanium can be observed in tissues surrounding implants, as well as in regional lymph nodes and pulmonary tissue (Wennerberg et al, 2004). Under unfavourable conditions: acidic pH occurring in a peri-implantitis for example, or excessive mechanical forces on the implant, or close contact of the implant with another metal (amalgam, gold alloy), titanium may corrode and release titanium ions or microparticles of titanium in the area of bone surrounding the implant, which can induce inflammation in affected tissues (Messer and Wataha, 2002). It has been suggested that this mechanism may play a role in loosening orthopaedic endoprostheses (Nakashima et al, 1999), but it has not yet been demonstrated as a factor in the failure of dental implants. Titanium has also been reported to activate macrophages, which may secrete cytokines involved in various disease processes (Muller and Valentine-Thon, 2006). Titanium has a high affinity for proteins, and titanium ions (haptens) released by corrosion may combine with endogenous proteins to form antigenic molecules, captured by Langerhans cells, presented to T-lymphocytes, which in turn can cause the patient to be sensitized to titanium. People are exposed to titanium through environmental sources. Numerous devices such as watches, jewellery and spectacle frames are made of titanium alloy. Most environmental exposure to titanium results from exposure to TiO2 (E171), which is used in cosmetics such as sunscreens, make-up and deodorants, and in food, medicines or toothpaste. It has been shown that our body can contain a concentration of 50 ppm of titanium (Forte et al, 2008). From then on, sensitization to titanium is possible, through environmental sources, and not necessarily from previous contact with dental implants.

3.1 Allergy to titanium

The first cases in which delayed sensitivity to titanium was suspected, with a local granulomatous reaction, have been described in patients wearing a cardiac pacemaker (Peeters et al, 1984, Yamauchi, 2000). In these cases, the diagnosis of a titanium allergy was made with, respectively, a positive patch test with a little square of the pacemaker placed in artificial perspiration (Peeters et al, 1984), and a positive intra-dermal reaction to an eluate of the surface of the pacemaker (Yamauchi et al, 2000).

More recently, a well documented case of type IV allergy to titanium contained in an osteosynthesis plate inserted for a fracture of the hand was described. The patient had developed eczema on the hand within a few weeks of the insertion of the plate, and an absence of bone healing. A lymphoblastic transformation blood test (LTT) proved positive, although the patch test for TiO2 was negative. Following the removal of the plate, the LTT gave negative results and the eczema disappeared (Thomas et al, 2006).

Admittedly, it may be difficult to extrapolate results in cases of dental and orthopaedic implants. The skin and the oral mucosa behave differently regarding their potential to develop an allergic reaction (the number of Langerhans cells is greater in skin, the vascular network is more highly developed in the oral mucosa, and the latter is less permeable to antigens). Moreover, implant prosthetic abutments are coated in the mouth with glycoproteins which act as a protective barrier hampering contact between the metal and the mucosa, and the intraosseous contact surface is smaller in dental implants than in orthopaedic ones (Fischer, 2008). In orthopaedic allergy cases, biopsies generally reveal a granulomatous reaction, with numerous macrophages in the vicinity of the prosthesis. This is not the case with dental implants, and different immunological mechanisms may be involved in the two cases (Messer and Wataha, 2002, Nakashima et al, 1999, Muller and Valentine-Thon, 2006).

The case of a patient with facial eczema suggestive of type IV allergy to titanium following the placement of a mandibular dental implant has been reported (Egusa et al, 2008). In this case, an allergy to titanium was diagnosed by the combination of clinical signs (appearance of eczema within a few weeks of implant placement), and a positive blood test (LTT). The diagnosis of allergy to titanium was confirmed by the disappearance of eczema following removal of the implants.

More recently, it has been demonstrated that clinically-relevant hypersensitivity to titanium can occur following exposure to titanium (Muller and Valentine-Thon, 2006). In that study, 56 patients had developed severe health problems (muscle and joint pain, chronic fatigue syndrome, neurological problems, depression, or acne-like facial inflammation) after receiving Ti-based dental implants, orthodontic braces or endoprostheses. The authors used the MELISA test, which had proved effective in the diagnosis of hypersensitivity to metals (Stejskal et al, 1994), as well as patch tests. Of the 56 patients tested with MELISA, 37.5% were positive, 28.5% ambiguous and 33.9% negative to titanium. Among the 33.9% negative to titanium, 57.9% showed lymphocyte reactivity to nickel or other metals. All 54 patch-tested patients were negative to titanium. Following removal of the implants, a remarkable clinical improvement was noticed and among the 15 retested patients this clinical improvement correlated with normalisation of MELISA reactivity.

In a prospective study over a three-year period (Sicilia et al, 2008), 1500 patients with dental implants were monitored. In that study, an allergy to titanium was diagnosed on the basis of clinical signs of an allergy appearing following implant placement, or on the basis of an unexplained failure of the implant, and a patch test positive for titanium, tested in the form TiO2, or for a titanium metal powder in aqueous solution. The results of this study show that 0.6% (1/800) of patients with dental implants have a patch-test positive for titanium, but 0% (0/35) of the patients without implants have this result. The epicutaneous tests are positive in 50% (8/16) and 62.8% (5/8) of the patients who show signs, respectively, of an allergy following implant placement, and unexplained early failure of one or more implants. In patients having allergies to one or more metals (nickel, chromium, cobalt, gold or mercury), 5.3% (1/19) have a patch test positive for titanium. It should be noted that the authors do not report the characteristics of the titanium in their patients (titanium alloy or commercially pure titanium?). The rate of corrosion is higher with titanium-aluminium-vanadium implants, which may have an influence on the prevalence of allergic reactions.

All these reports reflect the difficulty in evaluating suspected titanium hypersensitivity. It is known that the epicutaneous tests used in the diagnosis of an allergy to titanium are still not very sensitive, and there is no standardized valid patch-test preparation for this. Moreover, the lack of concordance between the results of patch-tests and blood tests (MELISA) is illustrated in the above study (Muller and Valentine-Thon, 2006). Given the difficulties of diagnosing a titanium allergy, studies probably underestimate the true prevalence of titanium allergies in patients having dental implants.

3.2 Diagnosis of a titanium allergy

The above studies demonstrate that titanium can induce clinically relevant hypersensitivity and other immune dysfunctions in certain patients chronically exposed to this metal. Titanium should no longer, therefore, be considered biologically inert. In implantology, it is reasonable to say that allergy testing for titanium is indicated in some cases.

3.2.1 Before implant placement

It has been shown that many patients suffer from multiple allergies (Forte et al, 2008), and that people with a history of allergy to metals or jewellery have a greater risk of developing a hypersensitivity reaction to a metal implant (Hallab et al, 2001).

Furthermore, although titanium allergy has a low prevalence rate, for patients with a previous history of allergies, it may be advisable to carry out a metal allergy assessment and allergy testing before placing permanent implants, in order to avoid a failure of the implant due to an allergic reaction to titanium.

3.2.2 After implant placement

The failure of implants has been widely studied, and the main causes of dental implant failure are infection and overload (Esposito et al, 1999a, 1999b, 1999c). However, some failures are difficult to explain, such as spontaneous rapid exfoliation of the implant, or the successive failure of implants in the same patients, known as "cluster phenomenon", without any infection or overload risk factor identified. Authors agree that in these cases, there must be a systemic determinant of failure that has not been identified or understood (Wood and Vermilyea, 2004, Chuang, 2005).

An allergic reaction can be reasonably suspected after dental implant placement, on the basis of signs or symptoms associated with allergy, such as rash, urticaria, pruritus, swelling in the orofacial region, oral or facial erythema, eczematous lesions of the cheeks, or hyperplastic lesions of soft tissue (the peri-implant mucosa) (Mitchel et al, 1990). In these cases, allergy testing should be performed.

3.2.3 Tests available for the diagnosis of an allergy to titanium

As described in chapter 3.2, there is no consensus on how a sensitization and/or allergic reaction to titanium should be explored. It is also difficult to compare the results from different studies related to titanium allergies, because some refer to the use of patch tests, while others use prick tests and/or blood tests (LTT, MELISA) (Sicilia et al, 2008, Valentine-Thon et al, 2006).

To date, no standard patch test for titanium has so far been developed, and positive reactions to titanium have only rarely been demonstrated with skin testing (Forte et al, 2008).

The sensitivity of patch tests has been shown to be about 75% for type IV metal allergy. Some authors have suggested that 0.1% and 0.2% titanium sulphate solution and 0.1% and 0.2% titanium chloride are successful reagents for the skin-patch tests and could be a valuable alternative to the titanium oxide normally used for patch testing (Okamura et al, 1999), but so far no study related to dental implants allergies has used the method.

The MELISA test has been validated to detect sensitization to titanium and other metals (Sjekstal et al, 1999, Muller and Valentine-Thon 2006), but there can be some lack of specificity in lymphocyte proliferation.

It would be valuable to have a sensitive and specific test that could help in the diagnosis of titanium sensitization or allergy.

3.2.4 Future prospects in the diagnosis of sensitization or allergy to titanium

Interleukin-17 and Interleukin-22 are produced by a subset of a recently defined T-cell line, known as Th-17. IL-17 has been associated with many inflammatory diseases in humans, including rheumatoid arthritis, organ rejection and asthma. It has been showed that the number of Th-17 cells and the expression of IL-17 was significantly increased in positive patch test biopsies, regardless of the nature of the antigen (Oboki et al, 2008, Zhao et al, 2009, Larsen et al, 2009).

IL-22 is a critical mediator in mucosal host defence, which has complex pro-inflammatory and anti-inflammatory and autoimmune effects. It has been shown that patients with contact dermatitis to nickel had a significantly higher IL-22 blood level, compared with control (Ricciardi et al, 2009), indicating a possible involvement of IL-22 in the pathogenesis of human allergic contact dermatitis.

It would be interesting to develop a blood test, based on the measurement of the production of IL-17 and/or IL-22 by lymphocytes, in order to be able to diagnose with certainty a sensitization to titanium.

Our team is currently trying to develop a technique, using flow cytometry, for the purpose of detecting the activation of lymphocytes stimulated by a metal, and measuring different mediators (cytokines, inflammatory mediators) released in response to the metal.

4. References

Alanko K., Kanerva L., Jolanki R., Kannas L. & Estlander T. *Oral mucosal diseases investigated by patch testing with a dental screening series.* Contact Dermatitis, 1996; 34 (4):263-267.

Axell T. *Hypersensitivity of the oral mucosa: clinics and pathology.* Acta Odontol. Scand.2001, 59:315-319.

Chuang S., Cai T., Douglass C., Wei L. & Dodson T. *Frailty approach for the analysis of clustered failure time observation in dental research.* J.Dent Res., 2005; 84: 54-58.

Egusa H., Ko N., Shimazu T. & Yatani H. *Suspected association of an allergic reaction with titanium dental implants: a clinical report.* J. Prosthet Dent. 2008, 100: 344-7.

Esposito M., Hirsch J., Lekholm U. & Thomsen P. *Differential diagnosis and treatment strategies for biologic complications and failing oral implants: a review of the literature.* Int J. Oral Maxillofac. Impl. 1999; 14: 473-90.

Esposito M., Lausmaa J;, Hirsch J; & Thomsen P. *Surface analysis of failed oral titanium implants.* J. Biomed. Mater res. 1999; 48: 559-68.

Esposito M., Thomsen P., Ericson L. & Lekholm U. *Histopathologic observations on early oral implant failures.* Int J Oral Maxillofac Impl. 1999, 14: 798-810

Evrard L. & Atash R. *Restauration de l'édentation complète mandibulaire dans le cas d'une crête osseuse fine, à l'aide de deux implants de faible diamètre en alliage Titane-Zircone stabilisant une prothèse en résine par l'intermédiaire de deux attachements Locator.* Dentist News, 2009, 19: 14-19

Evrard L., Waroquier D. & Parent D. *Allergies to dental metals. Titanium: a new allergen.* Rev. Med. Brux. 2010, 31: 44-9

Evrard L. & Parent D. *Oral allergies to dental materials. Review of the literature and report of three cases.* Bull. Group Int Rech Stomatol. Odontol., 2010; 49: 14-19

Fischer 's. *Allergy.* Eds. Spinger-Verlag. 2008: 684-5.

Forte G., Petrucci F. & Bocca B. *Metal allergens of growing significance: epidemiology, immunotoxicology, strategies for testing and prevention.* Inflammation and Allergy, 2008, 7: 1-18

Garhammer P., Schmalz G., Hiller K., Reitinger T. & Stolz W. *Patients with local adverse effects from dental alloys: frequency, complaints, symptoms, allergy*. Clin. Oral Invest. 2001;5:240-249.

Gawkrodger D J. *Investigation of reactions to dental materials*. Br. J. Dermatol.2005; 153:479-485.

Geetha M., Singh AK., Asokamani R. & Gogia AK. *Ti based biomaterials, the ultimate choice for orthopedic implants – A review*. Prog Mater Sci, 2009, 10: 1-29

Gell P. & Coombs R., *The classification of allergic reactions underlying disease*. In: R.R.A. Coombs and P.G.H. Gell, Editors, *Clinical Aspects of Immunology*, Blackwell Science (1963).

Grevers G. & Röcken M. *Atlas de poche d'allergologie*. 2002. Flammarion Médecine-Sciences.

Axell T. *Hypersensitivity of the oral mucosa: clinics and pathology*. Acta Odontol. Scand.2001;59:315-319.

Hallab M., Mikecz K., Vermes C., Skipor A. & Jacobs J. *Differential lymphocyte reactivity to serum-derived metal-protein complexes produced from cobalt-based and titanium-based implant alloy degradation*. J. Biomed Mater. Res. 2001; 56: 427-36.

Koch P. & Bahmer F. *Oral lesions and symptoms related to metals used in dental restorations: A clinical, allergological, and histological study*. J. Am. Acad. Dermatol. 1999; 41:422-430.

Laine J., Kalimo K. & Happonen RP. *Contact allergy to dental restorative materials in patients with oral lichenoid lesions*. Contact Dermatitis. 1997;36:141-146.

Larsen J., Bonefeld C., Poulsen S. & Geisler C. *IL-23 and IL-17-mediated inflammation in human allergic contact dermatitis*. J Allergy Clin Immunol. 2009; 123: 486-492

Leigh AS., Fowler JR., Morgan W. & Looney SW. *Dental metal allergy in patients with oral, cutaneous and genital lichenoid reactions*. Am. J. Contact Dermatitis. 2001;12 (3):146-150.

LeSueur BW. & Yiannias AJ. *Contact stomatitis*. Dermatol. Clin 2003;21:105-114.

Yiannias JA., el-Azhari RA., Hand JH., Pakzad SY. & Roger RS. *Relevant contact sensitivities in patients with the diagnosis of oral lichen planus*. J. Am Acad. Dermatol. 2000;42:177-182.

Lygre G. B., Gjerdet N. R., Grönningstraeter A. G. & Björkman L. *Reporting on adverse reactions to dental materials: intraoral observations at a clinical follow-up*. Community Dent Oral Epidemiol. 2003;31:200-206.

Messer & Wahata. *Dental materials: biocompatibility. In Encyclopedia of Materials: Science and Technology*. 2002. ISBN: 0-08-043152-6. pp 1-10

Müller K. & Valentine-Thon E. *Hypersensitivity to titanium: clinical and laboratory evidence*. Neuro Endocrinol Lett, 2006, 27: 31-35

Nakashima Y., Sun D., Trindade M., Maloney W., Goodman S. & Schurman D. *Signaling pathways for tumor necrosis – a and interleukin-6 expression in human macrophages exposed to titanium alloy particulate debris in vitro*. J Bone Joint Surg. 1999; 81: 603-15.

Oboki K., Ohno T., Saito H. & Nakae S. *Th17 and allergy*. Allergology International. 2008; 57: 121-134

Okamura T., Morimoto M,. Fukushima D. & Yamane G. J Dent res. 1999; 78: 1135.

Peeters MS., Schroeter AL., Van Hale HM., Broadbent JC. *Pacemaker contact sensitivity*. Contact Dermatitis, 1984, 11:218-218

Ricciardi L., Minciullo P., Saitta P., Trombetta D., Saija A. & Gangemi S. *Increased serum levels of IL-22 in patients with nickel contact dermatitis.* Contact Dermatitis. 2009; 60: 57-58

Scully C. *Oral and Maxillofacial Medicine.* Ed Elsevier, Edinburgh; 2004, ISBN 0723610746, PP194-204.

Sicilia A., Cuesta S., Coma G., Guisasola C., Ruiz E. & Maestro A. *Titanium allergy in dental patients: a clinical study on 1500 consecutive patients.* Clin. Oral Implants Res; 2008, 19: 823-35.

Steinemann S. *Titanium – the material of choice?* Periodontology; 2000; 17: 7-21.

Stejskal V., Cederbrant K., Lindvall A., Forsbeck M. &MELISA- *An in vitro tool for the study of metal allergy.* Toxicol in vitro. 1994; 8: 991-1000.

Thomas P., Brandl W., Majer S., Summer B. &, Przybilla B. *Hypersensitivity to titanium osteosynthesis with impaired fracture healing, eczema and T-cell hyperresponsiveness in vitro: case report and review of the literature.* Contact Dermatitis, 2006, 55: 199-202.

Vamnes J., Lygre G., Grönningstraeter A. & Gjerdet N. *Four years of clinical experience with an adverse reaction unit for dental biomaterials.* Comm. Dent. Oral Epidemiol. 2004;32:150-157.

Waroquier D., Evrard L., Nelis M. & Parent D. *Allergic contact dermatitis presenting as geographical tongue with pruritus.* Contact Dermatitis. 2009; 60: 106-119.

Waroquier D., Evrard L., Flamme M. & Parent D. *Apport des tests épicutanés dans la mise au point des stomatodynies.* Bull du GERDA, 2007

Wennerberg A., Ide-Ektessabi A., Hatkamata S., Sawase T., Johansson C., Albrektsson T., Martinelli A., Sodervall U. & Odelius H. *Titanium release from implants prepared with different surface roughness.* 2004. Clin. Oral Impl. Res. 15: 505-512.

Wood M., Vermilyea S. *A review of selected dental literature on evidence-based treatment planning for dental implants: reports of the committee on research in fixed prosthodontics of the academy of fixed prosthodontics.* J Prosthetic Dentistry. 94: 447-462.

Yamauchi R., Morita A., Tsuji T. *Pacemaker dermatitis from titanium.* Contact Dermatitis, 2000, 42: 52-53

Zhao Y., Balato A., Fishelevich R., Chapoval A., Mann D. & Gaspari A. *Th17/Tc17 infiltration and associated cytokine gene expression in elicitation phase of allergic contact dermatitis.* British J Dermatol; 2009, 161: 1301-1306

8

Dental Implant Surfaces - Physicochemical Properties, Biological Performance, and Trends

Ahmed M. Ballo[1,2], Omar Omar[1,2], Wei Xia[2,3] and Anders Palmquist[1,2]
[1]*Department of Biomaterials, Institute of Clinical Sciences, The Sahlgrenska Academy, University of Gothenburg*
[2]*Biomatcell VINN Excellent Center of Biomaterials and Cell Therapy*
[3]*Angstrom Laboratory, Department of Engineering Sciences, Uppsala University*
[1,2]*Gothenburg*
[3]*Uppsala,*
Sweden

1. Introduction

Pure titanium and titanium alloys are well established standard materials in dental implants because of their favorable combination of mechanical strength, chemical stability, and biocompatibility (Brunette *et al.*, 2001). Integration of titanium implants with the surrounding bone is critical for successful bone regeneration and healing of dental implant.

The concept of osseointegration was discovered by Brånemark and his co-worker and, has had a dramatic influence on clinical treatment of oral implants. The first generation of successfully used clinical titanium implants, which were machined with a smooth surface texture, now approach 50 years in clinical use. Since then, implant surfaces have long been recognized to play an important role in molecular interactions, cellular response and osseointegration, and scientists all over the world have developed the second generation implants with surfaces which can accelerate and improve implant osseointegration. These second generation of clinically used implants underwent mechanical blasting coupled or not, with acid etch, bioactive coatings, anodized and, more recently, laser modified surfaces. (Cochran et al., 1998; Jansen et al., 1993; Palmquist et al., 2010; Brånemark et al., 2010). These implants have been extensively documented in vivo, including long-term clinical studies and experimental histological and biomechanical evaluation in animal models. For more knowledge in clinical results of commercially available implants the reader is referred to the following literature (Esposito et al., 2005; Esposito et al., 2003; Albrektsson & Wennerberg, 2004b).

The main objective for the development of implant surface modifications is to promote osseointegration, with faster and stronger bone formation. This will likely confer better stability during the healing process, which, preferentially, will improve the clinical performance in the area of poor bone quality and quantity. Furthermore, such promotion may, in turn, accelerate the bone healing and thereby allowing immediate or early loading protocols.

Recently growing micro and nano- technology is rapidly advancing surface engineering in implant dentistry. Such advances in surface engineering technologies have resulted in more complicated surface properties from micro- and nanometer scales, including the morphology, chemistry, crystal structure, physical, and mechanical properties. Such surfaces, intentionally modified with respect to microscale and nanoscale features, may represent a next generation of oral implant systems if possible to transfer to complex three-dimensional geometries. Hitherto, micro- and nano-fabricated surfaces have not reached the clinical evidence stage. However, it is not known whether the improved bone response is due to surface roughness or the surface composition. Furthermore, somewhat surprisingly, there is yet not enough hard evidence (randomized clinical trials) to tell whether the second generation of the implants has a better clinical performance than the machined implants used earlier. Nevertheless, experimental evidence from in vitro and in vivo studies strongly suggests that some types of surface modifications promote a more rapid bone formation than machined surfaces.

It has been proposed that increasing osteoconductivity by these surface design strategies is related to the altered implant topography resulting in enhanced osteoblast and preosteoblast adhesion, thereby leading to accelerated bone formation (Chehroudi et al., 1992; Cooper et al., 1998). However, it is well known that titanium implantation in bone results in contact of the titanium surface with complex environment including blood components and other cells, not only the osteogenic ones. Recently, it has been shown that changes in the physico-chemical properties of the titanium results in significant modulation of cell recruitment, adhesion, inflammation and bone remodelling activities in addition to regulation on bone formation response (Omar, 2010).

These different methods for implant surface modification may lead to different and unique surface properties that might affect the host-to-implant response.

This chapter reviews the state of art of development in dental implant surfaces and current trends in surface modifications that aim to accelerate the osseointegration of dental implants. This chapter also contains an overview of the most popular surface textures, chemical modifications including nano-surface design based on nanoscale modification of the implant surface, but also briefly describe the interface biology of oral implant is also discussed. Finally, it concludes with a summary and future outlook.

2. Surface roughness of titanium implants

Surface roughness has been identified as an important parameter for implants and its capacity for being anchored in bone tissue. There exist a variety of different manufacturing methods to increase the surface roughness of the implant, where the most commonly used are: Machining, Sandblasting, Acid etching, Anodic oxidation, Laser modification or a combination of these. Further, commercially available implants have been categorized according to the roughness value (S_a) into 4 groups (Albrektsson & Wennerberg, 2004a), smooth (S_a < 0.5 μm), minimally rough (S_a = 0.5-1.0 μm), moderately rough (S_a = 1.0-2.0 μm) and rough (S_a > 2.0 μm). The S_a value represents the mean height of peaks and pits of the surface, while another important parameter is S_{dr}, which represents the developed surface area compared to a perfect flat area. With a larger surface area a larger contact to the bone tissue could be obtained. There exists another 50 some direct or combined surface roughness parameters (Gadelmawla et al., 2002) however, it is unknown to what extent these are important. For S_a measurements different factors will affect the outcoming result as the type of equipment used, the area of analysis, the filtering process of the raw data, the cut-off values as well as where on the implant the measurements are performed. To obtain more comparable values in the literature guidelines for measurements have been published (Wennerberg & Albrektsson, 2000). Further, it is important to acknowledge that the surface chemistry and surface phase composition of the implant surface will change by altering the surface roughness (Kasemo & Lausmaa, 1988).

2.1 Machined surface

The first generation of osseointegrated implants had a relatively smooth machined surface (Branemark et al. 1969). The machined implant surface is solely turned and considered to be minimally rough (Figure 1). Different roughness values have been published using different measuring techniques. Moreover, manufacturing tools, bulk material, lubricant and machining speed will influence the resulting surface topography. Typical S_a values for machined surfaces are 0.3-1.0 µm. The surface oxide consists of a 2-10 nm thick mostly amorphous layer of TiO_2 (Lausmaa, 1996). Depending on the sterilization method the oxide layer could be crystallized into rutile structure (Jarmar et al., 2008). Further, the thickness and temperature is important on the phase composition (Radegran et al., 1991).

The bone responses to machined surfaces have been extensively evaluated in different animal models as well as clinical trials. The machined surface was the first used surface in clinical dental applications and has excellent long time follow-up (Adell et al., 1981; Brånemark et al., 1977). Further, other extra oral applications with bone anchored implants use machined implants, such as bone anchored hearing aids (Brånemark et al., 2001) and bone anchored amputations prosthesis for major limbs as legs and arms (Robinson et al., 2004; Rydevik, 1997). The healing around the implant is characterized by an increase in bone-implant contact starting at the implantation while the biomechanical stability slightly decrease over the first weeks, possible due to inflammation and bone remodeling, and being fully recovered after 4 weeks in rat tibia (Brånemark et al., 1997). Endosteal down growth of bone tissue covering the implant threads occurs in the marrow cavity and reach up to 70% bone implant contact after 16 weeks in rat tibia which could be compared to clinically stable oral implants retrieved up to 16 year after implantation where the bone-implant contact was measured to 56-85% (Sennerby et al., 1991). Eighty-five % bone-implant contact was observed for a clinically stable bone anchored amputations prosthesis retrieved after 11 years (Palmquist et al., 2008). Further, in the latter study it was shown that hydroxyapatite forms directly at the implant surface shown in high-resolution transmission electron microscopy (TEM).

2.2 Sandblasted surface

Increased roughness of an implant could be achieved by blasting the surface by small particles, usually called sandblasting or grit blasting (Figure 2). When the particles hit the implant surface it will create a crater. The surface roughness is hence dependent on the bulk material, the particle material, the particle size, the particle shape, the particle speed and the density of particles. The resulting surface roughness is usually anisotropic consisting of craters and ridges and occasionally particles embedded in the surface.

The surface roughness increases with the size of the particles used (Wennerberg et al., 1992) where 25 µm particles blasted surfaces were rougher than the machined surface while smoother than 75 µm and 250 µm blasted surfaces. Typical S_a values are 0.5-2.0 µm. Further, implants blasted with 25 µm and 75 µm particles show higher removal torque compared to a machined implant surface after 12 weeks of healing in either rabbit tibia or femur (Wennerberg et al., 1995).

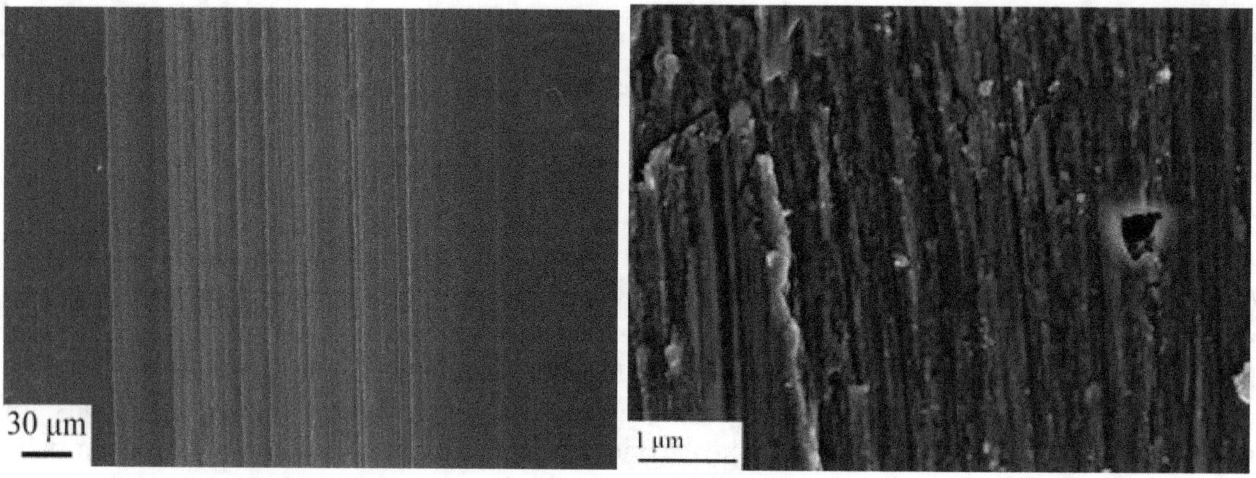

Fig. 1. Scanning electron micrograph of machined implant surface.

Significantly higher bone-implant contact was observed for the 25 μm blasted surface compared to machined surface while the bone area within the threads were significantly higher for the machined surface after 12 weeks (Wennerberg et al., 1995) and 1 year healing (Wennerberg et al., 1997). The blasting particle material, either TiO_2 or Al_2O_3 with a size of 25 μm, didn't show any difference in bone response with respect to removal torque, bone-implant contact and bone area after 12 weeks healing (Wennerberg et al., 1996a). Similar removal torque while significantly higher bone-implant contact and bone area was observed for implants blasted with 25 μm particles compared to 250 μm particles (Wennerberg et al., 1996b). The biological response to blasted implants show a optimal bone response with regards to removal torque values and bone implant contact to implants when a roughness of 1.5 μm is a achieved (Wennerberg, 1996). No ultrastructural studies of the interface between bone and implant surface have been found in the literature for blasted implants.

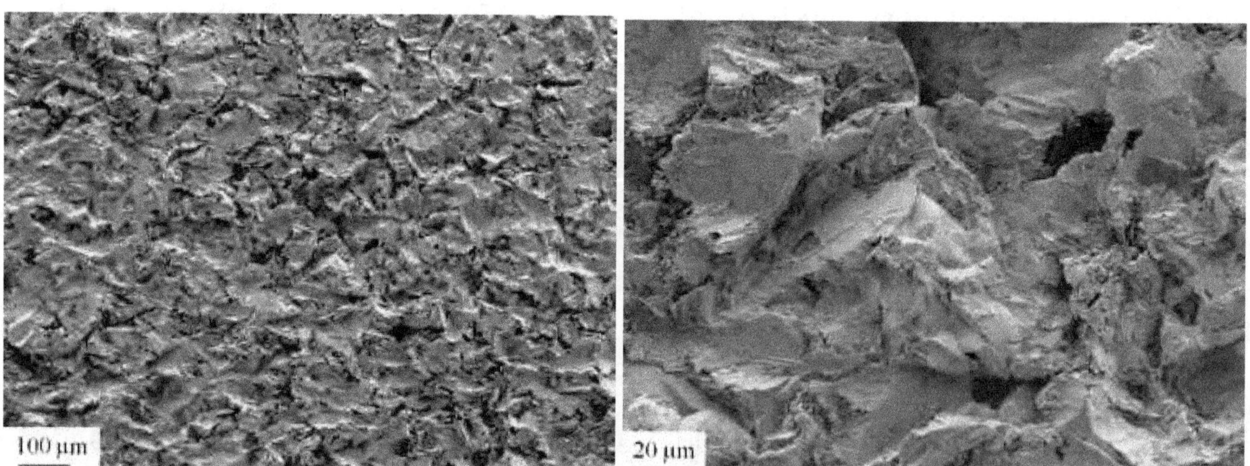

Fig. 2. Scanning electron micrograph of sandblasted surface.

2.3 Acid etched surface

With acid etching the surface is pitted by removal of grains and grain boundaries of the implant surface, as certain phases and impurities are more sensitive to the etching a selective removal of material is obtained (Figure 3). The resulting roughness is dependent on the bulk material, the surface microstructure, the acid and the soaking time. The surfaces are generally considered minimally rough as the typical S_a values are 0.3-1.0 μm. Few analyses of the surface layer have been found, but speculative a titanium hydride layer could form due to the presence of hydrogen ions in the acid. The surface oxide has been found to be a native amorphous titanium oxide with a thickness of around 10 nm (Sul et al., 2006). The dental implant with acid etching presented implant surface morphology similar to Master Plus R (Conexão Sistemas e Protese) and Frialit Plus R (Maillefer, Swaziland).

The bone response to acid etched implants has been compared to machined implants in animal models. Significantly higher bone-implant contact was observed for acid etched implants compared to machined implants in a rabbit model after 1 and 2 months, while no difference was found after 14 days (Celletti et al., 2006). Also significantly higher bone-implant contact was observed in a poor bone quality dog model after 4 months healing while no difference in bone area was obtained (Weng et al., 2003). Significantly increased removal torque was needed to remove acid etched implants compared to the machined implant after 1, 2 and 3 months healing in rabbit while significantly lower removal torque was needed when comparing to titanium plasma sprayed implants (Klokkevold et al., 2001). Significantly lower bone-implant contact, bone area and removal torque was observed when comparing acid etched implants to anodic oxidized implants in rabbit tibia after 6 weeks healing (Gottlow et al., 2000).

On the ultrastructural level a number of publications have utilized the fracture technique for sample preparation. The interfacial bone tissue was composed of an electron dense zone (20-50 nm) closest to where the implant had been in the section followed by either mineralized bone tissue or an intermediate layer of finely fibrilar mineralized zone (100 nm) which was found at areas with ongoing bone remodeling (Steflik et al., 1992, 1997, 1998). It was further found that osteocyte cellular processors was extending towards the implant surface (Steflik et al., 1994).

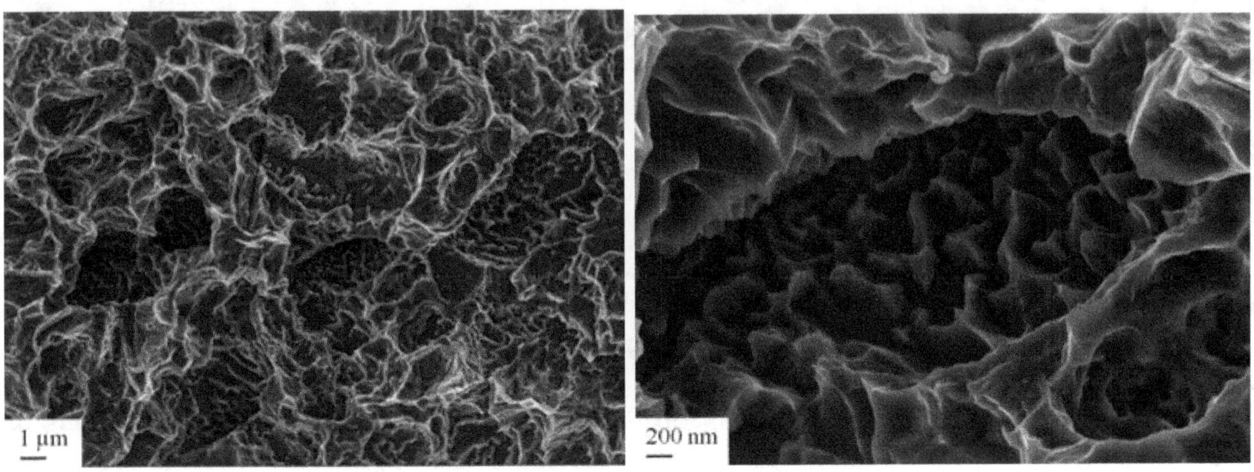

Fig. 3. Scanning electron micrograph of acid etched titanium surface.

2.4 Sandblasted and acid etched surface (SLA)

Commercially available dental implants are usually both blasted by particles and then subsequent etched by acids. This is performed to obtain a dual surface roughness as well as removal of embedded blasting particles. The etching reduces the highest peaks while smaller pits will be created and the average surface roughness will be reduced.

By the beginning of the 90s, intensive research had already shown that the sandblasted and acid etched surface had advantages compared to nearly every other type of implant surface, including the titanium plasma spray surface which, until that time, had been the standard for ITI implants (Buser et al., 1991, Schroeder et al. 1981).

Typical S_a values for blasted and acid etched implants are 1-2 μm. The chemical process of the acid etching will change the surface structure and it has been reported a creation of a titanium hydride layer with a thickness of 1-2 μm intermediate the surface oxide and the bulk metal (Conforto et al., 2004). Further, by rinsing the SLA implant in a nitrogen atmosphere and storing in saline solution until installation, the amount of carbon contamination could be reduced and improving the hydrophilicity of the implant surface (Rupp et al., 2006). The result of this procedure is creating a new hydrophilic surface (SLActive) (Figure 4). This procedure allows the SLActive to maintain a chemically active surface that conditioned to the human body.

Also the anions from the acid could be incorporated in the oxide layer such as fluoride ions if etched in hydrofluoric acid (Figure 5) (Cooper et al., 2006).

The bone response to blasted and etched implants has been compared to different implant surfaces. Higher removal torque was needed to unscrew the dual modified surface compared to solely acid etched implants in a pig model with 10 weeks of healing (Szmukler-Moncler et al., 2004).Significantly higher removal torque was obtained compared to machined surface while similar values compared to titanium plasma sprayed implants while no differences was observed in the bone density around the 3 different implant types (Buser et al., 1999). Significantly higher removal torque and higher bone-implant contact has been observed for blasted and fluoride modified implants compared solely blasted implants in a rabbit model after 1 and 3 months healing (Ellingsen et al., 2004).

Several studies have shown that SLActive implants achieve a higher bone contact and stability at earlier time points (6 weeks) when compared with SLA implants, and dramatically reduced healing times from 12 to 6 weeks (Buser et al., 2004; Schwarz et al., 2007). No ultrastructural studies of the interface to sandblasted and acid etched implant have been found in the literature.

2.5 Anodized surface

The anodized surface (TiUnite) is a partial crystalline and phosphate enriched titanium oxide characterized by a microstructured surface with open pores in the low micrometer range (Figure 6). Anodization or anodic oxidization as it's also called is an electrochemical process carried out in an electrolyte. The structural and chemical properties could be tailored by varying different process parameters, such as anode potential, electrolyte composition, temperature and current (Lausmaa, 2001). Further, depending on the electrolyte composition, different ions could be integrated in the oxide layer, such as phosphorous (Hall & Lausmaa, 2000), calcium (Frojd et al., 2008) and magnesium (Sul et al., 2005). At lower voltages, below the dielectric breakdown limit, a rather constant oxide growth is obtained, while at higher voltages, an increased gas evolution is obtained rendering the surface oxide porous (Lausmaa, 2001). The crystalline structures of anodized oxides are amorphous with crystalline grains of anatase (Jarmar et al., 2008).

The bone response to anodized implants has been evaluated in different species and healing times and most often compared to the original machined surface. Significant higher bone to implant contact has been reported as well as increased biomechanical removal torque values for phosphorous containing anodized surfaces compared to machined surfaces in dog and rabbit (Albrektsson et al., 2000; Henry et al., 2000). The phosphorous containing anodized

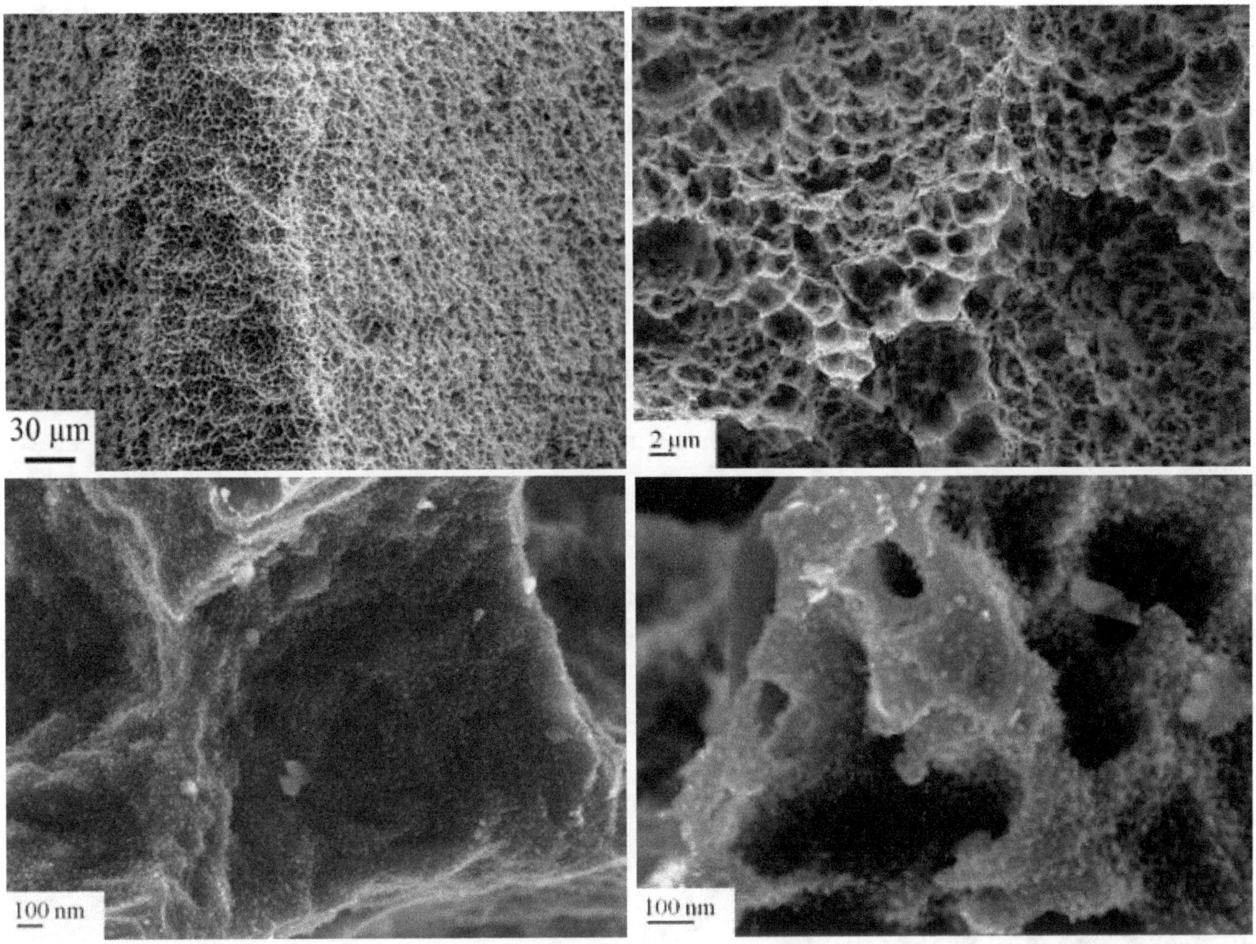

Fig. 4. Scanning electron micrograph of Straumann® Sandblasted and acid etched implant surface (SLA). Nanofeatures on the SLActive implant surface.

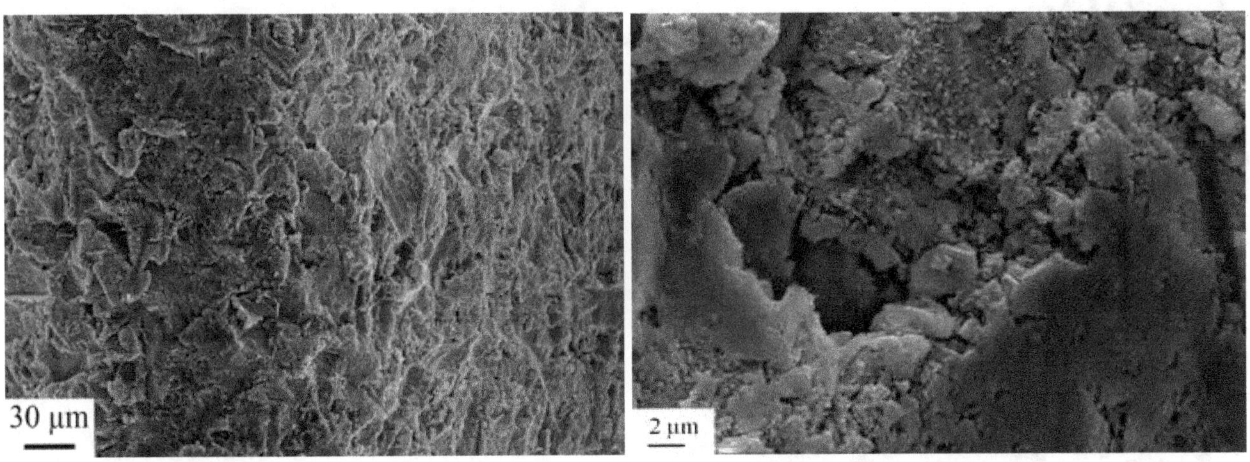

Fig. 5. Scanning electron micrograph of titanium dental implants in a fluoride modified surface (osseospeed® implant).

surface has also been shown to promote the early molecular events taking place at the immediate implant surface (Omar et al., 2010). Further, increased bone implant contact was obtained when calcium ions were incorporated in the anodized oxide compared to non calcium containing anodized oxide surface in the rabbit (Frojd et al., 2008) as well as higher removal torques were observed for magnesium incorporated oxides compared to non magnesium oxide surfaces (Sul et al., 2005a). One study have been performed on the ultrastructural level of oxidized implants, where a failed TiUnite (NobelBiocare) implant was removed prior to stage 2 surgery due to lack of osseointegration. TEM analysis of FIB prepared samples showed an amorphous zone between the bone tissue and the implant surface (Giannuzzi et al., 2007). Furthermore, in the later study, interdiffusion of titanium, phosphorus and calcium between the bone and the coating where intimate bone-implant contact was observed, suggested that chemical bonding also exists within this interface. The remove torque to anodized implants has been compared to sandblasted, acid etched, and machined implants in animal models. Significantly higher removal torque was observed for anodized implants compared other groups in a rabbit model after 12 weeks (Elias et al., 2008).

A higher clinical success rate was observed for the anodized titanium implants in comparison with turned titanium surfaces of similar shapes (Jungner et al., 2005). Two mechanisms have been proposed to explain this osseointegration: mechanical interlocking through bone growth in pores, and biochemical bonding (Schupbach et al., 2005; Sul et al., 2005b).

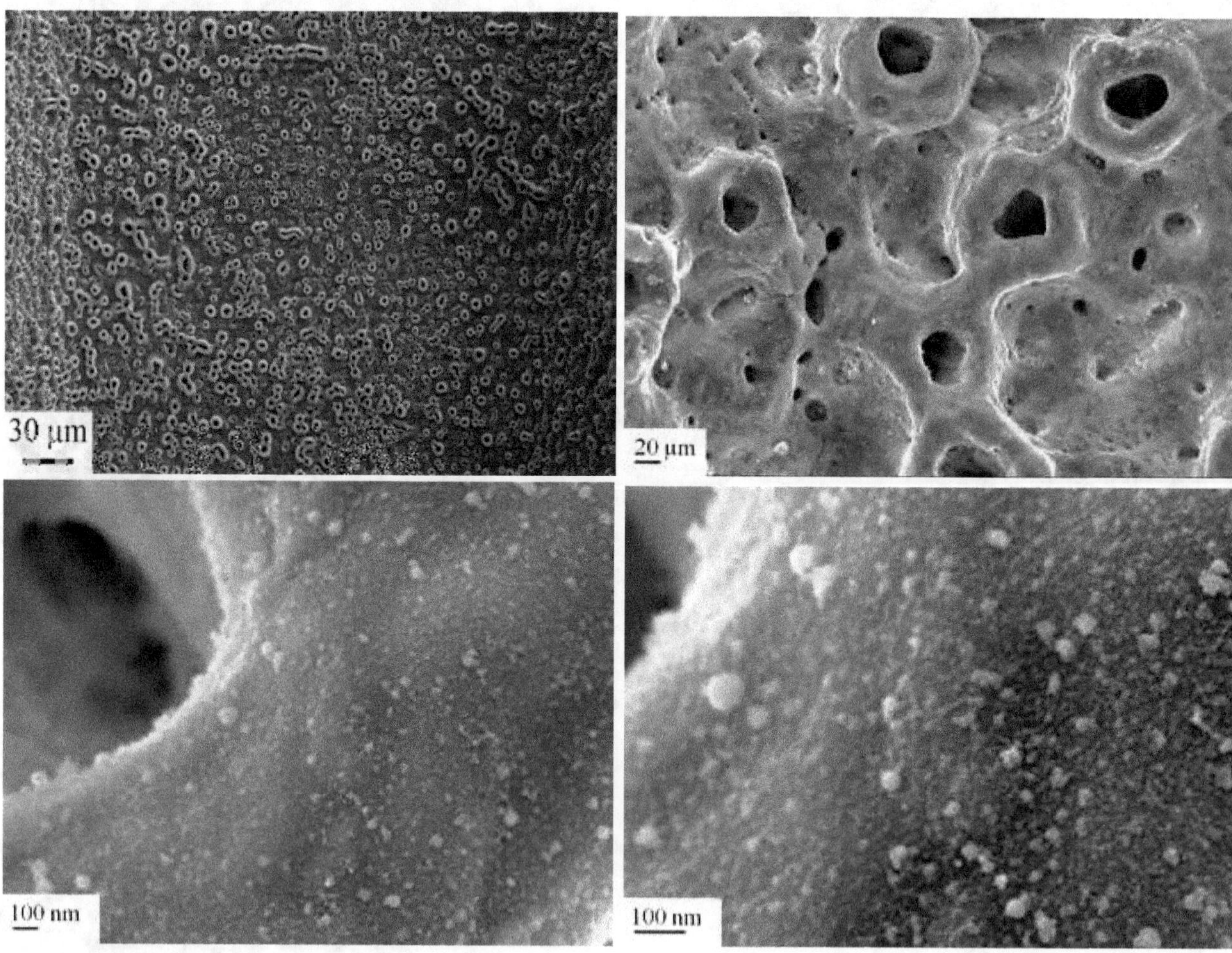

Fig. 6. A) Scanning electron micrograph of an anodized TiUnite® implant surface, B, C) the presence of pores with dimensions around 1-10 μm, and smaller pores with diameters below 1 μm, D) nanofeatures on the anodized implant surface.

2.6 Laser modified micro- and nano-structured surface

Laser is an emerging field for use as a micromachining tool to produce a 3-D structure at micrometer and nanometer level. The technique is a method of choice for complex surface geometries. The technique generates short pulses of light of single wavelength, providing energy focused on one spot. It is rapid, extremely clean, and suitable for the selective modification of surfaces and allows the generation of complex microstructures/ features with high resolution. These advantages make the technique interesting for geometrically complex biomedical implants.

The Brånemark BioHelix Implant (Figure 7) has surface modified with laser micromachining process to create micro- and nano-structured surface roughness in only the inner part of the thread. The inner part of the thread is believed to be more suitable for bone formation than the outer part (Thomsson & Esposito, 2008).

The laser technique has several advantages, add no chemicals and can be used in routine manufacturing. Only the valley and parts of the flank of the implant threads was laser treated while the remaining part was left as-machined. The idea behind this design is that the flack portion of the implant thread, which might have the higher risk to expose to the

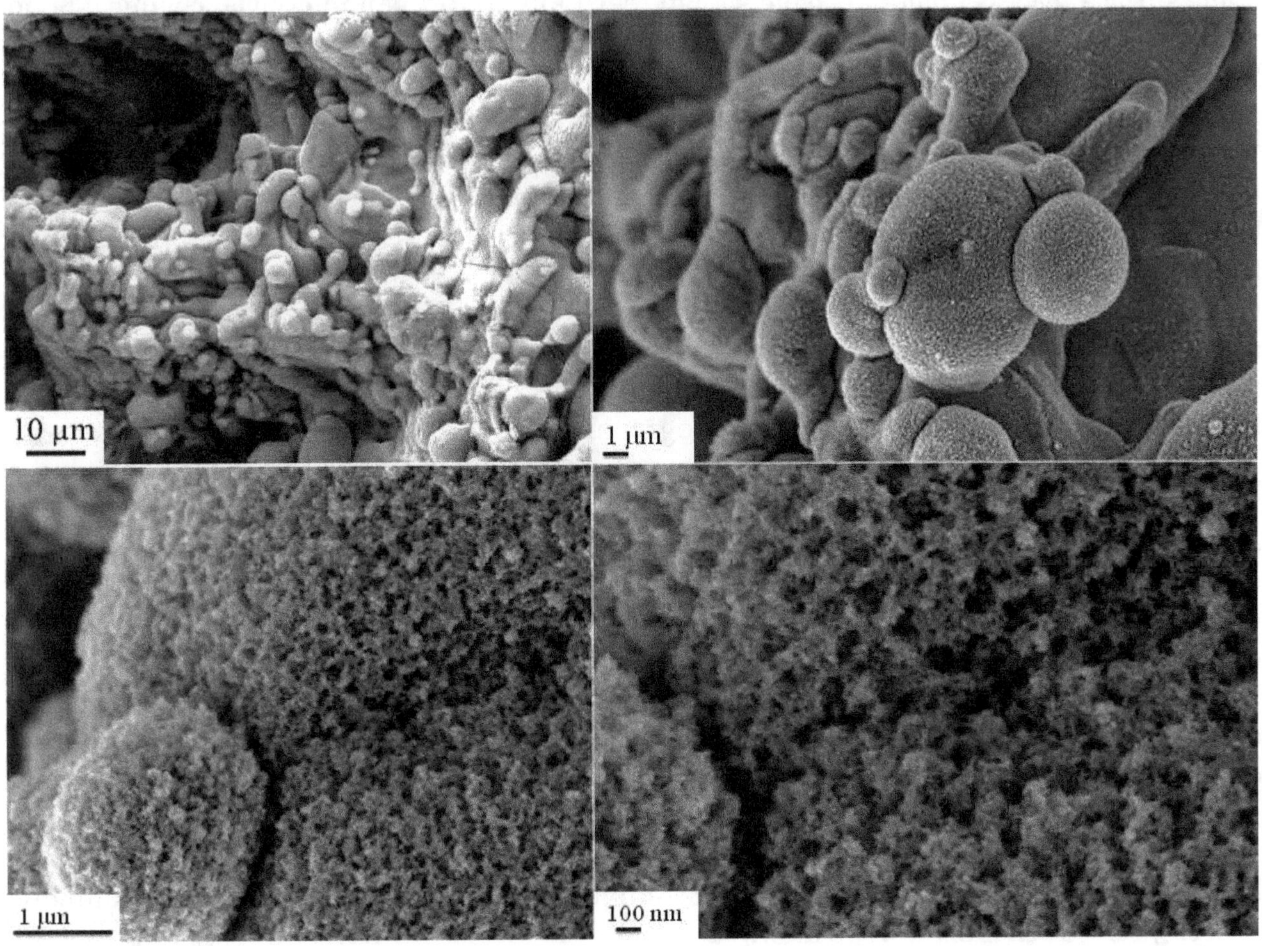

Fig. 7. Scanning electron micrograph of Brånemark BioHelix implant. The bottom portion of the threads is modified by laser processing, whereas the parts of the flanks and the tops are as machined. Higher magnification of the laser modified surface, showing the nanotopography.

microorganism and plaque, is characterised by relatively smooth surface to minimize the incidence of peri-implantitis, whereas the valley part of the implant threads has the rougher surface.

Short-term, experimental *in vivo* studies of laser-modified titanium implants with nano-scale surface topographical features have demonstrated a significant increase in removal torque and different fracture mechanisms (Palmquist et al., 2010; Brånemark et al., 2010). Of clinical importance is that nanostructured surfaces promoted long-term bone bonding and interface strength *in vivo* as determined by a coalescence between mineralized bone and the nanostructured surface and a substantial increase in removal torque (Palmquist et al., 2010).

One 1-year retrospective case series showed excellent clinical results of Brånemark BioHelix dental implants placed according to conventional procedures (Thomsson & Esposito, 2008). However, randomized clinical trials with suitable controls are needed to confirm these preliminary results.

3. Calcium phosphate coatings on titanium implants

Some surface reactive materials have shown the ability to form an interfacial chemical bond with surrounding tissues through a series of biophysical and biochemical reactions, causing 'bioactive fixation' of the implant (Cao & Hench 1996). Bioactive materials can be biostable (i.e. synthetic hydroxyapatite) or bioresorbable (i.e. bioactive glasses and glass-ceramics). Some bioactive ceramics like bioactive glasses of certain compositions have been claimed to have a real chemical bonding ability with soft tissues (Wilson et al., 1981). However, bioactive ceramics in the bulk form are not suitable for load-bearing applications as their flexural strength, strain-to-failure and fracture toughness are less than that of bone and their elastic moduli are greater than that of bone. For these reasons they are usually applied as coatings on metallic implants that possess superior mechanical properties. Calcium phosphates (CaP) are the most common family of bioceramics well-known for their use in biological application. CaP in the crystallographic form of apatite is an important mineral constituent of bone. Calcium phosphate ceramics are integrated within bone following a well known sequence of events (Frayssinet, et al. 1993). They are considered to be bioactive and osteoconductive. Bioactivity would be due to epitaxial nucleation of carbonated apatite crystals at the surface of ceramic grains. This layer of biological apatite might contain endogenous proteins and might serve as a matrix for osteogenic cell attachment and growth (Davies 2003).

Different types of methods have been introduced to prepare calcium phosphate coatings on dental implant (table 1 & 2). These methods can be divided to two groups: physical and chemical methods. Sometimes they can also be called dry and wet methods. Typically physical techniques include plasma spraying deposition, physical vapour deposition, magnetron sputtering deposition, ion beam assisted deposition, pulsed laser deposition, and hot isostatic pressing. Chemical techniques include sol-gel method, biomimetic process, electrochemical deposition, micro-arc oxidation (MAO) and electrophoretic deposition.

Physical techniques are widely used for preparation of calcium phosphate coatings. The bonding strength between coatings and implants is higher than those prepared by chemical methods. However, most of these methods have difficulties in coating of complex 3D geometries such as rough screw-shaped dental implants. Chemical methods can be used to treat the implants with complex geometries. The treating temperature of chemical methods is low. The most important thing is that bioactive molecules and drugs can be incorporate into calcium phosphate coatings via chemical methods, such as biomimetic process.

Technique	Characteristics	Properties
Plasma spraying deposition (PS)	(1). High temperature >1000°C (2). Reproducible (3). High deposition rate (4). Atmosphere: Air, vacuum (popular), low pressure	(1). 2D (2). No homogeneity of crystallnity (3). Promote fast and strong fixation and bone growth in vivo and clinically (4). Bacteria adhesion
Magnetron sputtering deposition (MS)	(1). High deposition rate (2). Metallic and non-metallic substrates (3). DC and RF	(1). 2D (2). Ion doped hydroxyapatite and composites coatings
Ion beam assisted deposition (IBAD)	(1). The coating is amorphous, and needed to be heat treated further (2) The final crystallinity is dependent on the time, temperature and amount of water vapour present during the coating. (3). Low deposition rate compared to PS	(1). 2D (2). High adhesive strength (3). Graded crystallinity
pulsed laser deposition (PLD)	(1). Fast deposition rate (2).Multi-component and metastable materials	(1). 2D (2) HA, OCP, α, β-TCP
Hot isostatic pressing (HIP)	(1). High temperature and pressure	(1). 2D

Table 1. Physical techniques for implant coatings

In the last four decades, continuous research on HA and CaP have not only focused on tissue-coating interface, but also on the problems associated with the coating process and optimization of coating properties for maximum tissue response (Sun et al., 2001). A major dilemma for evaluation the bone tissue response of CaP coating compare to uncoated titanium implants (Morris et al. 2000; Barrere et al. 2003), is that the process of surface chemical modifications are often associated changes in topography and visa-versa. In addition, several factors may have influenced the results of *in vivo* evaluation at the interface of CaP coated implants.

Technique	Characteristics	Properties
Sol-gel method	(1). Combine with different coating process, such as dip and spinning coatings, following sintering (2).Substrates with complex geometry (3).Metallic and non-metallic substrates (4). Thin film	(1). 3D (2). Easy to control the composition (3). High sintering temperature for HA coatings
Biomimetic process	(1). Low temperature (2). Different types of substrates which could induce HA formation, such as metallic implants, bioceramics, polymers	(1). 3D (2). Bone-like crystal structure (3). Ion doped HA (4). Low bonding strength (5) Porous structure (6). Incorporate bio-molecules and drugs
Electrochemical deposition	(1). Conducting substrates (2). Chargeable particles (3). Low temperature	(1).3D (2). Low boding strength between coatings and substrates (3). Composite coatings (4). (4). Thick and cracked coatings
Electrophoretic deposition	(1). Conducting substrates (2). Chargeable particles (3). Low temperature	(1). 3D (2). Low boding strength between coatings and substrates (3). Composite coatings (4). Thick and cracked coatings
Micro-arc oxidation (MAO)	(1). Ambient temperature (2). Substrates with complex geometry (3). Electrolytic oxidation	(1).3D (2). HA and ion doped HA
Ultrasonic spray pyrolysis	(1). Ambient temperature (2). Continuous and pulse spray	(1). 2D (2). Cracks in coatings (3). The bonding strength of coatings prepared by pulse spray is better than that by continuous spray

Table 2. Chemical techniques for implant coatings.

3.1 Plasma spraying

HA coatings were first introduced in the middle 1980s for improved fixation between bone and implant (Furlong and Osborn, 1991). Since that time, these materials have been extensively used in orthopaedic and dental implants. Plasma-spraying is commercially the most frequently used method for deposition of calcium phosphate coatings, such as HA, onto implant materials to improve their bioactivity.

The thickness of hydroxyapatite coatings produced by plasma-spray varies from 100 to 300 μm (Willmann, 1997). With plasma spraying processing the surface area of titanium implant has increased up to approximately six times than the original surface. The arithmetic average roughness (R_a) for hydroxyapatite coated by plasma-spraying process is 5.0 ± 1.0 μm.

The bone tissue responses to plasma sprayed hydroxylapatite (HA) coatings on titanium implant have been well documented. Several earlier experimental studies have shown a higher percentage of bone-implant contact for HA-coated implants when compared with titanium implants in different species and types of bone (De Groot et al., 1987; Denissen et al., 1990). The histological findings demonstrated that the cortical bone reaction to titanium and HA-coated titanium was similar, but the HA-coated surfaces induced more bone deposition in areas on non-cortical bone contact than uncoated surfaces. Based on findings of a substantial reduction of the HA coating thickness after 12 weeks (Jansen, et al., 1991). Other studies in animal model have shown that the chemical composition of HA coating has a positive influence on the bone response, while, the influence of roughness is less evident (Vercaigne, et al., 1998).

In reference to the interfacial strength, the HA-coated implants were reported to have higher push-out strength in compared to non-coated implants (Cook et al., 1987). HA coated implants have also exhibited a greater torque removal value compare to Ti screw implants (Carr et al., 1995).

On the ultrastructural level, newly formed acicular crystallites were adjacent to the larger HA crystals of the plasma-sprayed coating. Needle-like crystals seemed even to grow at the surface and in the smallest holes of the HA coating. Collagen fibrils were not observed in the bonding area. The tiny crystals of the newly formed mineralized tissue developing in the cavities of the implanted material appeared to be more or less randomly oriented, thus resembling woven bone (Hemmerle, et al. 1997).

However, despite clinical success, it has been recognized that the plasma-spraying method has several disadvantages, including poor long-term adherence of the coating to the substrate material, non-uniformity in thickness of the deposited layer, and variations in crystallinity and composition of the coating. Other significant factors causing implant failures include microbial infection (Rosenberg et al., 1991; Verheyen et al., 1993).

3.2 Sputter-deposition

Sputtering process has been shown to be a particularly useful technique for the deposition of bioceramic thin films (based on Ca–P systems), due to the ability of the technique to provide greater control of the coating's properties and improved adhesion between the substrate and the coating.

Scanning electron microscopy showed that the deposited films had a uniform and dense structure (Figure 8). The calcium phosphate has been reported to range from 1.5 and 2.6. The *in vitro* dissolution appeared to be determined by the degree of the coating's crystallinity

(Ong & Lucas, 1998; Ong et al, 1997). The disadvantages with sputter coating is extensive time consuming, produces amorphous coatings and Ca/P ration of the coating is higher than of synthetic HA.

The thickness of hydroxyapatite coatings produced by sputter process varies from 0.5 to 3.0 μm (Ding, 2003). With sputter processing the surface roughness of the coating depends on the roughness of the substrate (Hayakawa et al., 2000). The arithmetic average roughness (R_a) for hydroxyapatite coated by sputter process is 3.0 ± 1.2 μm.

In a study using TiO2-gritblasted and sputtered CaP implants, the sputtered CaP coatings showed improved initial fixation and healing response when implanted into the trabecular bone of the goat (Vercaigne et al., 2000; Hayakawa et al., 2000). In a separate study comparing sputtered CaP coatings to plasma-sprayed HA coatings, the ultimate interfacial strength observed for the sputtered CaP-coated implants (as-sputtered and sputtered followed by post- deposition heat treatment) was not significantly different from the plasma-sprayed HA coated implants 12 weeks after implantation, suggesting that sputtered CaP coatings are comparable to plasma-sprayed HA coatings with respect to ultimate interfacial strength. This was supported by the histological findings that indicated no statistical difference in percent bone contact length between plasma-sprayed HA-coated implants and the as-sputtered CaP-coated implants at 12 weeks after implant placement (Yang et al., 2005).

Further, sputtered calcium phosphate coated titanium implants have showed higher removal torque compared to control uncoated titanium implants after 3 weeks of healing. This difference in the removal torque strength was no longer evident after 12 weeks of healing (Ong et al., 2002).

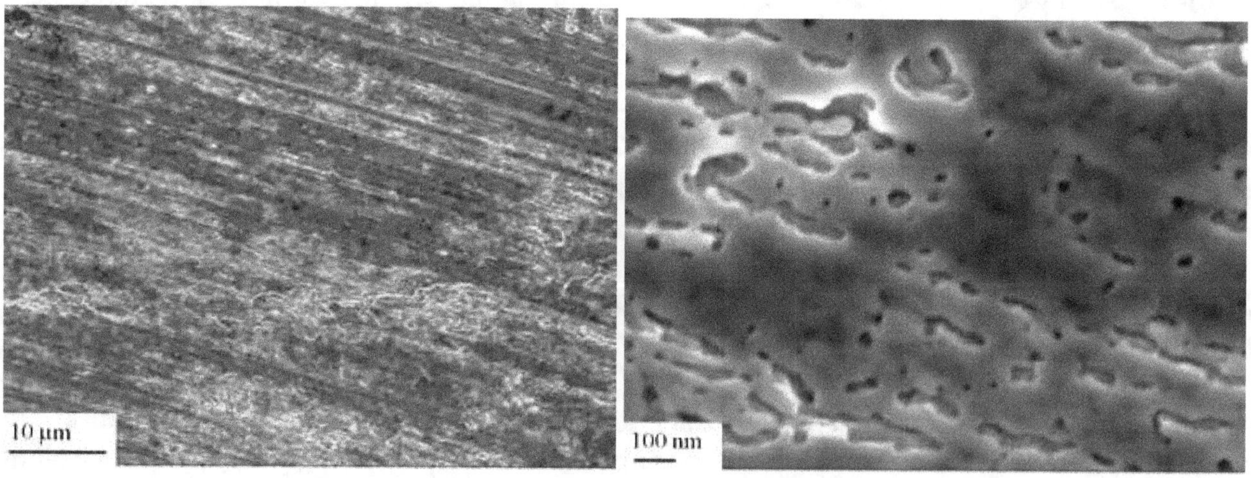

Fig. 8. Scanning electron micrograph of sputter CaP coated titanium implant.

3.3 Biomimetic precipitation

Biomimetic deposition of calcium phosphate onto surfaces of implant materials is a technique originally developed by Kokubo and co-workers (Kokubo et al, 1990). This method allows hydroxyapatite and other calcium phosphate surfaces to be deposited on substrates in a simulated body fluid (SBF) under physiological conditions of temperature and pH, on complex geometrical shapes.

The classical biomimetic Ca–P coating normally requires an immersion period of about 14–28 days with replenishment of SBF solution. It is observed that the thickness of the apatite layer increases as the immersion period increases. In very recent years efforts have been made (Habibovic et al., 2002; Ma et al., 2003; Barrere et al., 2004; Muller et al., 2004) to make this process fast to increase its practical utility.

In the biomimetic method, a layer of usually rough and porous, calcium-deficient apatite will grow on the surface of implants. The Ca/P ratio for HA biomimetic coating was 1.51 (He et al, 2007), and the thickness of HA coatings produced by biomimetic process varies from 20 to 25 μm (Yang et al., 2005).

It is well known that the tissue and cell response could be considerably influenced by the composition and topography of the implant surfaces.[14] Biomimetically produced apatite surfaces may, therefore, be useful in facilitating early bone ingrowth into porous surfaces without the potential for coating debris, macrophage infiltration, fibrous tissue encapsulation, and eventual coating failure as may occur with the plasma-sprayed hydroxyapatite coating.[15]

Little information is available on bone tissue responses to biomimetic coatings on titanium implant. Very few experimental studies have shown the biomimetic HA coating did not have any positive effect on new bone formation and on the shear strength at the early bone healing stage (Fuming, et al, 2008; He et al, 2009; Yang, et al, 2009).

Recently, it has been found that the morphology of the biomimetic apatite surfaces changed by adding ions as substitutes to HA such as strontium (Sr), and silicate (Si) ions (Zhang & Zou, 2009; Xia et al., 2010).

Adding Sr ion change the morphology of biomimetic apatite from plate-like for the pure HA to sphere-like (Figure 9). Surface analysis results showed that 10-33% of Ca ions in the apatite have been substituted by Sr ions, and that the Sr ions were chemically bonded with apatite and successfully incorporated into the structure of apatite (Xia et al., 2010).

Our recent findings have showed that biomimetically prepared Sr and Si-ion substituted apatite films deposited on Ti implants provide bioactive surfaces which promote early bone formation. The mechanisms behind these responses may be release of Sr ions, and the nature of bonding of Si ions in the HA structure, whose fast hydrolysis is deemed to contribute to the surface hydrophilicity, respectively (Ballo et al., 2010).

3.4 Bioactive glass coatings

Originally introduced by Hench (Hench et al., 1971), silica-based bioactive glasses are slowly resorbing synthetic osteoconductive materials which are able to form strong chemical bond with bone. Several methods have been applied to obtain a bioactive glass coating on the load bearing part of the implants (Hench & Andersson, 1993). Several attempts have been made to create bioactive glass coatings on alumina (Greenspan & Hench 1976), stainless steel (Schepers et al., 1989), Co-Cr-Mo alloy (Lacefield & Hench, 1986), fiber-reinforced composite (Ballo et al. 2009, 2011), and titanium alloys (West et al., 1990, Kitsugi et al., 1996). Application of a double glass coating has been suggested to solve the problem of differences in thermal expansion coefficients. Recently, several attempts were made to prepare bioactive glass coatings on titanium and Ti6Al4V (Bloyer et al., 1999, Saiz et al., 2002). Application of a ground layer prepared from inert glass with a thermal expansion coefficient close to that of Ti6Al4V provided good adhesion to the substrate (Oku et al., 2001). This ground coating can be used in combination with more surface reactive glass coatings (Gomez-Vega et al., 2000a), with embedded hydroxyapatite and/or bioactive glass particles (Gomez-Vega et al., 2000b), or a sol-gel-derived silica coating (Gomez-Vega et al., 2001). Reactive plasma spraying

(Schrooten et al., 2000) or processing with infra-red laser (Moritz et al., 2004) have also been attempted to create bioactive glass coatings on titanium and its alloys.

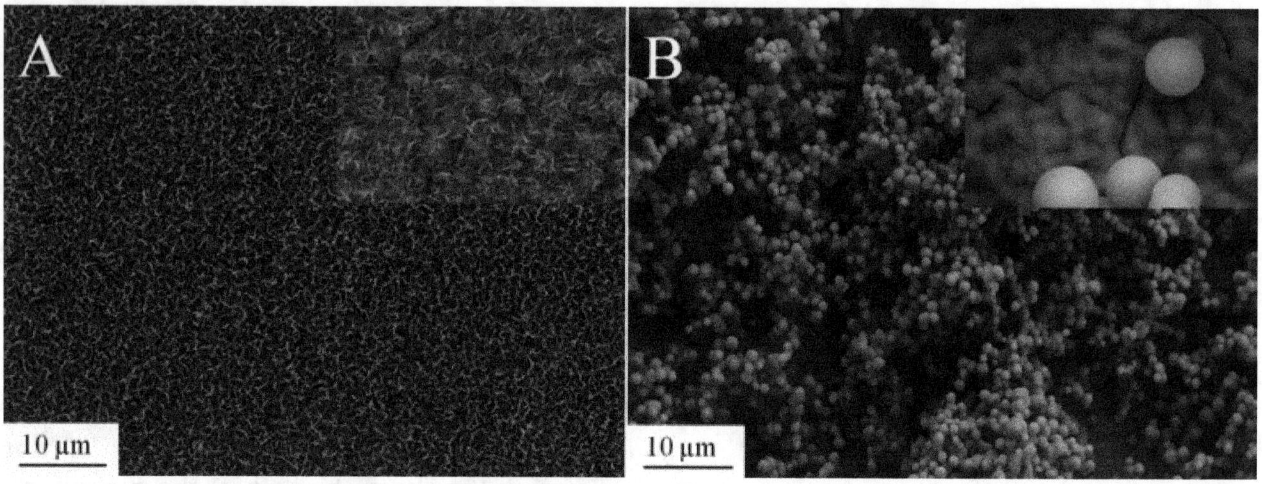

Fig. 9. Scanning electron micrograph of biomimetic apatite surface modification of titanium implants. A) Pure apatite with plate-like structure, B) Sr-HA with sphere-like structure.

Several experimental studies have shown that titanium implants coated with BAG were integrated into host bone without a connective tissue capsule and significantly greater osseointegration and high removal torque in compare to the control uncoated titanium implants (Moritz et al., 2004). Also significantly higher bone-implant contact was observed for BAG coated titanium implants than those in both the uncoated and HA coated titanium implants after 4, 12, and 24 weeks of healing (Xie et al., 2010).

Recently, one 1-year comparative clinical study showed that bioactive glass coated implants were as equally successful as hydroxyapatite in achieving osseointegration and supporting final restorations (Mistry et al., 2011). However, further clinical studies are needed to confirm these preliminary results.

4. Biological response to titanium implant surface modification

Osseointegration is the fortunate outcome of bone tissue healing around titanium implant. It is a biological process in which a direct anchorage is established by formation of bone tissue around the implant without the growth of fibrous tissue at the bone-implant interface (Branemark, Adell et al. 1969; Branemark, Hansson et al. 1977). Despite the wide use of osseointegrated titanium implants and the substantially growing research on the development of new titanium surfaces and/or modification of existing surfaces, a detailed understanding of the mechanisms of osseointegration is still lacking. The current knowledge on the process of healing at different titanium implants is predominantly gained from histological and biomechanical data and correlation with normal fracture healing. The histological and biomechanical studies strongly advocate that bone would respond differently by alteration of the implant surface properties (Larsson, Esposito et al. 2001).Consequently, great attention has been given to study, *in vitro*, the cellular and molecular activities on different substrates and to extrapolate the results to the actual interfacing between implant and living bone tissue. Based on results from the *in vitro* studies, the surface influences the initial sequences of protein adsorption, platelet adhesion and haemostasis, complement activation, inflammation and osteogenic cell response

(Nygren, Tengvall et al. 1997; Park and Davies 2000; Masaki, Schneider et al. 2005; Tan, Qian et al. 2006). Taking into account the important information acquired from these studies, however, they remain to large extent unrepresentative for the actual paradigm of the *in vivo* implantation scenario. For instance, early *in vivo* studies revealed that that the process of bone formation at titanium implants is preceded by recruitment of cells of different types and at different levels of morphological differentiation (Sennerby, Thomsen et al. 1993; Sennerby, Thomsen et al. 1993). However, the functional activities of the different cells and the roles of cells other than osteogenic ones in the healing process have not been clearly defined. A key question is how early molecular and cellular events are influenced by material surface properties *in vivo*, and how these early events influence the organization of the surrounding tissue and its interlocking or bonding with the material surface and, in turn, the capacity of this interface to adapt to long-term continuous load interactions.

The new advances in research technologies have made it possible to apply molecular techniques to analyze the interface between the living tissues and implant surface. Such tools can be used at high degree of precision to discover mechanisms that govern osseointegration including events of early inflammation, mesenchymal stem cells (MSCs) recruitment and cell-cell communication. Nevertheless, the advent of these approaches requires establishing reliable procedures to collect cell samples from within the *in vivo* interface in the way that their spatial distribution can be determined. Using the highly sensitive quantitative polymerase chain reaction (qPCR) in conjunction with the well documented rat tibia model, it has been revealed that gene expression of the interfacial implant-adherent cells is immediately and differently influenced by titanium implants depending on their surface properties (Omar, Lenneras et al. 2010; Omar, Svensson et al. 2010). The model was further combined with immunohistochemistry and SEM to confirm the presence of specific cell types at the interface. Ultimately, the regulations of inflammation, bone formation and bone resorption processes were correlated to the strength of the early formed bone-implant interface, by measuring the removal torque (Omar, Lenneras et al. 2011) (Table 3).

The inevitable early inflammation and the processes of cellular recruitment and adhesion to titanium implants in bone are obscure and have not received similar attention as that given during soft tissue integration. In soft tissue healing around titanium discs, higher release of tumor necrosis factor-alpha (TNF-α) was observed in response to porous titanium with and without plasma protein layer compared to machined titanium after 3 hours (Jansson, Kalltorp et al. 2002), as well as for machined titanium compared to copper after 12 hours of implantation (Suska, Esposito et al. 2003). The soft tissue data presented strong evidence on the modulation of inflammatory cell responses by titanium surface roughness and composition, respectively. The local releases of inflammatory mediators, in addition to the modulatory role of the implant surface, initiate the cascade that controls early inflammatory events. These events involve the release and regulation of primary acute phase cytokines. By activation of their target cells, these cytokines generate a second wave of cytokines, including members of the chemokine family.

In bone, higher expression of the chemokine, monocyte chemoattractant protein-1 (MCP-1), was revealed at machined implant surface compared to anodically oxidized implant (Omar, Lenneras et al. 2010). This was coupled with higher expression of pro-inflammatory cytokines TNF-α (3 hours and 1 day after implantation) and interleukin-1beta (IL-1β) (1 day and 6 days after implantation) at the machined implants (Omar, Lenneras et al. 2010; Omar, Svensson et al. 2010). The temporal expression profile for MCP-1 was similar to the expression of pro-inflammatory cytokines telling that the recruitment of inflammatory cells was accompanied by cytokine activity at both surfaces. The immunohistochemical sections for the same time period showed CD163-labeled monocytes/macrophages at both surfaces. However, a general SEM observation in all samples was that a large amount of fibrinous material covered the machined implants (Figure 10). Fibrin has been shown to enhance the pro-inflammatory response to biomaterials (Tang and Eaton 1993) which might explain the upregulated pro-inflammatory cytokine expression at the machined surface as early as 3 and 24 hours (Omar, Lenneras et al. 2010) and at later time periods (Omar, Svensson et al. 2010).

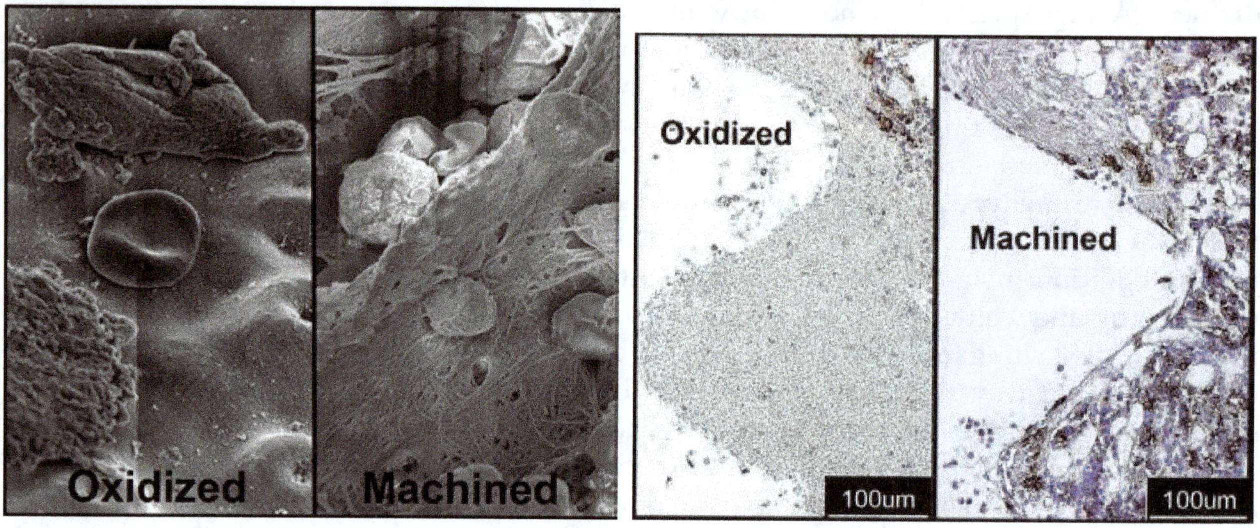

Fig. 10. Left, scanning electron microscopy images of oxidized and machined implant retrieved 24h after implantation. Right, immunohistochemical sections of the interface 24h after implantation showing CD163-positive monocytes/macrophages in the interface zone. Biological material adherent the machined implant was highly fibrinous with numerous erythrocytes and leukocytes compared to the oxidized implants.

One of the major observations during the initial 24 hours after implantation in bone was the significant modulation of the chemokine receptor CXCR4 (Omar, Lenneras et al. 2010). These results provided the first set of data on the role of this chemokine receptor at titanium implants in bone. After 12 hours of implantation, 11-fold higher CXCR4 expression was demonstrated at the oxidized implants compared to the level at machined implants. CXCR4 together with its exclusive ligand, stromal derived factor-1alpha (SDF-1α), has recently gained significant attention as a major axis for local and systemic recruitment of MSCs to sites of tissue repair and regeneration (Yu, Li et al. ; Ceradini, Kulkarni et al. 2004; Shichinohe, Kuroda et al. 2007; Wang, Deng et al. 2008). Blocking of CXCR4 significantly inhibited *in vivo* migration of circulating alkaline phosphatase (ALP) positive osteoblast progenitor cells to subcutaneously implanted BMP-2 containing collagen pellets (Otsuru, Tamai et al. 2008). Other studies have also demonstrated that MSC migration to a fractured tibia site is highly dependent on CXCR4 in a time- and dose-dependent manner (Granero-Molto, Weis et al. 2009). The revealed upregulation of the chemokine CXCR4 at the oxidized implant surface was corroborated by SEM and immunohistochemical observations showing the predominance of mesenchymal stem cells at that surface.

At the *in vivo* bone implant interface, the cellular attachment is meditated via protein rich layer to which cells adhere using variety of surface receptors, mainly form integrin family. The modulation of expression of specific integrins may reflect specific temporal and

conformational changes in protein adsorption influenced by the physico-chemical properties of the surface. T-shaped hollow titanium implants treated with sulphuric and hydrochloric acids showed higher expression and peak of β1 and β3 integrins in the surrounding bone after 1 week in rat femur compared to machined titanium and non implant defect (Ogawa and Nishimura 2003). Cells adherent to oxidized surfaces showed upregulation of integrin-β1 during the 24 hours of implantation (Omar, Lenneras et al. 2010). Since CXCR4 exhibited association with integrin-β1 at the oxidized implants, this together with the increased expression of osteogenic markers, such as ALP and osteocalcin (OC), and the higher number of mesenchymal cells, as shown in SEM observations, altogether suggested that the oxidized implant was associated with higher recruitment of MSCs through mechanisms which involve modulation of CXCR4 chemokine receptor and integrin-β1expression (Figure 11).
Integrin-β2, expressed mainly by leukocytes (Stewart, Thiel et al. 1995) and not by cells of osteoblastic lineage (Hughes, Salter et al. 1993), was higher at the oxidized implants after 12 hours of implantation. This integrin has also been shown to be expressed by osteoclast progenitors (Hayashi, Nakahama et al. 2008). Results showing a higher expression of osteoclastic marker (cathepsin K; CATK) at the oxidized surface (Omar, Svensson et al. 2010) suggested that the higher expression of β2 integrin may be due to the early presence of osteoclasts in the interface.

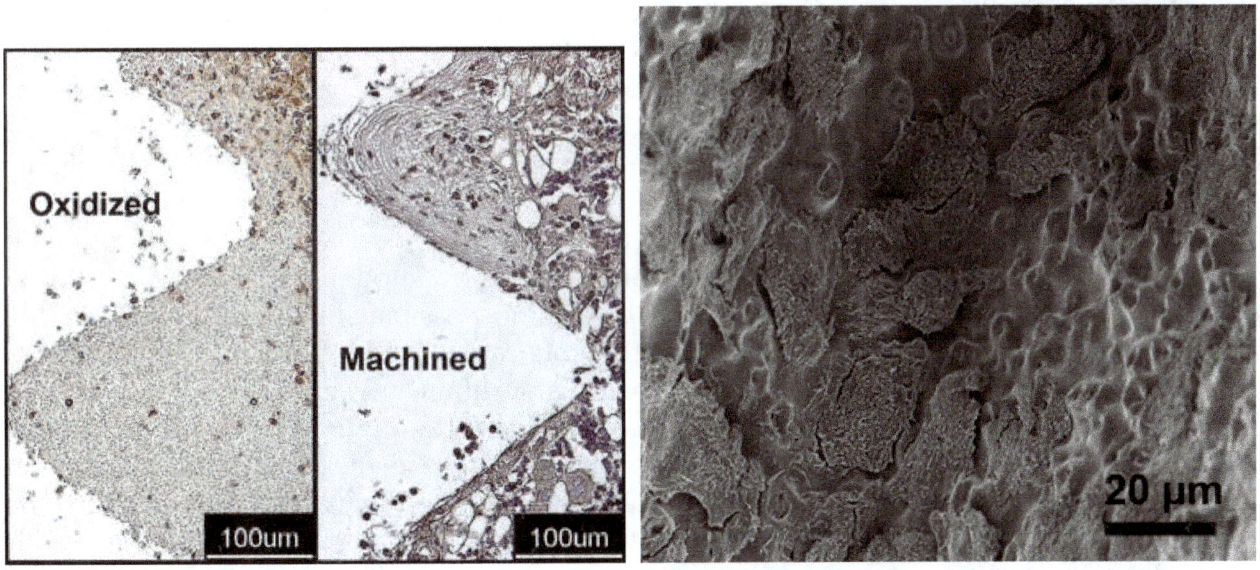

Fig. 11. Left, immunohistochemical sections of the interface 24h after implantation showing periostin positive mesenchymal and osteoprogenitor cells. Right, scanning electron microscopy of oxidized implant retrieved 24h after implantation. On the oxidized implants, mesenchymal cells were frequently seen.

Peak expression for ALP, OC, tartrate resistant acid phosphatase (TRAP) and CATK was detected 3 days after implantation in rat bone (Omar, Svensson et al. 2010). Previous studies in bone fracture model (without implants) in similar animal model have shown that ALP and OC expression attained their peaks after 5 and 11 days, respectively (Jingushi and Bolander 1990). Osteoclastic gene expression levels of TRAP and CATK have been shown to attain their earliest peaks between 7 - 14 days (Uusitalo, Hiltunen et al. 2000; Nagashima, Sakai et al. 2005). The observations that the peak expression of osteogenic and osteoclastic markers was detected as early as 3 days at the implant surface and that oxidized implants were associated with significantly higher levels than machined implants indicate, firstly, that bone remodeling around implants starts much earlier than what has previously been assumed (mainly based on conclusions from fracture models and *in vitro* experiments with one cell population), and, secondly, that the implant surface has an influence on the level of expression of bone differentiation and remodeling markers. Possible mechanisms for the accelerated implant-associated bone response include multiple cell participation and cross-talk, influenced by material surface physicochemical properties and topography of the implanted surfaces.

The regulation of gene expression at implant surfaces *in vivo* is a complex process. It is probably that material properties influence the gene expression of several factors, in addition to the secretion, organization and remodelling of the extracellular matrix components. Thereby these events may further affect key-factors, such as Runx2, which is crucial transcription factor for osteogenic differentiation and bone formation. The higher expression of osteoblast markers, (ALP) and (OC), and osteoclast marker, (CATK), was in parallel to a higher expression of Runx2 at the oxidized surfaces compared to machined ones after 3 days of implantation (Omar, Svensson et al. 2010). Similar results were demonstrated for hydrofluoric acid (HF) etched surface in comparison to similar surface without acid etching (Guo, Padilla et al. 2007). In the latter study, Runx2 expression was evident after 7 days in rat tibia and was associated with higher expression of ALP and bone sialoprotein (BSP). Regulatory effect on the expression of Runx2 was also confirmed for the HF surface in rabbit cortical bone concurrently with higher expression of collagen 1 and OC after 8 weeks of implantation (Monjo, Lamolle et al. 2008). At the implant surface, collagen-rich matrix organization together with increased expression of integrin-β1 may characterize an important pathway for Runx2 activation and consequently the downstream osteogenic activity and bone formation (Figure 12).

The performance of dental implants is best evaluated with respect to their stability into the implantation site. The *in vivo* interfacial gene expression model has been successfully combined with removal torsion analysis to determine possible relationship between the molecular events and torque strength at the interface (Omar, Lenneras et al. 2011). Significantly higher and constant increase in removal torque was registered for the oxidized implants throughout the period of 6 – 28 days of implantation (Figure 13). At the same time, the increased biomechanical strength at the interface of the oxidized implants was in association with higher expression levels of bone formation genes (OC and Runx2). The increased expression of bone formation genes during this period was coupled with upregulated expression of bone resorption genes (TRAP and CATK). The high expression of bone formation and bone resorption indicated an active remodelling throughout the time periods concomitant with an increasing biomechanical strength of the interface. In agreement, other studies compared the expression of different genes and pull-out force of coin-shaped implants with different hydrofluoric acid modification after 4 weeks in rabbit (Lamolle, Monjo et al. 2009; Taxt-Lamolle, Rubert et al. 2010). The test implant group that showed increased pull-out values, revealed higher expression of OC, collagen 1 and TRAP and decreased expression of TNF-α and IL-6.

On the other hand, low and unchanged values were observed in removal torque strength for the machined implants during the evaluation periods 6, 14 and 28 days. Machined implants were associated with an increased expression of pro-inflammatory cytokines (TNF-α and IL-1β) during the early (week) phase of osseointegration (Omar, Lenneras et al. 2010; Omar, Svensson et al. 2010), observations which were extended also to the later stages of osseointegration (Omar, Lenneras et al. 2011). It has previously been suggested that the

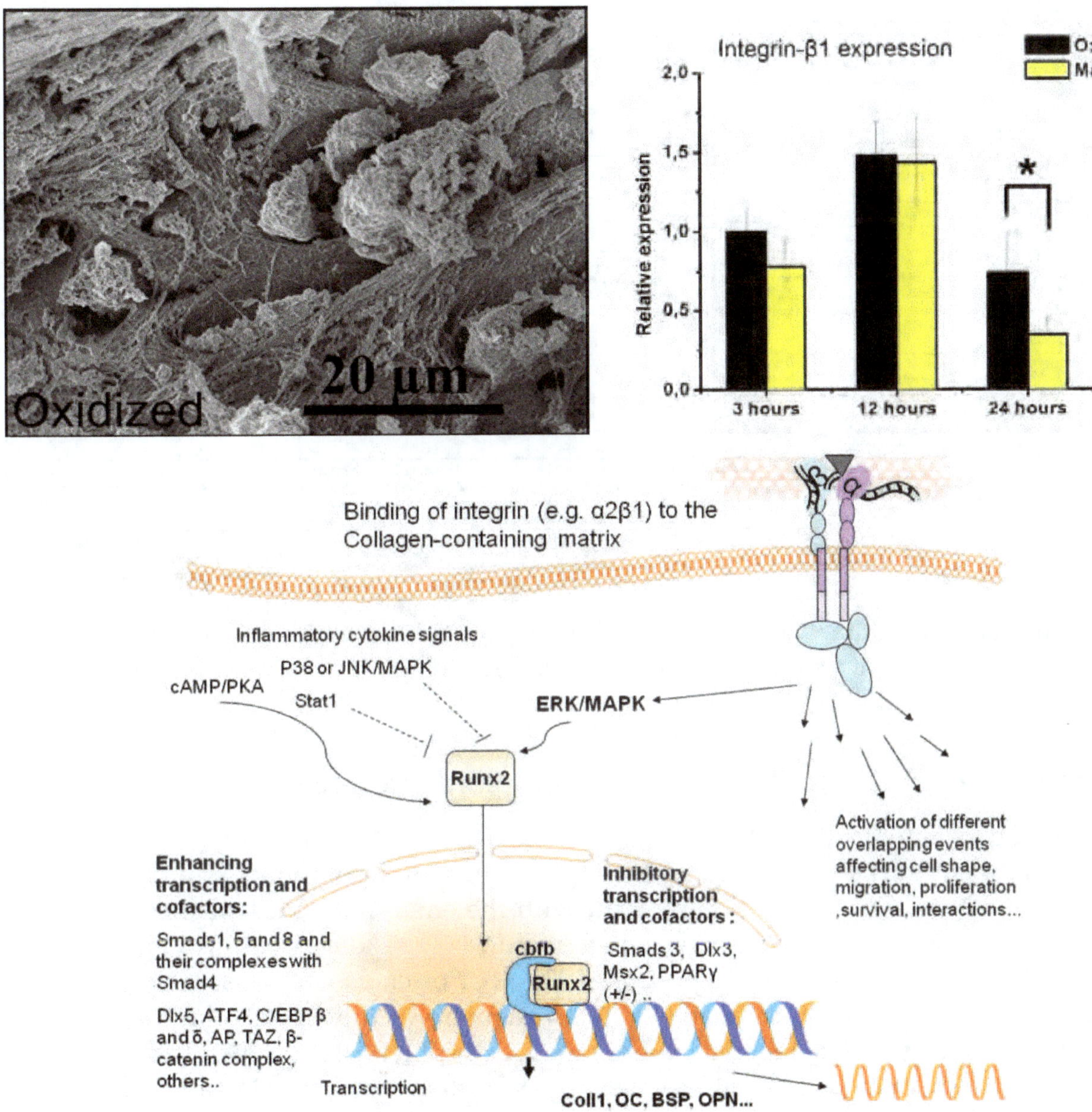

Fig. 12. Upper left, SEM image of oxidized implants retrieved 6d after implantation. Well-organized collagen network with numerous mesenchymal cells were observed on the oxidized implant. Upper right, a graph showing significantly increased expression of integrin-β1 at oxidized implant after 1d of implantation. The lower drawing illustrates activation of osteogenic response by mechanisms involving binding of integrin-α2β1 to collagen-rich matrix.

initial reduction and plateauing of the biomechanical strength of machined implants could be a manifestation of post-surgical inflammation and the remodelling activity (Branemark, Ohrnell et al. 1997). This is partly supported by the present results, given that machined implants, which were associated with higher expression of pro-inflammatory cytokines, did not reveal any increase in the biomechanical strength between 6 and 28 days. Whereas the increase in remodelling activity coupled with increased bone forming activity were in line with increased interface resistance for similar time periods.

		Initial phase		Early phase			Late phase	
		3h	12h	1d	3d	6d	14d	28d
qPCR	TNF-α	2-fold at machined	No differnce	2-fold at machined	No difference	3-fold at machined	No difference	3-fold at machined
	IL-β1	No difference	No differnce	5-fold at machined	No difference	3-fold at machined	2-fold at machined	2-fold at machined
	MCP-1	No difference	No difference	2-fold at machined	Not analyzed	Not analyzed	Not analyzed	Not analyzed
	CXCR4	No difference	12-fold at oxidized	No difference	Not analyzed	Not analyzed	Not analyzed	Not analyzed
	Intg-β2	No difference	2-fold at oxidized	2-fold at oxidized	Not analyzed	Not analyzed	Not analyzed	Not analyzed
	Runx2	Not analyzed	Not analyzed	No difference	6-fold at oxidized	No difference	No difference	2-fold at oxidized
	ALP	Not analyzed	Not analyzed	No difference	5-fold at oxidized	2-fold at oxidized	No difference	No difference
	OC	Not analyzed	Not analyzed	No difference	5-fold at oxidized	5-fold at oxidized	3-fold at oxidized	3-fold at oxidized
	CATK	Not analyzed	Not analyzed	No difference	4-fold at oxidized	2-fold at oxidized	2-fold at oxidized	No difference
	TRAP	Not analyzed	Not analyzed	No difference	2-fold at oxidized	2-fold at oxidized	2-fold at oxidized	2-fold at oxidized
Scanning electron microscopy (SEM) and backscattered SEM		-Higher proportion of fibrinous material adherent to machined. -Larger proportion of mesenchymal cells firmly anchoring to oxidized.		- Fibrinous material with entrapped leukocytes were evident throughout the 6 days at the machined. -Fairly organized collagenous network and many mesenchymal cells scattered all over the oxidized at days.			-mineralized lamellar bone and areas of newly formed bone for both. - Machined implant: separated from bone by a narrow gap. -Oxidized implant: direct contact with bone. Bone ingrowth into micropores.	
Histology and Immuno- -histochemistry		-Hematoma organization. -Prominent fibrin mesh at machined. - CD163 positive cells (Monocytes and macrophages) at both implants. -Periostin positive cells (mesenchymal and osteoprogenitors) at both implants.		-Tissue organization with different cellular populations. -Higher degree of vascularity and organization at oxidized. -CD163 positive (Monocytes and macrophages) at both. -Periostin reactivity (osteoprogenitors and osteoblasts) and throughout regenerated tissue at both implants. -Bone formation (woven bone)			-Woven bone remodeled. -Mature bone forming the interface.	
Biomechanical stability		Not analyzed		-Oxidized implant demonstrated higher magnitude and significant increase in biomechanical resistance during the first 28 days. -Machined implant showed lower magnitude and non-significant increase in biomechanical resistance during the first 28 days. - The oxidized implant showed a fracture-like breakpoint while the machined implant showed the typical curve with mainly separation in the immediate bone-implant interface.				
Biological processes		Clot formation, hematoma organization, initial inflammation, multiple cell chemotaxis and recruitment and adhesion		Downregulation of inflammatory phase, growth factor production, tissue organization, differentiation of osteogenic and osteoclastic cells, coupled bone formation and remodeling			Mature osteoclasts and osteoblasts, continuous coupled bone formation and remodeling (maturation), later abating of remodeling, Steady inflammatory milieu.	

Table 3. Summary of cellular and molecular activities at oxidized and machined implant during the first 4 weeks of implantation in rat tibia. The biological activities were correlated to the biomechanical stability of oxidized and machined implants in the same animal model.

5. Ultrastructure characterization of bone-implant interface

In order to further understand the bonding mechanisms that occur between living bone tissue and implant surface, analytical tools with sufficient resolution for ultrastructural analysis are needed. This especially important with the emerging nano-structured implant surfaces. Further, not only the structural aspect should be considered but also the chemical nature of the interface layer is of importance. The tool of choice is transmission electron microscopy (TEM) where various analytical tools often are readily used in high resolution. The electron-solid interaction generates different contrast phenomena, depending on crystal structure and atom number as well as interactions with the sample electrons generating energy-losses of the primary electron beam and secondary x-rays for chemical analysis. Further, elastic scattering and interference contrast could also be used for structural analysis. Hence, TEM is a versatile tool alloying structural and chemical analysis with high lateral and volumetric resolution. However, the literature of biomedical implants in bone tissue using TEM is scarce where the main reason is the sample preparation, especially for metallic implants. The sample should be around 100 nm thick to be electron transparent. Further a balance between contrast and overlapping information occurs, where less contrast is obtained when the sample becomes thinner, while the amount of overlapping information in the sample increases with the thickness.

5.1 TEM sample preparation methods

Different methods for sample preparation have been developed and are often optimized for each branch of research. Within the materials research field, polishing techniques, etching and broad ion milling are often employed, while the ultramicrotome is often used for

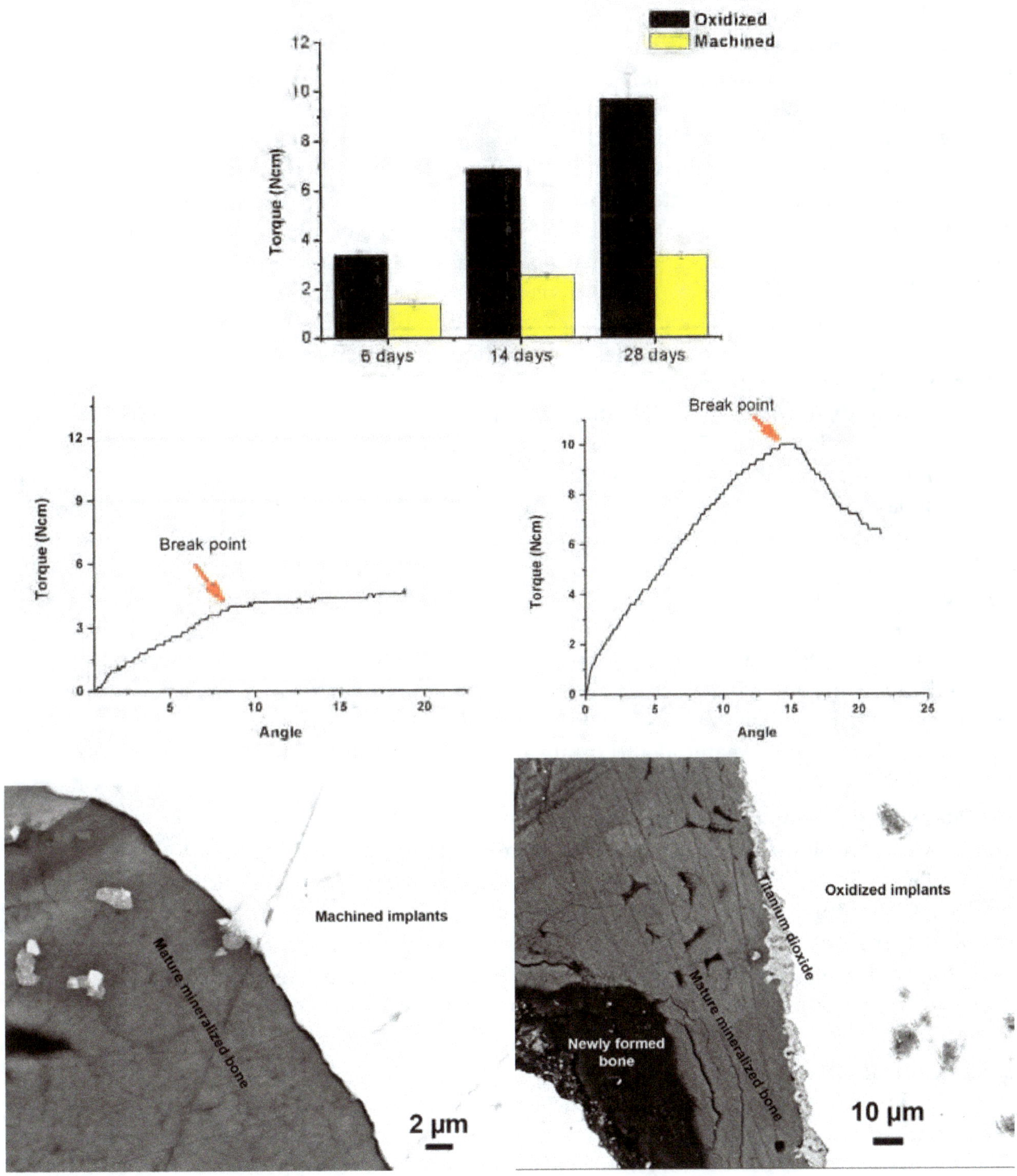

Fig. 13. Upper, a graph showing significant increase in the removal torque values for oxidized implants during early osseointegration. The middle graphs show the load-deformation curves of machined (left) and oxidized (right) implants after 28d of implantation. The deformation of the machined implant interface is mainly due to separation whereas a fracture-like pattern is registered for the oxidized implant. The lower backscattered SEM images show machined implant (left) was separated from bone by a narrow gap. Direct contact of the bone with the oxidized implant (right) was detected with generalized bone ingrowth into different sized micropores.

tissues. Within the field of biomaterials, the samples are composed of both hard materials as metals and ceramics and tissues as bone and soft tissue, therefore a different strategy has to be employed, as the diamond knife in the ultramicrotome could not cut through the hard implant material and the grinding, etching and broad ion milling will destroy the tissue.

Different strategies have been introduced where the main focus has been focused on removing the uncuttable implant material allowing the use of the ultramicrotome. One of these methods used experimental implants made of plastic which were coated with a thin enough layer of the material that was tested so it was still cuttable with the ultramicrotome. Different metal coating has been used such as titanium, zirconium, gold and steel (Albrektsson et al., 1985, 1982a, 1982b). This method was restricted to experimental studies, as the plastic implants did not posses clinically acceptable mechanical properties. Other methods were developed to be able to evaluate implants from clinical situations where different solutions to remove the implant were used. One method was based on gently fracture away the implant material either during the decalcification step (Steflik et al., 1992) or after resin embedding (Thomsen & Ericson, 1985). Uncertainties of the integrity of the interfacial tissue remained as the material was completely removed. A strategy for keeping the oxide layer intact, having an intact interface, while removing the bulk properties of the implant allowing ultramicrotome sectioning was developed. By electrochemical dissolution of the metallic titanium the oxide layer was still present in the section (Radegran et al., 1991), however, this technique demineralized the tissue (Sennerby et al., 1991). Another metod used was sawing and grinding to remove the bulk metal leaving the surface layer of the implant intact (Leize et al., 2000), this may be useful for thicker surface coatings as plasma-sprayed titanium, but with most commercially available dental implant rather thin oxides are present. With the use of focused ion beam (FIB) intact bone-implant interfaces could be prepared, allowing both material and tissue analysis (Engqvist et al., 2006).

5.2 Interface analysis of different surfaces

Quit few ultrastructural analysis of the bone-implant interface are presented in the literature as compared to the total amount of articles using bone anchored implants. The most published literature evaluates the machined surface or similar smooth surface using mainly the plastic implant replica model or the fracture method. The fracture method has also been used for acid etched implants, while the FIB has mainly been used for the laser-modified implant surface. Some articles evaluate plasma-sprayed surfaces and oxidized surfaces.

5.2.1 Smooth implant surface

Different interfaces have been described for machined implants, some dependent on the healing time and some depending on sample preparation method. Most of the analysis showed that an interposed amorphous electron lucent layer of approximalty 20-50 nm was found between the mineralized bone and implant surface (Albrektsson et al., 1985, 1982; Linder et al., 1983). This was often with a poorly mineralized zone of a few hundred nm containing collagen fibrils prior to the mineralized bone tissue (Albrektsson et al., 1985, 1986). Others found instead an electron dense layer of similar thickness prior to the mineralized bone tissue, either directly at the implant surface (Ayukawa et al., 1998) or with a larger amorphous zone in direct contact with the surface (Sennerby et al., 1991, 1992). Also a direct contact between mineralized bone tissue and implant surface has been reported using different sample preparation techniques (Albrektsson et al., 1981; Brunette et al., 1991;

Meyer et al., 2004). By the use of high-resolution TEM crystalline hydroxyapatite was found precipitated directly at the implant surface of a machined titanium implant retrieved after 11 years of clinical loading (Palmquist et al., 2008). The sample preparation technique seem to be essential where plastic implant replicas seem to show a predominance for an intervening electron lucent layer, while the fracture technique show a predominance for an electron dense layer and a thicker amorphous zone. With FIB difficulties in sample preparation for smoother implant surfaces is separation between the tissue and implant (Palmquist et al., 2009)., most likely due to shrinkage of the tissue during dehydration (Lawton et al., 1995) and resin embedding, on the other hand this suggests that the separation for the fracture technique occurs at the immediate interface, and it has been shown that low amount of remnants were found on the implant after fracture (Lausmaa & Linder, 1988).

5.2.2 Roughened implant surface

The most studies have been performed using an acid etched surface, increasing the roughness by pitting and the creation of craters in the surface. The results using the fracture technique of acid etched surfaces showed an electron dense layer interposed between the implant surface and the mineralized bone tissue (Steflik et al., 1992a, 1992b, 1998). Further, at areas of less mature bone tissue a zone of mineralized collagen fibril layer was found between the mineralized bone and the electron dense layer (Steflik et al., 1992b, 1998). Further, the use of high-voltage TEM has enabled tracking of the canaliculus which reach the implant surface (Steflik et al., 1992a, 1994). For plasma-sprayed implants and plastic implant replicas of plasma-sprayed implants a direct bone-implant contact has been described at most places as well as an intervening layer with indistinct structure reaching up to 1 µm in thickness (Leize, 2000; Hemmerle & Voegel, 1996). By combining micro and nano topography by the use of laser ablation, an intimate contact between mineralized bone tissue and implant surface oxide has been described (Palmquist et al., 2010) using the FIB technique. Further, elemental analysis showed the presence of calcium and phosphorous in the nano structured surface oxide (Palmquist et al., 2011). The FIB has also been used to analyse the bone-implant interface of a failed dental implant retrieved with smaller amount of bone tissue, the results showed an electron lucent layer closest to the implant surface as well as bone ingrowth in the porous oxide (Giannuzzi et al., 2005, 2007).

5.2.3 Bioactive implant surface

The use of bioactive coating may enable a chemical bond between the implant surface and surrounding bone tissue. Most frequently used bioactive coating is hydroxyapatite. Thin sputtered and Plasma-sprayed HA coatings has been shown to form an intimate contact with bone tissue (Engqvist et al., 2006; Grandfield et al., 2011a, 2011b) with minor resorption of the coating. The use of calcium aluminate coating showed also an intimate contact with bone tissue, where different crystalline phase was observed in the coating while the outermost layer of the coating facing the bone tissue was calcium deficient (Palmquist, et al., 2009). Ultrastructural analyses of hydroxyapatite scaffolds and bone tissue have shown the formation of an apatite layer between the collagenous bone and implant surface (Grandfield et al., 2010a). Further, this layer was shown to have a distinct difference in crystal direction from the crystals in the collagenous bone tissue with the used of electron tomography (Grandfield, et al., 2010b). Further, the incorporation of ions in the hydroxyapatite has shown to influence the rate of dissolution and also the rate of bone formation (Porter et., 2004a, 2004b, 2005).

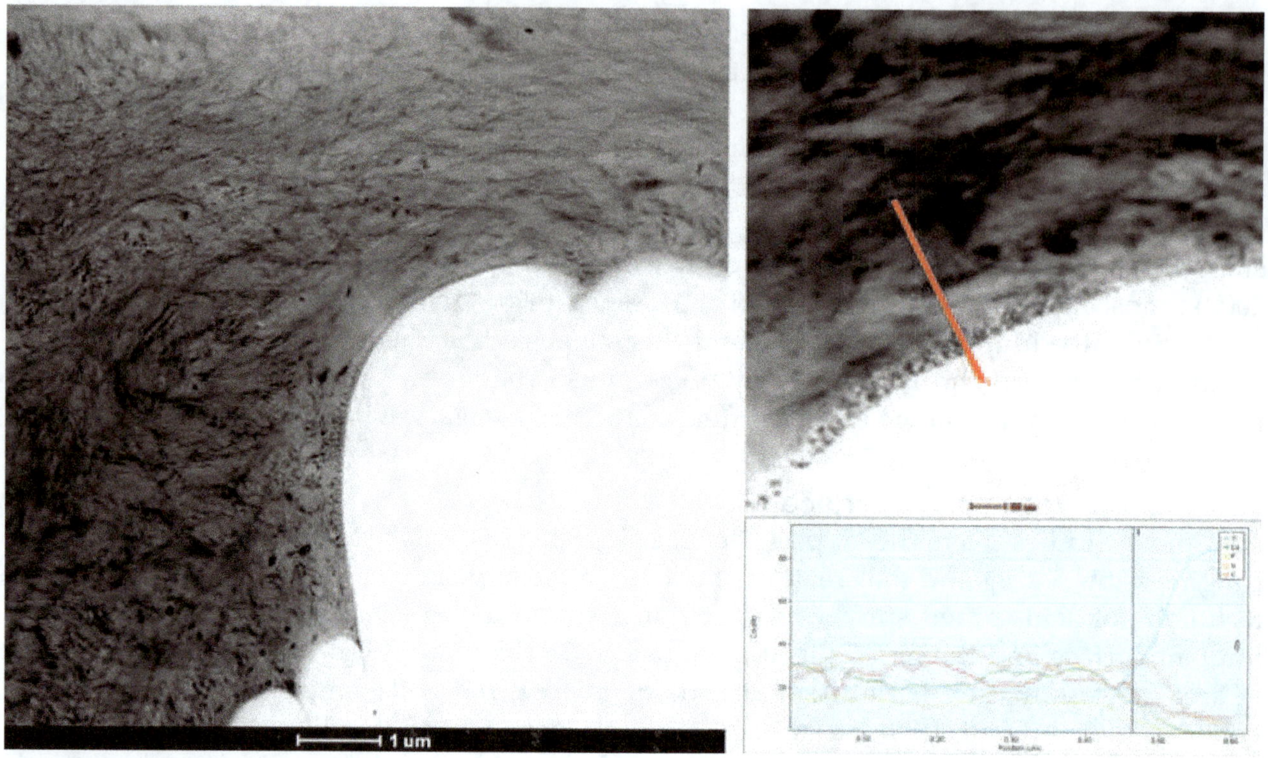

Fig. 14. HAADF-STEM micrographs of laser modified titanium implants after 6 months healing in rabbit, the left image show an overview where bone tissue are found with an intimate contact to the implant surface, collagen banding is observed close to the implant surface. Right, a closer view of the interface, where the enlarged surface oxide is clearly observed with intimate contact to the bone tissue. The EDS line scan along the red line show the presence of Calcium and Phosphorous in the bone tissue, and Titanium in the bulk metal. An overlap zone observed where calcium, phosphorous, titanium and oxygen are seen simultaneously indicating bone ingrowth in the nano structured surface oxide.

6. Summary

The new generation dental implants exhibit a large variation in surface properties, both in terms of structural and chemical compositions. The selection criteria for the first generation of dental implants were mainly based on their mechanical properties and corrosion resistance under physiological conditions. The current surfaces have mainly underwent topographical modification and, to a lesser extent, alteration in chemical composition. The aim of surface modifications was to achieve an enhanced biological response. Experimental studies and clinical experience provided extensive empirical knowledge about the role of such surface modifications for biological responses. However, comprehensive understanding of the biological response at the bone-implant interface is still lacking and further research is required to understand the biological processes taking place at the interface, and how these are influenced and can be controlled by specific surface properties.

7. Future prospective in dental implant surfaces

Future development of the next, third generation of dental implants should be based on increased knowledge about the interface biology on cellular and molecular levels. The development of future generations of oral implants for compromised tissue conditions will, most probably, entail tailored modifications of material surfaces. Implant surfaces, selectively, designed for drug and/or cell releases represent promising candidate strategy. Other surface modifications, such as selective ion substitutions of biomimetic surfaces may further improve the biological response to those surfaces. Further, as the bacterial infection is a major challenge which may jeopardize the success of osseointegrated implants, implant modification resulting in antibacterial activity might be of importance to reduce such complications.

8. References

Adell, R; Lekholm, U; Rockler, B. & Branemark, PI. (1981). A 15-year study of osseointegrated implants in the treatment of the edentulous jaw. Int J Oral Surg, 10, 387-416.

Albrektsson, T; Brånemark PI; Hansson, HA. & Lindström, J. (1981). Osseointegrated titanium implants. Requirements for ensuring a long-lasting, direct bone-to-implant anchorage in man. Acta Orthop Scand, 52, 155-170.

Albrektsson, T. (1982). Ultrastructural Analysis of the Interface Zone of Titanium and Gold Implants, in Advances in biomaterials, T. Albrektsson, A.J.C. Lee, and P.I. Brånemark, Editors. Wiley: Chichester. p. 167-177.

Albrektsson, T; Hansson, HA. & Ivarsson B. (1985). Interface analysis of titanium and zirconium bone implants. Biomaterials, 6, 97-101.

Albrektsson, T. & Hansson, HA. (1986). An ultrastructural characterization of the interface between bone and sputtered titanium or stainless steel surfaces. Biomaterials, 7, 201-205.

Albrektsson, T; Johansson, C; Lundgren, AK; Sul, YT. & Gottlow J. (2000). Experimental Studies on Oxidized Implants: A histomorphometrical and biomechanical analysis. Applied Osseointegration Research, 1, 21-24.

Albrektsson, T. & Wennerberg, A. (2004a). Oral implant surfaces: Part 1--review focusing on topographic and chemical properties of different surfaces and in vivo responses to them. Int J Prosthodont, 17, 536-543.

Albrektsson, T. & Wennerberg, A. (2004b). Oral implant surfaces: Part 2--review focusing on clinical knowledge of different surfaces. Int J Prosthodont, 17, 544-564.

Ayukawa, Y., et al., (1998). An immunoelectron microscopic localization of noncollagenous bone proteins (osteocalcin and osteopontin) at the bone-titanium interface of rat tibiae. J Biomed Mater Res, 41, 111-9.

Ballo, AM; Xia, W; Lindahl, C; Lausmaa, J; Engqvist, H. & Thomsen, P. (2010). Bone responses to ions-substituted apatite/titanium dioxide coating on titanium implants. 88th General Session & Exhibition of the IADR, Barcelona, Spain, July, 2010.

Ballo, AM; Närhi, TO; Akca, EA; Ozen, T; Syrjänen, SM; Lassila, LV. & Vallittu, PK. (2011). Prepolymerized vs. in situ-polymerized fiber-reinforced composite implants--a pilot study. J Dent Res, 90, 263-267.

Ballo, AM; Akca, EA; Ozen, T; Lassila, L; Vallittu, PK. & Närhi TO. (2009). Bone tissue responses to glass fiber-reinforced composite implants--a histomorphometric study. Clin Oral Implants Res, 20, 608-15.

Barrere, F; Snel, MME; van Blitterswijk, CA; de Groot, K. & Layrolle, P. (2004). Nano-scale study of the nucleation and growth of calcium phosphate coating on titanium implants. Biomaterials, 25, 2901-2910.

Barrere, F; van der Valk, CM; Meijer, G; Dalmeijer, RA., De Groot, K. & Layrolle, P. (2003). Osteointegration of biomimetic apatite coating applied onto dense and porous metal implants in femurs of goats. Journal of Biomedical Materials Research 67: 655–665.

Bloyer, DR; Gomez-Vega, JM; Saiz, E; Mcnaney, JM; Cannon, RM. & Tomsia, AP. (1999). Fabrication and characterization of a bioactive glass coating on titanium implant aloys, Acta mater, 47, 4221-4224.

Brånemark, R; Brånemark, PI; Rydevik, B. & Myers RR. (2001). Osseointegration in skeletal reconstruction and rehabilitation: a review. J Rehabil Res Dev, 38, 175-181.

Brånemark, PI; Hansson, BO; Adell, R; Breine, U; Lindstrom, J; Hallen, O. & Ohman A. (1977). Osseointegrated implants in the treatment of the edentulous jaw. Experience from a 10-year period. Scand J Plast Reconstr Surg Suppl, 16, 1-132.

Brånemark, R; Emanuelsson, L; Palmquist, A. & Thomsen, P. (2010). Bone response to laser-induced micro- and nano-size titanium surface features. Nanomedicine. (In press)

Brånemark, R; Ohrnell, LO; Nilsson, P. & Thomsen, P. (1997). Biomechanical characterization of osseointegration during healing: an experimental in vivo study in the rat. Biomaterials, 18, 969-978.

Brånemark, PI; Adell, R; et al. (1969). Intra-osseous anchorage of dental prostheses. I. Experimental studies. Scand J Plast Reconstr Surg, 3, 81-100.

Brunette, DM; Ratkay, J. & Chehroudi B. (1991). Behaviour of Osteoblasts on Micromachined Surfaces, in: The bone-biomaterial interface, J.E. Davies, Editor , Univ. of Toronto Press: Toronto. p. 425-437.

Brunette, DM; Tengvall, P; Textor, M. & Thomsen, P. *(eds)* (2001). Titanium in medicine: material science, surface science, engineering, biological responses, and medical applications. Berlin, Germany: Springer.

Buser, D; Broggini, N; Wieland, M; Schenk, RK; Denzer, AJ; Cochran, DL; Hoffmann, B; Lussi, A. & Steinemann, SG. (2004). Enhanced bone apposi-tion to a chemically modified SLA titanium surface. J Dent Res, 83, 529–533.

Buser, D; Schenk, RK; Steinemann, S; Fiorellini, JP; Fox, CH. & Stich, H. (1991). Influence of surface characteristics on bone integration of titanium implants. A histomorphometric study in miniature pigs. J Biomed Mater Res, 25, 889-902.

Buser, D; Nydegger, T; Oxland, T; Cochran, DL; Schenk, RK; Hirt, HP; Snétivy, D. & Nolte, LP. (1999). Interface shear strength of titanium implants with a sandblasted and acid-etched surface: a biomechanical study in the maxilla of miniature pigs. J Biomed Mater Res, 45, 75-83.

Cao, W. & Hench, LL. (1996). Bioactive Materials. Ceramics International, 22, 493-507.

Carr, AB ; Larsen, PE ; Papazoglou, E. & McGlumphy, E. (1995). Reverse torque failure of screw-shaped implants in baboons: baseline data for abutment torque application. Int J Oral Maxillofac Implant, 10, 167-174.

Celletti, R; Marinho, VC; Traini, T; Orsini, G; Bracchetti, G; Perrotti, V, et al. (2006). Bone contact around osseointegrated implants: a histologic study of acid-etched and machined surfaces. J Long Term Eff Med Implants, 16, 131-143.

Ceradini, DJ; Kulkarni, AR et al. (2004). Progenitor cell trafficking is regulated by hypoxic gradients through HIF-1 induction of SDF-1. Nat Med, 10, 858-864.

Chehroudi, B; Ratkay, J. & Brunette, DM. (1992). The role of implant surface geometry on mineralization in vitro and in vivo: a transmission and electronmicroscopic study. Cells Mater, 2, 89-104.

Cook, SD; Kay, JF. & Thomas, KA. (1987). Interface mechanics and histology of titanium and HA-coated titanium for dental implant applications. Int J Oral Maxillofac Implants, 2, 15-22.

Cooper, LF; Masuda, T; Yliheikkila, PK. & Felton, DA. (1998). Generalizations regarding the process and phenomenon of osseointegration. Part 2: in vitro studies. J Oral Maxillofac Implants, 13, 163-174.

Cooper, LF; Zhou, Y; Takebe, J; Guo, J; Abron, A; Holmen, A, et al. (2006). Fluoride modification effects on osteoblast behavior and bone formation at TiO2 grit-blasted c.p. titanium endosseous implants. Biomaterials, 27, 926-936.

Conforto, E; Caillard, D; Aronsson, BO. & Descouts, P. (2004). Crystallographic properties and mechanical behaviour of titanium hydride layers grown on titanium implants. Philosophical Magazine, 84, 631-645.

Cochran, DL; Schenk, RK; Lussi, A; Higginbottom, FL. & Buser, D. (1998). Bone response to unloaded and loaded titanium implants with a sandblasted and acid-etched surface: A histomorphometric study in the canine mandible. Journal of Biomedical Materials Research, 40, 1–11.

Davies, JE. (2003). Understanding peri-implant endosseous healing. Journal of Dental Education, 67, 932–949.

De Groot, K; Geesink, R; Klein, CP. & Serekian, P. (1987). Plasma sprayed coatings of hydroxylapatite. J Biomed Mater Res, 21, 1375-1381.

Denissen, HW; Kalk, W; De Nieuport, HM; Maltha, JC. & Van de Hooff, A. (1990). Mandibular bone response to plasma-sprayed coating of hydroxyapatite. Int J Prosthodont, 3, 53-58.

Ding, S. (2003). Properties and immersion behavior of magnetrons puttered multi-layered hydroxyapatite/titanium composite coatings. Biomaterials, 24, 4233–4238.

Ding, S; Ju, C. & Lin, JC. (1999). Characterization of hydroxyapatite and titanium coatings sputtered on Ti-6Al-4V substrate. J Biomed Mater Res, 44, 266–279.

Elias, CN; Oshida, Y; Lima, JH. & Muller, CA. (2008). Relationship between surface properties (roughness, wettability and morphology) of titanium and dental implant removal torque. J Mech Behav Biomed Mater, 1, 234-42.

Ellingsen, JE; Johansson, CB; Wennerberg, A. & Holmen, A. (2004). Improved retention and bone-tolmplant contact with fluoride-modified titanium implants. Int J Oral Maxillofac Implants, 19, 659-666.

Engqvist, H., et al., (2006). A novel tool for high-resolution transmission electron microscopy of intact interfaces between bone and metallic implants. J Biomed Mater Res A, 78, 20-24.

Esposito, M; Coulthard, P; Thomsen, P. & Worthington, HV. (2005). The role of implant surface modifications, shape and material on the success of osseointegrated dental implants. A Cochrane systematic review. Eur J Prosthodont Restor Dent, 13, 15-31.

Esposito, M; Worthington, HV; Thomsen, P. & Coulthard, P. (2003). Interventions for replacing missing teeth: different types of dental implants. Cochrane Database Syst Rev, CD003815.

Frayssinet, P ; Trouillet, JL ; Rouquet, N ; Azimus, E. & Autefage, A. (1993). Osseointegration of macroporous calcium phosphate ceramics having a different chemical composition. Biomaterials, 14, 423-429.

Frojd, V; Franke-Stenport, V; Meirelles, L. & Wennerberg, A. (2008). Increased bone contact to a calcium-incorporated oxidized commercially pure titanium implant: an in-vivo study in rabbits. Int J Oral Maxillofac Surg, 37, 561-566.

Fuming, H; Guoli, Y; Xiaoxiang, W. & Shifang, Z. (2008). The removal torque of titanium implant inserted in rabbit femur coated with biomimetic deposited Ca-P coating. J Oral Rehabil. 35, 754-65.

Furlong, RJ. & Osborn, JF. (1991). Fixation of hip prostheses by hydroxyapatite ceramic coatings. J Bone Jt Surg, 73, 741-745.

Gadelmawla, ES; Koura, MM; Maksoud, TMA; Elewa, IM. & Soliman, HM. (2002). Roughness parameters. Journal of Materials Processing Technology, 123, 133-145.

Giannuzzi, LA; Giannuzzi, NJ. & Capuano, MJ. (2005). FIB, SEM, and TEM of Bone/Dental Implant Interfaces. Microscopy and Microanalysis, 11, 998-999.

Giannuzzi, LA; Phifer, D; Giannuzzi, NJ. & Capuano, MJ. (2007). Two-dimensional and 3-dimensional analysis of bone/dental implant interfaces with the use of focused ion beam and electron microscopy. J Oral Maxillofac Surg, 65, 737-747.

Gomez-Vega, JM; Hozumi, A; Saiz, E; Tomsia, AP; Sugimura, H. & Takai, O. (2001). Bioactive glass-mesoporous silica coatings on Ti6Al4V throgh enameling and triblock-copolymer-templated sol-gel processing, J Biomed Mater Res, 56, 382-389.

Gomez-Vega, JM; Saiz, E; Tomsia, AP; Marshall, GW. & Marshall, SJ. (2000a). Bioactive glass coatings with hydroxyapatite and Bioglass particles on Ti-based implants. I. Processing, Biomaterials, 21, 105-111.

Gomez-Vega, JM; Saiz, E; Tomsia, AP; Oku, T; Suganuma, K; Marshall, GW. & Marshall, SJ. (2000b). Novel bioactive glass functionally graded coatings on Ti6Al4V, Adv Mater, 12, 894-898.

Gottlow, J; Johansson, C; Albrektsson, T. & Lundgren, AK. (2010). Biomechanical and Histological Evaluation of the TiUnite and Osseotite Implant Surfaces in Rabbits after 6 Weeks of Healing. Applied Osseointegration Research, 1, 25-27.

Grandfield, K., et al. (2011a)., Ultrastructural characterization of the hydroxyapatite-coated pedicle screw and human bone interface. Int J Nano and Biomaterials. Accepted for publication.

Grandfield, K., et al. (2011b)., Free form fabricated features on CoCr implants with and without hydroxyapatite coating in vivo: a comparative study of bone contact and bone growth induction. J Mater Sci Mater Med. Accepted for publication

Grandfield, K., et al. (2010a)., Bone Response to Free-Form Fabricated Hydroxyapatite and Zirconia Scaffolds: A Transmission Electron Microscopy Study in the Human Maxilla. Clinical implant dentistry and related research. Accepted for publication.

Grandfield, K., et al., (2010b). Visualizing biointerfaces in three dimensions: electron tomography of the bone-hydroxyapatite interface. J R Soc Interface, 7, 1497-1501.

Greenspan, DC. & Hench, LL. (1976). Chemical and mechanical behavior of bioglass-coated alumina. J Biomed Mater Res, 10, 503-509.

Granero-Molto, FJA; Weis, et al. (2009). Regenerative effects of transplanted mesenchymal stem cells in fracture healing. Stem Cells, 27, 1887-1898.

Guo, J., R. J. Padilla, et al. (2007). The effect of hydrofluoric acid treatment of TiO2 grit blasted titanium implants on adherent osteoblast gene expression in vitro and in vivo. Biomaterials, 28, 5418-5425.

Habibovic, P; Barrère, F; van Blitterswijk, CA; Groot, K. & Layrolle, P. (2002). Biomimetic Hydroxyapatite Coating on Metal Implants. J. Am. Ceram. Soc, 85, 517-522.

Hayashi, H; Nakahama, K; et al. (2008). The role of Mac-1 (CD11b/CD18) in osteoclast differentiation induced by receptor activator of nuclear factor-kappaB ligand. FEBS Lett, 582, 3243-3248.

Hall, J. & Lausmaa, J. (2000). Properties of a new porous oxide surface on titanium implants. Applied Osseointegration Research, 1, 5-8.

Hayakawa, T; Yoshinari, M; Nemoto, K; Wolke, JGC. & Jansen, JA. (2000). Effect of surface roughness and calcium phosphate coating on the implant/bone response. Clin Oral Implant Res, 11, 296–304.

He, F; Liu, L; Zhao, S; Zhao, S; Chen, S. & Wang, X. (2007). Fast formation of biomimetic apatite coatings on pure porous titanium implant's surface. Sheng Wu Yi Xue Gong Cheng Xue Za Zhi, 24, 806–811.

He, F; Yang, G; Wang, X. & Zhao, S. (2009). Bone responses to rough titanium implants coated with biomimetic Ca-P in rabbit tibia. J Biomed Mater Res B Appl Biomater, 90, 857-63.

Hemmerle, J; Onçag, A. & Ertürk S. (1997). Ultrastructural features of the bone response to a plasma-sprayed hydroxyapatite coating in sheep. J Biomed Mater Res, 36:418-425.

Hemmerle, J. & Voegel, JC. (1996). Ultrastructural aspects of the intact titanium implant-bone interface from undecalcified ultrathin sections. Biomaterials, 17, 1913-1920.

Hench, LL; Splinter, RJ; Allen, WC. & Greenlee, TK. (1971) Bonding mechanisms at the interface of ceramic prosthetic materials. J Biomed Mater Res Symposium, 2, 117–41.

Hench, LL. & Andersson, ÖH. (1993). Bioactive glass coatings. In Hench LL and Wilson J editors. An introduction to bioceramics, World Scientific, 239.

Henry, PJ; Tan, AES; Allan, BP; Hall, J. & Johansson C. (2000). Removal Torque Comparison of TiUnite and Turned Implants in the Greyhaound Dog Mandible. Applied Osseointegration Research, 1, 15-17.

Hughes, DE; Salter DM;, et al. (1993). Integrin expression in human bone. J Bone Miner Res, 8, 527-533.

Jansen, JA; van de Waerden, JP; Wolke, JG. & de Groot, K. (1991). Histologic evaluation of the osseous adaptation to titanium and hydroxyapatite-coated titanium implants J Biomed Mater Res, 25, 973-989.

Jansen, JA; Wolke, JGC; Swann, S; van der Waerden, JPCM. & de Groot K. (1993). Application of magnetron-sputtering for producing ceramic coatings on implant materials. Clinical Oral Implants Research, 4, 28–34.

Jansson, E; Kalltorp, M; et al. (2002). Ex vivo PMA-induced respiratory burst and TNF-alpha secretion elicited from inflammatory cells on machined and porous blood plasma clot-coated titanium. Biomaterials, 23, 2803-2815.

Jarmar, T; Palmquist, A; Branemark, R, Hermansson, L; Engqvist, H. & Thomsen, P. (2008). Characterization of the surface properties of commercially available dental implants using scanning electron microscopy, focused ion beam, and high-resolution transmission electron microscopy. Clin Implant Dent Relat Res, 10, 11-22.

Jingushi, S. & Bolander ME. (1990). Biological Cascades of Fracture Healing as Models for Bone-Biomaterial Interface. The Bone-Biomaterial Interface. J. E. Davies. Toronto, University of Toronto Press: 250-262.

Jungner, M; Lundqvist, P. & Lundgren, S. (2005). Oxidized titanium implants (Nobel Biocare TiUnite) compared with turned titanium implants (Nobel Biocare mark III) with respect to implant failure in a group of consecutive patients treated with early functional loading and two-stage protocol. Clin Oral Implants Res, 16, 308–312.

Kasemo, B. & Lausmaa, J. (1988). Biomaterial and implant surfaces: a surface science approach. Int J Oral Maxillofac Implants, 3, 247-259.

Kitsugi, T; Nakamura, T; Oka, M; Senaha, Y; Goto, T. & Shibuya, T. (1996). Bone-bonding behavior of plasma-sprayed coatings of BioglassR, AW-glass ceramic, and tricalcium phosphate on titanium alloy. J Biomed Mater Res, 30, 261-269.

Klokkevold, PR; Johnson, P; Dadgostari, S; Caputo, A; Davies, JE. & Nishimura, RD. (2001). Early endosseous integration enhanced by dual acid etching of titanium: a torque removal study in the rabbit. Clin Oral Implants Res, 12, 350-357.

Kokubo, T; Kushitani, H; Sakka, S; Kitsugi, T. & Yamamuro, T. (1990). Solutions able to reproduce in vivo surface-structure changes in bioactive glass-ceramic A-W. J Biomed Mater Res, 24, 721–734.

Lacefield, WR. & Hench, LL. (1986). The bonding of Bioglass to a cobalt-chromium surgical implant alloy. Biomaterials, 7, 104-108.

Lamolle, SF ; Monjo, M ; et al. (2009). Titanium implant surface modification by cathodic reduction in hydrofluoric acid: surface characterization and in vivo performance. J Biomed Mater Res A, 88, 581-588.

Larsson, C; Esposito, M; et al. (2001). The Titanium-Bone Interface In Vivo. Titanium in Medicine. D. M. Brunette, P. Tengvall, M. Textor and P. Thomsen. New York, Springer, 587-648.

Lausmaa, J. & Linder, L. (1988). Surface spectroscopic characterization of titanium implants after separation from plastic-embedded tissue. Biomaterials, 9, 277-280.

Lausmaa J. (1996). Surface spectroscopic characterization of titanium implant materials. Journal of Electron Spectroscopy and Related Phenomena, 81, 343-361.

Lausmaa J. (2001). Mechanical, Thermal, Chemical and Electrochemical Surface Treatment of Titanium. In: Brunette DM, editor. Titanium in medicine : material science, surface science, engineering, biological responses and medical applications. Berlin: Springer, 1019.

Lawton, DM; Oswald, WO. & McClure, J. (1995). The biological reality of the interlacunar network in the embryonic, cartilaginous, skeleton: a thiazine dye/absolute ethanol/LR White resin protocol for visualizing the network with minimal tissue shrinkage. J Microsc, 178, 66-85.

Leize, EM; Hemmerle, J. & Leize, M. (2000). Characterization, at the bone crystal level, of the titanium-coating/bone interfacial zone. Clin Oral Implants Res, 11, 279-288.

Linder, L., et al., (1983). Electron microscopic analysis of the bone-titanium interface. Acta Orthop Scand, 54, 45-52.

Ma, J; Huifen, W; Kong, LB. & Peng, KW. (2003). Biomimetic processing of nanocrystallite bioactive apatite coating on titanium. Nanotechnology, 14, 619-623.

Masaki, C ; Schneider, GB ; et al. (2005). Effects of implant surface microtopography on osteoblast gene expression. Clin Oral Implants Res, 16, 650-656.

Meyer, U., et al., (2004). Ultrastructural characterization of the implant/bone interface of immediately loaded dental implants. Biomaterials, 25, 1959-1967.

Mistry, S; Kundu, D; Datta, S. & Basu, D. (2011). Comparison of bioactive glass coated and hydroxyapatite coated titanium dental implants in the human jaw bone. Aust Dent J, 56, 68-75.

Monjo, M ; Lamolle, SF ; et al. (2008). In vivo expression of osteogenic markers and bone mineral density at the surface of fluoride-modified titanium implants. Biomaterials, 29, 3771-3780.

Morris, HF; Ochi, S; Spray, JR. & Olson, JW. (2000). Periodontal-type measurements associated with hydroxyapatite-coated and non-HA-coated implants: uncovering to 36 months. Annals of Periodontology/the American Academy of Periodontology, 5, 56–67.

Muller, FA; Jonasova, L; Helebrant, A; Strnad, J. & Greil, P. (2004). Biomimetic apatite formation on chemically treated titanium. Biomaterials, 25, 1187.

Nagashima, M; Sakai, A; et al. (2005). Bisphosphonate (YM529) delays the repair of cortical bone defect after drill-hole injury by reducing terminal differentiation of osteoblasts in the mouse femur. Bone, 36, 502-511.

Nygren, H; Tengvall, P. et al. (1997). The initial reactions of TiO2 with blood. J Biomed Mater Res, 34, 487-492.

Ogawa, T. & Nishimura I. (2003). Different bone integration profiles of turned and acid-etched implants associated with modulated expression of extracellular matrix genes. Int J Oral Maxillofac Implants, 18, 200-210.

Oku, T; Suganuma, K; Wallenberg, LR; Tomsia, AP; Gomez-Vega, JM. & Saiz, E. (2001). Structural characterization of the metal/glass interface in bioactive glass coatings on Ti-6Al-4V, J Mat Sci Mat Med, 12, 413-417.

Omar, O. (2010). Mechanisms of Osseointegration: Experimental Studies on Early Cellular and Molecular Events in vivo [Doctoral thesis]. Göteborg: University of Gothenburg.

Omar, O; Svensson, S; Lennerås, M; Zoric, N; Suska, F; Hall, J; Nannmark, U, & Thomsen, P. (2010). In vivo gene expression at anodically oxidized versus machined titanium implants. J Biomed Mater Res, 92, 1552-1566.

Omar, O ; Lenneras, M. et al. (2010). Integrin and chemokine receptor gene expression in implant-adherent cells during early osseointegration. J Mater Sci Mater Med, 21, 969-980.

Omar, O; Lenneras, ME. et al. (2011). The correlation between gene expression of proinflammatory markers and bone formation during osseointegration with titanium implants. Biomaterials, 32, 374-386.

Ong, JL; Raikar, GN. & Smoot, TM. (1997). Properties of calcium phosphate coatings before and after exposure to simulated biological fluid. Biomaterials, 18, 1271-1275.

Ong, JL. & Lucas, LC. (1998). Auger electron spectroscopy and it use for the characterization of titanium and hydroxyapatite surfaces. Biomaterials, 19, 455-64.

Ong, JL; Bessho, K; Cavin, R. & Carnes, DL. (2002). Bone response to radio frequency sputtered calcium phosphate implants and titanium implants in vivo. J Biomed Mater Res, 59, 184-190.

Otsuru, S; et al. (2008). Circulating bone marrow-derived osteoblast progenitor cells are recruited to the bone-forming site by the CXCR4/stromal cell-derived factor-1 pathway. Stem Cells, 26, 223-234.

Palmquist, A; et al., (2009). Calcium aluminate coated and uncoated free form fabricated CoCr implants: A comparative study in rabbit. J Biomed Mater Res B Appl Biomater, 91, 122-127.

Palmquist, A; et al., (2010). Biomechanical, histological, and ultrastructural analyses of laser micro- and nano-structured titanium alloy implants: A study in rabbit. J Biomed Mater Res A, 92, 1476-1486.

Palmquist, A; et al., (2009). Morphological studies on machined implants of commercially pure titanium and titanium alloy (Ti6Al4V) in the rabbit. J Biomed Mater Res B Appl Biomater, 91, 309-319.

Palmquist, A; Jarmar, T; Emanuelsson, L; Branemark, R; Engqvist, H. & Thomsen P. (2008). Forearm bone-anchored amputation prosthesis: a case study on the osseointegration. Acta Orthop, 79, 78-85.

Palmquist, A., et al., (2011). Biomechanical, Histological and Ultrastructural Analyses of Laser Micro- and Nano-structured Titanium implant after 6 months in rabbit. J Biomed Mater Res B Appl Biomater, Accepted for publication.

Park, JY; & Davies., JE. (2000). Red blood cell and platelet interactions with titanium implant surfaces. Clin Oral Implants Res, 11, 530-539.

Porter, A., et al., (2005). Effect of carbonate substitution on the ultrastructural characteristics of hydroxyapatite implants. J Mater Sci Mater Med, 16, 899-907.

Porter, AE; Best, SM. & Bonfield, W. (2004). Ultrastructural comparison of hydroxyapatite and silicon-substituted hydroxyapatite for biomedical applications. J Biomed Mater Res A, 68, 133-41.

Porter, AE; et al., (2004). Ultrastructural comparison of dissolution and apatite precipitation on hydroxyapatite and silicon-substituted hydroxyapatite in vitro and in vivo. J Biomed Mater Res A, 69, 670-679.

Radegran, G; Lausmaa, J; Mattsson, L; Rolander, U. & Kasemo, B. (1991). Preparation of ultra-thin oxide windows on titanium for TEM analysis. J Electron Microsc Tech, 19, 99-106.

Robinson, K; Brånemark, R. & Ward, D. (2004). Future Developments: Osseointegration in Transfemoral Amputees. In: Smith D, Michael J, Bowker J, editors. Atlas of Amputations and Limb Deficiencies: Surgical, Prosthetic and Rehabilitation Principles. Third Edition ed, 673-681.

Rosenberg, ES; Torosian, JP. & Slots, J. (1991). Microbial differences in 2 clinically distinct types of failures of osseointegrated implants. Clin Oral Implants Res, 2, 135-144.

Rupp, F; Scheideler, L; Olshanska, N; de Wild, M; Wieland, M. & Geis-Gerstorfer, J. (2006). Enhancing surface free energy and hydrophilicity through chemical modification of microstructured titanium implant surfaces. J Biomed Mater Res A, 76, 323-334.

Rydevik. B. (1997). Amputation prostheses and osseoperception in the lower and upper extremity. In: Brånemark P-I, Rydevik B, Skalak R, editors. Osseointegration in skeletal reconstruction and joint replacement. London: Guintessence Books, 175–182.

Saiz, E; Goldman, M; Gomez-Vega, JM; Tomsia, AP; Marshall, GW. & Marshall, SJ. (2002). In vitro behaviour of silicate glass coatings on Ti6Al4V, Biomaterials, 23, 3749-3756.

Schepers, E; Ducheyne, P; De Clerq, M. (1989). Interfacial analysis of fiber-reinforced bioactive glass dental root implants, J Biomed Mater Res, 23, 735-752.

Schrooten, J. & Helsen, JA. (2000). Adhesion of bioactive glass coating to Ti6A14V oral implant. Biomaterials, 21, 1461-9.

Schroeder, A; van der, Zypen, E; Stich, H. & Sutter, F. (1981). The reactions of bone, connective tissue, and epithelium to endosteal implants with titanium-sprayed surfaces. J Maxillofac Surg, 9, 15-25.

Schupbach, P ; Glauser, R ; Rocci, A; Martignoni, M; Sennerby, L; Lundgren, A. & Gottlow, J. (2005). The human bone-oxidized titanium implant interface: a light microscopic, scanning electron microscopic, back-scatter scanning electron microscopic, and energy-dispersive X-ray study of clinically retrieved dental implants. Clin Implant Dent Relat Res, 7, 36–43.

Schwarz, F; Herten, M; Sager, M; Wieland, M; Dard, M. & Becker, J. (2007). Bone regeneration in dehiscence-type defects at chemicallymodified (SLActive) and conventional SLA titanium implants:A pilot study in dogs. J Clin Periodontol, 34, 78–86.

Shichinohe, H; Kuroda, S ; et al. (2007). Role of SDF-1/CXCR4 system in survival and migration of bone marrow stromal cells after transplantation into mice cerebral infarct. Brain Res, 1183, 138-147.

Sennerby, L; Ericson, LE; Thomsen, P; Lekholm, U. & Astrand, P. (1991). Structure of the bone-titanium interface in retrieved clinical oral implants. Clin Oral Implants Res, 2, 103-111.

Sennerby, L; Thomsen, P; et al. (1993). Early tissue response to titanium implants inserted in rabbit cortical bone. Part I Light microscopic observations. Journal of Materials Science: Materials in Medicine, 4, 240-250.

Sennerby, L; Thomsen, P; et al. (1993). Early tissue response to titanium implants inserted in rabbit cortical bone. Part II Ultrastructural observations. Journal of Materials Science: Materials in Medicine, 4, 494-502.

Sennerby, L; Thomsen, P. & Ericson, LE. (1992). Ultrastructure of the bone-titanium interface in rabbits. Journal of Materials Science: Materials in Medicine, 3, 262-271.

Steflik, DE; Corpe, RS; Lake, FT; Sisk, AL; Parr, GR; Hanes, PJ; et al. (1997). Composite morphology of the bone and associated support-tissue interfaces to osseointegrated dental implants: TEM and HVEM analyses. Int J Oral Maxillofac Implants, 12, 443-453.

Steflik, DE; Corpe, RS; Lake, FT; Young, TR; Sisk, AL; Parr, GR; et al. (1998). Ultrastructural analyses of the attachment (bonding) zone between bone and implanted biomaterials. J Biomed Mater Res, 39, 611-620.

Steflik, DE; Parr, GR; Sisk, AL; Hanes, PJ. & Lake, FT. (1992). Electron microscopy of bone response to titanium cylindrical screw-type endosseous dental implants. Int J Oral Maxillofac Implants, 7, 497-507.

Steflik, DE; Sisk, AL; Parr, GR; Lake, FT; Hanes, PJ; Berker; DJ; et al. (1994). Transmission electron and high-voltage electron microscopy of osteocyte cellular processes extending to the dental implant surface. J Biomed Mater Res, 28, 1095-1107.

Steflik, DE; et al., (1992). High-voltage electron microscopy and conventional transmission electron microscopy of the interface zone between bone and endosteal dental implants. J Biomed Mater Res, 26, 529-45.

Stewart, M; Thiel, M; et al. (1995). Leukocyte integrins. Curr Opin Cell Biol, 7, 690-696.

Sul, YT; Johansson, C; Byon, E. & Albrektsson, T. (2005a). The bone response of oxidized bioactive and non-bioactive titanium implants. Biomaterials, 26, 6720-6730.

Sul, YT; Johansson, C; Wennerberg, A; Cho, LR; Chang, BS. & Albrektsson, T. (2005b). Optimum surface properties of oxidized implants for reinforcement of osseointegration: surface chemistry, oxide thickness, porosity, roughness, and crystal structure. Int J Oral Maxillofac Implants, 20, 349–59.

Sul, YT; Johansson, C. & Albrektsson, T. (2006).Which surface properties enhance bone response to implants? Comparison of oxidized magnesium, TiUnite, and Osseotite implant surfaces. Int J Prosthodont, 19, 319-328.

Sun, L; Berndt, CC; Gross, KA. & Kucuk, A. (2001). Materials fundamentals and clinical performance of plasma-sprayed hydroxyapatite coatings: a review. J Biomed Mater Res (Appl Biomater), 58, 570-92.

Suska, F; Esposito, M; et al. (2003). IL-1alpha, IL-1beta and TNF-alpha secretion during in vivo/ex vivo cellular interactions with titanium and copper. Biomaterials, 24, 461-468.

Szmukler-Moncler, S; Perrin, D; Ahossi, V; Magnin, G. & Bernard, JP. (2004). Biological properties of acid etched titanium implants: effect of sandblasting on bone anchorage. J Biomed Mater Res B Appl Biomater, 68, 149-159.

Tan, KS; Qian, L; et al. (2006). The role of titanium surface topography on J774A.1 macrophage inflammatory cytokines and nitric oxide production. Biomaterials, 27, 5170-5177.

Tang, L. & Eaton, JW. (1993). Fibrin(ogen) mediates acute inflammatory responses to biomaterials. J Exp Med, 178, 2147-2156.

Taxt-Lamolle, SF; Rubert, M; et al. (2010). Controlled electro-implementation of fluoride in titanium implant surfaces enhances cortical bone formation and mineralization. Acta Biomater, 6, 1025-1032.

Thomsen, P; Ericson, LE. (1985). Light and transmission electron microscopy used to study the tissue morphology close to implants. Biomaterials, 6, 421-424.

Thomsson, M; Esposito, M. (2008). A retrospective case series evaluating Branemark BioHelix implants placed in a specialist private practice following 'conventional' procedures. One-year results after placement. Eur J Oral Implantol, 1, 229-234.

Uusitalo, H ; Hiltunen, A ; et al. (2000). Expression of cathepsins B, H, K, L, and S and matrix metalloproteinases 9 and 13 during chondrocyte hypertrophy and endochondral ossification in mouse fracture callus. Calcif Tissue Int, 67, 382-390.

Vercaigne, S; Wolke, JG; Naert, I. & Jansen, JA. (1998). Bone healing capacity of titanium plasma-sprayed and hydroxylapatite-coated oral implants. Clin Oral Implants Res, 9, 261-271.

Vercaigne, S; Wolke, JGC; Naert, I. & Jansen, JA. (2000). A histologicalevaluation of TiO2-gritblasted and Ca-P magnetron sputter coated implants placed into the trabecular bone of the goat: Part 2. Clin Oral Implant Res, 11, 314–324.

Verheyen, CC; Dhert, WJ; Petit, PL; Rozing, PM. & de Groot, K. (1993). In vitro study on the integrity of a hydroxylapatite coating when challenged with staphylococci. J Biomed Mater Res, 27, 775-781.

Wang, Y; Deng, Y; et al. (2008). SDF-1alpha/CXCR4-mediated migration of systemically transplanted bone marrow stromal cells towards ischemic brain lesion in a rat model. Brain Res, 1195, 104-112.

Weng, D; Hoffmeyer, M; Hurzeler, MB. & Richter, EJ. (2003). Osseotite vs. machined surface in poor bone quality. A study in dogs. Clin Oral Implants Res,14, 703-708.

Wennerberg, A. & Albrektsson, T. (2000). Suggested guidelines for the topographic evaluation of implant surfaces. Int J Oral Maxillofac Implants, 15, 331-344.

Wennerberg, A; Albrektsson, T; Ulrich, H, & Krol, JJ. (1992). An optical three-dimensional technique for topographical descriptions of surgical implants. J Biomed Eng, 14, 412-418.

Wennerberg, A; Albrektsson, T; Andersson, B. & Krol, JJ. (1995). A histomorphometric and removal torque study of screw-shaped titanium implants with three different surface topographies. Clin Oral Implants Res, 6, 24-30.

Wennerberg, A; Ektessabi, A; Albrektsson, T; Johansson, C. & Andersson, B. (1997). A 1-year follow-up of implants of differing surface roughness placed in rabbit bone. Int J Oral Maxillofac Implants, 12, 486-494.

Wennerberg, A; Albrektsson, T; Johansson, C. & Andersson, B. (1996). Experimental study of turned and grit-blasted screw-shaped implants with special emphasis on effects of blasting material and surface topography. Biomaterials, 17, 15-22.

Wennerberg, A; Albrektsson, T. & Andersson, B. (1996). Bone tissue response to commercially pure titanium implants blasted with fine and coarse particles of aluminum oxide. Int J Oral Maxillofac Implants, 11, 38-45.

Wennerberg, A. On the surface roughness and implant incorporation. Göteborg: Göteborg University; 1996.

West, JK; Clark, AE; Hall, MB. & Turner, GE. (1990). In vivo bone-bonding study of Bioglass-coated titanium alloy. In Yamamuro T, Hench LL, Wilson J. editors. Handbook of bioactive ceramics, Vol I, CRC Press: Boca Raton FL, 161-166.

Willmann, G. (1997). Bioceramics, 10, 353-356.

Wilson, J; Pigoit, HH; Schoen, FT. & Hench, LL. (1981). Toxicology and biocompatibility of bioglass. J Biomed Mater Res, 15, 805.

Xie, XH; Yu, XW; Zeng, SX; Du, RL; Hu, YH; Yuan, Z; Lu, EY; Dai, KR. & Tang, TT. (2010). Enhanced osteointegration of orthopaedic implant gradient coating composed of bioactive glass and nanohydroxyapatite. J Mater Sci Mater Med, 21, 2165-2173.

Xia, W; Lindahl, C; Lausmaa, J; Borchardt, P; Ballo, A; Thomsen, P. & Engqvist, H. (2010). Biomineralized strontium-substituted apatite/titanium dioxide coating on titanium surfaces. Acta Biomater, 6, 1591-1600.

Yang, GL; He, FM; Hu, JA; Wang, XX. & Zhao, SF. (2009). Effects of biomimetically and electrochemically deposited nano-hydroxyapatite coatings on osseointegration of porous titanium implants. Oral Surg Oral Med Oral Pathol Oral Radiol Endod. 107, 782-9.

Yang, Y; Kim, KH. & Ong, JL. (2005). A review on calcium phosphate coatings produced using a sputtering process--an alternative to plasma spraying. Biomaterials, 26, 327-37.

Yu, J; Li, M; et al. SDF-1/CXCR4-mediated migration of transplanted bone marrow stromal cells towards areas of heart myocardial infarction via activation of PI3K/Akt. J Cardiovasc Pharmacol.

Zhang, E. & Zou, C. (2009). Porous titanium and silicon-substituted hydroxyapatite biomodification prepared by a biomimetic process: characterization and in vivo evaluation. Acta Biomater, 5, 1732-1741.

9

Biological Reactions to Dental Implants

Lucian Toma Ciocan[1], Florin Miculescu[2],
Marian Miculescu[2] and Ion Patrascu[1]
[1]*"Carol Davila" Medicine and Pharmacy University*
[2]*University "Politehnica"*
Bucharest
Romania

1. Introduction

Generally, the cells' isolated systems are more sensitive than the tissues of the body at the contact with material outside the natural system. Although, the research by applying some viable methods *in vitro* is constantly growing, because the cellular mechanism of the toxicity assessment materials can be described through some simple and cheep experiments, that could represent viable alternatives for testing *in vivo* on animals bio bases and, finally, on people. Using these testing methods, the materials can be classified according to their degree of toxicity and chosen, if necessary, for further testing *in vivo*. To appreciate the materials' biocompatibility for implantation in human body and to provide their functionality *in vivo* in the maximum safety for the patient represent a rigorous complex process, with two important distinct steps (Black, 1992): conducting preliminary assessment tests such as cytotoxicity, awareness, the irritant potential, intracutaneous reactivity, systemic toxicity (acute), subchronic toxicity (subacute), genotoxicity, implantation, hemocompatibility, or conducting tests for complementary evaluation, that consist in testing the chronic toxicity, the carcinogenicity, the toxicity of reproduction and development (growth) and the biodegradation.

Through the process of testing *in vitro* the biomaterials can be assessed in a number of functions and characteristics of cells, as: integrity of membrane, cytoskeleton, viability, proliferation, proteins synthesis, oxidative response, mobility, secretion, response to growth factors, cell-cell interactions. To prepare the materials for testing the cytotoxicity has a great importance, because those physical and chemical properties strongly influence the cells response and the entire experimental system. Testing standards and how to prepare samples for testing *in vitro* are present at all professional bodies, including International Organization for Standardization (ISO), Ente Nazionale Italiano di Unificazione (UNI), British Standards Institute (BSI), Deutsches Institut fur Normung (DIN), Swiss Association for Standardization (SNN), Association Francaise de Normalisation (AFNOR), American Society for Testing and Materials (ASTM), American Dental Association (ADA). In such a standard are presented the requirements for physical and chemical form of materials, sterilization procedures, form and size of samples and any treatment required to obtain a sample suitable for cytotoxicity testing. The adoption of these specifications is recommended when pursued some comparisons between different laboratories or when you need a report for a manufacturer; application of those standards among other things ensure that the material or its properties are not impaired by the procedure of preparation of samples for testing. In case of testing *in vitro*, solid materials are usually used when tested biomaterial surface affects the cell response clearly. In these cases, the combination of solid material - formed cell experimental system that reproduces the best situations arising *in vivo*. It is very important to know that only the mere change in form and the sample size studied can make the difference between obtaining as result a nontoxic effect or a very cytotoxic one (Brodbeck et al., 2001). Obtaining cell adhesion on biomaterials is considered a positive phenomenon in order to continue the test for studying the biomaterial behaviour after implantation. To assess cell adhesion to foreign surfaces is mainly used cell counting, and electron microscopy techniques and computer assisted measurements are used to assess the distribution and morphology.

2. Materials and methods for evaluation

The most popular standard of testing the biomaterials, ISO 10993, in the section dedicated to the *in vitro* tests (the 5ft part), does not specify the most important parameters for cytotoxicity testing, but only lists certain characteristics and properties that can be pursued during the course of the evaluation of biomaterials in vitro behaviour, to permit the research laboratories to determine their own steps to make on the cell type, duration of exposure, assessment method, etc. According to this standard, to be performed cytotoxicity tests must be met several conditions:

a. The tests must be performed on finished product or representative samples of the finished product or materials;
b. Choosing the testing methods must take account into:
   - nature, extent, duration, frequency and conditions of exposure or contact with the human body surface in normal use devices provided;
   - physical and chemical nature of the finished product;
   - toxic potential of chemical components of the finished product formula;
   - relationship between body size and device surface to which it is applied
   - existing information based on literature, experience and clinical trials;
   - protect humans and animals to perform experiments;

For the use in cytotoxicity testing of biomaterials are offered several types of cells and cell lines. At this point, it is still debated question of use *in vitro* testing fresh cells selected from explants, primary cells, or selected cellular lines. Likewise, it is not indicated the duration of cell exposure to materials / devices, as, generally, it is dictated by the test method applied, but it can be taken into account the average duration of implantation of the tested biomaterial. (Kilburn et al., 2003)

Currently, testing the cytotoxicity needs 24 hours, but, in many cases, this exposure can be diminished or extended. The duration of contact with the materials may be restricted to 1-2 hours, as it is recommended for the testing of some types of dental materials that will be applied to the oral mucosa only for a few minutes. This reduction in testing time in cell culture is because, having gone through a period of 24 hours of investigation can be obtained for a highly toxic material / device tested, which could lead to rejection due to raise awareness. If this material has unique properties and optimal performance *in vivo* short exposures, the benefit obtained by its use may be higher than the risk of patient.

The ISO 10993 standard indicates that for testing the cytotoxicity "the assessment type is at free choice". The Standard are presented in four categories of assessment types, including which we find a cell morphology one and some measurements of cell parameters. The same standard is specified also that, for original cataloging of materials, methods adopted by the laboratory must be technically simple, reproducible, and applicable to a broad spectrum. The initial cataloging of biomaterials, cell viability, or the number of dead cells and to determine cell growth inhibition are common parameters. Using the assessment of these factors can be measured the tests' toxicity, as the biomaterials are classified according to their cytotoxic effect. Although their cell viability and growth are clearly defined, the distinction becomes less clear when it used the same test method to measure both parameters.

If cell growth, although time consuming, cell counting hemocytometer or Coulter counter is still widely used. The cell counting methods have a high risk of inaccuracy, mainly because of the steps needed to obtain cells in suspension, including repeated washing and cell transfer. Since there is no need for a transfer cell after contact with the biomaterial, the staining procedure of microplates cultures of cells is used to quantify their DNA's. Currently, dye fixing cell cultures are used substances such as amido black, crystal violet and methylene blue, later on being obtained the solubilisation of the cell adsorbed color, as the absorption of blue color can be measured with a specific wavelength of color used (Puleo & Nanci, 1999).

The best demonstration of the ability of cells to grow *in vitro* in case of biomaterials testing consists of trying to form colony cells. The main limitation of this technique consists of the experiment duration: the results of an experiment can be obtained after two three weeks, since the materials that temporarily blocks cell division can be classified as cytotoxic if cells are prematurely processed. (Yan et al., 1997) To achieve ranking as cytotoxicity of biomaterials, it is necessary to apply quantitative methods. They are necessary also if biomaterials' cataloguing is required, but if it is imperative to have an answer for validation or invalidation of a product, while the morphological and qualitative methods provide important information, and can not dictate such a decision; qualitative methods can be used only to characterize the biomaterials. In the study of biomaterials' cytotoxicity should be measured the damages caused by them in cellular cultures, in order to define a limit of nontoxicity. The cytotoxic effect is expressed in terms of the proportion of surviving cells after the contact with the biomaterial; using the values expressed in percentages may be compared to the results of various test methods. (Dekker, 1994). In none of the documents mentioned above, any limit is established for estimating the maximum acceptable value of toxicity. Some authors classify materials as cytotoxic when the cell survival is less than 50% or 75%, while others resort to statistics to detect a significant difference between the materials and tests. A material can be used clinically, even if it has a relatively high toxicity, due to a lack of valid alternatives. From this point of view, especially for clinical applications may be chosen the least toxic materials available.

By analyzing the cellular inhibition' growth induced by biomaterial and the cellular cycle of used culture, the toxicity' grade was expressed as percentage depending the cellular proliferation inhibition (CPI%), by the formula: CPI% = 1 when the number of sample cells/the number of control cells equalizes 100. Using CPI%, 4 different levels of toxicity have been identified, namely: "high toxicity" (CPI%=50), "medium toxicity" (CPI%<50% & >25%), "low toxicity" (CPI%<25%) and nontoxicity (CPI%=0). (Hazan, 1993).

Currently, the apoptosis is detected by flow cytometry in most cases and only rarely by conventional electronic microscopy techniques or DNA electrophoresis site, which can be complementary techniques. The flow cytometry with complementary techniques such as optical microscopy, confocal fluorescence, scanning or transmission fully covers all the biochemical and morphological aspects that need to be taken into account in the biocompatibility of materials.
The release of high concentrations of implants and prosthetic components in the body, due to the occurrence of corrosion phenomenon, may favour the appearance of the necrotic phenomena and the inflammatory reactions of the surrounding tissue. However the release of these elements in the body may be followed by toxic effects, characterized by apoptotic phenomena: this situation is less serious, because the tissue adaptation to the implant is not seriously affected. In conclusion, although theoretically simple, the applicable to cellular culture tests to assess the biocompatibility requires a number of factor limits that are determined after a thorough analysis. As mentioned, the main items to consider include the preparation and handling of material, test methods and quantitative assessments. It is also very important the conclusion that the mechanism of occurrence of cell death induced by the material is uncertain, the final conclusions regarding the interactions between the biomaterials and implants or prosthesis can be explained by studying the reactions of tissues observed after *in vivo* implantation.
The compatibility with blood or the hemocompatibility materials and medical devices is determined by using uncurled blood (a major limitations of these test) and the evaluation of blood clots on the surface of test samples, and also the activation of the coagulation cascade, the adhesion of platelets, the complement system activation and the erythrocytes. Depending on the ultimate goal of biomaterial use, the hemocompatibility tests must be conducted in static or dynamic conditions. (Anselme et al., 2000).
The *in vitro* cellular culture models can be used to determine the effects of chemical compounds (the concentration of ions released during the corrosion of metals or molecules released during the degradation of polymers) on the body. The materials that do not meet the toxicity should not be further considered. Even if the materials pass the test of cellular culture, must be taken into account also the effects caused by the products resulting of degradation on cellular morphology, proliferation and other cell functions.

2.1 Biomaterials *in vitro* testing methods

As it has been previously described, the *in vitro* cellular culture models can be used in the preliminary assessment of biocompatibility of materials. As with other models, measures must be taken in interpreting the data correctly and avoid risks that may result from an incorrect extrapolation. Without doubt, these models are very useful in studying the cell functions, but still, this approach has its limitations. These results must be combined with those from *in vivo* tests to reveal all the aspects of biocompatibility.
Determining the safety of a biomaterial and its efficacy as a implanted device is finally made after its implantation on animals. Such studies, realized on an animal material correctly chosen, have been shown to be directly applicable in human subjects. The most biological processes, in particular wound healing, are also compatible. The specialized literature is replete with descriptions of animal models that were used to evaluate various materials and devices. Unfortunately, there are deficiencies in terms of the pathological data from the observations made on materials and implanted devices in human subjects. This deficiency is

linked to issues of recovery and histological evaluation of an implanted device when a patient's death was not caused by its presence. The choice of an animal species relies more on its cost and / or availability than on the relevance for the human situation. As provided in the ISO rules, the first phase of testing a new material is best performed in a tissue culture. The second phase of testing for any application is the subcutaneous or intramuscular implantation in rodents, with a histopathological evaluation of the tissue that develops around the test material. If you want to use it for orthopedic purposes, the material should be implanted into the rabbit femoral intramedullary cavity. The animal model chosen for the third phase of the complete testing the device depends on its final application. (Ilin & Skvortsova, 2002)

The ideal animal model should have many reproducible features to simulate an analogue or counterpart condition in which the material would find use in humans. The scientific criterion for selection of the animal model depends on the intention of applying the biomaterial. More specifically, should be taken into account the anatomical, biochemical, physiological, pathological and/or psychological characteristics. Over the years, it has been found through trial and failure that human systems resemble with different animal species. In addition to anatomic, pathologic and physiologic similarities with humans, that should be taken into account when choosing an animal model, the researcher conducting the experiment may be limited in choice, because practical considerations. The size and conformation of the animal may be one of the limits. The small animals cost less and are easier to handle. However, surgical procedures on large animals are easier to perform.

The bone healing and its reactions with biomaterials in goats, showed a similarity to those of humans on the type of cell, collagen structure, the structure of the soft and hard tissue, but also on the time of occurrence of the specific biological phenomena. In addition to management considerations, goats and sheep, as well as rats tend to develop ectopic ossifications in these structures, highlighting them as unviable models for researching the characteristics of artificial tendon healing. The rabbit represents an often test system used in Orthopedics. Even if an important part of special publications support the inadequacies of animal model in predicting similar behaviour of biomaterials implants in humans, it is still widely used. The reasons are probably more historical and economic. (Wennerberg et al., 2003)

The dental implants have been studied in dogs, monkeys, baboons and pigs. Although the specific anatomy of these species is quite different from that of human, the tissue responses to periodontal disease and gingival withdrawals are quite similar. This research area resembles Orthopedics.

The wound healing studies performed to observe the effectiveness of different treatments wounds are best performed on young domestic pig. The animals' use into laboratory for *in vivo* testing should be responsibly done and only after have been met the other conditions of preliminary biocompatibility, eventually after using computer simulation models and *in vitro* experiments. The main concern in using animals for *in vivo* testing is not to produce to the animal an unnecessary suffering or harm. Therefore, the researchers should carefully select the animals that will test and make a detailed planning investigation. All these things should be realized taking into account the national and international laws.

2.1.1 Classification of *in vivo* tests

The animal tests used to assess biocompatibility are classified into three main categories (Black, 1992):

- *The nonfunctional tests* can be applied in various forms, the implants being usually inserting into the soft tissue (subcutaneous, intramuscular or intraperitonal) with minor incisions, or into the hard tissue, through the practice of geodes or resection of the femoral head and the insertion of intramedullary implants. These studies are of short duration (days to months) and provide valuable information about local interactions between the implant and surrounding tissue, data being obtained in the absence of mechanical loads.
- *The ex vivo tests*, as arterio - venous and vein - venous suture type, are used to divert a portion of the blood of an animal to a material, and back into the circulatory system. In this case, vital information for determining the blood compatibility to the used materials is the accumulation of proteins, cell adhesion and clots' formation on the material' surface.
- *The functional tests* involve implantation into the animal organism of some reduced scale prostheses, for example hip or heart prostheses implantation in similar conditions to those in the human body. These tests are lengthy; require special conditions regarding the design, production, testing of various types of prostheses, while being complex and expensive.

The use of materials for implants and medical devices applied on animals provide valuable information on the complex interactions that occur between the implant and the body, the chronic and acute inflammatory responses and all the problems throughout the process. It also can cause pyrogenic, immunological and toxicological animals' responses to implants. Detailing the methods and procedures is available in the specialized literature and publications of standards institutions. Compared to scientific standards, the medical evaluations should be carried out lawfully. Furthermore, *in vivo* and *ex vivo* tests must meet

Location	Influence factor
Material	Chemical volume and chemical surface properties Surface roughness Superficial Porosity Superficial energy Surface charge Chemical and physical stability Chemical properties of degradation products The physical characteristics of breakdown
Implant	Size and Shape The elasticity mode / stiffness
Host Organism	Species (in animal experiments) Tissue type and location Age Genre General health Medications
Implantation method	Surgical techniques Fixing the tissue implant Infection

Table 1. Factors that may influence implant-tissue interaction (Black, 1992).

the requirements of empowered institutions. After received the acceptance of these institutions, the medical devices can be implanted in a small number of patients that will be closely monitored.

In all cases of testing the biomaterials, the ethical considerations are very important. The identity of those who take part in these tests must be kept confidential. The animal tests can provide very important information about materials and medical devices, the tissues in which they have been implanted, but also the implant acceptance by human or animal body. To conduct practical experiments necessary to evaluate the interactions occurring at the tissue implant interface, we chose the rabbit as animal model study, because it is an often used animal for clinical studies, has enough dimensions and does not involve special surgical conditions, and the postoperative monitoring and maintenance costs are relatively low. (Moiseev, 2004)

By performing the implantation tests, it seeks global response, the result of the interaction between implant and host tissue, the role of the phenomena on the tissue implant interface. Their progress may depend on the properties and characteristics of volume and shape of the implant, and its surface roughness. Generally, by evaluating tissue reactions at the implant interface may be a distinction between bioinert, biotolarated and bioactive materials and also can get information on biofunctionality, biocompatibility, biodegradation, and bioactivity. The overall response of the body, considered as a measure of biocompatibility is determined by reference to the factors presented in Table 1.

3. Experimental study on tissue biomaterial interaction

3.1 Determination of chemical composition of biomaterials

The first step in evaluating any biomaterial, metal or not, is up to the identification and characterization in terms of its chemical composition. Currently, it is available for conducting such investigations a variety of compositional characterization methods. To make the characterization in terms of chemical composition, the research presented in this paper, we used the following energy spectrometry (EDS), method that allows the materials assessment with sufficient precision for characterization and classification of selected biomaterials into specific ASTM standards groups. For the study of the interactions that occur at the interface implant tissue to cover as wide a range, we selected the most representative class of biomaterials and used metal groups, as follow: commercially pure titanium, titanium alloy Ti6Al4V type, CoCrMo alloy, and austenitic stainless steel to a medical purpose. The quantitative chemical determinations made by EDS spectrometry have allowed cataloging tested materials, see Figure 1, and their classification in terms of the compositional type in ASTM marks of the biomaterials. To avoid the phenomenon of contamination of samples, they were cleaned by ultrasonic in methanol at 50° C for 15 minutes and then doubly distilled pure water at 90° C, 30 minutes and dried in hot air.

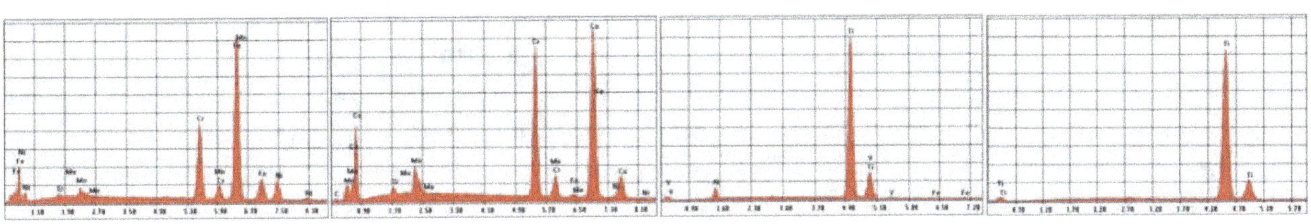

Fig. 1. EDS spectra characteristic chemical compositional analysis of the main classes of metallic biomaterials.

The experimentally determined values are within the limits imposed by ASTM standards, in the following classes: commercially pure titanium covered in ASTM F67; Ti6Al4V alloy type fall in ASTM F136; CoCrMo alloy type fall in ASTM F75; Type 316 austenitic stainless steel covered in ASTM F138.

3.2 Micro structural characterization of metallic biomaterials

The characterization of biomaterials in terms of micro is a particularly important factor in the interaction of the implant tissue interface due to at least three respects:

- corrosion resistance of biomaterial is correlated with its microstructure;
- microscopic surface inhomogenity, such as crystal grain boundaries or secondary phase precipitates, could be important in protein adsorption on metal surfaces uneven;
- formation of mineralized bone tissue is dependent on bone cells' activity, activity influenced by the superficial topography of the substrate.

The existence of conflicting results in terms of material influence on short-term interactions between bone cells and the various surface layers, may have as a possible explanation the fact that the correlations between various factors that manifest themselves such as umectability and topography of the substrate surface, respectively, the chemical processes at the interface implant biological environment. At a microscopic scale, the surfaces of biomaterials can act differently. On the surface of the biomaterials, can be portions or areas of different functionality, and they may interact differently with biomolecules. For example, many metallic biomaterials contain at least two different phases. Not only that reacts differently with molecules of different phases, and grain boundaries behave differently from the middle of grains. (Smith et al., 1992)

The selected samples were directly analyzed by light microscopy for evaluation according to ASTM standards for each biomaterial in part, in terms of the incluzionary status. After evaluation and compliance with standards in this regard, the samples were subjected to the metallographic attack by chemical reagents specific for each material. Whenever necessary, the metallographic attack was carried out electrochemically. Due to limited space, this paper presents a few representative images (see figure 2).

The sample type 316L austenitic stainless steel was obtained by implementing the solution hardening (1050°C/water) and plastic deformation at cold, with a degree of deformation of 30%. The chemical composition of type 316L steel falls within ASTM F138 limit, the determined percentage of molybdenum (2.19%) is to the lower limit, thus ensuring a low tendency of formation of δ ferrite. In the chemical composition of this steel, copper has not been detected (detection limit of copper by EDS method being 0.1% by weight), which is recommended by ASTM standard F138. The percentage of nickel located at the lower level (12.33%), in conjunction with a sufficiently low percentage of manganese (1.79%) led to the avoidance of appearance of the δ ferrite traces according ASTM F138. Metallographic speaking, the standard recommends the lack of the δ ferrite phase in its structure and also the average of the grain size not exceeding 5, which is a dimension of the grain size with a high degree of uniformity, less or equal than to 100μm. In accordance with the quantitative analysis obtained by the Underwood method (interception method), it has result a grain size according to ASTM E112, of 11.0, which shows a much smaller grain and more uniform than the maximum permissible value in the standard. The structure consists of austenite grains, relatively deformed in longitudinal section and stronger macle than the cross sectional. Following electrolytic attack, both in longitudinal section and cross-sectional, deformation lines can be observed, where the attack occurred more stressed, which is obvious what is noticed in the images obtained through interferential phase contrast. The lack of compounds (carbides of Cr and Mo) in the structure leads to the assertion that the heat treatment of hardening of formal solution (1050°C/water) was well chosen and leaded. The hardness determinations have been registered a medium value of 341HB, which complies with the requirements of ASTM F138.

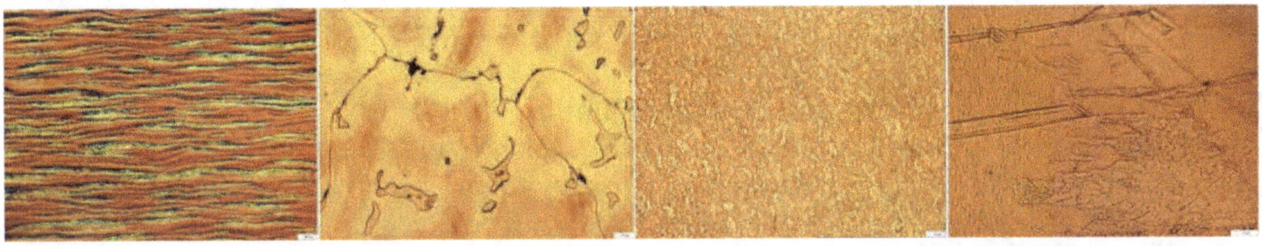

Fig. 2. Bright field optical microscopy images on the analyzed samples surface (from left to right - 316L austenitic stainless steel type, CoCrMo alloy type, Ti6Al4V and CP Titanium).

The examined CoCrMo alloy fits the ASTM F75 standard, both in terms of chemical composition and structural point of view. The able cast microstructure consists of a matrix rich in cobalt, alpha-phase strongly segregated, with interdendritic and limit grain separately compounds. These compounds are mainly formed with one of the carbons: Co, Cr or Mo (which is according date of the specialized literature). (Stanford et al., 2003) Carbide content may decrease the same time with a homogenization of alpha phase, by thermal annealing treatment later realized. According ASTM F75, strength criterion in selecting material for use in making medical implants is not recommended to be important for its rejection. The area occupied by a grain is about 4mm^2, the dendrites' orientation in the grain is predominantly by the grain growth direction. The samples were taken from a 30mm diameter ingot, which is why, because the relatively low speed of solidification, the grain size has large and irregular values. For the characterization of dendritic structure, it has been made measurements of the distances between their axes, resulting in values of maximum 86mm and minimum 4µm.

The Ti6Al4V alloy samples type "ELI" (Extra Low Interstitial) were plastically deformed by hot rolling at 900°C heat treated at 720°C for one hour / air cooling. The resulting structure consists of elongated grains of alpha phase, light, in a matrix of transformed beta phase. Alpha ASTM F136 is finely dispersed, as is the beta one. The Alpha phase is slightly distorted plastic, and the resulting structure after heat treatment is a typical one, which has been taken into account the temperature "beta transus". The quantitative microscopy studies have led to the identification of a score of the grain size of about 12, which shows a degree of advanced finishing the grain size, using the same analytical method as previously investigated biomaterial; this score has a direct effect on increasing resistance to fatigue of the material. The inclusionary state was characterized by measuring the length of the inclusions, resulting in minimum values of 1.44/1.07µm and maximum 37.87/14.25µm. In terms of distribution, it is noted that over 70% of the inclusions have a size smaller than 4.7µm. The average area occupied by inclusions is about 1%, which is an inclusionary state falling standard. The commercial purity titanium has been used to perform experiments covered in ASTM F67 standard and in terms of chemical composition of interstitial content elements that affect decisively technological and operating characteristics is corresponding to the three grade/level. The used biomaterial is in plastic deformed state, with a strain of about 30%, the grains having diameters between 10 and 100μm, which is consistent with moderate plastic deformation undergone material; the grain size was determined by computerized quantitative analysis, ASTM E112 - Underwood interception method, resulting in a score equal to 11. Also, in the grains that have suffered a stronger deformation, it is noted the presence of slip lines parallel and straight, specific to the compact hexagonal crystallization system, characteristically of this metal; otherwise, it has also been the order of surface corrosion prepared by the attack of the Kroll reagent, used to highlight the structure: parallel slip lines, grain boundaries and ultimately subgrain limit.

3.3 Corrosion resistance of biomaterials evaluation

Based on current knowledge, it is impossible to provide the behaviour of metallic biomaterials in the biological environment, unlike to providing corrosion behaviour of metals in an inorganic fluid. Also, it is very difficult to track the details of the in vivo experiments or in real time. Most times the obtained results represent a collection of snapshots realized under very different conditions. The appreciation potential of the electrode and the variation in time can be determined by the corrosion resistance of a biomaterial. Based on the records can draw variation diagrams of stationary potential in time. A comparative study of curves obtained for the four metallic biomaterials (see figure 3), previously characterized micro structural, reveals that, in terms of stationary potential value, the most electropositive (so the best in terms of general corrosion) is titanium, followed in descending order of Ti6Al4V alloy type, alloy type 316L austenitic stainless steel, and CoCrMo alloy. Studying the potential variation over time, it notes that the first two alloys are stabilized by a relatively small active area, the potential remaining stationary and not representing sudden changes that indicate some form of localized corrosion.
Larger active zones present 316 and the CoCrMo alloys, but steady change in the potential of the two alloys is different in time. Thus, stainless steel has a stable and more electropositive steady potential in time, while in case of CoCrMo alloy (cast) occur sudden changes of the potential. These variations have as the main cause the presence of casting

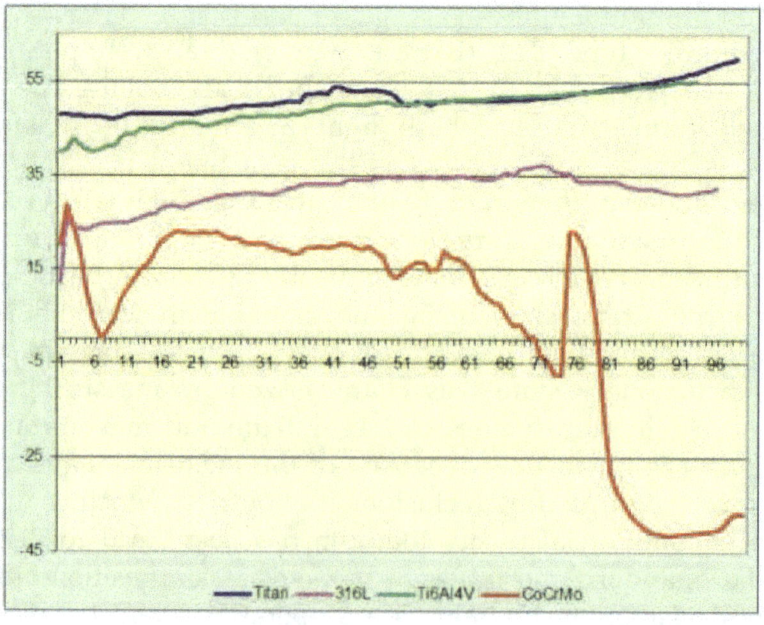

Fig. 3. Tabulated results of benchmark tests for stationary potential variation over time.

defects. A comparative study of the corrosion cycles indicates that all the alloys present a field of passivation, but the value curve of passivation and the potential area in which appears this field is different.

The lowest intensity of corrosion and passivation current is presented by the titanium. In the case of CoCrMo alloy, which despite having a potential range of passivation current lower, both current corrosion intensity and current passivation intensity are below that of Ti6Al4V alloy and steel 316L, the latter showing values of these parameters higher than those of other materials. In the case of titanium and titanium alloy, the surface is unaffected by corrosion. In the case of type 316L stainless steel immersed surface is frosted, and with points of corrosion. The analysis of the distribution of chemical elements in a direction, the wren area, shows a decrease in iron concentration, in that area is identified chromium oxicarbure, which confirms the results of tests of the same type presented in the specialized literature. The CoCrMo alloy, after corrosion test, also shows a frosted surface on which it can be observed the presence of corrosion products with different shapes and morphologies. At the core configurations, molybdenum corrosion is found, surrounded by chromium carbide. The emergences of these formations that allow the release of large amounts of alloy elements contained in the test environment are due to obtain the worst results in terms of corrosion resistance.

Through the assessment of the corrosion tests, very important results have been achieved for the study of biomaterial - biological environment interaction, which fully comply with the data presented in the specialized literature and provide us a first qualitative ordering of classes of the studied metallic biomaterials (Miculescu et al., 2007). Thus, in descending order in terms of corrosion resistance, we can arrange biomaterials as fallows: commercially pure titanium, titanium alloy Ti6Al4V type, austenitic stainless steel, CoCrMo alloy respectively, results correlate with those obtained from microstructural measurements, which can be seen, in contested areas, the presence of the generating compounds of specific forms of corrosion. The bridging the electrochemical tests by scanning electron microscopy imaging and EDS microanalysis is an important factor in further developments of research because it provides certainty of correctness and validity testing.

3.4 *In vitro* evaluation of metallic biomaterials cytotoxicity

By using cell culture techniques, it can cause lysis (death) of cells, cell growth inhibition, and some specific effects on cells caused by the devices, materials and / or their extracts. By *in vitro* testing of biomaterials we can appreciate a number of functions and characteristics of cells, such as membrane integrity, cytoskeleton, viability, proliferation, protein synthesis, oxidative response, mobility, secretion, response to growth factors, cell-cell interactions.

For cytotoxicity testing of the shown biomaterials, we have prepared polished samples as disks with 5mm diameter and 2mm height. The purpose of processing in this manner is to ensure the unity of biomaterials surface reaction, without surface roughness becomes a factor influencing the behaviour of cell culture. After preparation, biomaterials have been cleaned with organic solvents and washed with distilled and doubly distilled water to eliminate any possibility of foreign elements or metal ions that come into reactive contact with the analyzed materials. Afterwards, the materials were subjected to dried sterilization at 1800° C for one hour, being manipulated in sterile conditions. The elaborated and used experimental models have persuaded the possibility to realize some multifactorial and monofactorial analysis which allow the correlation into a unified system of the needed results to evaluate the implantable biomaterials quality and the effect on the biological

environment. Determining the influence of various metal samples above the fibroblast culture has been done by direct observation using the optical microscopy.
In the short term cytotoxicity tests, it was used a VERO cell line containing fibroblast-like cells. Cells were seeded in sterile polymer plates with a density of 600,000 cells / well. The cells were grown like in some evolving cultures of the monolayer Eagle environment, Dulbeco modified (DMEM), supplemented with 10% fetal bovine serum (FBS) and with added antibiotics (PSN). The atmosphere in the cell culture chamber was 5% CO2 in humidified air. The extraction test (MEM) maintained the report between the outer surface of the material and fluid volume (average) and was constant in all series of materials placed in the experiment. After harvesting the environment (MEM), 2 - 3 washes were done with FBS, pH 7.2 and then were fixed in methanol for 2 3 minutes at 4° C. 10% Giemsa stain was used for staining. The evaluation of cell cultures was performed at 24, 48, 96 hours respectively. After completing 96 hours of the cell culture' development, the metal samples were taken from the culture plates, then they were washed with FBS and fixed in 0.1 M phosphate buffer, to analyze them by light microscopy and scanning electron microscopy, so we can evaluate the follow parameters: monolayer confluence, cells floating degree, morphological changes. The percentage growth inhibition was determined by counting the cells, and the measurements were corrected for control with a negative filter. As a reference experiment, we took a fibroblast culture in which no metallic sample was immersed, the culture being kept under the same conditions of the experiments in which were immersed metallic samples.
The optical microscopy images (see figure 4), during light phases' contrast, have aimed the cellular culture at the limit between cellular culture and immersed sample. At all the studied experiments, a cellular monolayer was obtained, without being registered any free spaces, in which fully lack the cellular culture. In the case of the cellular culture without metallic sample (blank), the fibroblast cells of the culture highlight morph-structural fairly uniform characteristics. Covering the well with cellular formation is about 90%, being obviously the cells' compaction and the appearance of the phenomenon of forming a multilayer culture.

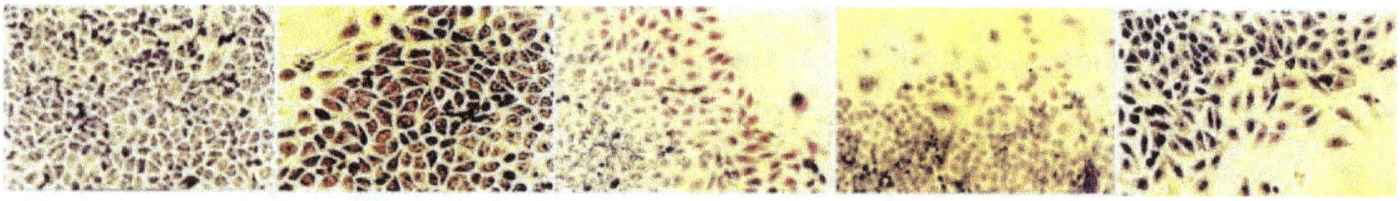

Fig. 4. Cell culture optical microscopy image of the analyzed samples (from left to right - blank, CP Titanium, Ti6Al4V, CoCrMo alloy type and 316L austenitic stainless steel type).

Maintaining the titanium in the presence of the fibroblasts has as result a normal behavior of cells development and a positive chemotactism/chemo attraction related to the material, expressed through the migration and adherence of cells to its surface. The cellular culture joins and forms monolayer, considered as a clear indicator of a favorable biomaterial cell interaction. It can be observed flattening of cell shape and appearance of the cytoplasm emissions which prove the adherence and movement on the biomaterial surface. Significant is the tendency to establish intercellular contacts through extensions, gradually becoming close contacts and cells forming a single compact layer. In all cases, the cells have normal appearance with kernel and obvious nucleoli, the cytoplasm is dense and rich in cellular organelles, and the peripheral cytoplasmic area leads to monolayer formation. This area, with recognized vesicles in the cytoplasm, shows an intense functional activity, related to the synthesis and secretion of active substances that are necessary for the cells to migrate and establish the implant and other cells interrelations. Covering the studied area with cells is about 85%.

The fibroblast cultures maintained in the presence of Ti6Al4V alloy sample has coverage of 75% of the well area in which the study has been made. The fibroblasts morphology is still normal, the cell-cell and cell-biomaterial attachment being high. The cells' orientation towards the immersed sample in the fibroblasts culture confirms the results presented in the specialize literature on the increased biocompatibility of this alloy. (Futami et. al, 2000)

The cellular culture aspect studied in the presence of the sample made of CoCrMo alloy type is uniform and lighter, covering the well with cells being about 65%, similar to the results presented by many authors. (Puleo & Nanci, 1999). The cellular culture compactibility is hight till an appreciate distance from the biomaterial, in its closures being observed a small number of cells uniformly dispersed throughout the perimeter samples. Sample type 316L austenitic stainless steel has a high degree of toxicity, comparatively with other cells, the fact being highlighted by a reduce cells viability, confirmed by the specialized literature (Kocijan et al., 2004). Even though cell layer density represents approximately 55% from the analyzed surface, the fibroblasts' morphology is normal and uniform. The cells' attachment is manifesting also on the cell-cell interface, but on the biomaterial-cell interface. Finally, depending on the studied biomaterial type, we obtained the monolayer formation which had varied from 90 to 55% of the surface, in some cases, being noticed the pluristratification trend.

Watching the cellular culture *in vitro* tests during 96 hours of investigation, in witness and parallel groups in the presence of the metallic samples, demonstrated the evolution of evolution of cell populations in percentage of proliferating, mobility and adhesion which, even though they had presented some variations, were within general acceptable biocompatibility terms. Obtaining these results can be correlated with the release of ions and particles in the structure and composition of the material in the environment, which would be consistent with the results of corrosion tests. It was also noted that the fibroblasts reached the level of metallic biomaterials surfaces generally tend to migrate onto those surface, and the function of intercellular adhesion is slower (inhibited). The results experimentally obtained are similar to data of the specialized literature where it is presented the same order of the metallic biomaterials' cytotoxicity. (Brodbeck et al., 2001).

3.5 *In vivo* nonfunctional studies on animals

The implant surface structure has a significant influence, both for joining tissue and the strength of adhesion to tissue. As this force is defined as a fraction of the pressing force of the area on which it is exerted, loading in real conditions may be even greater as the surface area is bigger. From this simple consideration, it is clear that a soft surface of the implant, with small area of contact with tissue, presents a lower adhesive strength than a structured surface. The biomaterials' surface properties are commonly grouped into three categories: geometric, chemical and electrical. Geometrically speaking, the substrates with more pronounced topographical features will exhibit a bigger surface for the interaction with proteins.

If it should be used an implant which geometry included angles and edges, the interaction between it and the biological tissue would be influenced, because undesired tensions would be introduced into the system. To avoid such problem we got implants with rounded edges. Since the rabbit is a relatively small animal, the implants were proportional, but with sufficient large areas that provide qualitative information and allow the production of normal phenomena and processes for such experiments. Given that the chemical, topographical, mechanical and electrical properties can affect the interaction between proteins and cells with the material, it requires a careful characterization of the surface.

The interaction of the intraosseous and intramuscular metal implants is influenced by their chemical composition and surface roughness. The design shape and size of implants was carried out primarily at obtaining nonfunctional specimens with surfaces that offer the possibility to investigate after conducting biological sampling, with many different preparation degrees in terms of roughness and smallest dimensions as possible, so the in vivo test could be done on small animals, cheep, easily maintained and monitored after surgery.

In vivo research undertaken on animals has focused on two areas:

- *The processes evolution of osseointegration of titanium implants,* goal in which have been made three samples of 99.99% pure titanium, metal considered by the specialized studies, as first on the biocompatibility scale, the samples having the parallelepiped shape with equal sides 2,5/2,5/5mm (L/l/h) transcortical implanted in the femoral head of three adult rabbits, according to the ISO 10993indications;
- *Osseointegration of metal implants by the degree of surface preparation;* of human functional prostheses were made rectangular samples with dimensions above mentioned. Each axial face of the sample was prepared by grinding on emery paper of different roughness: P1000 (metallographic polishing), P800, P600 P320 respectively. The samples thus prepared were transcortical implanted in the tibia same subject, an adult rabbit.

Before the implant, the samples prepared by the above methodology were sterilized with γ ray to be biological measured, also being ensured their protection until the implant surgery. To achieve the surgery, it had opted for the rabbit's tranquilization with 1% Vetranquil, followed by general intramuscular anesthesia by administration of 5mg / kg body of Ketamine. This administration was performed before preparing the operative field and about 15 minutes before surgery.

After the antiseptization and isolation of the operative field, it was performed a longitudinal incision along the antero-medial face of the calf for about 4,5cm. With the Pean forceps The Pean forceps the tegument was taken off till the muscular plane level obtaining two flaps "envelope" on both sides of the incision line.

After exposure and longitudinal incision of the tibial cranial muscle fascia, the site had been penetrated, with a Pean forceps, perpendicular to the muscle plan till the bone plane, among the fibers of this muscle. Selling the forceps' arms and its removal permitted the access towards the anterior medial tibia. After the dezinsertion of the muscular fibers the periosteum was taken off, exposing the diaphy bone plate up to the cranial epiphysis. At this level, with the help of rotary instruments at a speed of 5000rpm and under continuously irrigation with saline, are created the geodes, with shapes and sizes about equal to those of the transverse surfaces of implants. The implants are perpendicular inserted in geodes, by percussion. After hemostasis, the wounds are sutured with catgut wire in deep planes and with synthetic yarns in tegument plane.

The antibiotic prophylaxis was realized according standard norms, in unique doze, with cefazolin (cephalosporin generation I) - Lyzolin, which had been intramuscular administrated 50mg/kg body 30 minutes before the surgery and 6 hours after surgery. 10 days after surgery, the sutures wires were removed.

3.5.1 Biological material sampling

The sampling was realized by sacrificing the subjects, at 2, 4 and 6 months after implantation (titanium implants), 2 months respectively after implantation (the type Ti6Al4V alloy and austenitic stainless steel type 316L) (see figure 5). To be investigated, the samples had been kept 6 hours in saline, had been fixed with 30% glutaraldehyde solution, after that being rewashed with normal saline and ultra pure deionized water, in order to remove organic particles resulting from the soft and hard tissue sectioning.

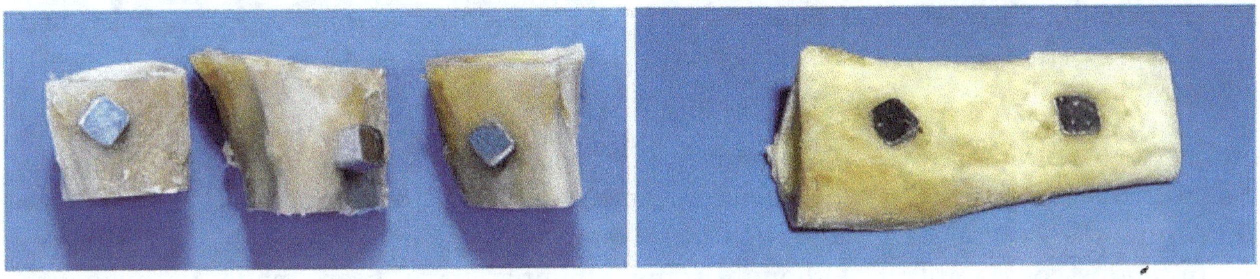

Fig. 5. The biological materials aspect after sampling: left-Ti 99,99% at 2, 4 and 6 months after implantation; right Ti6Al4V and 316L respectively, two months after implantation.

3.5.2 The osseointegration process evolution of the titanium implants

It was analyzed the morphology and topography of the periimplantary bone surface under which it could be systematized the gradual evolution of biological osseointegration processes of the titanium implants. There has been initially formed a periimplantar blood clot from the blood derived through the interruption of the continuity of the haversiene vessels from the edge of the bony defect created by drilling. This blood clot consisted of the figurative elements of blood (erythrocytes and platelets) situated in eyes of network or mesh of fibrin. The elements observed and described through the ESEM images demonstrate the existence of a complex process of periimplantar healing. In the neighbouring tissues of the implant, there are initially produced modifications of the inflammatory type represented by hyperaemia, plasmexodia and formation of a leukocyte and macrophagocyte infiltrate.

Alike bone fracture healing, in the peri-implant healing the blood vessels are damaged, and this results in haemorrhage and the formation of a blood clot, or hematoma. In the bone fracture healing the amount of blood loss from the circulation depends on the location of the fracture. In the femoral shaft, up to one litre of blood can be lost due to extravasation (Cormack, 1987) whereas the amount lost in dental implant placement is significantly less, with the healing site volume measured in millilitres (Davies, 2005). A few days after the implantation, a proliferation of two types of cells become visible: the fibroblasts that will form a periimplantar fibrous callus and endothelial cells that will generate a capillary network of new-formation observed by ESEM as a periimplantar vascular plexus (see figure 6).

This periimplantar well developed vascular network appears to be the result of the angioformation activity of the bone red marrow from the spongious bone. According other studies, angiogenesis is initiated predominantly from post-capillary venules, where endothelial cells degrade the subendothelial basement membrane and migrate and

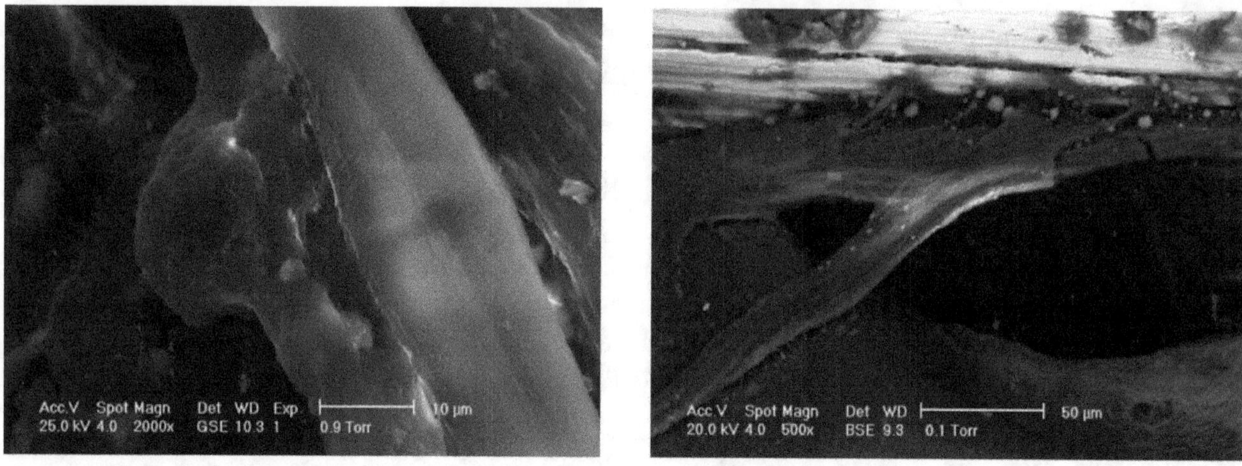

Fig. 6. Left - Extravasation of a blood cell at the level of the periimplantar bony tissue; right - ESEM microscopy image of the peri-implantar vascular plexus.

proliferate to form hollow capillary buds or sprouts. We now know a great deal concerning the molecular mechanisms of angiogenesis, (Lakey at al, 2000) but, at present, we still do not know how the patterns of angiogenesis may be affected by the presence, or surface design, of an endosseous implant, although some attempts have been made to image the vasculature that develops around endosseous implants. (Murakami, 1995;)
Interestingly, (Matsuo et al., 1999) showed some differences in the neovasculature in cortical bone around machined and plasma-sprayed implants that exhibited distance osteogenesis. Other works (Davies, 2005) has also demonstrated that implant surfaces, which are known to promote contact osteogenesis, also exhibit a richer immediate periimplant vascular supply within the healing compartment. The apparition of the neoformation vessels appearance is an important moment of the healing due to the fact that the bloodstream within periimplantar rennet being accomplished, it becomes possible both a number of cellular changes and the acceleration of the metabolism. Our observations showed that through the processes of proliferation of fibroblasts and vascular endothelium, the periimplantar clot is replaced by granulation tissue during 14 days from the surgical

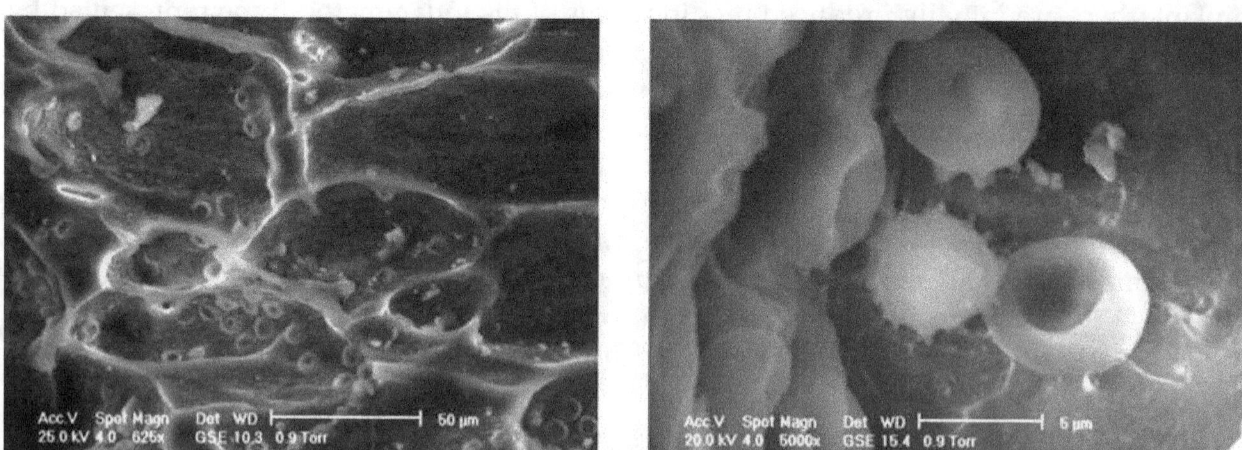

Fig. 7. ESEM image of the mature spongious bone tissue at the edge of bone defect created by drilling: osteoide trabeculae which delimit areoles filled with marrow blood tissue (left); platelets and hematite cells (right).

procedure. At the same time, a process of osteoclasis resorption at the edges of bone defect begins. ESEM technique, the unconditioning of the preliminary preparation of the biological specimen, and implicitly their deterioration, permitted the identification of a very intense cellular activity at the level of the implant-tissue interface. Immediately after implantation, the immune response triggered a proliferation of local macrophages.

While erythrocytes are clearly important in oxygen transport (see figure 7), they can reasonably be assumed to be of little importance in the mechanisms of early peri-implant healing. Platelets, however, are of considerable importance since their activation leads to a rearrangement in cell shape and to centralization of storage granules followed by the release of their contents into the extracellular environment (degranulation); and platelet degranulation releases a number of growth factors, such as platelet-derived growth factor (PDGF) and transforming growth factor beta (TGF-b), together with vasoactive factors such as serotonin and histamine. (Davies, 2005). Conventional wisdom holds that these factors play an important role in the regulation of the wound-healing cascade, (Park et al., 2001) based on in vitro and in vivo evidence of their stimulatory effects on the proliferation and migration of various cell types. (Gruber et al., 2002) For example, both PDGF and TGF-b have been shown to be not only mitogenic for fibroblasts but also chemotactic factors for fibroblasts, neutrophils, and smooth muscle cells, (Lucas et al., 1988) as well as osteogenic cells. (Lind, 1998) Indeed, not only has PDGF been shown to stimulate the proliferation of human osteoblasts, (Tsukamoto et al., 1991) but also is able to stimulate the recruitment, migration, and profileration of bone marrow-derived cells. (Oprea et al., 2003) Following platelet degranulation, arachidonic acid metabolites are secreted that cause vasoconstriction. Within the surrounding tissue, factors VII and III (tissue factor) in the extravasated blood cause the activation of factor X that, together with factor V, causes the conversion of prothrombin to thrombin, which cleaves the fibrinopeptides from fibrinogen to produce the fibrin of the clot (Colman et al., 1987).

Since fibrin, which is the reaction product of thrombin and fibrinogen released into the healing site, can be expected to adhere to almost all surfaces, osteogenic cell migration may be expected towards any implanted material. However, as is well known in dermal wound healing models, connective tissue cell migration is concomitant with wound contraction, which usually begins around the fifth day postwounding. (Peacock, 1984) Indeed, the migration of fibroblasts has been recognized as responsible for wound contraction, with individual cell adhesive contacts transducing a contractile force. (Galbraith et al., 1997) This ability of cells to contract the matrix through which they migrate can be modeled in vitro (Oprea et al., 2003;) and, in the bony peri-implant site could possibly cause retraction of the transitory fibrin scaffold away from the implant surface. The fact that primary osteogenic cells can cause fibrin contraction can be demonstrated by treating primary osteogenic cell cultures with cytochlasin-D, which blocks actin-dependent cell processes, such as cell migration, by capping actin filaments. (Pederson et al., 2001) Thus, the ability of an implant surface to retain fibrin during this wound contraction phase of healing is critical in determining if the migrating cells will reach the former (see figure 8). The implant surface design will play an important role in this fibrin retention. (Dumitru et al., 2005) Indeed, if implants are recovered a few days after implantation, the adhesion of this transitory matrix to some surfaces can be easily visualized. (Ciocan et al., 2010) In our research, after a period of several weeks the replacement of the granulation tissue with immature conjunctive (fibrous) tissue begins.

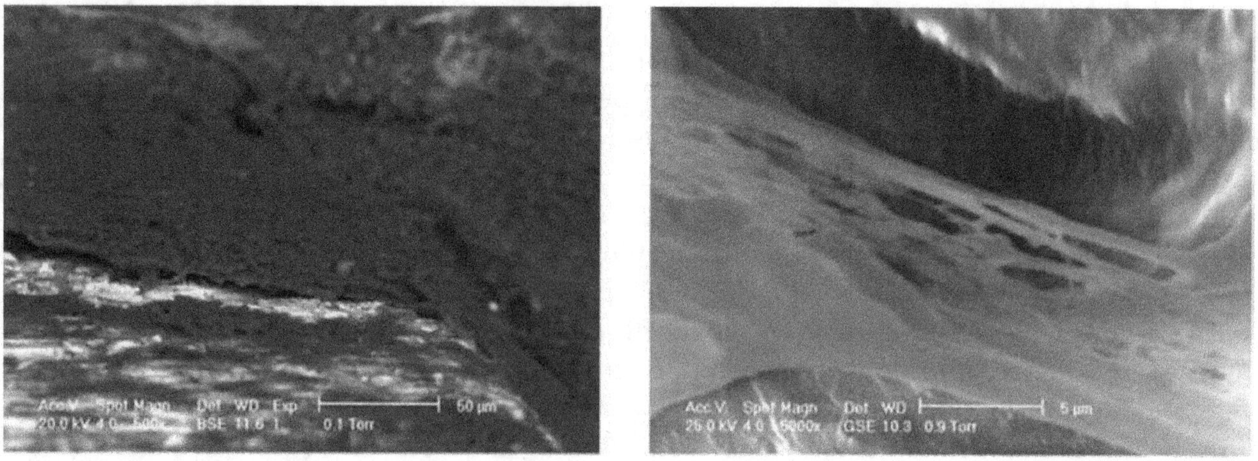

Fig. 8. ESEM images showing replacement of the granulation tissue with the periimplantar fibrous tissue (left) and continuous aspect of connective fibers and fibrocitary intense activity presence (right).

The conjunctive fibers (collagen) form a continuous texture on the implant surface in which there is identified a rich capillary vascularization while the cell population, dominantly of a fibrocitary nature, is much richer in younger elements. The most intense cellular activity was found in the area of biological tissue-implant interface. In the same period, the very first fine trabeculae of neoformation bone begins to appear.

Around endosseous implants, osteoblasts may lay down bone on the old bone surface or on the implant surface itself. This distinction was explored from the early 80'th as two phenomena, distance and contact osteogenesis, by which bone can become juxtapose to an implant surface. The periimplantar osteogenesis mechanism is still not completely elucidated. According to some authors, for about one month after the implantation, a partial bone marrow necrobiosis phenomenon occurs; similar biological phenomena are taking place for the heterotopy transplants. (Hutchinson, 2005) This mechanism seems to be responsible for the development of inductors, which determine the transformation of the mesenchymal cells from the receptor bed into osteoblasts. This phenomenon was confirmed by the image observations from this study. First, bone matrix is synthesized by only one cell: the osteoblast. While some would argue that osteoblasts from different anatomical sites represent different end members of this osteogenic differentiation pathway, the outcome remains the same: it is the osteoblast that makes bone matrix. Indeed, like most secretory cells, osteoblasts are polarized cells, and the direction of their secretory activity is away from the nuclear end of the cell (this is also true for the so-called reverse polarization of ameloblasts). Since the matrix secreted by osteoblasts becomes mineralized as bone tissue, the cell processes of osteoblasts become surrounded by mineralized matrix (and, with their canaliculi, form the only means of vital communication between surface osteoblasts and those that have become completed surrounded by matrix as osteocytes). Thus the osteoblast is irrevocably attached to the bone-forming surface.

The experimental results obtained have validated also the biomineralization three-phased experimental model described by Urist, 1965. According to this theory, the calcium ion is bounded to a protein in the first phase, it is associated in the second phase with phosphate forming Ca-PO_4 protein complex and finally in the third phase, there takes place the formation of the geometric configuration of a nucleation center. The degree of mineralization of conjunctive matrix around implant was counted by EDAX analisys (see

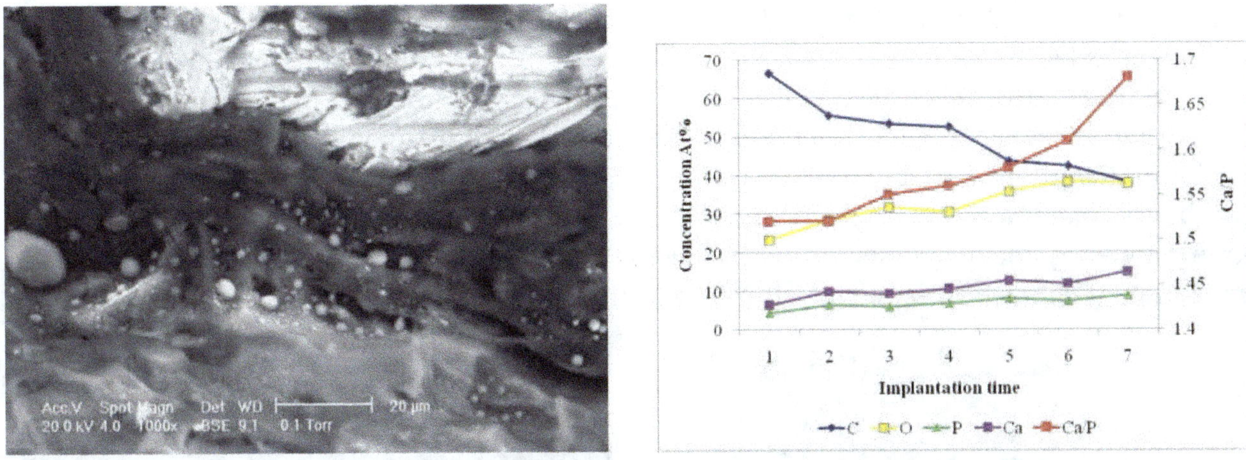

Fig. 9. Periimplantar phosphocalcic precipitations at the level of the vascular walls (left); Basic elements concentration (At%) variation with time after Ti implant insertion (right).

figure 9). The results of this analysis show the continuous mineralisation of the implant surrounding tissue during 6 month after implantation. This graphics presents the variation of the basic elements from the chemical composition of the bone in the "de novo" tissue that surrounds the titanium implants.

Although the concentration of the mineral elements (Ca, P) brought at the peri-implant healing site remain similar during time, the hydroxiapatite precipitations are continuous growing in the same time with reduction of organic fibrous tissue (see table 2). The inflection point of the curve appear at the second half of the 3rd month after insertion when the mineral content of the tissue around implant exceeds the organic matrix one. After about two months from the implantation, the periimplantar tissue consists of a conjunctive fibrous tissue rich in cell population, which suffers intense bony neotransformation processes.

Time	C%	O%	P%	Ca%	Ca/P
7 days	66,34	23,1	4,23	6,34	1,52
14 days	55,48	28,33	6,4	9,79	1,52
1 month	53,32	31,61	5,91	9,16	1,55
2 month	52,5	30,33	6,71	10,46	1,56
3 month	43,66	35,76	7,98	12,6	1,58
4 month	42,45	38,33	7,36	11,85	1,61
6 month	38,36	37,9	8,86	14,88	1,68

Table 2. Concentration (At%) of the chemical elements at the implant-bone interface

At four months from the intervention, the periimplantar fibrous tissue is almost disappeared while the newbone has already started the functional remodelling (see figure 10), while after 6 months from the implantation, the newly formed bone is matured and functional remodeled so that the boundaries of the original bony defect can be hardly seen by the help of the electronic microscope (see figure 11).

Intimate biological mechanisms adherence of bone tissue on the surface of the pure titanium implant is cohesively demonstrated by bone substrate. Contact osteogenesis relies upon osteoconduction, (Osborn et al., 1980) or the recruitment and migration of differentiating osteogenic cells to the implant surface, together with "de novo" bone formation by those cells on the implant surface. Osteoconduction also occurs during normal tunneling remodeling in bone. In such remodeling, differentiating osteogenic cells are derived from undifferentiated peri-vascular connective tissue cells (pericytes), just as soft tissue fibroblasts have long been recognized as being derived from the mesenchymal cell populations of blood vessel adventia. (Ross et al., 1970) However, a more complex environment characterizes the peri-implant healing site.

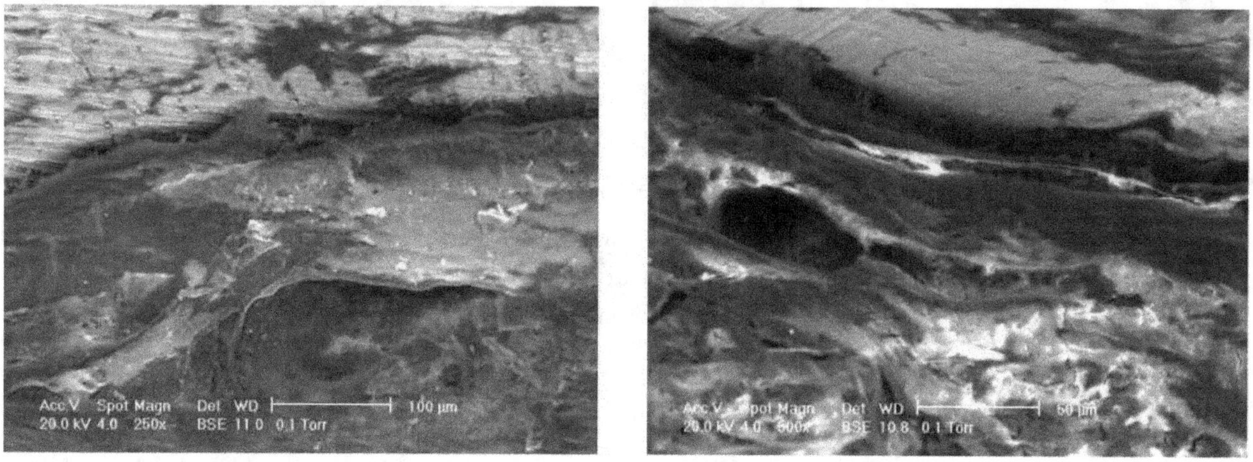

Fig. 10. Periimplantar fibrous tissue transformed into neoformation bony tissue after 3 month (left); after 4 month (right).

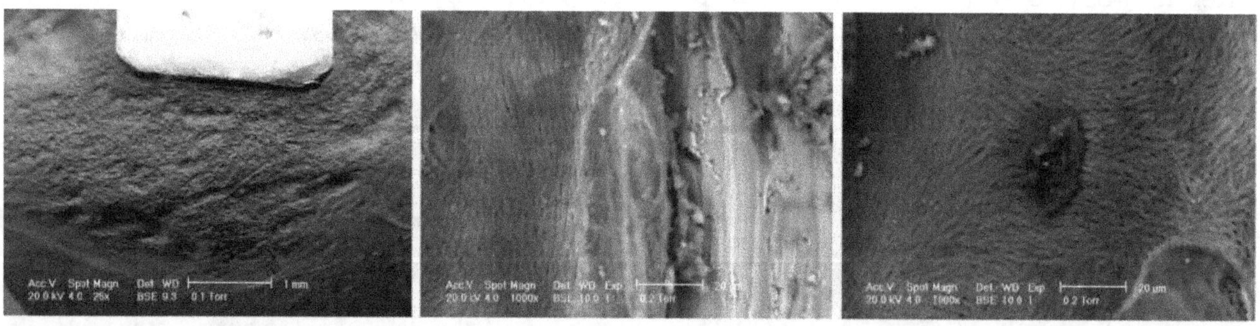

Fig. 11. ESEM macrography at 6 month- periimplantar new bone tissue in the full process of functional remodelling: left - bone wound healed around implant; center - mature bone connected to implant; right - osteon formatted in the periimplant new bone.

3.5.3 Osseointegration according to the roughness of the implant surface

Every samples was analyzed by electron microscopy (ESEM), using secondary electron detector in water vapor environment (GSE), retro scattered electron detector (BSE), respectively by qualitative and quantitative compositional analysis EDAX type. During the analysis by electron microscopy ESEM, it was identified the roughness of the surface, periimplantary hiatus sizes and periimplantary vascular plexus. It was also observed the thickness of the periimplantary fibrous callus under calcification and the morphology of the bone tissue neoformation (see figure 12). During an analysis of the sample of Ti6Al4V alloy under axial incidence, it was macroscopic (X20) noticed both filling the periimplantary defect with neoformation bone tissue and covering the implant with this one, on some areas. Afterwards, the bone implant interface was examined on each side of the sample.

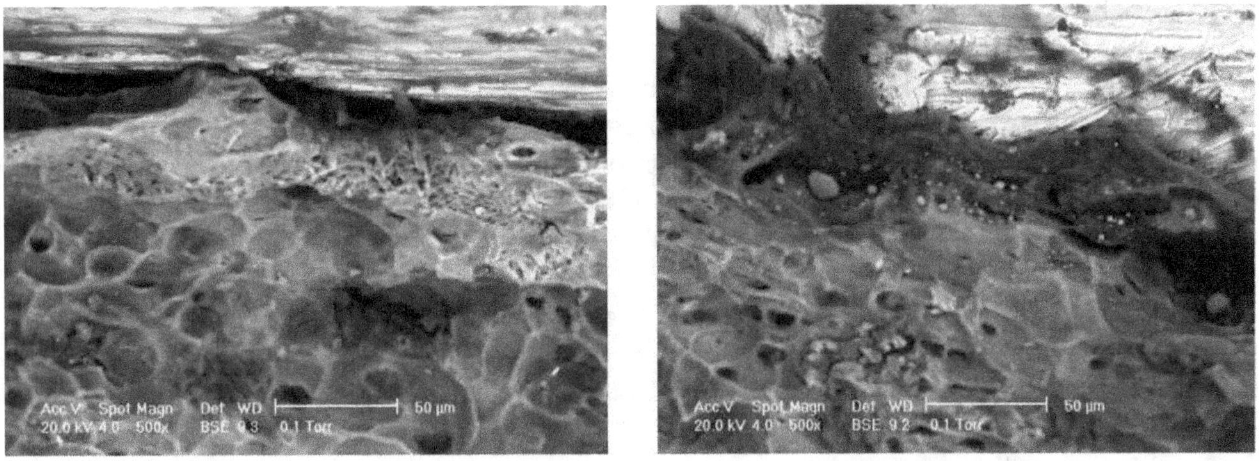

Fig. 12. Interface morphology of newly formed bone and the face 1 of the implant (left), and face 2, respectively (right).

The ESEM imaging identifies roughness surfaces. If training with roughness P600, the periimplantary hiatus has small dimensions, 5µm on average, the vascular plexus being absent. It is also noticed the lack of the fibrous tissue. The new formation of bone tissue presents a remodeling aspect. The surface roughness at this level (P320) (side 2) was the determining factor of the maximum neo-bony adhesion for this implant. However, the mineralization processes of the protean organic matrix are delayed from those presented in the side 1.

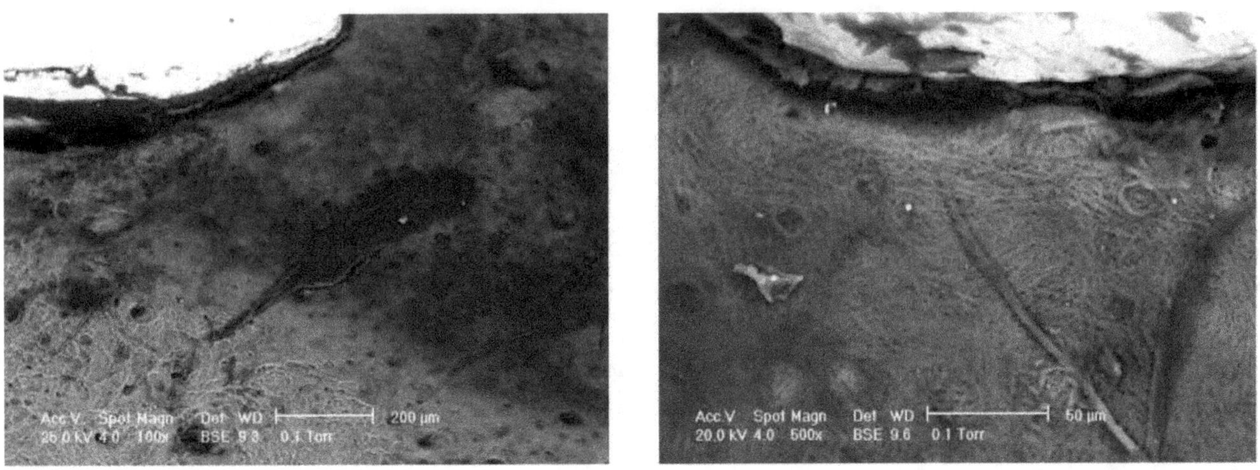

Fig. 13. Interface morphology of newly formed bone and the face 3 of the implant (left), and face 4, respectively (right).

At a roughness obtained with P1000 paper (face 3), on the periimplatary hiatus of 15µm large dimension, it is noticed the presence of a rich vascular plexus (see figure 13). The neoformation bone tissue presents Havers large and remote channels. At a roughness obtained with P800 paper (face 4), the hiatus is 10µm, periimplementary, being observed the presence of uncalcifying fibrous tissue, with thickness of 20 to 25µm. The image captures vascular axis of some Havers collateral channels.

4. Conclusion

In the context of the complexity of implant surfaces, due to the different structures and theirs roughness, also to different chemical compositions, the purpose of this study was to examine the processes of tissue implant interface. To achieve this desideratum, I performed, in this order, determinations regarding the biomaterials' microstructure, their resistance to the corrosion, their behavior and influence above the cellular cultures and, finally, *in vivo* tests on animals. I approached the interaction of implants made of metal biomaterials, with different structures and the surface roughness, with biological tissues, which included discussions on the mechanism of implants' incorporation and on the development and changes of living tissues during remodeling after insertion.

The surfaces of different implants were measured and compared to the bone surface, as it is known that these surfaces are covered, in many cases, with new bone deposits and therefore they serve as fixing points for newly formed bone. The structures' surfaces of the implants were characterized, measured and correlated to the morphometrical evaluations of the tissue - biomaterial contact.

By using cell culture techniques, it can cause lyses (death) of cells, cell growth inhibition, and some specific effects on cells caused by the devices, materials and / or their extracts. The percentage of the growth inhibition was determined by counting cells, and the measurements were corrected for control with a negative filter. As a reference experiment, we took a fibroblast culture in which no metallic sample was immersed, the culture being kept under the same conditions of the experiments in which were immersed metallic samples. It may be noted that a cellular monolayer was obtained, at all the studied experiments, without being registered any free spaces, in which fully lack the cellular culture. After analyzing the obtained images, it may be presented some important characteristics of the studied cellular cultures. In the case of the cellular culture without metallic sample (blank), the fibroblast cells of the culture highlight morph-structural fairly uniform characteristics. Covering the well with cellular formation is about 90%. It is obviously the cells' compaction and the appearance of the phenomenon of forming a multilayer culture. Finally, depending on the studied biomaterial type, we obtained the monolayer formation ranged from 90 to 55% of the surface, in some cases being noticed the pluristratification trend. The main indicators taken into account under the regulations existing standards were: cells' number, proliferation, cell adhesion to the substrate, cells' viability. The cellular culture system appears to be sensitive to the *in vitro* evaluation of metallic biomaterials with cells interactions and cellular response features. The experimental models, developed for investigations on cellular cultures, have been based on the overall assessment and namely that the cellular culture system is a useful means for testing the biomaterials' cytotoxicity and helps to reduce the experiments' number on animals.

The *in vivo* experimental study on animals regarding the interactions of the biomaterial-tissue interface showed that, whatever the samples' type was, it was macroscopically and microscopically found the bio-integrity of all implants. The speed of transforming the periimplantary fibrous tissue into a neo-differentiated bone tissue, respectively the "calcification" of the periimplantary fibrous tissue was significantly higher in terms of quality and quantity for the samples on which hydroxyapatite has been filed.

The observed and described imagistic elements allowed the real appreciation of the influence of metal surface preparation method on the bio-integrity complex process. For none of the samples were observed periimplantary osteolysis processes, which proves the existence of a favorable interaction between the implanted biomaterial and the biological structure (bone tissue). Whatever the implant type, it was noticed a direct proportionality between the preparation degree of implant surface (mechanical preparation, blasting, chemical attack) and the degree and speed of transforming the periimplantary tissues into mature bone tissue (tissue neoformation inflammatory vascular plexus, fibrous tissue, bone tissue neoformation). The development and periimplantary organic matrix mineralization degree was closely correlated with biochemical changes at the interface. The neoformation bone tissue was intensely mineralized in the case of pure titanium implant, less mineralized in the case of the TiAl64V implant, poorly mineralized for the implantation of Co-Cr-Mo and scarcely mineralized for stainless alloy implant.

By the help of the scan electronic microscopy, using an ESEM XL 30 electronic microscope, it was possible the observation and standardization of the biointegration processes from the interface of the titanium implants. The images presented, show the intimate evolution of the healing processes from this level and represent the fundamental base for the theory for the metallic implant osseointegration.

This study made possible the understanding of the intimate cellular and tissue bony integration mechanisms of the titanium metal implants. A few days after the implantation, a proliferation of two types of cells become visible: the fibroblasts that will form a periimplantar fibrous callus and endothelial cells that will generate a capillary network of neoformation observed by ESEM as a periimplantar vascular plexus. Through the processes of proliferation of fibroblasts and vascular endothelium, the periimplantar clot is replaced by granulation tissue during 7 days from the surgical procedure. At the same time, a process of osseoclastic resorption at the edges of bone defect begins. In two weeks, around implant it will be developed an immature conjunctive fibrous tissue. After about two months from the implantation, the periimplantar tissue consists of a conjunctive fibrous tissue rich in cell population, which suffers intense bony neotransformation processes. At four months, the periimplantar fibrous tissue is almost disappeared while the newbone has already started the functional remodelling. In 6 months from the implantation moment, the newly formed bone is matured and functional remodelled so that the boundaries of the original bony defect can be hardly seen by the help of the electronic microscope.

Based on image observations for the surrounding tissues unaffected by the experiment, the validation of the results obtained was possible. The degree of mineralization of conjunctive matrix around implant was counted by EDAX analysis. Our results showed that the concentration of the mineral elements (Ca, P) brought at the peri-implant healing site remain similar during time, while hydroxiapatite precipitations are continuous growing and organic fibrous tissue is reducing. The inflection point of the curve appear at the second half of the 3rd month after insertion when the mineral content of the tissue around implant exceeds the organic matrix one.

There are still many aspects of peri-implant healing that need to be elucidated. According to the authors, there should be rigorously investigated further the chemical-enzymatic mechanisms underlying the osseointegration biological processes.

5. Acknowledgment

This work was supported by CNCSIS-UEFISCSU (UEFISCDI); project number PN II-RU 104/2010.

6. References

Anselme K, Bigenelle M, Noel B, Dufresne E, Judas D, Iost A, Hardouin P., 2000, Qualitative And Quantitative Study Of Human Osteoblast Adhesion On Materials With Various Surface Roughnesses, *Journal of Biomed Mater Res*, 49, pp. 155-166.

Black J., 1992, *Biological Performance of Materials: Fundamentals of Biocompatibility*, 2nd ed., Marcel Dekker, ISBN 0-82-478439-1;

Branemark PI, Chien S, Grondahl HG, Robinson K., 2006, *The Osseointegration Book: From Calvarium to Calcaneus*, Quintessence Publishing, ISBN 1850970904.

Brodbeck WG, Shive MS, Colton E, Nakayama Y, Matsuda T, Anderson JM., 2001, Influence Of Biomaterial Surface Chemistry On The Apoptosis Of Adherent Cells, *Journal of Biomedical Mater Res.*, 55, pp. 661-668.

Ciocan LT, Miculescu F, Miculescu M, Patrascu I., 2010, Retrieval analysis on dental implants biointegration phases, *Romanian Journal of Morphology and Embryology*, 51, pp. 117-122.

Colman RW, Marder VJ, Salzman EW, Hirsh J. Overview of hemostasis. In: Colman RW, Hirsh J, Marder VJ, Salzman EW, eds., 1987, *Hemostasis and thrombosis/basic principles and clinical practice*, 2nd ed. Philadelphia: Lippincott, pp. 3-17.

Cormack DH., 1987, Bone. In: *Ham's histology*, 9th ed. Philadelphia: Lippincott, pp. 273-323.

Davies JE, 2005, Understanding Peri-Implpant Endosseous healing, *J Dent Edu*, Re-issued in Transfer of Advances Sciences into Dental Education, Toronto: Em squared Inc., 67, pp. 932-949.

Dekker A, Panfil C, Valdor M, Pennartz G, Richter H, Mittermayer Ch, Kirkpatrick CJ., 1994, Quantitative Methods For In Vitro Cytotoxicity Testing Of Biomaterials, *Cells Mater.*, 4, pp.101-112.

Dumitru N, D. Bunea D, Patrascu I, Ciocan LT, F. Miculescu F., 2005, Chemical Composition and Surface Preparation Level Influence on Metallic Implants Biointegrability, *European Cells and Materials*, 9, pp. 27-28.

Futami T., Fujii N., Ohnishi H., Taguchi N., Kusakari H., Ohshima H., Maeda T., 2000, Tissue Response To Titanium Implants In The Rat Maxilla: Ultrastructural And Histochemical Observations Of The Bone–Titanium Interface, *Journal of Periodontol*, 71, pp. 287–298.

Galbraith CG, Sheetz MP., 1997, A micromachined device provides a new bend on fibroblast traction forces. *Proc Natl Acad Sci USA*, pp. 9114-9118.

Gruber R, Varga F, Fischer MB, et al., 2002, Platelets stimulate proliferation of bone cells: involvement of platelet-derived growth factor, microparticles and membranes, *Clin Oral Impl Res*, pp. 529-535.

Hazan, R., Brener, R., and Oron, U., 1993, Bone Growth To Metal Implants Is Regulated By Their Surface Chemical Properties, *Biomaterials*, 14, pp. 570-574.

Hutchison J., 2005, The fate of experimental bone autografts and homografts, *British Journal of Surgery*, 39, pp. 552-561.

Ilin A.A., Skvortsova S.V., 2002, Titanium and Titanium Alloys, Effect of Thermohydrogen Treatment on the Structure and Properties of Titanium Alloy Castings, *Metal Science and Heat Treatment*, 44, pp. 5-6.

Kasemo B & Lausmaa J., 1991, The Biomaterial-Tissue Interface And Its Analogues In Surface Science And Technology, In Davies JE (editor) *The bone-biomaterial interface*, University of Toronto press, Toronto, pp. 19-32.

Kilburn M.R., Lewis A., Papageorgiou I., Allen G.C., Case C.P., 2003, Surface Characterization And Matal Ion Release From CoCr Alloy Used In Orthopaedic Implants, Proceeding of 18th European Conference on Biomaterials.

Kocijan A., Milosev I., Merl D.K., Pihlar B., 2004, Electrochemical Study Of Co-Based Alooys In Simulated Physiological Solution, *Journal of Applied Electrochemistry*, pp. 7.

Lakey L, Akella R, Ranieri JP, 2000, Angiogenesis: implications for tissue repair. In: Davies JE, ed. *Bone engineering*. Toronto: em squared Inc., pp. 137-142.

Lind M., 1998, Growth factor stimulation of bone healing: effects on osteoblasts, osteomies, and implant fixation, *Acta Orthop Scand Suppl.*, pp. 283:2-37.

Lucas PA, Caplan AI., 1988, Chemotactic response of embryonic limb bud mesenchymal cells and muscle-derived fibroblasts to transforming growth factor-beta. *Connect Tissue Res*, 18, pp. 1-7.

Matsuo M, Nakamura T, Kishi Y, Takahashi K., 1999, Microvascular changes after placement of titanium implants: scanning electron micrscopy observations of machined and titanium plasma-sprayed implants in dogs, *J. Periodontol*, 70, pp. 1330-1338.

Miculescu F, Bojin D, Ciocan LT, Antoniac I, Miculescu M, Miculescu N., 2007, Experimental researches on biomaterial-tissue interface interactions, *Journal of Optoelectronics and Advanced Materials*; 9, pp. 3303-3306.

Moiseev V.N., 2004, Titanium Alloys-Structural Titanium Alloys in Modern Mechanical Engineering, *Metal Science and Heat Treatment*, 46, pp. 3-4.

Murakami I., 1995, Scanning electron microscopic study on bone and microvasculature surrounding titanium implants, *J Jpn Prosthodont Soc*; pp. 123-134.

Oprea WE, Karp JM, Hosseini MM, Davies JE. 2003, Effect of platelet releasate on bone cell migration and recruitment in vitro, *J Craniofac Surg*, 14, pp. 292-300.

Osborn JF, Newesely H., 1980, Dynamic aspects of the implant-bone interface. In: Heimke G, ed. *Dental implants: materials and systems*. Muunchen: Carl Hanser Verlag, pp. 111-123.

Park JY, Gemmell CH, Davies JE., 2001, Platelet interactions with titanium: modulation of platelet activity by surface topography, *Biomaterials*, 22, pp. 2671-2682.

Peacock EE., 1984, Wound repair. In: Peacock, EE, ed. *Wound repair*. Philadelphia: Saunders, pp. 38-55.

Pederson SF, Hoffmann EK, Mills JW., 2001, The cytoskeleton and cell volume regulation. *Comp Biochem Physiol A Mol Integr Physiol*, 130, pp. 385-399.

Puleo, D.A. and Nanci, A., 1999, Understanding And Controlling The Bone-Implant Interface, *Biomaterials*, 20, pp. 2311-2321.

Ross R, Everett NB, Tyler R., 1970, Wound healing and collagen formation: VI. The origin of the wound fibroblast studied in parabiosis, *J Cell Biol*, 44, pp. 645.

M.D. Smith, J.C. Barbenel, J.M. Courtney, M.H. Grant, 1992, Novel quantitative methods for the determination of biomaterial cytotoxicity, *International Journal of Artificial Organs*, 15, pp. 191-194.

Stanford C.M., Schneider G., Keller J.C., Midura R., 2003, *Biomedical Implant Surface Topography And Its Effects On Osteoblast Differentiation, Bio-implant interface – Improving biomaterials and tissue reactions*, pp. 141-164, ISBN 0-8493-1474-7.

Tsukamoto T, Matsui T, Fukase M, et al., 1991, Platelet-derived growth factor B chain homodimer enhances chemotaxis and DNA synthesis in normal osteoblast-like cells (MC3T3-E1), *Biochem Biophys Res Commun*, 175, pp. 745-751.

Urist MR., November 1965, Bone: Formation by autoinduction, *Science*, 150, pp. 893 – 899.

Wennerberg A., Ide-Ektessabi A., Hatkamata S., Sawase T., Johansson C., Albrektsson T., Martinelli A., Sodervall U., Odelius H., 2003, Titanium Release From Implants Prepared With Different Surface Roughness- An in vitro and ex vivo study, *Proceeding of 18th European Conference on Biomaterials.*

Yan, W., Nakamura, T., Kobayashi, M., Kim, H., Miyaji, F., Kokubo, T., 1997, Bonding Of Chemically Treated Titanium Implants To Bone, *Journal of Biomed. Mater. Res.*, 37, pp. 267-275.

10

Implant Stability - Measuring Devices and Randomized Clinical Trial for ISQ Value Change Pattern Measured from Two Different Directions by Magnetic RFA

Jong-Chul Park, Jung-Woo Lee,
Soung-Min Kim and Jong-Ho Lee
*Department of Oral and Maxillofacial Surgery,
School of Dentistry, Seoul National University,
Seoul,
Korea*

1. Introduction

Implant stability plays a critical role for successful osseointegration, which has been viewed as a direct structural and functional connection existing between bone and the surface of a load-carrying implant(Bränemark, et al. 1977, Sennerby & Roos 1998). Achievement and maintenance of implant stability are prerequisites for successful clinical outcome(Sennerby & Meredith 2008). Therefore, measuring the implant stability is an important method for evaluating the success of an implant. Implant stability is achieved at two different stages: primary and secondary. Primary stability of an implant comes from mechanical engagement with cortical bone. It is affected by the quantity and quality of bone that the implant is inserted into, surgical procedure, length, diameter, and form of the implant(Meredith 1998).

Secondary stability is developed from regeneration and remodeling of the bone and tissue around the implant after insertion but is affected by the primary stability, bone formation and remodeling(Sennerby & Roos 1998). The time of functional loading is dependent upon the secondary stability. It is, therefore, of an utmost importance to be able to quantify implant stability at various time points and to project a long term prognosis based on the measured implant stability(Atsumi, et al. 2007).

2. Measuring analyses of implant stability

Presently, various diagnostic analyses have been suggested to define implant stability. Primary implant stability can be measured by either a destructive or a non-destructive method. Histomorphologic research, tensional test, push-out/pull-out test and removal torque test are classified as destructive methods. Non-destructive methods include percussion test, radiography, cutting torque test while placing implants, Periotest®(Siemens AG, Benshein, Germany), and resonance frequency analysis(RFA)(Meredith 1998).

2.1 Tensional test

The interfacial tensile strength was originally measured by detaching the implant plate from the supporting bone(Kitsugi, et al. 1996). Bränemark later modified this technique by applying the lateral load to the implant fixture(Bränemark, et al. 1998). However, they also addressed the difficulties of translating the test results to any area- independent mechanical properties(Chang, et al. 2010)(Fig. 1a).

2.2 Histomorphometric analysis

Histomorphometric analysis is obtained by calculating the peri-implant bone quantity and bone-implant contact(BIC) from a dyed specimen of the implant and peri-implant bone. Accurate measurement is an advantage, but due to the invasive and destructive procedure, it is not appropriate for long-term studies. It is used in non-clinical studies and experiments.

2.2 Push-out/pull-out test

The 'push-out' or 'pull-out' test is the most commonly used approach to investigate the healing capabilities at the bone implant interface(Brunski, et al. 2000). In the typical push-out or pull-out test, a cylinder-type implant is placed transcortically or intramedullarly in

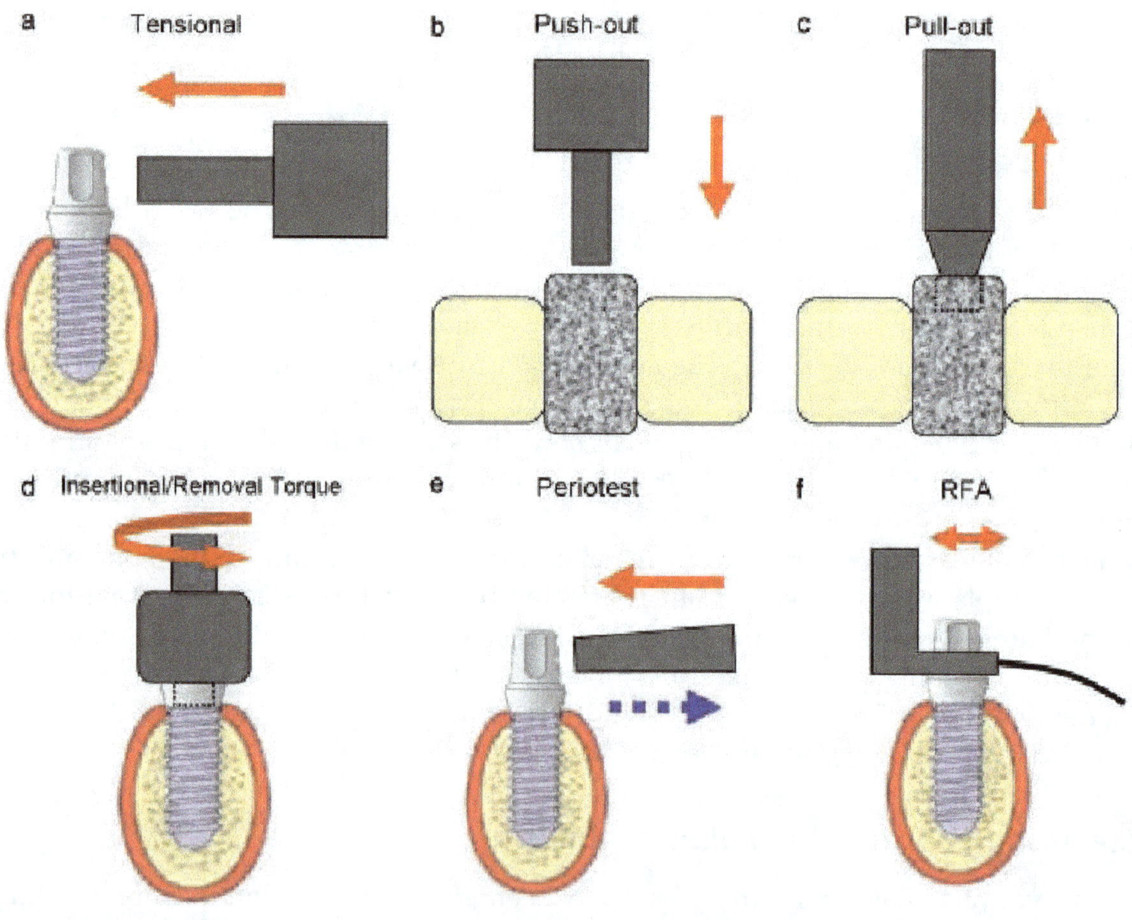

Fig. 1. Stability analyses for oral implant osseointegration from Chang, P. C., Lang, N. P. & Giannobile, W. V. (2010). "Evaluation of functional dynamics during osseointegration and regeneration associated with oral implants." Clinical Oral Implants Research 21: 1-12. (a) tensional test, (b) push-out test, (c) pull-out test, (d) insertional/removal torque test, (e) Periotest, and (e) resonance frequency analysis (RFA).

bone structures and then removed by applying a force parallel to the interface. The maximum load capability (or failure load) is defined as the maximum force on the force–displacement plot, and the interfacial stiffness is visualized as the slope of a tangent approximately at the linear region of the force–displacement curve before breakpoint (Brunski, et al. 2000, Lutolf, et al. 2003). Therefore, the general loading capacity of the interface (or interfacial shear strength) can be measured by dividing the maximum force by the area of implant in contact with the host bone(Berzins, et al. 1997). However, the push-out and pull-out tests are only applicable for non-threaded cylinder type implants, whereas most of clinically available fixtures are of threaded design, and their interfacial failures are solely dependent on shear stress without any consideration for either tensile or compressive stresses(Brunski, et al. 2000, Chang, et al. 2010)(Fig. 1b-c).

2.3 Removal torque analysis

Application of a reverse or unscrewing torque has also been proposed for the assessment of implant stability at the time of abutment connection(Sullivan, et al. 1996), however, implant surface in the process of osseointegration may fracture under the applied torque stress(Ivanoff, et al. 1997)(Fig.1d).

2.4 Percussion test

The test is carried out by a simple percussion with the handle of a dental instrument on the implant abutment and listening to the resulting sound. However, this method may be subjective according to the examiner and give inaccurate measurements for implants because of the high rigidity of implants and the lack of periodontal ligaments.

2.5 Insertion torque measurement

Insertion torque values have been used to measure the bone quality in various parts of the jaw during implant placement(O'Sullivan, et al. 2004). Insertion torque alone may be used as an independent stability measurement, but it may also act as a variable, affecting implant stability. In a different light, insertion torque is a mechanical parameter generally affected by surgical procedure, implant design and bone quality at implant site(Beer, et al. 2003). However, it cannot assess the secondary stability by new bone formation and remodeling around the implant. So it cannot collect longitudinal data to assess implant stability change after placement. Also, an increase in insertion torque may signify an increase in primary stability, but maximum insertion torque is produced by the pressure of implant neck on the dense cortical bone of the alveolus. Furthermore, it has been reported that if maximum insertion torque doesn't signify increased general bone density, it may indicate the insertion torque itself during tapping (Calandriello, et al. 2003)(Fig.1d).

2.6 Radiography

Radiography provides useful information for evaluating the quantity and quality of bone in the area for an implant before placing the fixture. It is also helpful in predicting implant stability by observing the process of osseointegration or peri-implant lesions. However, there is a limitation in image resolution and standardized X-rays are difficult to achieve due to the distortion of images, making quantitative measurements more challenging. In addition, it is difficult to perceive changes in the bone structures and morphology of the implant-bone interface unless over 30% bone loss occurs. Although the accuracy of the diagnosis is low, radiography is the major method used clinically to evaluate osseointegration and implant stability because of its convenience. (Albrektsson, et al. 1986).

2.7 Periotest®

Periotest® (Siemens AG, Benshein, Germany) was originally devised by Dr. Schulte to measure tooth mobility(Fig.2). Teerlinck, et al.(1991) used this method to overcome destructive methods in measuring the implant stability. Periotest® evaluates the damping capacity of the periodontium. It is designed to identify the damping capacity and the stiffness of the natural tooth or implant by measuring the contact time of an electronically driven and electronically monitored rod after percussing the test surface. Periotest value(PTV) is marked from -8(low mobility) to +50(high mobility). PTV of -8 to -6 is considered good stability.

Periotest® can measure all surfaces such as the abutment or prosthesis, but the rod must make contact at a correct angle and distance. If the perpendicular contact angle is larger than 20 degrees, or if the parallel contact angle is larger than 4 degrees, the measured value is invalid. Also, the rod and the test surface must maintain 0.6-2.0mm distance and if the distance is over 5mm, the measured value may be insignificant. (Ito, et al. 2008, Schulte 1988). Periotest® has limited clinical use since it cannot measure the mesiodistal mobility and the position and angle of the rod affects the measured value. Also, it cannot detect the small changes in the implant-bone surface. The most failing point of this method is that the percussing force on the implant may deteriorate the stability in poor initial stability implants.

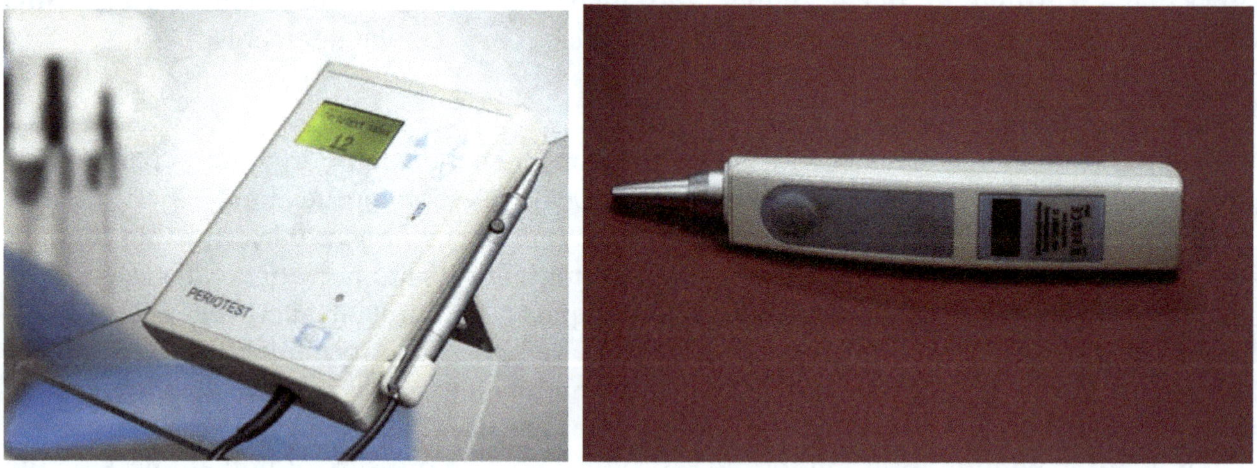

(a) (b)

Fig. 2. Periotest® (Siemens AG, Benshein, Germany) measures tooth mobility and implant stability by periotest value(PTV). (a) Periotest®, (B) Periotest®M.

2.8 Resonance Frequency Analysis(RFA)

In 1998, Meredith suggested a non-invasive method of analyzing peri-implant bone by connecting an adapter to an implant in an animal study. The experimented resonance frequency analysis system was commercially produced as Osstell™ (Osstell AB, Göteborg, Sweden).

A measurement of Osstell™ is displayed as implant stability quotient(ISQ) from 1 to 100, where 100 signifies the highest implant stability. Osstell™ was later followed by Osstell™ Mentor, and Osstell™ ISQ.

3. RFA principle and application

3.1 Introduction

Meredith et al.(1996) reported the use of resonance frequency analyzer to evaluate implant stability by applying architectural engineering, and proved in early in vitro test the ability of the device in evaluating the stiffness change of the surface. RFA uses the principle of when a frequency of audibility range is repeatedly vibrated onto an implant, the stronger the bone-implant surface, resonance occurs in a higher frequency. The first commercial product of the resonance frequency analyzer(RFA) was Osstell™(Osstell AB, Göteborg, Sweden)(Fig.3), followed by Osstell™ Mentor and recently Osstell™ ISQ was introduced. Osstell™ uses electronic technology and other devices(Osstell™ Mentor, Osstell™ ISQ) use magnetic technology (Fig.5).

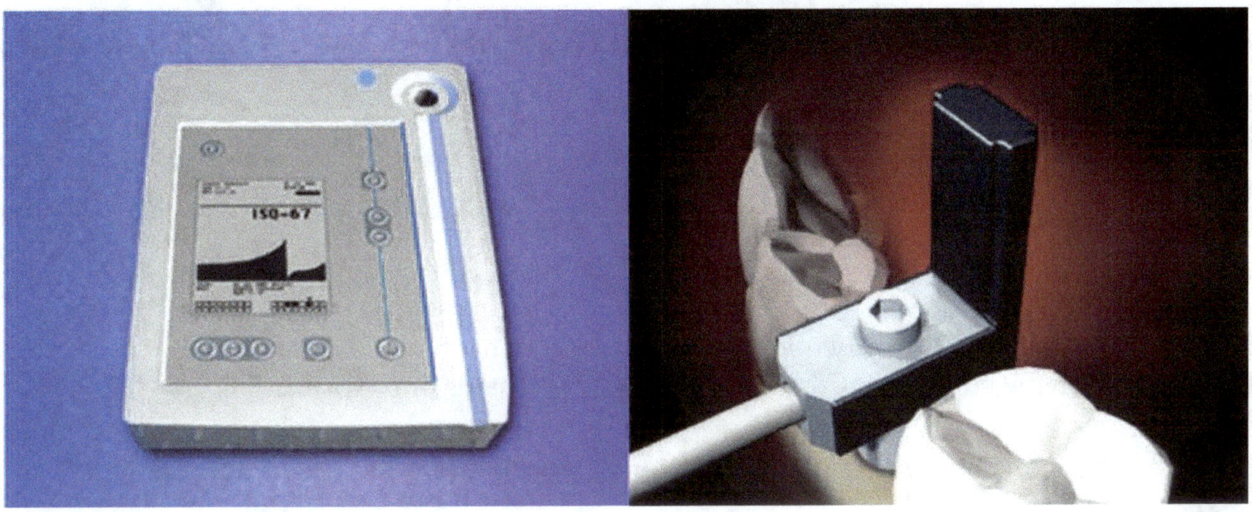

(a) (b)

Fig. 3. Pictures showing the first commercial products of resonance frequency analyzer. (a) the Osstell™ and (b) the application of the Osstell™ electronic transducer to the implant.(The figure and illustration are cited with permission from Osstell website, www.osstell.com, April, 2011)

3.2 Electronic technology resonance frequency analyzer(Osstell™)

The primary model Osstell™ produces alternating sine waves in a specific frequency range by uniform amplitude and makes the transducer connected to the implant or abutment vibrate under 1mm like an electronic tuning fork. A cantilever small beam is connected to the transducer and on this beam, 2 piezo-ceramic elements are attached. (Fig.3,4). One of them receives the signal and vibrates the transducer, and the other passes this vibration to the resonance frequency analyzer. Values on the monitor are displayed from 0-100 so that it can be conveniently used clinically. The value of 100 signify the highest stability state. Generally ISQ values for successfully integrated implants are reported from 57 to 82. These values can be displayed by graphs on the computer monitor or be expressed by values between 4500-8500Hz. The obtained output can be calculated by the equation below.

$$fn = \alpha\sqrt{\frac{EI}{\rho l^4}}$$

fn is the RF of the beam, l is the effective vibration length of the beam, E is the Young`s modulus, I is the moment of inertia, ρ is the mass, α the constant that increases as peri-implant bone density increases. Therefore, when osseointegration is achieved, RF increases since α value increases. 'l' signifies the length of implant above the bone. So as bone is resorbed, this value increases and thus RF decreases. In other words, ISQ is affected by the effective implant length, type of bone at implant site and bone density(Huang, et al. 2003, Huang, et al. 2003, Meredith, et al. 1996).

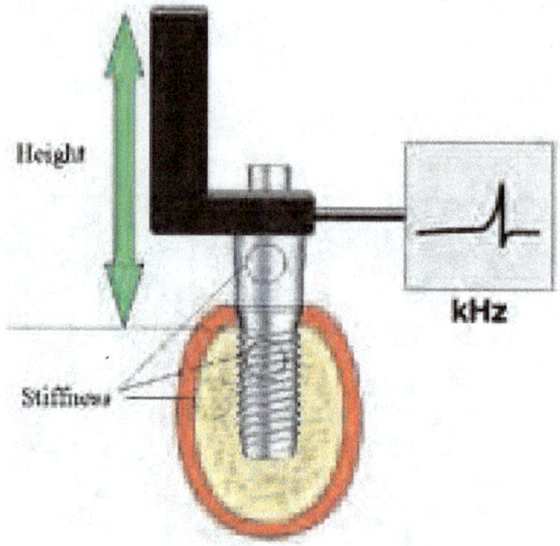

Fig. 4. Picture showing the principle of electronic resonance frequency analyzer. (The figure and illustration are cited from Osstell website, www.osstell.com, April, 2011)

3.3 Magnetic technology resonance frequency analyzer(Osstell™ Mentor, Osstell™ ISQ)

Resonance frequency between 3.5 KHz and 8.5 KHz formed from the magnetic field is converted into ISQ values by Osstell Mentor™(Fig. 5, 6). The transducer of Osstell Mentor™

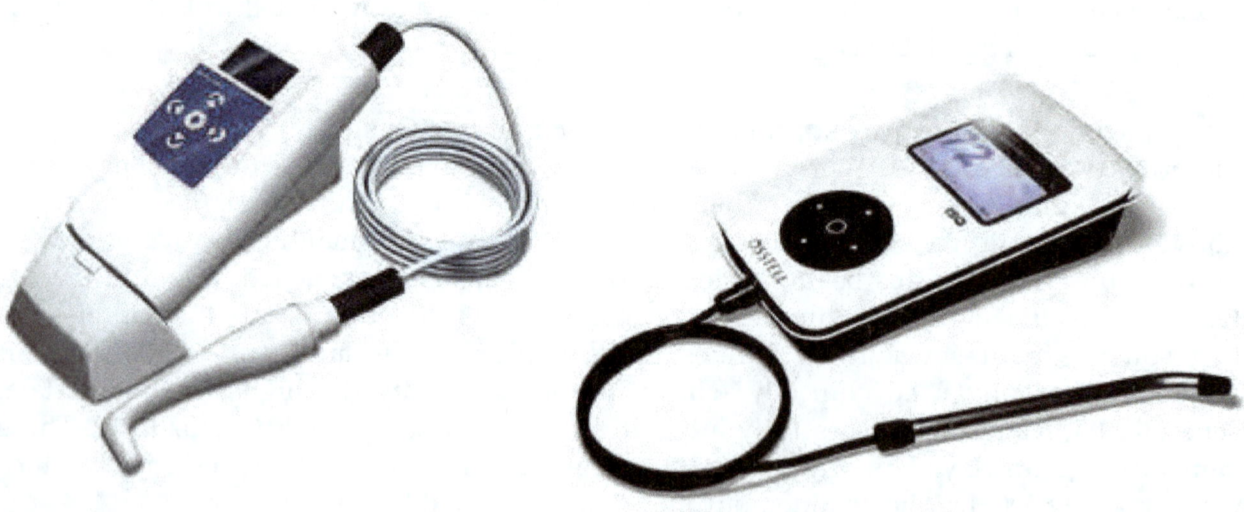

(a) (b)

Fig. 5. Osstell Mentor™ and Osstell ISQ™, both of devices measure ISQs by the magnetic technology. (The pictures are cited from Osstell website, www.osstell.com, April, 2011)

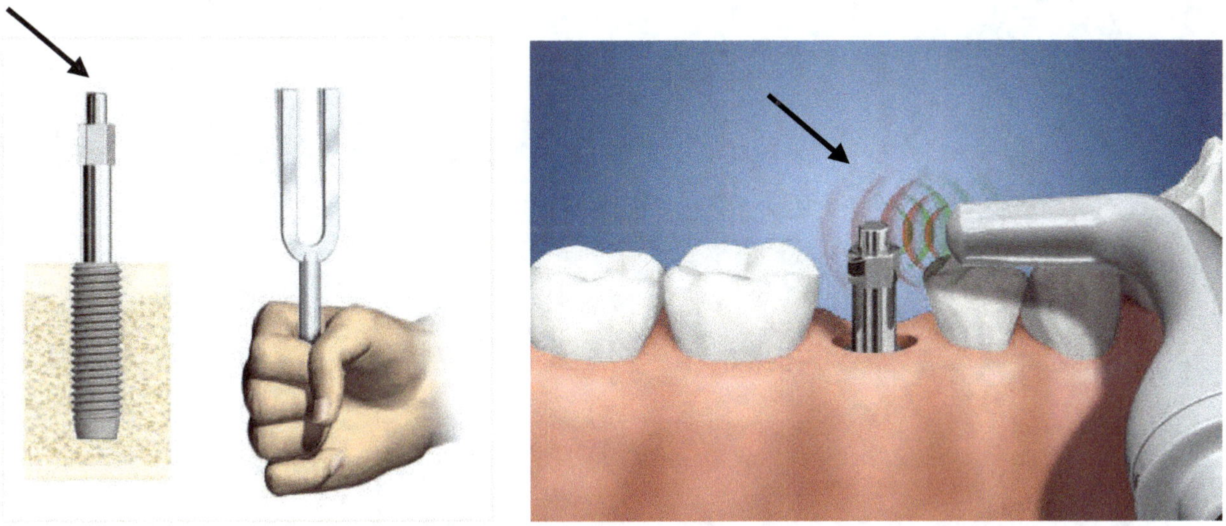

(a) (b)

Fig. 6. Principle of the Osstell Mentor™. Magnetic peg(Smart peg™) works like a tuning fork. Red arrow is the Smart peg™. (The figure and illustration are cited from Osstell website, www.osstell.com, April, 2011)

has a magnetic peg on the top and is fixed to the implant fixture or abutment by a screw below. When magnetic resonance frequency is released from the probe, the magnetic peg is activated. The activated peg starts to vibrate, and the magnet induces electric volt into the probe coil and the electric volt is sampled by the magnetic resonance frequency analyzer (Fig. 6). The values are expressed as numbers between 1-100 in ISQ as Osstell™ (Valderrama, et al. 2007).

The device is relatively expensive, and each implant system requires the respective transducer for Osstell™ and magnetic peg for Osstell Mentor™. The restricted use of the transducer and the magnetic peg is a great disadvantage. Also, evaluation is impossible in a prosthesis state or when the magnetic peg is damaged or when in contact with the soft tissue. Therefore, when using Osstell Mentor™, the Smart peg™ must maintain a distance of approximately 1-3 mm, angle of 90 degrees, and 3 mm above the soft tissue, otherwise the measured value may be affected (Fig. 7). Valderrama et al.(2007) reported in a study experimenting the correlation between Osstell™ and Osstell Mentor™ that the two devices had high significant correlation.

3.4 Influencing factors of Implant Stability Quotient(ISQ)

In many literature, it has been reported that ISQ is affected by implant diameter, surface, form, bone contact ratio, implant site, implant system, surgical procedure, bone quality and bone height (Atsumi, et al. 2007). RFA is determined by the changes in the interface stiffness, and it is affected in three aspects. First, bone-implant surface stiffness affects RFA and it increases through bone healing and remodeling. Secondly, the stiffness of bone itself, and bone density as well as the ratio of cortical and cancellous bone affects RFA. Finally, the stiffness of implant components can acts as a variable and it is affected by the interlocking structures, and the composing elements of the materials. Bone and implant surface stiffness may be affected by using a small-diameter final drill, changes in surgical techniques such as

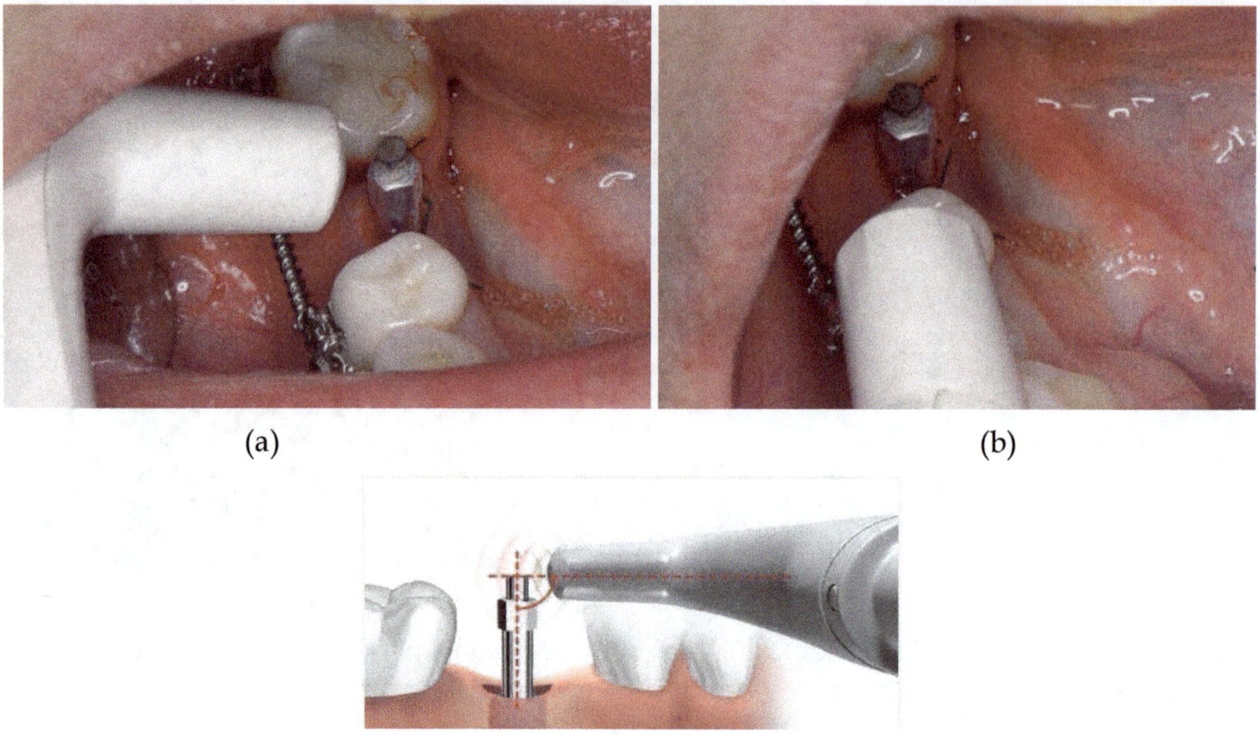

(a) (b) (c)

Fig. 7. Application of magnetic RFA(Osstell™ Mentor) after immediate implant installation. The manufacturer recommends that the probe be held perpendicular to the alveolar crest(a) for the first measurement, and in line with the crest for the other measurement(b). And the Smart peg™ must maintain a distance of approximately 1-3 mm, angle of 90 degrees, and 3 mm above the soft tissue(c).

bone compaction technique, self-tapping design implants and wide tapered implants, but not by implant length. In a histomorphologic study, it was reported that the resonance frequency value is highly correlated with the bone-implant contact amount(Friberg, et al. 1999, Meredith, et al. 1997). There are reports showing a correlation between RFA and the histomorphometric analysis, and other reports claim that the correlation between the bone density and ISQ is not significant. Therefore RFA signifies the bone anchorage of implants but the relation of RFA and bone structure is not yet clear (Alsaadi, et al. 2007, Huwiler, et al. 2007, Rasmusson, et al. 1998, Zhou, et al. 2008). Such diverse results showed RFA value decreases during the first 2 weeks after implant placement, and this change can be related to early bone healing such as biological change and marginal alveolar bone resorption. Bone remodeling reduces primary bone contact and in the early stage after implant placement, the formation of bony callus and increasing lamellar bone in the cortical bone causes major changes in bone density. Thus, in the healing process, primary bone contact decreases and secondary bone contact increases (Barewal, et al. 2003, Zhou, et al. 2008). Also, the 3-dimensional implant-bone contact is displayed 2 dimensionally in the histological sample and BIC has possibility of inaccuracy to signify bone-implant contact (Perrotti, et al. 2010). The relationship of bone structure and RFA is not fully understood. Since primary stability is affected by bone volume or bone trabecula structure as well as cortical bone thickness and density, the effect of bone quality on implant stability cannot be explained by bone microstructure alone (Huwiler, et al. 2007).

4. Which device is more accurate to determine the stability of dental implants - recent literature review

There are two groups of non-invasice devices. One is the RFA analyzer group and the other is the mobility measuring device. The Osstell™ is the commercial name of the RFA analyzer group. This device has a cable which is linked a electronic transducer (Fig. 3). The later version of the Osstell™ is the Ossetell™ mentor which has no cable and uses of magnetic resonance frequency (Fig. 5). Periotest® is the commercial name of the mobility measuring device. Periotest® M is the newer device of the Periotest® and it is a wireless version (Fig. 2).

4.1 PTV and ISQ

Many studies have indicated the presence of correlation between PTVs(the values of Periotest®) and ISQ (the values of Osstell™ and Ossetell™ mentor). However, the correlation of implant stability and each value are still the controversial issue. Aparicio et al. (2006) presentd that the validity and relevance of both ISQ and PTVs for clinical use have to be questioned in their review article. Lachmann et al. (2006) compared Osstell™ and Periotest® by in vitro study and demonstrated that both methods are useful in the evaluation of implant stability but the Osstell™ was more precise than the Periotest® to determine the actual dental implant stability at peri-implant defects. Zix et al. (2008) studied with controlled clinical trial and concluded that Periotest® values appear to be more susceptible to clinical conditions and the Osstell™ instrument seemed to be more precise than the Periotest®. Winter et al.(2010) investigated the correlation between the two devices through the finite element study and demonstrated that Periotest® values had only good correlation with implant stability in case when there's no bone loss. Oh et al.(2009) reported that the Periotest® and Osstell™ Mentor were useful and comparably reliable, showing a strong association with each other in assessing implant stability in their experimental study. In summarizing the literature, it is generally accepted that the RFA is more accurate than the mobility measuring device, but the mobility measuring device is more convenient in clinical usage than RFA (Fig.8).

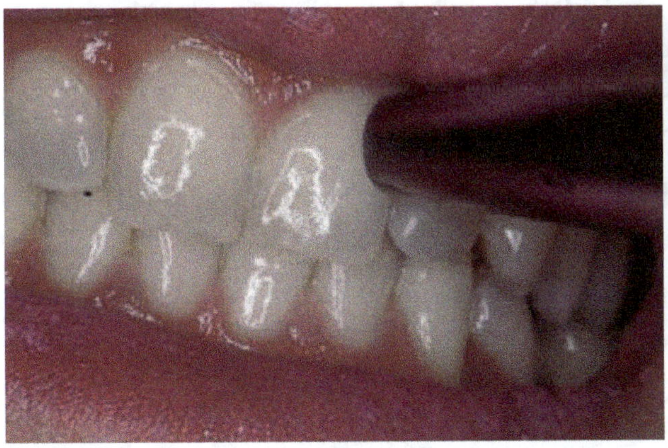

(a)

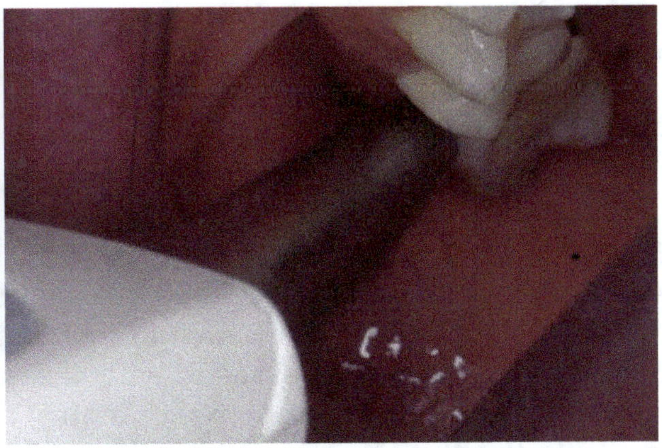

(b)

Fig. 8. Application of Periotest® M. This device can measure the implant stability and mobility of natural teeth without special device, for example magnetic peg. (a) is the application of Periotest® M to natural tooth. (b) is the measurement of implant stability during follow-up period without implant crown removal.

4.2 Electronic resonance frequency and magnetic resonance frequency

Valderrama et al.(2007) performed clinical research using electronic- and magnetic-based devices on 34 non-submerged titanium dental implants in 17 patients and demonstrated that changes in implant stability measured with the magnetic device correlate well with those found with the electronic device. Both devices confirmed the initial decreases in implant stability that occur following placement and identified an increase in stability during the first 6 weeks of functional loading. Tozum et al.(2010) compared three devices which are RF with cable, RF wireless and wireless mobility measureing device using 30 dental implants in human dried cadaveric mandibles. The authors demonstrated that both RF with cable and RF wireless seem to be suitable to detect peri-implant bone loss around implants. But wireless mobility measureing device may not be suitable to detect the 1 mm peri-implant bone changes.

5. ISQ change pattern measured at different direction using magnetic RFA

Data from a conventional piezoelectric RFA are generally obtained with the transducer in the buccolingual position, because the shape of the transducer restricts its orientation when adjacent teeth remain. The measurement of the stiffness of the bone/implant complex in one direction by the use of piezoelectric RFA reflects the stability of an implant only partially, because implant–bone fusion occurs at 360° around a fixture and implant stability is a general reflection of this fusion. According to studies that used piezoelectric RFA, the ISQ of the mesiodistal(MD) measurement was 10 points higher than that of the buccolingual(BL) measurement(Fischer, et al. 2008, Veltri, et al. 2007). Unlike piezoelectric RFA, magnetic RFA(Mentor™: Ostell AB) is recommended to measure two ISQs, using the vibrations that occur in the directions of the higher and lower resonance frequency as a basis(Sennerby & Meredith 2008), because magnetic RFA can provide multi-directional measurements and it is known that the orientation of the transducer (mesiodistal or buccolingual) may affect the measurement of the implant stability quotient (ISQ). If the numerical difference of these two values is more than three ISQ units, both of them are displayed simultaneously. To ensure that both values are measured, the manufacturer of Mentor™ recommends that the probe be held perpendicular to the alveolar crest for one measurement, and in line with the crest for the other measurement. However, it is not known whether the ISQs estimated using Mentor™ vary with the direction of measurement in the same way as estimates measured using piezoelectric RFA. For this reason, the authors performed an randomized clinical trial to determine whether it is necessary to take measurements in both the mesiodistal(MD) and buccolingual(BL) directions in order to assess changes in bone–implant stiffness when such measurements are made using magnetic RFA.

5.1 Study design, methods and materials

A prospective clinical trial was completed, in a total of 53 patients, on 71 non-submerged dental implants that were inserted to replace the unilateral loss of mandibular molars. Two non-submerged implant systems with the same diameter (4.1mm), length (10mm), and collar height (2.8mm) were used in this clinical study. Standard Straumann® Dental Implants (Institut Straumann AG, Basel, Switzerland) were used for 32 of the implants. Osstem SSII Implants (Osstem Implants, Seoul, Republic of Korea) were used for the remaining 39 implants. Mentor™ (Ostell AB, Göteborg, Sweden) was used for to make magnetic RFA measurements. In addition, Type 4 Smartpeg™ (Osstell AB. Göteborg, Sweden) pegs were used during magnetic RFA. The ISQs were measured during the surgical procedure and at 4 and 10 weeks after surgery. Measurements were taken twice in each direction: in the buccolingual direction from the buccal side (BL) and in the mesiodistal direction from the mesial side (MD). The mean of the two measurements in each direction was regarded as the representative ISQ of that direction. The higher and lower values of the buccolingual and mesiodistal ISQs were also classified separately. In other words, the ISQ of each implant was estimated using four measures at each time: the ISQ measured from the direction perpendicular to the alveolar crest on the BL; the ISQ from the direction parallel to the alveolar crest on the MD; the ISQ showing the higher value of the BL and MD (MX); and the ISQ showing the lower value of the BL and MD (MN). Discrepancies in ISQ were calculated by subtracting the BL from the MD in each period. The variation in ISQ was quantified by subtracting the MN from the MX during surgery; it was found to be the same as the absolute value of the ISQ discrepancy. The implants tested were classified into two groups: a group with variation in ISQ of three or more (3+Group) and a group with variation of less than 3 (3-Group).

5.2 Result of the study

During the surgical procedure, the ISQ discrepancies measured from 2 different directions were 0.36 to 1. Ten weeks later, the discrepancies had decreased to -0.14 to 0.42. Eight out of the 53 implants were classified in the 3+Group, accounting for 15.1% of the total(Table 1). The bone width at the insertion area was 6.89mm for the 3+Group and 6mm for the 3-Group (P=0.171). The average age of the 3+Group was 51.88 years, whereas that of the 3-Group was only 47.6 years. However, the difference was not statistically significant (P=0.398).

No differences were found between the BL and MD, but significant differences between MX and MN were observed at every measurement point for each implant system. The average BL during surgery showed a significant difference between the 3+Group and the 3-Group (P=0.002). No significant differences were observed in the MD values (P=0.177). The average MN during surgery showed a significant difference (P<0.001). In contrast, there were no significant differences in the MX values (P=0.417)(Table 2, 3). The ISQs were compared between the 3+Group and the 3-Group to determine whether there was a change in the values over time. A significant difference between the two groups was observed for the MN values (P=0.001). However, no significant differences were found for the MX values between the two groups (P=0.597). With respect to the BL and MD values, a significant difference was found between the two groups only for the BL value (P=0.001 for BL, P=0.392 for MD; Fig. 9).

5.3 Conclusion

The variation in ISQ obtained using magnetic RFA measurements from the two different directions was lower than that reported using piezoelectric RFA. The mean of the discrepancy in ISQ that was calculated from data obtained using magnetic RFA was <1 point. This showed that the discrepancy in ISQ was not skewed to the MD in such an extreme manner as the discrepancy of 10 points found using piezoelectric RFA. With this respect, two- directional measurement is not meaningful. However, our study demonstrated the possibility of observing a different pattern of change between the higher and lower values in a single implant. A significant difference was observed between the 3+Group and the 3-Group in the lower value (MN) of the change in ISQ during the initial healing period. This suggests that a longitudinal comparison of the higher and lower values may improve the evaluation of implant stability, in comparison with the use of a single directional measurement. This suggests that the follow-up observation of scale-based ISQ (lower and higher) values may detect a significant change in the ISQ pattern more readily than the direction-based observations (MD and BL).

Variables	ISQ variation		*P*-value*
	<3	≥3	
Implant based (N=71)			
Implant number	60	11	
Location			1
molar	30	6	
2nd molar	30	5	
Age (mean±SD)	47.00 ± 12.47	53.09 ± 10.27	0.123
Age			
10-50	33	3	0.111
>50	27	8	
Sex			
male	37	7	1
female	23	4	
Smoking			
Yes	26	4	0.75
No	34	7	
Width(mean±SD) †	6.93 ± 2.02	6.09 ± 0.30	0.12
Implant type			
Straumann	27	5	1
SSII	33	6	
Insertion depth (mean±SD) ‡			
Proximal	1.81 ± 0.56	1.85 ± 0.86	0.844
Distal	2.10 ± 0.59	1.91 ± 0.84	0.34
Participant based (N = 53)			
Participant number	45	8	
Location			
molar	20	4	0.771
2nd molar	25	4	
Age (mean±SD)			
Age			
10-50	24	3	0.486
>50	21	5	
Sex			
male	28	6	0.583
female	17	2	
Smoking			
Yes	17	3	0.99
No	28	5	
Width(mean±SD) †	6.89 ± 1.9	6 ± 0	0.171

Implant type			
Straumann	21	4	0.862
SSII	24	4	
Insertion depth (mean±SD) ‡			
Proximal	1.71 ± 0.53	2.03 ± 0.86	0.547
Distal	2.03 ± 0.6	2.13 ± 0.86	0.841

Data unit, except for continuous variables, are presented as the number. The units of age, width, and insertion depth are year, mm, respectively.
**P*-values were calculated by a χ2-test for nominal variables, and Mann-Whitney test for continuous for continuous variables.
†Width was measured in the buccolingual direction using a microcompass, after implant insertion.
‡Insertion depth was checked by measuring the distance between the implant shoulders and the alveolar bone using a UNC periodontal probe.

Table 1. Comparison of demographic data between the two groups of patients with implants showing different levels of implant stability quotient (ISQ) variation during implant surgery (Cited from Park et al, 2010)

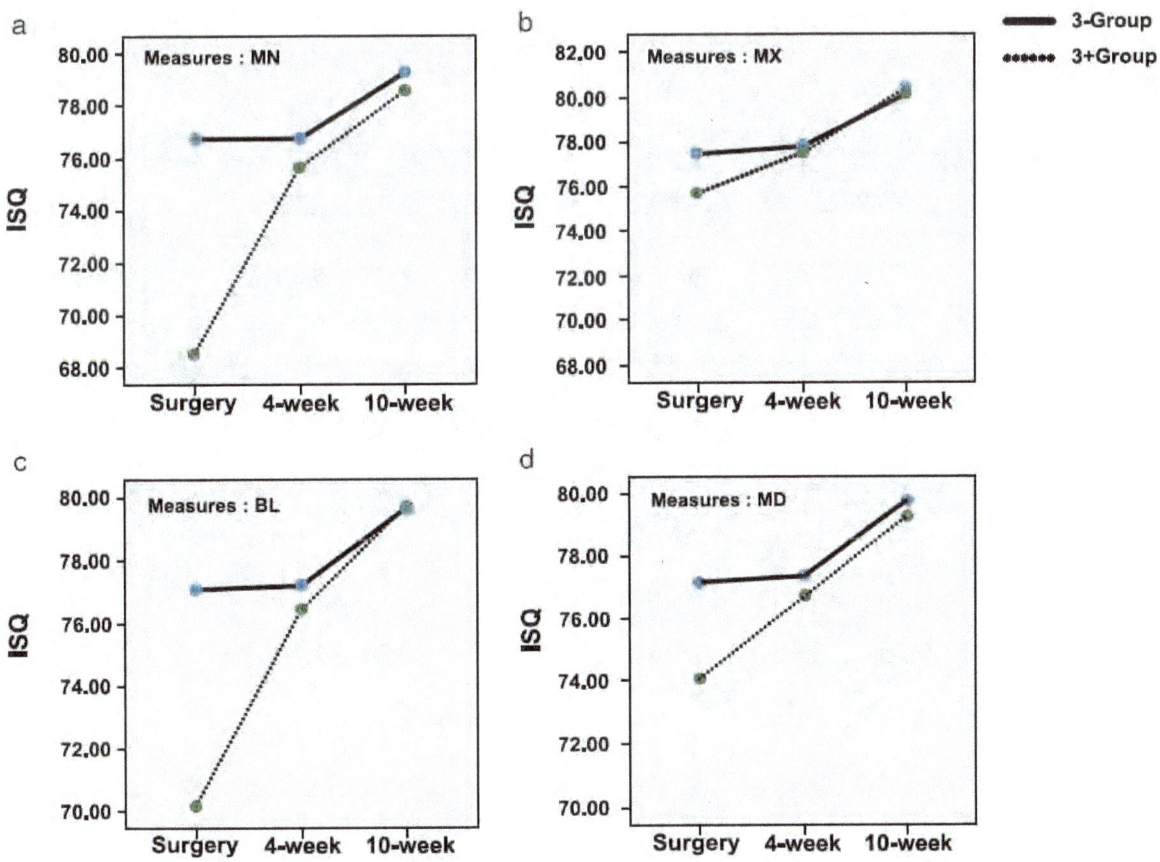

Fig. 9. The comparison of the pattern of change in the implant stability quotient (ISQs) obtained from the four measures from surgery to 10 weeks after surgery. 3+Group=the group with ISQ variation of 3 or more. 3-Group=the group with ISQ variation of < 3. (a) Pattern of change of minimum. (b) Pattern of change of maxilmum. (c)Pattern of change of buccoligual. (d) Pattern of change of mesiodistal.

	ISQ (mean ± SD)		ISQ (mean ± SD)	The difference of the paired data (mean ± SD)	**P**-value *
All implants (N=53)					
During surgery					
BL†	76.01 ± 6.57	MD‡	76.69 ± 6.26	0.71 ± 3.21	0.063
MX§	77.2 ± 6.13	MN‖	75.51 ± 6.6	1.72 ± 2.79	<0.001
At post-operative week 4					
BL	77.09 ± 5.59	MD	77.28 ± 5.58	0.19 ± 1.82	0.469
MX	77.72 ± 5.52	MN	76.3 ± 5.6	1.11 ± 1.46	<0.001
At post-operative week 10					
BL	79.65 ± 3.98	MD	79.69 ±3.97	0.01 ± 1.76	0.671
MX	74.56 ± 6.19	MN	73.04 ± 6.2	1.58 ± 2.47	<0.001
Straumann (N=25)					
During surgery					
BL	73.28 ± 6.38	MD	74.32 ± 6.02	1.10 ± 2.72	0.056
MX	74.56 ± 6.19	MN	73.04 ± 6.2	1.58 ± 2.47	<0.001
At post-operative week 4					
BL	74.8 ± 4.52	MD	75.22 ± 4.28	0.42 ± 1.48	0.199
MX	75.54 ±4.23	MN	74.48 ±4.54	1.06 ± 1.1	<0.001
At post-operative week 10					
BL	78.1 ± 3.65	MD	78.34 ± 3.76	0.24 ± 1.98	0.732
MX	78.78 ± 3.51	MN	77.66 ± 3.8	1.12 ± 1.64	0.001
SSII (N=28)					
During surgery					
BL	78.45 ± 5.82	MD	78.8 ± 5.78	0.36 ± 3.6	0.523
MX	79.55 ± 5.17	MN	77.71 ± 6.24	4.84 ± 3.09	<0.001
At post-operative week 4					

BL	79.14 ± 5.72	MD	79.13 ± 6.02	-0.02 ± 2.07	0.861
MX	79.66 ± 5.86	MN	78.5 ± 5.87	1.16 ± 1.74	0.001
At post-operative week 10					
BL	81.04 ± 3.8	MD	80.89 ± 3.82	-0.14 ± 1.54	0.71
MX	81.43 ± 3.69	MN	80.5 ±3.88	0.93 ± 1.23	0.001

**P*- value was calculated using a Wilcoxon signed ranks test between BL and MD, or between MX and MN
†BL is the ISQ measured from the direction perpendicular to the alveolar crest at the buccal side
‡MD is the ISQ measured from the direction parallel to the alveolar crest at the mesial side
§MX is the ISQ of the direction that showed the higher value between BL and MD
‖MN is the ISQ of the direction which show the lower value between BL and MD

Table 2. Comparison of four different measures of implant stability quotient (ISQ) (Cited from Park et al, 2010)

Period	Mode	ISQ Variation				*P*-value †
		< 3 (N=45)		≥ 3 (N=8)		
		ISQ (mean ± SD)	*P*-value*	ISQ (mean ± SD)	*P*-value*	
All implants (N=53)						
During surgery	BL	77.08 ± 5.97	0.567	70 ± 6.95	0.161	0.002
	MD	77.17 ± 5.8		73.94±8.48		0.177
	MX	77.48 ± 5.85	<0.001	75.56±7.97	0.012	0.417
	MN	76.78 ± 5.9		68.38±6		<0.001
At post-operative week 4	BL	77.23 ± 4.81	0.663	76.31±9.26	0.553	0.650
	MD	77.4 ± 4.95		76.63±8.75		0.722
	MX	77.78 ± 4.86	<0.001	77.38±8.81	0.018	0.862
	MN	76.79 ± 4.87		75.56±9.1		0.551
At post-operative week 10	BL	79.66 ± 3.99	0.471	79.63±4.14	0.553	0.639
	MD	79.78 ± 3.83		79.19±4.93		0.731
	MX	80.16 ± 3.81	<0.001	79.86±3.93	0.018	0.866
	MN	79.28 ± 3.97		78.5±4.8		0.645

**P*- value were calculated using a Wilcoxon signed ranks test between BL and MD, or between MX and MN in each group based on ISQ variation
† *P*- value were calculated using a two-way analysis of variance between the two groups based on ISQ variation.

Table 3. Comparison of four different measures of implant stability quotient (ISQ) between the two implant groups based on the level of ISQ variation during implant surgery (Cited from Park et al, 2010)

6. Acknowledgement

This work was supported by Seoul Research & Business Development (PA100004), granted by Seoul Metropolitan Government, Republic of Korea.

7. References

Albrektsson, T., Zarb, G., Worthington, P. & Eriksson, A. R. (1986) The long-term efficacy of currently used dental implants: A review and proposed criteria of success. *The International journal of oral & maxillofacial implants* 1: 11-25.

Alsaadi, G., Quirynen, M., Michiels, K. & van Steenberghe, D. (2007) A biomechanical assessment of the relation between the oral implant stability at insertion and subjective bone quality assessment. *J Clin Periodontol* 34: 359-366.

Aparicio, C., Lang, N. P. & Rangert, B. (2006) Validity and clinical significance of biomechanical testing of implant/bone interface. *Clinical oral implants research* 17 Suppl 2: 2-7.

Atsumi, M., Park, S. H. & Wang, H. L. (2007) Methods used to assess implant stability: Current status. *The International journal of oral & maxillofacial implants* 22: 743-754.

Barewal, R. M., Oates, T. W., Meredith, N. & Cochran, D. L. (2003) Resonance frequency measurement of implant stability in vivo on implants with a sandblasted and acid-etched surface. *The International journal of oral & maxillofacial implants* 18: 641-651.

Beer, A., Gahleitner, A. & Holm, A. (2003) Correlation of insertion torques with bone mineral density from dental quantitative ct in the mandible. *Clinical oral implants research* 14: 616-620.

Berzins, A., Shah, B., Weinans, H. & Sumner, D. R. (1997) Nondestructive measurements of implant-bone interface shear modulus and effects of implant geometry in pull-out tests. *Journal of biomedical materials research* 34: 337-340.

Bränemark, P., Hansson, B., Adell, R., Breine, U., Lindstrom, J., Hallen, O. & Ohman, A. (1977) Osseointegrated implants in the treatment of the edentulous jaw. Experience from a 10-year period. *Scandinavian journal of plastic and reconstructive surgery. Supplementum* 16: 1-132.

Branemark, R., Ohrnell, L. O., Skalak, R., Carlsson, L. & Bränemark, P. I. (1998) Biomechanical characterization of osseointegration: An experimental in vivo investigation in the beagle dog. *Journal of orthopaedic research : official publication of the Orthopaedic Research Society* 16.

Brunski, J., Puleo, D. & Nanci, A. (2000) Biomaterials and biomechanics of oral and maxillofacial implants: Current status and future developments. *The International journal of oral & maxillofacial implants* 15: 15-46.

Calandriello, R., Tomatis, M. & Rangert, B. (2003) Immediate functional loading of branemark system implants with enhanced initial stability: A prospective 1- to 2-year clinical and radiographic study. *Clinical implant dentistry and related research* 5: 10-20.

Chang, P. C., Lang, N. P. & Giannobile, W. V. (2010) Evaluation of functional dynamics during osseointegration and regeneration associated with oral implants. *Clinical oral implants research* 21: 1-12.

Fischer, K., Stenberg, T., Hedin, M. & Sennerby, L. (2008) Five-year results from a randomized, controlled trial on early and delayed loading of implants supporting full-arch prosthesis in the edentulous maxilla. *Clinical oral implants research* 19: 433-441.

Friberg, B., Sennerby, L., Meredith, N. & Lekholm, U. (1999) A comparison between cutting torque and resonance frequency measurements of maxillary implants. A 20-month clinical study. *International journal of oral and maxillofacial surgery* 28: 297-303.

Huang, H. M., Chiu, C. L., Yeh, C. Y. & Lee, S. Y. (2003) Factors influencing the resonance frequency of dental implants. *Journal of oral and maxillofacial surgery* 61: 1184-1188.

Huang, H. M., Chiu, C. L., Yeh, C. Y., Lin, C. T. & Lee, S. Y. (2003) Early detection of implant healing process using resonance frequency analysis. *Clinical oral implants research* 14: 437-443.

Huwiler, M. A., Pjetursson, B. E., Bosshardt, D. D., Salvi, G. E. & Lang, N. P. (2007) Resonance frequency analysis in relation to jawbone characteristics and during early healing of implant installation. *Clinical oral implants research* 18: 275-280.

Ito, Y., Sato, D., Ito, D., Kondo, H. & Kasugai, S. (2008) Relevance of resonance frequency analysis to evaluate dental implant stability : Simulation and histomorphometrical animal experiments. *Clinical oral implants research* 19: 9-14.

Ivanoff, C. J., Sennerby, L. & Lekholm, U. (1997) Reintegration of mobilized titanium implants. An experimental study in rabbit tibia. *International journal of oral and maxillofacial surgery* 26: 310-315.

Kitsugi, T., Nakamura, T., Oka, M., Yan, W. Q., Goto, T., Shibuya, T., Kokubo, T. & Miyaji, S. (1996) Bone bonding behavior of titanium and its alloys when coated with titanium oxide(tio2) and titanium silicate (ti5si3). *Journal of biomedical materials research* 32: 149-156.

Lachmann, S., Laval, J. Y., Jager, B., Axmann, D., Gomez-Roman, G., Groten, M. & Weber, H. (2006) Resonance frequency analysis and damping capacity assessment. Part 2: Peri-implant bone loss follow-up. An in vitro study with the periotest and osstell instruments. *Clin Oral Implants Res* 17: 80-84.

Lutolf, M. P., Weber, F. E., Schmoekel, H. G., Schense, J. C., Kohler, T., Muller, R. & Hubbell, J. A. (2003) Repair of bone defects using synthetic mimetics of collagenous extracellular matrices. *Nature biotechnology* 21: 513-518.

Meredith, N. (1998) Assessment of implant stability as a prognostic determinant. *The International journal of prosthodontics* 11: 491-501.

Meredith, N., Alleyne, D. & Cawley, P. (1996) Quantitative determination of the stability of the implant-tissue interface using resonance frequency analysis. *Clinical oral implants research* 7: 261-267.

Meredith, N., Book, K., Friberg, B., Jemt, T. & Sennerby, L. (1997) Resonance frequency measurements of implant stability in vivo. A cross-sectional and longitudinal study of resonance frequency measurements on implants in the edentulous and partially dentate maxilla. *Clinical oral implants research* 8: 226-233.

O'Sullivan, D., Sennerby, L., Jagger, D. & Meredith, N. (2004) A comparison of two methods of enhancing implant primary stability. *Clinical implant dentistry and related research* 6: 48-57.

Oh, J.-S., Kim, S.-G., Lim, S.-C. & Ong, J. L. (2009) A comparative study of two noninvasive techniques to evaluate implant stability:Periotest and osstell mentor. *Oral surgery, oral medicine, oral pathology, oral radiology, and endodontics* 107: 513-518.

Park, J.C., Kim, H.D., Kim, S.M., Kim, M.J. & Lee, J.H.(2010) A comparison of implant stability quotients measured using magnetic resonance frequency analysis from two directions: a prospective clinical study during the initial healing period. Clinical oral implants research 21:591-597.

Perrotti, V., Piattelli, A. & Iezzi, G. (2010) Mineralized bone-implant contact and implant stability quotient in 16 human implants retrieved after early healing periods: A histologic and histomorphometric evaluation. *The International journal of oral & maxillofacial implants* 25: 45-48.

Rasmusson, L., Meredith, N., Kahnberg, K. E. & Sennerby, L. (1998) Stability assessments and histology of titanium implants placed simultaneously with autogenous onlay bone in the rabbit tibia. *International journal of oral and maxillofacial surgery* 27: 229-235.

Schulte, W. (1988) The new periotest method. *Compendium (Newtown, Pa.). Supplement*: S410-415, S417.

Sennerby, L. & Meredith, N. (2008) Implant stability measurements using resonance frequency analysis: Biological and biomechanical aspects and clinical implications. *Periodontology 2000* 47: 51-66.

Sennerby, L. & Roos, J. (1998) Surgical determinants of clinical success of osseointegrated oral implants: A review of the literature. *The International journal of prosthodontics* 11: 408-420.

Sullivan, D. Y., Sherwood, R. L., Collins, T. A. & Krogh, P. H. (1996) The reverse-torque test: A clinical report. *The International journal of oral & maxillofacial implants* 11: 179-185.

Tozum, T. F., Bal, B. T., Turkyilmaz, I., Gulay, G. & Tulunoglu, I. (2010) Which device is more accurate to determine the stability/mobility of dental implants? A human cadaver study. *Journal of oral rehabilitation* 37: 217-224.

Valderrama, P., Oates, T. W., Jones, A. A., Simpson, J., Schoolfield, J. D. & Cochran, D. L. (2007) Evaluation of two different resonance frequency devices to detect implant stability: A clinical trial. *Journal of periodontology* 78: 262-272.

Veltri, M., Balleri, P. & Ferrari, M. (2007) Influence of transducer orientation on osstell stability measurements of osseointegrated implants. *Clinical implant dentistry and related research* 9: 60-64.

Winter, W., Mohrle, S., Holst, S. & Karl, M. (2010) Parameters of implant stability measurements based on resonance frequency and damping capacity: A comparative finite element analysis. *The International journal of oral & maxillofacial implants* 25: 532-539.

Zhou, Y., Jiang, T., Qian, M., Wang, J., Shi, B., Xia, H., Cheng, X. & Wang, Y. (2008) Roles of bone scintigraphy and resonance frequency analysis in evaluating osseointegration of endosseous implant. *29* 4: 461-474.

Zix, J., Hug, S., Kessler-Liechti, G. & Mericske-Stern, R. (2008) Measurement of dental implant stability by resonance frequency analysis and damping capacity asessment: Comparison of both techniques in a clinical trial. *The International journal of oral & maxillofacial implants* 23: 525-530.

Permissions

All chapters in this book were first published in IDAREP, by InTech Open; hereby published with permission under the Creative Commons Attribution License or equivalent. Every chapter published in this book has been scrutinized by our experts. Their significance has been extensively debated. The topics covered herein carry significant findings which will fuel the growth of the discipline. They may even be implemented as practical applications or may be referred to as a beginning point for another development.

The contributors of this book come from diverse backgrounds, making this book a truly international effort. This book will bring forth new frontiers with its revolutionizing research information and detailed analysis of the nascent developments around the world.

We would like to thank all the contributing authors for lending their expertise to make the book truly unique. They have played a crucial role in the development of this book. Without their invaluable contributions this book wouldn't have been possible. They have made vital efforts to compile up to date information on the varied aspects of this subject to make this book a valuable addition to the collection of many professionals and students.

This book was conceptualized with the vision of imparting up-to-date information and advanced data in this field. To ensure the same, a matchless editorial board was set up. Every individual on the board went through rigorous rounds of assessment to prove their worth. After which they invested a large part of their time researching and compiling the most relevant data for our readers.

The editorial board has been involved in producing this book since its inception. They have spent rigorous hours researching and exploring the diverse topics which have resulted in the successful publishing of this book. They have passed on their knowledge of decades through this book. To expedite this challenging task, the publisher supported the team at every step. A small team of assistant editors was also appointed to further simplify the editing procedure and attain best results for the readers.

Apart from the editorial board, the designing team has also invested a significant amount of their time in understanding the subject and creating the most relevant covers. They scrutinized every image to scout for the most suitable representation of the subject and create an appropriate cover for the book.

The publishing team has been an ardent support to the editorial, designing and production team. Their endless efforts to recruit the best for this project, has resulted in the accomplishment of this book. They are a veteran in the field of academics and their pool of knowledge is as vast as their experience in printing. Their expertise and guidance has proved useful at every step. Their uncompromising quality standards have made this book an exceptional effort. Their encouragement from time to time has been an inspiration for everyone.

The publisher and the editorial board hope that this book will prove to be a valuable piece of knowledge for researchers, students, practitioners and scholars across the globe.

List of Contributors

Tatsuo Shirota, Masashi Hatori, Masanori Nakamura and Satoru Shintani
Showa University, Japan

Atsushi Nakamura
Yamato Tokushukai Hospital, Japan

Yoshiro Matsui
Kagawa University, Japan

S. Anil
Department of Periodontics and Community Dentistry, College of Dentistry, King Saud University, Riyadh, Saudi Arabia
Dental Implant and Osseointegration Research Chair, King Saud University, Riyadh, Saudi Arabia

P.S. Anand
People's College of Dental Sciences & Research Centre, Bhanpur, Bhopal, Madhya Pradesh, India

H. Alghamdi and J.A. Jansen
Radboud University Nijmegen Medical Center, HB Nijmegen, The Netherlands
Dental Implant and Osseointegration Research Chair, King Saud University, Riyadh, Saudi Arabia

Umit Karacayli
Department of Oral and Maxillofacial Surgery, Gulhane School of Medicine, Ankara

Nuket Mas
Department of Anatomy, Faculty of Medicine, Afyon Kocatepe University, Afyonkarahisar Turkey

Su-Gwan Kim
Dept. of Oral and Maxillofacial Surgery, School of Dentistry, Chosun University Republic of Korea

José Mauricio dos Santos Nunes Reis, Lígia Antunes Pereira Pinelli, Nicolau Conte Neto, Marcelo Silva Monnazzi and José Cláudio Martins Segalla
UNESP - Univ Estadual Paulista / Araraquara Dental School Brazil

Samira Faegh, Hsuan-Yu Chou and Sinan Müftü
Northeastern University, Department of Mechanical Engineering Boston, Massachusetts USA

Laurence Evrard
Stomatology and Maxillo-facial Surgery Department Hopital Erasme - ULB Brussels Belgium

Ahmed M. Ballo, Omar Omar and Anders Palmquist
Department of Biomaterials, Institute of Clinical Sciences, The Sahlgrenska Academy, University of Gothenburg
Biomatcell VINN Excellent Center of Biomaterials and Cell Therapy, Gothenburg

Wei Xia
Biomatcell VINN Excellent Center of Biomaterials and Cell Therapy, Gothenburg
Angstrom Laboratory, Department of Engineering Sciences, Uppsala University, Uppsala, Sweden

Lucian Toma Ciocan and Ion Patrascu
"Carol Davila" Medicine and Pharmacy University

Florin Miculescu and Marian Miculescu
University "Politehnica" Bucharest Romania

Jong-Chul Park, Jung-Woo Lee, Soung-Min Kim and Jong-Ho Lee
Department of Oral and Maxillofacial Surgery, School of Dentistry, Seoul National University, Seoul, Korea

Index

www.ingramcontent.com/pod-product-compliance
Lightning Source LLC
LaVergne TN
LVHW081021210926
848485LV00004B/917

Ghost Words and Invisible Giants

H.D., Djuna Barnes, and the Language of Suffering

Lheisa Dustin

FAIRLEIGH DICKINSON UNIVERSITY PRESS
Vancouver • Madison • Teaneck • Wroxton

Published by Fairleigh Dickinson University Press
Copublished by The Rowman & Littlefield Publishing Group, Inc.
4501 Forbes Boulevard, Suite 200, Lanham, Maryland 20706
www.rowman.com

6 Tinworth Street, London SE11 5AL, United Kingdom

Fairleigh Dickinson University Press gratefully acknowledges the support received for scholarly publishing from the Friends of FDU Press.

British Library Cataloguing in Publication Information Available

Library of Congress Cataloging-in-Publication Data

Names: Dustin, Lheisa, 1973- author.
Title: Ghost words and invisible giants : H.D., Djuna Barnes, and the language of suffering / Lheisa Dustin.
Description: Vancouver ; Madison : Fairleigh Dickinson University Press ; Lanham, Maryland : The Rowman & Littlefield Publishing Group, Inc., [2021] | Includes bibliographical references and index. | Summary: "Lheisa Dustin describes "language of suffering" of iconic modernist authors H.D. and Djuna Barnes, tracing psychic splitting and virulent thought patterns in their creative works. She argues that this language, where word and meaning are disconnected, signals breaks in consciousness haunted by spectral objects of fear and desire"—Provided by publisher.
Identifiers: LCCN 2021009756 (print) | LCCN 2021009757 (ebook) | ISBN 9781683932307 (cloth) | ISBN 9781683932314 (epub)
Subjects: LCSH: H. D. (Hilda Doolittle), 1886-1961—Criticism and interpretation. | H. D. (Hilda Doolittle), 1886-1961—Language. | Barnes, Djuna—Criticism and interpretation. | Barnes, Djuna—Language. | Suffering in literature. | Psychoanalysis and literature. | Modernism (Literature)—United States.
Classification: LCC PS3507.O726 Z625 2021 (print) | LCC PS3507.O726 (ebook) | DDC 811/.52—dc23
LC record available at https://lccn.loc.gov/2021009756
LC ebook record available at https://lccn.loc.gov/2021009757

For my mother

Contents

Acknowledgments

My gratitude to Abdul Gabbar Al Sharafi of Sultan Qaboos University for supporting my research leave to finish this book; to the University of Delaware Special Collections librarians, for sending a copy of Barnes's 1934-5 correspondence with Emily Holmes Coleman all the way to Dubai; to Lonnie Weatherby from the McGill University library, who helped me find and hold on to the books I needed; to Stephen Ross, University of Victoria, who first got me thinking about psychoanalysis and spectrality; to Andre Furlani and Manish Sharma, for inviting me back to Concordia University's English department as a visiting researcher; to Chris Fox, for her excellent feedback and encouragement; to Adrian Williams, for his beautiful cover art; to James Gifford and Zachary Nycum, for their editorial savvy; to Moishe Dolman, for his moral support; to Mu Soeng, for guiding me to the passages I needed in Buddhist and Hindu scriptures; to Alain and Rachel Lepine, Chokyi Nyima Rinpoche, Sister Chân Không, Andrew Harvey, David Loy, Adyashanti, and Ajahn Sucitto, for inspiration. Most of all, thank you to Luke Carson for your ongoing generosity, responsiveness, and wisdom.

Introduction

I. THOUGHT PATTERNS, PSYCHIC STRUCTURES, ONENESS

The language of suffering, as I render it through psychoanalytic linguistic theory, is language in which there is a more than usual disconnect between the sounds and images of words (signifiers), and their meanings (signifieds). Such language has a spectral quality and may take many forms, sometimes simultaneously, manifesting as words that have lost their meanings, but still whirl and repeat, as if searching for links to these lost meanings. These words occur in speech, writing, and thought, which when closely examined, also consist of distinct words. The language of suffering haunts our conscious or pre-conscious minds and manifests in our speech and writing as enigmatic formal characteristics that suggest fragmentation, or as repeating words and phrases, or as strangely complex and unending articulations. It may for some of us come with a sense that someone else may understand it better than we do, or even that it comes from a source outside ourselves, though this source may not be apparent to other people. I use "invisible giants" to refer to a subject's sense of an outside agent who may understand the meaning of, or is the source of, their words and thoughts and the imperative charge they carry. With "ghost words," I refer to words whose real meanings are shameful or unacceptable to the subject who holds them. These ghost words are presented to the world as having other, innocuous meanings, but they tend to repeat insistently, as if they could by repetition completely express the meanings they encrypt. The language of suffering may appear as thoughts and phrases whose meanings we already know, but that are no longer vivid or connected to any ongoing experience; they have a dead but compelling quality. Though these words and thoughts usually do not refer to a present situation, they call up habituated affective charges, trauma responses, and preoccupations and behaviors that are not optimal for the wellbeing of the subjects they haunt.

This book traces the ways that the language of suffering appears in works by modernist American writers Djuna Barnes (1892–1982) and H.D. (Hilda Doolittle, 1886–1961), who also identifies by her spiritual and pen name Delia Alton in some texts. Though many factors contribute to Barnes's and

H.D.'s writing styles, I focus on the connections of the disconnected and repetitive articulations in their work to personal suffering and confusion. I also suggest possible correlations of such language to unusual object relations in their lives, relational patterns that may contribute to their characteristic textual patterns. My interest is in exploring the psychic terrain in which words unconsciously or half-consciously mingle with perceptions and actions—and take forms that may be agonizing as well as beneficial, stabilizing, or creative. For Barnes and H.D., I argue, the repetitive patterns that appear in their work shore up a more consistent sense of selfhood, but also create suffering.

H.D.'s and Barnes's writings suggest unusual complications in their sense of difference from others. In a seeming paradox, the experience of difference from others, which generally enables individuation, seems to turn inside out for them. Instead of being a positive source of definition, difference instead becomes the impetus for a harrowing and traumatic union with the perceived other or others. I speculate that oneness, in its sense as differentiation, reverses into oneness as non-differentiation for H.D. and Barnes because their sense of difference may have been less than normally established in early life—though H.D. also intentionally cultivated unbounded states when she became interested in spiritualism and occultism, and Barnes describes them as central to her creative process. In any case, porous psychic boundaries in adulthood, though contributing to their innovative poetics, also made them more vulnerable to others who came to represent for them a negation, boundary, or difference. These tenuous boundaries may also correlate to a difficulty in disidentifying with their thoughts: that is, recognizing thoughts as only thoughts and not necessarily authoritative—especially when these thoughts pertain to the others who represented difference. Thus, the feedback loops of re-articulation that appear in H.D.'s and Barnes's creative works reflect and reinforce habitual patterns of affect, but may also circumvent direct encounters with both lack and lack's flip side, oneness, by recasting this paradoxical lack/oneness as an external event or relationship, which it calls up in indirect, dramatic form (for Barnes) or which it seeks to relate to all other signifiers (for H.D.). This externalization of lack/oneness, and the proliferation of disconnected thoughts pertaining to it, replaces the nonreferential awareness of lack or oneness that comes with a hiatus in thought. H.D. imagines the language of suffering to have potential meanings, not yet signified but perhaps known to enigmatic deities—invisible giants—that may in the future grant clarity, completion, and individuation to the seeker who follows her thoughts. For Barnes, ghost words, words whose meanings are disavowed, do not promise anything, but may enable a sense of individuation that requires repetition to be maintained.

I draw most on psychoanalyst Jacques Lacan's (1901–1981) conceptual framework to study the language of suffering because Lacanian theory opens out into, and I think contributes to, contemporary discussions of consciousness. Though Lacan's work has been criticized in feminist, queer, and poststructuralist discourses, it is also true that radical interventions in the discourses of mental health—critical psychiatry,[1] anti-psychiatry,[2] postpsychiatry,[3] the mad pride movement,[4] and disability studies[5] – claim Lacan as an intellectual precursor who energetically defended the truth-value of so-called psychotics' testimonies from the invalidation of psychiatric approaches.[6] They point out that unlike his contemporaries, Lacan takes his ideas about what psychotics are experiencing from what they are actually saying, and that he destigmatizes their suffering by ascribing it, like everyone else's, to early family dynamics and circumstantial triggers rather than to organic pathology.

Lacan further suggests that so-called psychotics are not the only deluded ones, arguing instead that their delusions evidence a different relationship to language, the social order, and the unconscious than the delusions that most people share—for instance, the delusion of freedom and autonomy. In Lacan's terminology, every psyche has a structure either neurotic, perverse, or psychotic. The perverse and psychotic discourses of capture by another appear to Lacan to pertain to the actual state of the modern subject's capture and occupation by the "big Other" (*l'Autre*): the forces of language, the social order, and the unconscious that constitute and propel all of us in one way or another.[7] So-called neurotics hold a delusion of personal freedom in relationship to Lacan's big Other,[8] although, as Lacan suggests in later theory, the reality of an Other who guarantees meaning is part of their delusion. On the other hand, so-called psychotics directly experience their subjugation, but perceive it as subjugation not by the big Other but by "small," particular persecuting others: for instance God, or the Devil, or the CIA.[9] So-called perverts imagine themselves in somewhat more socially credible ways as the instrument of the other's enjoyment—where the other is envisioned paradoxically as both big and small—and sometimes stage this in sadomasochism, or as social theorist Slavoj Žižek (b. 1949) first elaborated, collectively in totalitarianism.[10]

The signifier of One, Lacan writes, is the signifier of difference that is foreclosed and denied in so-called psychotic and perverse psychic structures.[11] Thus, its appearance in personal relationships is perceived as threatening and traumatic, as the "ferocious *jouissance* [enjoyment]" of the other.[12] The signifier of oneness as singularity and autonomy here heralds anxiety regarding a perceived threat to autonomy. In Lacan's terminology, the other who first represents the subject's lack and thereby inaugurates subjectivity—the father figure—shifts into the other who represents inundating unity and threatens subjectivity—the mother figure.[13]

My idea of oneness as non-differentiation differs from Lacan's descriptions in that direct awareness of it could also be positive, as in what are called mystical or transcendent experiences. I speculate, however, that this direct awareness may come with particular hurdles for subjects who did not at any time form strong psychic boundaries. Perhaps, as some teachers and theorists of meditation and mindfulness suggest, many or all subjects who experience the dissolution of psychic boundaries through these practices experience similar hurdles at times.[14] I speculate that a subject's habitual sense of oneness as personal separateness—the assimilation of what Lacan calls the signifier One, or the "One-father" (*Un-père*) – may ease the threat of experiences of oneness as dissolution, or non-differentiation.[15] On the other hand, these experiences may be harrowing at times for anyone, since the sense of bounded selfhood may be altered or destroyed, and the unconscious forces that it kept at bay may appear to close in.

Lacan suggests, as do psychoanalyst collaborators Nicolas Abraham (1919–1975) and Maria Torok (1925–1998), that our ways of negating the sense of wrongness and lack that we all experience shape our perception of the relation between language and meaning—and thus structure the way we think, speak and write. This sense that something is wrong and lacking, and should or must be different, is sometimes called the imperative. For Lacan it is instilled in a child by its initial encounter with a father figure that represents a boundary between the child and the mother, or primary caregiver, and thus both mother's and child's lack as such. In Lacan's view, the sense of subjugation to an order and an imperative comes not necessarily from the actual father, but from the object, identified with the name or "no" of the father, that first draws the mother's desire away from the child and bars their union.[16] The child hereafter knows absence and difference, and thus understands how a sound (or later, an image) can stand for something not present. This encounter thus inaugurates the initial split, for the child, between signifiers (sounds or images) and signifieds (concepts), and precedes the child's first words. Often this is the word for "mother," an evocation of the primary caregiver who is no longer experienced as fully present, and who thereby becomes the first object of desire.[17] The child now unconsciously internalizes language as a synchronic system in which words take their meanings through their difference from other words.[18] It enters what Lacan calls the symbolic order: the order of set limits, shared language and meanings, and differing perspectives, that governs social relationships and structures.[19] This is, at least, how neurotic subjects develop.

In H.D.'s and Barnes's work, however, father figures suddenly appear as invasive and inundating. Barnes's and H.D.'s repeated literary enactments of the lack and difference imposed by the father figure seem to reverse, becoming union or non-differentiation from the (m)other figure's ferocious *jouissance*: an excessive, intolerable pleasure that straddles the threshold into pain.[20] An encounter with difference and lack, which Lacan calls castration, is perhaps not assimilated, but rather externalized in what Lacan calls the imaginary register as a personalized other who dominates or threatens the subject's very identity.

Since the parental (for Lacan, paternal) imperative is already a negation, an initial childhood apprehension of loss and limitation, "denegation" (*dénégation*) denotes the psychic negation of negation. Here, a particular pattern of thinking and relating ongoingly pushes away, by repressing or externalizing, the subject's sense of something lacking. I follow Lacan and Abraham and Torok in arguing that our patterns of negating this sense of lack also appear in our subsequent relations to love objects and parent figures, and in the way we connect language to meaning. I trace particular patterns in H.D. and Barnes's creative work, where the relationships of language to meaning, agency to authority, and the protagonist to the supernatural or divine, follow characteristic patterns.

The symmetry in these sets of imagined relations suggests a resonance among the fraught family dynamics depicted in their work and letters, their habitual responses to parent figures and love objects, and the ways that they use language to evoke meaning. Extreme devastation, whirling ghost words, and invisible giants follow in textual wakes when loved and parental others betray trust or withhold love, interest, engagement. Although most people respond to such situations with grief, endless interpretive replays of the rejection or betrayal, and even a sense of disconnectedness from the world, I suggest that the thought patterns that appear in H.D's and Barnes's work in response to such losses are particularly persistent. This may be because the thoughts also serve to hold back the shattering experience of personal negation attendant on this loss or lack—its shift into the sense of obliterating non-differentiation from another or from others. Indeed, the thought patterns may represent traumatic experience (of separation that is also annihilating union) in repetitive ways in part to achieve, through repetition, a semblance of difference and distinct identity.

For Lacan the first encounter with the imperative, which signifies difference and lack, normally places the subject in the symbolic order that governs language and meaning. Within this order words take meaning through their differentiation from other words and can thus indicate distinct concepts in thought, speech and writing. Correlatively, the subject takes their sense of identity through their perceived difference from others and their uncertainty regarding what others desire. In Lacan's theory, neurotic subjects are most individuated: they most apprehend their mother's lack and desire and their own inability to completely fulfill her, which implies their own lack and desire.[21] In 1960, Lacan describes the initial question that structures the subject as "*Chè Vuoi?*": "What do you want?" This question follows the recognition that there is something that the (m)Other lacks and desires, and that the subject too must lack something, since they cannot completely fulfill the mother. Neurotic subjects enter into symbolic language, or it enters into them, when this lack and difference are unconsciously internalized, or repressed.

However, instead of repressing it, the subject may negate the imperative through disavowal or foreclosure, and thus understand language differently. In Lacan's rather bleak tripartite model of psychic structures, the neurotic or castrated subject represses this encounter with the imperative, which the perverse subject disavows, or denies, and the psychotic subject forecloses, or excises as though it had never occurred.[22] Foreclosure, which conditions the psychotic subjective structure, is a mode of thought and language that does not reliably differentiate words, thoughts, and people from one another. Thus, the psychotic delusion involves asymbolic words whose meaning "essentially refers to nothing but itself" and therefore "can't be exhausted by reference to another meaning," as normally happens in the process of signification.[23]

Lacan insists that a subject's speech and writing negate unacceptable meanings and ideas in different ways according to their own mode of negating lack.[24] Unlike neurotic subjects, whose communications show the ability to clearly distinguish signs from one another, perverse or psychotic subjects, for whom the mother figure's demand (for the subject) is not checked by a father figure who recasts her demand as desire, show more difficulty in distinguishing one sign from another, and self from others. Their communications are dominated by speech in the imaginary, not the symbolic, register.

H.D.'s and Barnes's relationships to their senses of difference can be read in their writing and personal lives as perpetuating their suffering as well as igniting their creativity. In Lacan's terminology, the symbolic castration that inaugurates difference is not fully experienced but returns in "the real," as a repeating traumatic event in life and art, where it manifests itself in a beloved other's perceived or real violence, betrayal, and/or abandonment. In H.D.'s and Barnes's work the lack of lack spawns repeating patterned cycles in which lack is violently or cruelly thrust upon female protagonists—and then worse, withdrawn. The horror of scenes that stage castration, though hardly bearable, is still imagined as a better alternative than the meltdown into unboundedness that each writer portrays with both fear and longing. However, what Lacan calls castration (oneness as singularity and lack) and castration's reversal (oneness as non-differentiation or unboundedness) are by a strange logic one and the same; at least they are not reliably different. Their indistinguishability demands the restaging of castration-union in order to maintain a sense of difference. Correlative to these dramatic cycles in H.D.'s and Barnes's oeuvres is the disconnection between signifier and signified in the language that composes the literary work, and the looping recurrence of ghostly signifying chains within it. Thus, the attacks and betrayals by loved others depicted in these works, that seemingly drive their narratives and shape and define their characters, also occasion the characters' and narrators' seemingly compulsive citation of these traumatic events and others. These depictions call into question simple divisions between interiority and exteriority, agency and conditioning, in considering traumatized subjectivity. If conscious or unconscious memories of others constitute us, where is the distinction between self and other? What remains of us if we forget—or if we remember?

I read Barnes's and H.D.'s creative indeterminacy in light of their familial and romantic histories and their broader social visions and involvements or noninvolvement (for instance, H.D.'s occult practices and psychoanalytic sessions, Barnes's fascination with spectacle and physical exhibition, followed by her later reclusion). I seek to delineate the different modes of splitting, separateness, and oneness that appear in their work, and suggest the internalized negations that may give rise to them. Psychoanalytic theory that addresses the effects of object relations on signification allows me to read how the psychic movements in these works, the views of temporality, the supernatural, and relationship itself depicted in them, may mirror the relation between signifier and signified implied by their styles and contents.

II. SELF-AWARENESS AND PATHOLOGY: FRAMES OF REFERENCE

Lacan writes in 1953–1954 that the imperative "is consonant with the register and the idea of the law, that is to say with the totality of the system of language." However, the imperative that sets the law in place is also "the destruction of the law"[25]:

> One should also emphasize . . . its senseless, blind character, of pure imperativeness and simple tyranny . . . the law is entirely reduced to something, which cannot even be expressed, like the '*You must*,' which is speech deprived of all its meaning. It is in this sense that it ends up being identified with whatever is most devastating, most fascinating, in the primitive experiences of the subject. It ends up being identified with what I call the *ferocious figure*, with the figures that we can link to primitive traumas the child has suffered, whatever these are.[26]

The imperative—for Lacan instilled in the child by the father figure—may be repressed, disavowed, or foreclosed. In the latter two reactions, it is less integrated into the subject as a social order including language, and more projected onto the outside world as the malignant, encroaching, or controlling intentions of real or imagined others toward the subject.

I use psychoanalyst Melanie Klein's (1882–1960) theory alongside Lacan's to give my work on subjectivity some independence from the father figure, and because Klein's more evidently process-oriented accounts of the lifelong dynamics of splitting, projection, and incorporation invite open-ended readings of H.D.'s and Barnes's writing patterns. Imperatives appear in Klein's writing as projections that stem more from an infant's innate anxiety than from internalized encounters with others. For Klein they develop in two ways: first from destructive and controlling impulses toward an other arising from the infant's own death instinct, which it projects onto the other as the other's persecutory intention toward it, and later as fear that the other has been harmed by these impulses and desire to make reparation.[27] Klein uses the terms "persecutory anxiety" and "depressive anxiety," respectively, to describe the functioning of imperatives.

The persecutory anxiety of early infancy gives rise to primary defense mechanisms, splitting and projection, by which the infant diffuses the anxiety generated by its own destructive impulses. This phase, which Klein calls the "paranoid-schizoid position," is characterized by the splitting of both self and others into good and bad part-objects and the projection of aggressive and controlling impulses onto the bad parts.[28] In the paranoid-schizoid position, impulses to control or destroy early "bad objects" (e.g., the breast, the penis) are projected by the infant and later the adult subject onto the bad objects, and experienced as the persecutory or dominating intentions of others toward the subject. Primarily paranoid-schizoid subjects consistently mistake their own violent impulses for the violent intentions directed at them by others.[29] While it may alleviate primordial anxiety, however, this splitting of external objects into good and bad also fragments the ego, thoughts, feelings and relationships.[30]

In the next stage, which Klein terms the "depressive position," the infant begins to fear that its violent fantasies have harmed its objects and to wish to repair this damage. It moves from splitting and projection to a reverse movement, a melancholic incorporation of others and identification with them. In the depressive position, the split between good and bad objects is to a greater or lesser extent repaired. Good and bad part-objects knit together somewhat within the subject's ego to form whole objects.

For Klein, paranoid and schizophrenic processes in adulthood proceed from the incomplete transition from the paranoid-schizoid position to the depressive position in infancy. This uncompleted transition inhibits normal development throughout life, which Klein describes bleakly as an unending oscillation between the paranoid-schizoid position, in which subjects manage overwhelming anxieties with splitting and projection, and the depressive position, in which they remorsefully incorporate and integrate their damaged part-objects. Painful as this appears, Klein's alternative is even worse. If a subject's persecutory anxiety is too strong, external objects appear too threatening and their incorporation is imagined, not as repairing damaged objects, but as being "forcefully entered" and "ruled" by malignant objects.[31] This inability to internalize objects in a reparative way gives rise to excessive and rapid processes of psychic fragmentation.[32] Because the internalization of external objects is experienced as an attack, the depressive position too quickly reverts to the paranoid-schizoid position—to further splitting and projection. In this way, a "vicious circle" is created where the imperative toward control and destruction sabotages the imperative toward reparation and integration, and integration reverses into fragmentation.[33]

I want to make it clear here that my use of psychoanalytic theory does not imply my agreement with the stigmatization of subjects that sometimes accompanies it. Instead, contemporary contemplative practice and theory also influence my analysis of the language of suffering in H.D.'s and Barnes's literary work. These frames of reference may seem surprisingly disparate. However, in different ways Lacan, Abraham and Torok, and Klein all describe models of negation of variously imagined imperatives that resonate for me with Buddhist and *advaitic,* or non-dual, analyses of mind and meditative practices. A correlative to the processes theorized in psychoanalytic literature, where traumatic content is often understood to pattern and drive thought, can for me be found in popular texts by and for contemporary practitioners of formal meditation, where such drives and thought patterns are ascribed to everyone. When engaged in intensive practice meant, in the terminology of many modern teachers, to heal the psyche by making unconscious content conscious,[34] meditators often report the onslaught of repetitive, sometimes trivial and sometimes terrifying thoughts, and experiences of the dissolution or groundlessness of self that can leave them shaken as well as liberated. Some contemplative teachers and scriptures suggest that these thought onslaughts inevitably attend the meditative contemplation of dissolution.[35] Likewise, contemporary advaitic meditation teacher Adyashanti (b. 1954) describes the arising of powerful thought forms as attendant on what he calls *awakening*, where it is revealed that we are not separate but rather "that which manifests as all things, as all experiences, as all personalities."[36] Writes Adyashanti,

> Part of what happens when we awaken is that the top gets ripped off our ability to suppress, and we find it very hard to hold anything at bay. In the aftermath of an awakening, some very powerful thought forms may arise—things we pushed down very deeply, that we tried very hard to keep unconscious.[37]

Although experiences of dissolution would at first glance seem the opposite of identity with everything, Buddhist historian and philosopher David Loy (b. 1947) speculates that these may be simply two ways, developed and elaborated in various contemplative traditions, of languaging the experience of nonduality.[38] In my reading, Barnes and H.D.'s work, and Lacan's theory, also suggest that subjective dissolution and nondifferentiation may be profoundly interconnected experiences.

My attempt to map common ground between psychoanalytic and religious discourses has precedents. Modern and contemporary contemplative or spiritual discourses often use psychoanalytic terminology to describe unusual experiences, such as dissolution of "the ego" into nothingness or mystical union, or the surfacing of "unconscious" thought patterns into "the conscious mind" as a result of meditation.[39] *Trauma*, too, has become a household word in contemporary Buddhist discourse, where it is understood as common, if not universal.[40] More obscure psychoanalytic terms can also be read in this cross-disciplinary, cross-cultural spirit as perhaps describing common processes, since psychic fragmentation and looping by means of thought and language can presumably occur in anyone who uses language, whether these are called negation (Lacan), suppression (Adyashanti), or repression, disavowal, or foreclosure (Sigmund Freud, 1856–1939). Hence I borrow Freud's and Lacan's terms "disavowal" and "foreclosure," Abraham and Torok's "cryptophoria" and "psychic crypt," and Klein's still popular "splitting" and "projection" to detail the patterns that appear in Barnes's and H.D.'s writing and ways of relating to others, focusing on literary language that correlates to specific patterns and processes of managing what appears as unbearable to them. Yet I wish these patterns to be understood as fluid, contingent, and broadly relevant.

Language, such as that in this book, can only roughly approximate its source and flow in, and among, subjects. The pattern is new at every moment, and the fixed structures that mid-twentieth-century psychoanalysis describes strain to hold the more fluid, data-driven, and/or context-oriented formations in contemporary relational models like attachment theory, relevance realization theory, and speculative realism.[41] Yet I believe that it can find ways to communicate with varied disciplines such as psychology and psychiatry, mindfulness studies, cognitive science, neuroscience, linguistics, and cultural and religious studies, all of which are joining in conversations about consciousness, thought and feeling patterns, and personal agency. Psychoanalysis, seeking the places where language encounters awareness, can contribute to these inquiries while opening to their emphasis on process and contingency. The thought patterns I read as imbricated in suffering may also be seen in terms of transpersonal states and creative experimentation, as shaping our creativity, impinging on what we believe to be true, and influencing how we relate to others. They may be seen as exemplary of the kinds of split subjectivity that appear in modernity's and postmodernity's texts generally, whether religious, contemplative, literary, critical, confessional, scientific, or propagandizing. The language of suffering, and the indeterminacies it frames, may be received as literary or as mad, or in other, less value-fraught ways. My reading of the psychic structures suggested by H.D.'s and Barnes's work explores how certain habits of pushing away difference (the foundation of conceptual understanding) can shape texts and lives, but let me be clear: this inquiry neither pathologizes nor celebrates Barnes and H.D., even if it is tempting to think in these terms.

To me the imperative, as a sense that something is wrong or lacking which our thought and communication works to manage or negate, might come from an early parent figure or configuration of object relations—or from something else. While painful encounters with subsequent parent figures and love objects have been found to trigger effects in a subject's language and consciousness, I offer early parent figures as playing a limited role in the psychic patterns that much psychoanalysis sources in them. I use Lacan's, Klein's, and Abraham and Torok's theories to describe "disorders" (i.e., types of thought and language that psychoanalysis implicates in interminable human suffering) and a correspondence between H.D.'s and Barnes's modes of asymbolism and their ways of suffering. However, I do not imagine that all experiences that align with asymbolic language must involve suffering, that all language with a rift between signifier and signified must be language of suffering, or that Barnes and H.D. do not intentionally use asymbolism to disrupt, affirm, and otherwise comment on society, language, and life.

The terrible history of the mental health industry, and the history of H.D. and Barnes studies, where these authors were painstakingly reclaimed from obscurity into today's literary canons, weigh on discussions of pathologization in literary studies today, and on this book. Pathologization is often considered synonymous with dehumanization, invalidation, and social othering, a destruction of physical and mental autonomy. Daniel Paul Schreber (1842–1911), author of *Memoirs of My Nervous Illness*[42] and the subject of Freud's only extended investigation of psychosis as well as Lacan's, and Gilles Deleuze (1925–1995) and Félix Guattari's (1930–1992) famous studies of psychosis—though none of them ever met Schreber—called this destruction of autonomy *soul murder* (*Seelenmord*).[43] The argument that another person is behaving or thinking in a way that causes them confusion and suffering when they may not self-identify as doing so, especially when they are not there to speak for themselves, must be made carefully. However, I believe that it is important that this argument be possible in literary studies, and that it does not invalidate the person or their work. The current depathologizing trajectory in literary criticism, when it involves a sole focus on the empowering or anti-patriarchal effects of psychic processes such as trauma or schizophrenia, which involves great anguish for many people, comes with its own problems, creating strange aporias and closing off fields of study, and individual voices, that suggest that a psychic process or behavior may invoke suffering.[44] I hope that, in time, the theoretical systems I use may be translatable into other discourses—perhaps cognitive science, mindfulness studies, trauma studies, philosophy, or psychology—that can address H.D.'s and Barnes's questions about agency and differentiation in less controversial ways.

Contemporary spiritual teachers of many stripes argue that suffering and, synonymously (as they construct them), pathology are ubiquitous, though this view is contested in religious studies.[45] I believe this, and thus I do not argue that normally symbolic language indicates freedom from suffering or from the self-destructive and repetitive trajectory of the symbolic order(s) in which it takes meaning. The word *pathology*, as popular spiritual teacher Eckhart Tolle (b. 1948) notes, comes from the Greek word *pathos*, or suffering.[46] Tolle characterizes our civilization as pathological:

> If the history of humanity were the clinical case history of a single human being, the diagnosis would have to be: chronic paranoid delusions, a pathological propensity to commit murder and acts of extreme violence and cruelty against his perceived "enemies"—his own unconsciousness projected outward.[47]

This vision is not so far from H.D.'s and Barnes's literary renderings of the social world. H.D. depicts masculine and "scientific" (or objectifying) forces and men that rule civilization, who project their unconscious content onto feminine protagonists, then react to their projections with violence. Barnes depicts humanity as always already suffering from a "universal malady" imbricated in power, language and desire, locked in a dance of ruin.[48] Observations regarding the suffering inherent in our condition abound in ancient through contemporary religious and contemplative teachings. The Sanskrit word *māyā* is often translated as *illusion* and, in Hinduism, denotes the state of individual and collective delusion (particularly, the delusion of separateness and autonomy) that results in *samsāra*, the endless looping round of birth and death fueled by *karma*, actions whose results perpetuate rebirth. Hindu scriptures like the *Bhagvata Purana* prophesy that this collective delusion will eventually bring about extreme social degradation, fiery apocalypse, and the near decimation of life on earth.[49] The idea of freedom from this samsāric round through personal and world transformation, as prophesied by Hindu scholar and mystic Aurobindo (1872–1950) has indeed been taken up by the mad pride movement and identified with the messianic "delusion," here envisioned in positive terms.[50]

Buddhism also emphasizes the ubiquity of suffering in the human condition. As Buddhist scripture renders it, the first of the Four Noble Truths discovered by the Buddha is the truth of *dukkha*, a Pali word most often rendered into English as *suffering*, or, more recently, *unsatisfactoriness* or *stress*.[51] The Second Noble Truth of Buddhism identifies the cause of suffering as *taṇhā*, translated in the modern era as *desire* and usually now as *craving*.[52] Early Buddhist scriptures predict that human mental defilement leading to suffering, which I understand in Tolle's sense as normative pathology, will eventually result in the destruction of each "world-cycle," either by water, air, or, as with our particular world-cycle, by fire.[53] While I do not necessarily anticipate this, the social and environmental crises of our times—as well as H.D.'s and other modernists' sometime apocalypticism, and insistence on the connection between personal and social madness and redemption—call for us to re-admit the consideration of pathology into literary and modernist studies.[54] H.D. herself drew on religious understandings of patterned selfhood. Buddhist and Hindu-influenced occult doctrines of *karma* and *samsara*, Christian-toned legends of sacrifice and martyrdom, and psychoanalytic theory all impact her depictions of her devastating encounters with male authority figures and love objects. Though she came to see these encounters as redemptive cycles of mystical initiation,[55] they also opened questions for her about how to think about therapeutic, healing, or redemptive experiences and processes as distinct from "mad" or compulsive ones.

Desire (*désir*) is for Lacan predicated on the apprehension of separateness and lack, and caught in language and the play of signification.[56] Loy explains our "sense-of-lack," as he calls it, as the result of our failed attempts to "ground" our sense of self in the thoughts and objects we identify with it. This failure results in the perceived need for more complex symbolizations of ourselves, such as artworks.[57] Lacan, similarly, describes most of what any analysand [patient] says in analysis as "merely a response to the failure of his silence, when faced with the perceived echo of his own nothingness."[58] From a simplified Buddhist-Lacanian perspective, then, the language of suffering might be all language, all our books and articles attempts to firm up our identities. I view suffering as imbricated in language and differentiated identity, though I acknowledge the varying magnitudes of anguish or psychic complexity that subjects may experience. My inquiry is admittedly influenced by the belief that greater mental freedom is possible, and that it requires us to first notice our mental bondage. To me, this freedom would involve an easing of dissociation and the compulsive thought and behavior patterns associated with it, a clearer and more vivid lived awareness, and an ability to endure the sense that there is something wrong or lacking without projecting this sense onto an external cause. I imagine a measure of freedom from the imperative rooted in philosopher and gender theorist Judith Butler's (b. 1956), description of agency: a "hiatus in . . . the compulsion to install an identity through repetition." However, I hope that such agency might also result in changes to the patterns of affect, thought, and relationship that underlie our actions.[59]

Many self-awareness practices encourage us to observe that thoughts proliferating in our minds distract from this deep sense of something lacking, something not being as it should be, which I identify with Lacan's understanding of castration and the imperative. Teachers of these practices suggest that the more we can be aware of this sense of lack as such, the less we tend to get caught up in thoughts (where "caught up" means losing awareness that these are only thoughts, not necessarily true, and losing awareness of ourselves in the present).[60] Loy asserts that this direct awareness of lack as such, which he calls *primordial lack-as-anguish*, eventually leads to the destruction of what he calls the *sense-of-self*, or the ego, as well as the *sense-of-lack*.[61] This, writes Loy, "for psychoanalysis is a definition of psychosis. For Buddhism, it may describe enlightenment. . . . The issue becomes whether the subject-object distinction can break down in different ways: if the mystic can swim in the same sea that drowns the psychotic."[62] Though Lacan describes what is not signifiable—what is not assimilated into the symbolic order—as "the real" and describes the encounter with it in negative terms as a psychotic break,[63] it may be possible to relate to whatever is not symbolized in more positive ways. However, the encounter with the nonreferential may have destabilizing effects, or even activate alternate modes of referentiality, particularly for those of us whose experiences of the world are less than normally mediated by stable boundaries and systems of signification.

H.D. and Barnes evidence particular trouble disidentifying with thoughts and becoming aware of them as such. However tormenting the thoughts, they seem to offer protection from something worse—which I call after Lacan the "*nom du père*," the name or "no" of the father, which summons the subject to a place of lack.[64] Self-protective thought and language accompanies such threats to identity in H.D. and Barnes's work, though as well as working as a buffer against subjective dissolution, it may also be a way of recasting subjectivity, as suggested by Jonathan Flatley's discussion of modernist literary work as a means of "self-estrangement" and empowerment.[65]

Flatley draws on the aesthetic theory of philosopher Theodor Adorno (1903–1969) to support his argument that, as the affect that present others evoke in us is traced by psychoanalysis to ghostly others from the past, and so denaturalized, likewise the affect of the author, "mapped" in modernist literature onto its broader sociohistorical context, estranges the reading subject from their usual objects and from themselves, while simultaneously calling forth their affective response.[66] This estrangement and invocation of affect denaturalizes their usual attachments, exposing the contingency of the identifications underlying them.[67] Flatley writes of aesthetic self-estrangement as produced by our "return to the 'self,'" after reading a modernist literary work: "the subjectivity as we find it in our everyday lives, and its disjuncture with the affects and the mood we have experienced *without* a self, in a nonself."[68]

Such works thus enable a melancholic, but therapeutic, "self-distancing that allows one to see oneself as if from outside."[69] Mediated by the rendering of the author's affective life within a shared sociohistorical context, the reader's own emotional life is estranged, not only by being distanced, but also "in the sense of defamiliarization," where "one's range of moods, set of structures of feeling, and collection of affective attachments . . . appear weird, surprising, unusual, and thus capable of a new kind of recognition, interest, and analysis." Though one might argue that modernist writers may experience differently the aesthetic self-estrangement that their own affective maps make possible for readers—especially if they identify strongly with their characters and scenes, as H.D. and Barnes do—Flatley argues that self-estrangement functions for the author as well, transmuting depressive melancholy, where affect and interest are withdrawn from the world, into a new "way to be interested in the world."[70] Accordingly, he describes modernist literary works as expressions of an "active, transformative, ultimately antidepressive melancholia," which, like psychoanalysis itself, reconstructs lost object-cathexes (lost histories, lost hopes) by historicizing and socializing the affects associated with them.[71] Modernist melancholizing—Flatley borrows the term from Barnes's favorite book, Robert Burton's *The Anatomy of Melancholy* (1621)—thus becomes an active enterprise by means of which the gaps between the "promises and the social processes of modernity" are revealed.[72] The literary mapping of affects in modern psychic terrain spanning past and present, Flatley argues, enables a subject's return to the actual present by means of ghosts from the past.[73]

Ghosts from the past may not always, however, enable a return to consciousness. A ghostly other can also mask the particularity of an embodied other, as psychoanalytic theory suggests and as many who have been transference objects know. This is especially true when the subject whose affect is evoked by an other becomes caught in thought patterns whose function, as I argue, is to shape, manage, even evoke, the affect's intensity. Affects then get entangled within ghostly thought and language patterns at the expense of clear and vivid engagements with present others—as may have been the case for H.D. and Barnes, especially in later life.

III. PSYCHIC NEGATIONS, SPIRITUAL OPENINGS?

In his earlier writing on psychosis, Lacan insists that "the nucleus of psychosis has to be linked to a relationship between the subject and the signifier in its most formal dimension, in its dimension as a pure signifier."[74] What Lacan refers to as pure signifier, or the signifier disconnected from signified (which for him marks psychosis), in my view represents an extreme instance of an otherwise normal process of getting caught up in signification—in thought—to the point that we have less sense of anything that is not thought. Thus, we have less ability to disidentify with thought and to experience ourselves, and what we perceive, without reference to anything else.[75] Following the call of the pure signifier, we try to think something more that will bring our thoughts to a conclusion, but instead rehash the thoughts in a circular way with slight permutations. If we are writing, perhaps alone in a room with a computer and many books, our words may seem meaningful to us at the time, at least potentially; however, it may be difficult for someone else, or even ourselves, to read them later and be sure of our intentioned meanings. Or, just as possibly given the recent "mindfulness revolution" and explosion of interest in meditation and spirituality, we may be engaged in some contemplative technique meant to quiet our minds.[76] Instead, as meditation teachers describe, we may find ourselves caught in a Möbius strip of thought.[77] At such times, the words we are conjuring often compose thoughts unconnected to anything more vivid than the words themselves. I suggest that awareness of the vivid arises when the signifier is connected to a signified, as well as to other signifiers.

The experiences of ferocious, determining, inundating otherness that Barnes and H.D. describe may involve more than split off and projected internal content—as transpersonal psychology, object oriented ontology, some spiritual teachers, and Lacan himself, especially in later work, suggest. Transpersonal psychologist Stanislav Grof (b. 1931) describes a state he calls "spiritual emergency" that is often misdiagnosed as psychosis,[78] but which proceeds from an opening of the subject to "transcendence of the ordinary boundaries of personality [including] many experiences that have been called spiritual, mystical, religious, occult, magical, or paranormal."[79] Spiritual emergency may involve past life visions, communication with spirit guides, channeling (spirits) and "sacred marriage" with "an imaginary archetypal partner" in what Grof understands as a "dramatic psychic opening."[80] Here, writes Grof, "our personal boundaries may appear to melt and we can become identified with other people, groups of people, or all of humanity."[81] Likewise, transpersonal psychotherapist John Weir Perry (1914–1998) writes of a process of spiritual renewal that involves the experience of changing gender, a "heavenly marriage" with a "divine figure," and assuming a "messianic role" in the world.[82] H.D.'s descriptions of channeling and of sacred erotic encounters with larger than life partners, her belief in her messianic destiny, and her sorting of objects and identities, fit into Lacan's symptomatology, but also accord with the experiences of spiritual opening to a transpersonal reality that Grof and Perry describe. Erotic or sexual engagements with supernatural beings, abundant in texts both pathologized and sanctified, perhaps represent encounters with what has not been admitted into a subject's psychic life, whether in the personal realm (a father figure, a mother figure) or in the broader social realm (what is alienated in the subject because it is abjected or repressed by society). Perhaps something "out there" may be summoned in response to this psychic vacuum, as many, including H.D. and psychologist and philosopher William James (1842–1910), speculate: more individuated supramundane others that only some subjects perceive—or there may sometimes be less distinction than we suppose between projections and outer forces or entities.[83] We do not have to choose between, on the one hand, the pure projection described in most psychoanalytic theory and, on the other, academically disreputable accounts of turbulent encounters with something real beyond accepted categories. There is room for both, and more, in the complexity of lived experience. However, such real or imagined encounters do not necessarily integrate the excluded content into the subject's psychic life: they may be so traumatic as to result in more fragmentation and rapid cycles of recurrence rather than integration, as I argue is often the case for H.D. and Barnes. Lacan's 1960 description of gods as "a mode by which the real is revealed" can also be read as supporting this view.[84]

In addition to whatever supramundane beings or intensities which we may imagine it possible to relate, mundane objects and things in contemporary theory also explode modern notions of object relations and behave like dystopic gods with bad boundaries. Eco-theorist Timothy Morton (b. 1968), for instance, describes *hyperobjects*: massive, viscous, nonlocal, differently temporal, multidimensional objects such as global warming, and radioactive and plastic waste, which transcend the spatial-temporal boundaries of objects imagined in modernity and impinge into everyone's psychic space, though we may not be aware of them.[85] Hyperobjects, like Schreber's God, upset and disobey the spatial and temporal world order we know, and impinge on and eviscerate our bodies and thoughts. Such accounts may reflect an awareness of objects, intensities, and possibilities whose magnitudes and affective charges most of us repress in order to function as individuals in society.

Lacan's idea that the negation of the name, or *no*, of the father determined psychic structure was a characteristically modern one. If anything held together modern Western civilization it was this heightened sense of subjective separateness, lack, and alienation, and subjection by regulating powers that were, as Michel Foucault (1926–1984) argues, much more intimate and invasive than those in pre-modern times.[86] In modernism, the shadow of the father figure that determines the subject's mode of spatial and temporal connectedness with everything outside its own skin falls more heavily, so that theorists like Lacan and Foucault imagine modern subjectivity as a function of regulatory power. Those on whom the shadow of the father falls differently are cast as mad—not really subjects at all. However, for Lacan, they notice something that neurotics miss: their psychic capture and circular trajectory, though they misunderstand this capture by the big Other as capture by specific "imaginary others."[87] Lacan suggests that delusions and fixations, and their circular forms in thought and text, reflect not an alterity to the social order, but rather the truth of our capture by it. In contrast, the imagined freedom of the neurotic subject—autonomous, self-contained, exerting their will on passive, securely bounded objects, textually rendered perhaps in a plotted narrative arc where characters' choices seem to determine their fates—may elide this truth. H.D. and Barnes, and other experimental modernists like Gertrude Stein, James Joyce, and Virginia Woolf, as well as choosing to depict experiences of alterity, may also speak from experiences and explorations of a more looping, inadvertent, other-inflected consciousness.

Along with the possible influence of unusual states of consciousness, these authors' portrayals of nonlinear, unbounded, or predetermined time, being, fate, and consciousness were, as critics have noted, influenced by spiritualism, occultism, and even mainstream religious traditions. Along with W.B. Yeats's and H.D.'s fairly credulous engagements with the supernatural and esoteric, Ezra Pound, Virginia Woolf, T.S. Eliot, D.H. Lawrence, and many others are known within literary studies to have drawn, with varying reflexive distances, on occultist, spiritualist, Christian, Jewish, Buddhist, and Hindu cosmological systems.[88] Barnes numbers among them, in my view, as one who disguises her engagement. Her childhood was séance-saturated, and her late work, Catherine Setz argues, resonates with "submerged" affirmations of spirituality when read through its profound influence by the metaphysical poets, revealing her as "a poet melding Christian, pagan, even Eastern spirituality with a secular and stark appraisal of modernity expressed in old and new forms."[89] Though her persona is hard-bitten and her works salty regarding religious faith and spirit visitations, Christian-toned references and images of spirits, haunting, and possession abound in her earlier as well as later writing and often signal disavowal itself. Conversely, H.D., though considered alongside Yeats as the most credulous of modernism's occultists, might be said to be haunted by the incredulity that is given voice, as I will discuss, by the men who called her vision into doubt.[90] Avowed or disavowed beliefs, alongside experiential states of consciousness, likely contribute to both Barnes's and H.D.'s understandings of interpersonal boundaries, and hence of language, as unstable and perhaps permeable.

Though both authors respond to these uncertain limits with formal aporias and aphasias, proliferations, and figurations of violence—in the broad sense—in their work, their responses could hardly contrast more sharply in other respects. While each experiences difference as tenuous, Barnes's writing suggests a somewhat intentional though ingrained and compulsive shoring up of difference, whereas H.D.'s writing after the Second World War suggests a more inadvertent and confusing encounter with difference, a strong wish to end this confusion, and a growing sense that the only means to do so may be to be destroyed by the one who represents difference. Indeed, H.D.'s beliefs during and after the Second World War resonate with convictions that reappear like slighted ghosts in records of "mad" communications: that the world will soon end or disruptively transform; that this coming cataclysm necessitates psychic or bodily transformation; and that her role in an erotic union may save humanity, perhaps with a miraculous birth.

In our time, as apocalypticism becomes mainstream and scientific findings increasingly validate it, we must of course ask ourselves—as the mad pride movement points out—whether these ideas are madder than our habit of living as though our global civilization and perhaps life on earth, were not gravely at risk.[91] The subject-object boundaries suggested in works by H.D., Barnes, other experimental modernists, and even Schreber, may be read as gesturing toward relationships with objects whose magnitudes cannot be known in the modern symbolic order except by the traces they leave. I draw on Schreber's work, in part, to suggest how Schreber, as the original exemplar of the category of psychosis, might push back against psychoanalytic notions of "sane" relatedness. If we compare psychoanalytic formulations of object relations in psychosis to emerging theorizations of subject-object relations, such as thing theory, object-oriented ontology or speculative realism, we may, as Morton speculates, find symmetrical visions of relationship, difference and identity.[92] Morton's call to a subjectivity in which our impressions are recognized as the "footprints of hyperobjects" and our situatedness as "uncanny" opens a space where Schreber's discourse, like H.D.'s and Barnes's, calls us toward a different vision.[93]

IV. "FORECLOSURE," "DISAVOWAL," AND H.D.'S AND BARNES'S WORK

In H.D.'s later work, labyrinths of asymbolic words and patterns are presumed to lead to the final answer and meaning often oscillates between ambiguous significance and formulaic repetition: the modes of "intuition" and "formula" with which Lacan, in 1955–1956, describes two types of neologism in psychotic language:

> The delusional intuition is a full phenomenon that has an overflowing, inundating character for the subject. It reveals a new perspective . . . one whose stamp of originality, whose characteristic savor, he emphasizes. There, the word . . . is the soul of the situation. At the opposite pole there is the form that meaning takes when it no longer refers to anything at all. This is the formula that is repeated, reiterated, drummed in with a stereotyped insistence.[94]

H.D. presents in these modes of intuition and formula a meaning that remains irreducible to concepts since lacking lack it excludes nothing. Yet it is largely her wish to find some way to limit, close, and finalize this meaning that drives these later works.

Like psychosis, perversion, understood by Lacan as a subjective "structure" rather than a behavior, results from the child's incomplete entry into the symbolic order where metaphor operates. Fetishism represents a subject's attempt to strengthen their sense of separation from the mother figure by supplementing the paternal bar with material objects or behaviors, thus calling a symbolic order into being.[95] In Freud's foundational discussions of perverse "disavowal," the emerging subject simultaneously avows and denies the mother's lack, or "castration," which for Freud is the mother's lack of a penis, and for Lacan, her lack of the phallus or her limited power (over the subject). The subject experiences itself as the mother's (later the other's) phallus, the thing that completes the other. In fetishism, particular objects and scenarios stand for castration, the (m)other's desire and its (other) objects. The (m)other's unconditional demand for the subject is thereby limited.

In perverse disavowal, a dominant pattern that I identify in Barnes's writing, the subject seeks both to affirm and to deny the separation from the (m)other by utilizing a fetish, or sometimes fetishized words. Though Lacan's discussion of perverse language is meagre, I expand on his remarks using other psychoanalytic theory, especially that of Nicholas Abraham and Maria Torok. Building on theories of melancholia and incorporation/introjection pioneered by Karl Abraham (1877–1925) and Sándor Ferenczi (1873–1933) and elaborated by Klein and Freud, Abraham and Torok elaborate on parental imperatives in a more individuated register, theorizing the splitting effects of both familial and broader social relations on psychic formation and language use in children. They suggest that imperatives can be imposed by any family member or by the broader social world in which certain scenes or memories are taboo and unspeakable. Shameful memories are symptomized by "cryptophoria": dysfunctional, anti-symbolic patterning in a subject's language and behavior that is meant to enclose internalized love objects and the secret, affect-charged words associated with them. I read cryptophoria as a permutation of fetishistic disavowal, since it both stages barred content and supplements the bar itself. Abraham and Torok write that through "antimetaphoric" behaviors, described as "taking literally what was meant figuratively," the cryptophore attempts to strip fetish word(s) of "figurativity," the metaphoricity that occurs in symbolic language.[96] The fetish works as a "symbol-cover" for the cryptophore's "fetish word," the word that is key to the secret, by presenting the word with another, purely literal, meaning.[97] Here, the substitution of literal for metaphoric meanings is more a form of self-protection, a banishment of the affect that metaphor can invoke, than the error of a psyche that has not internalized the difference necessary to metaphor.

Abraham and Torok's "psychic crypt" is an imaginary formation that intrapsychically preserves a love object whose loss cannot be spoken of because an imperative coming from this object—and from social taboos—renders the love socially unacceptable or shameful.[98] The secret love is not repressed (made unconscious), but is disassociated from its full affective meaning by changing the symbolism of the words associated with it. The cryptophore's history is hidden in full view in signs that are filled with other significations. Cryptophoria involves inexhaustible allusions to the encrypted content, whether in language or behavior. While the words' and behaviors' literal meanings and functions appear to be the going concern, the reverse is true in the cryptophore's psychic economy. Their fleeting, ghostly connotations are what remain and return, looping back into whatever context presents itself, while their apparent denotations are incidental.

For instance, the word *leche*, Spanish for "milk" (similar to lécher, French for *lick*, and to English *lechery*), evocative of the white, milky semen spilled during ejaculation, comes to be the fetish word of Abraham and Torok's "man of milk."[99] Since the encrypted secret of the man of milk is that his sister gave their *(lecherous) father hand jobs during a vacation in Spanish South America, he regales his analyst with free-associative words and fantasies that pertain to milk and milking (lait de chèvre*, "goat's milk"), as well as traction and pulling. He also admits to being an avid performer of cunnilingus (*lécher*, "to lick").[100] Similarly, another analysand encrypts his memories of incestuous desire between himself and his mother while she washed him as a boy in frequent references to water, washerwomen, and inundation.[101] In a nonverbal register, the sister of Freud's famous patient known as the Wolf Man (1886–1979) commits suicide by ingesting liquid mercury (*rtut* in Russian), an act intended by cryptophoric logic to neutralize the shameful connotation of the homophonic *teret* (to rub) by pretending that it is appetizing. *Teret* is the word she associates with her incestuous relationship with her father.[102]

The psychic phantom, on the other hand, consists of fragments of the unspoken knowledge of a love object, closed off in the subject's psyche and restricting full communication. For instance, a woman's unspoken knowledge that her father was denounced to the Nazis by her mother and died in a concentration camp appears as a transgenerational phantom in her son's hobbies and professional pursuits, which include splitting rocks and gassing butterflies.[103]

Both crypt and phantom are split off from the subject's sense of self, and are often outside their consciousness, disabling rather than enabling the integration of perceptions and memories into a coherent sense of self.[104] Consequently, crypt and phantom affect the subject's relationship to language, interfering with its metaphorical function, which is perceived as threatening because metaphor has the power to invoke the shameful and affective connotations of certain words. Fetish words deny this power by seeming, literally, to pertain to something else. Thus they both invoke and deny some erotically charged scene in which, often, the cryptophore's desire met with that of a family member, as I suggest may be the case for Barnes. Cryptophoric subjects know that the fetishized object, word or behavior is not identical to the unspeakable lost object and scene. Yet they paradoxically persist in the belief that it is, and so simultaneously shore up and deny difference. In this way, Barnes's work invokes erotically charged imperatives—and the ferocious figures associated with them—through fetish words, while simultaneously denying them by referencing these words to other signifieds. The repetition and resistance to interpretation that characterize the Barnesian *tableau* also characterize fetishism as Abraham and Torok describe it,[105] where the fetishist fixes the symbolic history of the fetish in signs that are filled with another signification.

In the works I focus on, H.D.'s *The Sword Went Out to Sea* (2007) and *Helen in Egypt* (1961) and Barnes's *Ryder* (1928) and *Nightwood* (1936), the authors use characters and figures of speech to portray psychic splitting and supernatural life. Ghosts, gaps and dualities, the living dead, strange gods, individuals whose subjecthood is also dual—even multiple—appear at the boundaries of Barnes's and H.D.'s thought and language. These supernatural figures embody the meaning is excluded by the negations that structure ghostly language, and sometimes also represent lost familial love objects of the works' authors and characters. Modes of negation of parental imperatives, then, as well as literary and otherworldly modernism, impact the formal and stylistic elements of these works and the social and supernatural worlds that they evoke. Barnes's and H.D.'s modes of expressing meaning—cryptic, formulaic or ineffable—correlate to the ways that the social and supernatural function in their work.

According to this model, H.D.'s work evidences foreclosure, a mode of thought and language that sabotages signification. This incapacity can endanger the psyche with the hallucinatory return of (haunting by) that which cannot be symbolized. The paternal signifier of castration, which Lacan first calls the *nom du père* and later the phallus, is imagined as returning from outside in embodied, threatening, and eroticized forms.[106] When father figures, who represent the symbolic order to H.D., undermine the vision that she offers them, she struggles endlessly to make sense of these invalidations. She does so by placing them within a broad, vaguely imagined system, formula or pattern, but that never remains stable. It is not that she cannot find reasons for their perceived rejections that make sense—she can—but she cannot settle on anything because she cannot exclude anything from possible, if unclear, relevance. She constantly finds new associations—objects, myths, legends, other worlds, otherworldly beings, cosmic cycles, associates, historical figures, divine plans—that appear significant in some enigmatic, vaguely intuited way. These provide "traces of direction," as she calls this unclear significance, that if pursued could, she hopes, eventually lead her to a sense of closure.[107] This sense of closure is prevented because *Sword* and *Helen in Egypt*, in their lack of a lack of associations that are considered possibly relevant to an enigmatic, never complete meaning, evidence what Lacan calls foreclosure. H.D. will not or cannot limit the re-branching associations and unclear questions, which appear to her to concern both her rejection by a male authority figure and love object, and her key importance to the entire world and the course of history.

The betraying father figure and love object appears in *Sword* and *Helen* as a multiplicity of fatal heroes based primarily on Lord Hugh Caswall Tremenheere Dowding (1882–1970), retired Royal Air Chief Marshall, hero of the Battle of Britain, séance practitioner, and author of the spiritualist volumes, *Many Mansions* (1943) and *Lychgate* (1945). Dowding refused, in 1946, to receive and take seriously the spirit messages that H.D. had been communicating to him, chiefly in letters, since 1945. His repudiation triggered a breakdown and her internment, beginning in May 1946, in Klinik Brunner, a "private hospital for nervous cases" owned by Dr. Theodore Brunner, in Küsnacht, Switzerland.[108] H.D.'s literary work following Dowding's rejection becomes a quest for a satisfying explanation of it within her own psyche. She finds, instead, ever more traces of direction: events, things, and beings that may be associated with it in some way as yet to be determined. Perhaps to forestall this proliferation of unclearly relevant associations, she attempts also to establish in *Sword* and *Helen* that the rejection is its own meaning, that H.D. herself is, quite literally, the ultimate meaning of everything and, therefore, signs and events need not have coherent meanings.

If after the Second World War, H.D. attempts unsuccessfully to find the conclusion of her haunting thoughts through writing, Barnes, in contrast, imagines no positive conclusion. In contrast to H.D.'s foreclosure, Barnes's work suggests disavowal, hiding unspeakable meanings in plain view. The mode of meaning that Barnes employs puts the interpreter into a different position than does clear language, or clearly disorganized language: readers are less certain, less able to achieve closure of any kind, and perhaps this is part of the point, though, as Elizabeth Pender and Catherine Setz have argued, it marginalized her work by placing it at a distance from postwar critical formulations of modernist literary value.[109] Barnes imagines, perhaps, a reader whose interpretive flailing and bungled certainties she dances around, a reader whose confusion is necessary to the meaning of Barnes's writing—for Barnes. The reader's uncertain engagement with Barnes's meaning may be crucial to the author's sense of self, perhaps not only by bearing witness to her traumatic memories, as Julie Taylor suggests, but also by misunderstanding her.[110] Since more conventional people believe in stable limits and, therefore, believe that certain words, objects or behaviors really signify what they only appear to signify, Barnes can both invoke and hide her "real" meanings by means of the (castrated) other's credulity. Her cryptic invocations of content outside the boundaries of the speakable suggest a psychic structure in which limits, and the symbolic meanings they enable, are fragile. She shores up these boundaries through aesthetically gorgeous and affect-charged indirectness.

The fragmentation, resistance to interpretation, and repetition in Barnes's work are characteristic of cryptophoric modes of expression, which fix meanings in enigmatic, repetitive patterns. Her writing orbits particular hidden meanings with words and scenes that both establish and transgress the limits of symbolic communication. Here, limits are not so much limits to what may be done to a person within a literary world she imagines as lawless, as Rachel Potter also notes, but rather limits to what may be clearly communicated.[111] Thus, these "limits" are themselves psychic transgressions, since they forbid the subjects' free disclosure of their experience (e.g., "this must not be spoken of"). Understood through Abraham and Torok's discussion of cryptophoria, this invocation of the boundary between parentally and socially sanctioned speech and unspeakable content is motivated by multiple and conflicting desires. On one hand, the subject wishes to exorcise the ghost words, to dispel the affective charges of the unspeakable scenes she cites. However, complete discharge would require the clear articulation of the encrypted content to another person or to a community of others. On the other hand, the subject wants to perpetuate the affective charges that the ghost words call up (or at least the erotic components of those charges) and to maintain the boundary that their cryptic indirection establishes between herself and others: both the loved and lost other, and the other as reader. The latter desires are served by cryptophoric patterns; however, the desire to exorcise the ghosts is sabotaged by these patterns, since it is in them that the ghosts subsist.

In Barnes's universe of "hunter, hunting hunter," limits do not enable an impartial and consistent (however harsh) social order in which autonomy can be claimed.[112] Rather, Barnes's ghost words haunt a lawless and perverse universe and compel fetishistic behavior. They suggest not repression, not the unconscious, but rather disavowal, the half-known that is at once accepted and rejected by being staged with another ostensible meaning. Barnes's cryptic tableaux attempt to create a textual "unconscious" by presenting, yet forbidding, knowledge to the reader. This simultaneous invocation and concealment—the double movement of disavowal—supplement Barnes's sense of separation from what she invokes and hides. The meanings that are both invoked and dispelled (but never completely) by her tableaux resonate compellingly with the violations in her family relationships. Permeable personal boundaries allow, perhaps drive, her to describe madness, envisioned as total possession by an imperative, in words. Her descriptions themselves may reinforce the boundary between the enunciator and the madness enunciated.

Barnes's main preserved object is perhaps the strangely sexualized relationship that she had with her grandmother, Zadel Barnes Gustafson (1841–1917), a mother figure with whom she shared a bed for fifteen years. Zadel's 1909 letters to her young granddaughter are sexually explicit, depicting horniness in response to her letters and implying a sexual relationship between them.[113] No overtly sexual act, beyond playing with her grandmother's breasts, appears in Barnes's writing; if they had other secrets (as I suggest they did), Barnes writes around them. Barnes avowedly loved Zadel "as a child usually loves its mother."[114] Zadel's and Barnes's explicitly sexual correspondence, the many references to incest in Barnes's work, the sexually ambiguous, untrustworthy mother—and grandmother—figures, and the ghostly grandmother in *Nightwood*, have suggested to several critics that their intimacies were more erotically charged and traumatic than Barnes's biographer Phillip Herring surmises.[115] If their intimacies appeared to the young Barnes, as they did to Herring, as mere "fondling"[116] and "bawdy humor,"[117] or, as Mary Lynn Broe argues, as a lesbian alliance against the patriarchal order, Zadel's collusion in Barnes's other sexual violations, by family friend Percy Faulkner and perhaps by her father Wald Barnes, as well as Barnes's entry into the broader world where these activities were tacitly recast as shameful, may have heightened the traumatic charge of their earlier encounters.[118]

Some of Barnes's writing implies (as she also told George Barker) that her father raped her. Opinions vary as to whether this rape occurred. Early biographer Andrew Field argues that it did and it is hidden in Barnes's writing behind a more presentable betrayal, the sexual encounter arranged by Zadel and Wald, when Barnes was sixteen, with the much older Percy Faulkner. Writes Field, "It did happen, and the outrage was the shadow-play behind all her art."[119] Conversely, Herring suggests that Barnes's literary depictions of father-daughter rape result from her sense that her father vicariously participated in her violation by Faulkner or perhaps in an earlier violation by another man.[120] Barnes's longtime friend and correspondent, Emily Coleman (1899–1974), reports in her diary that Wald propositioned Barnes sexually before this abuse.[121] Herring writes that Wald beat Barnes, as a child, with a horsewhip, and once lowered her into a well and gloated over her fear.[122] Music producer and photographer Hank O'Neal (b. 1940), sometime friend to Barnes in the last years of her life and author of a memoir of these years, also recalls Barnes telling him that her father "enjoyed beating her with a whip."[123] Both recount that, according to Barnes, her grandmother endeavored to protect her from her father's wrath. If we believe that there was ever a sexualized relationship between grandmother and granddaughter, the fact that Barnes sometimes verbally accused her father, but never her grandmother, of sexual violations might support my argument that *Nightwood* evidences a psychic crypt containing Barnes's grandmother, but not her father: what can be spoken of directly, in Abraham and Torok's theory, can be unearthed from the psychic crypt and ceases to reappear in indirect allusions.[124] Perhaps tellingly, *Ryder* does not undercut its grandmother figure Sophia's power by exposing her desire as successfully as it does with its father figure, Wendell; and it is the grandmother, not the father, whose presence most haunts the pages of *Nightwood*.

V. READING H.D. AND BARNES

H.D. and Barnes scholars have understood their work as contributing to queer, feminist, anti-patriarchal, and anti-imperialist modernism in both content and style. For many readers, both authors oppose patriarchy and hegemony, not only at the level of literary content by depicting patriarchal aggression and suggesting other modes of sociality through image and narrative, but also by way of parody (in Barnes's case) and with intentionally enigmatic literary styles that resist transparency of meaning and the possibility of certainty, both of which come to be seen as ethically problematic in modernity. H.D. and Barnes are seen to elect instead an open-ended, nonconceptual, uncertain, nonnarrative, and/or pluralistic approach to meaning.[125] Barnes's readers have rightly asserted that her work refuses determinate meaning in favor of uncertainty and layered or broken meanings, in order to empower herself, or to resist or critique her sociopolitical context and its ideological and legitimating apparatuses. While these approaches have much value, they have in the past sometimes cooperated overly with Barnes's agenda by assuming the place of a credulous reader, who takes the literary work's images and scenes at surface value. Likewise, H.D.'s readers sometimes attempt to establish meaningful networks of associations, instead of conclusions, and to experience her texts in immediate, participatory, nonconceptual, or alternative ways, and to arrive at the most "complete picture" of what she meant.[126] The nearness of these approaches to their source texts enables brilliant and aesthetically beautiful readings, but has sometimes extended to an over-reproduction in literary criticism of Barnes's and H.D.'s styles of denegation. Especially in the case of H.D. scholarship, there is a large body of scholarly work that affirms its heterodoxy, indeterminacy, and positive affirmation of alternative modes of being and consciousness with a consistency that feels almost orthodox.

I read patterns of thought and affect into works that have often been described as intentionally resisting meaning, to argue that H.D.'s and Barnes's scintillating and indeterminate literary language can also be seen to reflect and reinforce particular kinds of suffering, confusion, and self-described lack of fulfillment in their lives and relationships. Since literary studies of Barnes, and especially H.D., have sometimes unequivocally celebrated the perceived ethical and epistemological triumphs of the authors' language, which in such studies represent a counter to patriarchy, authoritarianism, war, oppression of gender and sexuality, rational certainty, totality, and similar negatively charged terms, my argument may seem to gainsay much that has come before. I believe, though, that my work is an extension of the scholarship that has reclaimed these authors from the literary margins, since it examines how marginalizing categories of "literary," "mystical," and "pathological" can melt and dance in patterns that many or all of us can, perhaps, recognize as intimate. My goal is to move forward into acknowledging that there has been an aporia in H.D. and Barnes criticism into which the elephant of their mental suffering has been stuffed, perhaps prey to critics' own desires for exuberance, self-empowerment, or ethical high ground. I suggest that Barnes's work evidences cryptophoria, to be taken here as a patterning in creativity and agency rather than as a clinical category. Further, the patterns I trace in H.D.'s life and writing can be interpreted in terms of what Lacan and others have called psychotic processes—formulations that I draw on, but which I also call into question.[127] Much agency, intentionality, and social engagement have already been attributed to Barnes and H.D.'s work; I expand the critical field by seeking the unconscious or semi-conscious processes, rather than the fully intentional ones, that may be at play in it.

What emerges in the various critical approaches to questions of agency and pathology that we see in psychoanalytic theory, in feminist responses to it, in trauma theory, in anti-psychiatry and the mad pride movement, and in literary studies of H.D. and Barnes, are a variety of implicit stances toward the ethics and meaning of pathologization and depathologization. I believe that it is ethical to acknowledge the suffering and disempowerment that may attend what we call trauma, splitting, or disassociation—our negation of experience, affect and knowledge, which patterns our psychic lives. My view is that we do abandon parts of ourselves and our potential relational fields in response to developmental traumas or later threatening experiences. Though this abandonment may help us adapt to our social environments in the short or even the long term, it also entails personal and social challenges that are dangerous to ignore. Though many of psychoanalysis's early clinical methods have been shown to be less than effective—to say the least—and much of its theory has been called into question, it seems to me helpful (and interesting!) to correlate such negations to behaviors, beliefs, and communication styles—the sliding of our desires along signifying chains.[128]

NOTES

1. Turkle, "French Anti-psychiatry." Turkle reads Lacan's theory in light of mid-century French psychoanalysis's radical opposition to the French psychiatric establishment, pointing out the subversive impact of his view of the self as a misidentification based on a composite of misrecognitions, and his view of madness as a limit point to human freedom, rather than as a lesser or opposite state to normality (153–7). She argues that Lacan's thought profoundly influenced both Marxist and anti-psychiatric theory (158, 160–2).

2. Lacan, though predating the anti-psychiatry movement, is often considered alongside Michel Foucault as its forebear since he inveighed against psychiatry and offered an account of "madness" as socio-linguistically determined, rather than biological. See for instance Lifton, *The Protean Self*, where Lifton discusses Lacan alongside R.D. Laing (1927–1989), a founder of the anti-psychiatry movement, as a proponent of the fluid, unfixable self (26–7). Psychiatrist Mervat Nasser, too, puts Lacan at the source of anti-psychiatry: "[Anti-psychiatry] can be traced back to the writings of Jacques Lacan who was probably the first to glorify madness and regard it as the road to freedom. In a statement extracted from *Propos sur la Causalité psychique* Lacan says 'madness is not an insult to liberty but follows liberty like its shadow.' Lacan was also the first to launch an attack on established psychiatric thought and demand that psychoanalysis re-examine its concepts, with particular reference to explaining paranoia. He thought that the psychotic experience could be psychoanalytically understood in the same way as psychoanalysis offers an explanation for neurosis. In his rebellion he undermined genetic disposition and dismissed the possibility of any organic pathology" ("Rise and Fall," 743).

Other prominent figures in anti-psychiatry include David Cooper (1931–1986), Gilles Deleuze (1925–1995), Félix Guattari (1930–1992), and Thomas Szasz (1920–2012).

3. See Lewis, *Moving Beyond Prozac*, 174–9.

4. See Shimrat, "Meeting With Hilda Fernandez." Shimrat quotes Fernandez, psychotherapist and heroic figure in mad pride: "The beauty of Lacanian psychoanalysis . . . is that it is not based on psychopathology—the idea that aberrant thoughts and behaviors are disease symptoms" (7). See also Hejazi, "After Illness," 13.

5. See Prendergast, "The Unexceptional Schizophrenic." Prendergast points out that Lacan defends the self-determination of so-called schizophrenics, writing, "The problem according to Lacan is that these great observers [psychiatrists] thought that what schizophrenics were saying could not be what they were actually saying" (244). She quotes Lacan's words: "Wasn't it because they didn't go far enough in listening to the insane that the great observers who drew up the first classifications impoverished the material they were given—to such an extent that it appeared problematic and fragmentary to them?" (236, from Lacan, *Seminar III, The Psychoses*, 206).

6. Writes Lacan, "Why stigmatize in advance, as null and void, what issues from a subject who is presumed to be in the order of the meaningless, but whose testimony is more unusual or, even, entirely original?" (*Seminar III, The Psychoses*, 208).

7. Lacan (1960) describes the Other as "the locus in which speech is verified as it encounters the exchange of signifiers, the ideals they prop up, the elementary structures of kinship, the metaphor of the father considered as a principle of separation, and the ever reopened division in the subject owing to his initial alienation—on this side [the side of the Other] alone and by the pathways I have just enumerated, order and norms must be instituted which tell the subject what a man or a woman must do" ("Position of the Unconscious," 720).

8. Writes Lacan, "A certain mental breathing space seems indispensable to modern man, one in which his independence not only of any master but also of any god is affirmed, a space for his irreducible autonomy as individual, as individual existence. Here there is indeed something that merits a point-by-point comparison with delusional discourse. It's one itself" (*Seminar III, The Psychoses*, 133).

9. Writes Lacan, "Psychoanalysis . . . gives a curious endorsement to the psychotic's delusion because it legitimates it in the same sphere as the one in which analytic discourse usually operates [the unconscious] and because it rediscovers in his discourse what it usually discovers as the discourse of the unconscious . . . it could be said that the psychotic is a martyr of the unconscious, giving the term martyr its meaning, which is to be a witness. It's an open testimony. The neurotic is also a witness to the existence of the unconscious, he gives a closed testimony that has to be deciphered. The psychotic . . . seems arrested, immobilized, in a position that leaves him incapable of authentically restoring the sense of what he witnesses and sharing it in the discourse of others" (*Seminar III, The Psychoses*, 132).

10. Lacan, *Seminar XI*, 183–6; "Kant With Sade." See also Žižek, (1998) "Kant and Sade: The Ideal Couple" (*Lacanian Ink*, 13).

11. In psychosis, writes Lacanian scholar Ellie Ragland, "the signifier One (the phallic signifier or S1) for difference has not been inscribed, thus carving lack into the narcissistic ideal image. While lack sends most beings in search of another person to complement them, the psychotic subject seeks a literal image of him or herself in others, not a supplement to a lack. When the psychotic subject is threatened by another person's distance (difference), he treats that other as a persecutor, like the superego Lacan described as an agent of ferocious *jouissance* . . . a gaze to flee, a voice to obey, or someone to attack, but never a being of lack with whom one negotiates desire" (*Pleasures*, 49). Writes Lacan (1972), "If the unconscious is truly . . . structured like a language, it is at the level of language that we must investigate this One. . . . We must begin with the fact that this 'There's such a thing as One' is to be understood in the sense that there's One all alone [which] allowed us to isolate . . . the formulation 'the subject supposed to know'" (*Seminar XX*, 67).

12. *Jouissance* is Lacan's term for the excessive, intolerable enjoyment that is prohibited for the castrated subject who enters the symbolic order. Lacan writes (1960), "We must keep in mind that *jouissance* is prohibited to whoever speaks, as such—or, put differently, it can only be said between the lines by whoever is a subject of the Law, since the Law is founded on that very prohibition . . . But it is not the Law itself

that bars the subject's access to *jouissance*—it simply makes a barred subject out of an almost natural barrier. For it is pleasure that sets limits to *jouissance*, pleasure as what binds incoherent life together, until another prohibition . . . arises from the regulation that Freud discovered as the primary process and relevant law of pleasure" ("Subversion," 696).

13. This seeming paradox, in which an event constitutive of autonomous identity at the same time throws autonomy into question, recalls theorist Ruth Leys's discussion of the rhetorical conundrum that she finds in theories of trauma past and present. On one hand, Leys notes, "antimimetic" theories render trauma as proceeding from an external, originary event, outside of consciousness, memory, or socio-symbolic mediation, and correlatively see the resolution of trauma in terms of remembering. On the other hand, "mimetic" theories construct traumatic enactments as socio-symbolically mediated and auto-suggestive, involving some degree of consciousness, memory, and conditioning, and thus imagine resolution in terms of forgetting (*Trauma, passim*).

14. Psychologist and meditation teacher Mark Epstein, writes, "The experiences of terror [resulting from deep meditation] tend to reveal just how precarious the sense of self actually is, and just how groundless the soil of narcissistic craving can be. They have the effect of pulling the rug out from under us, of shaking the foundation on which we have constructed our accepted vision of ourselves" (*Thoughts*, 132). See also psychiatrist Willoughby Britton, "Messy" and *Dangers*, on the contemporary phenomena of psychic breakdowns at intensive meditation retreats.

15. Lacan, "On a Question," 481.

16. Lacan explains: "It is in the *name of the father* that we must recognize the basis of the symbolic function which, since the dawn of historical time, has identified his person with the figure of the law. This conception allows us to clearly distinguish . . . the unconscious effects of this function from the narcissistic relations, or even real relations, that the subject has with the image and actions of the person who embodies this function; this results in a mode of comprehension that has repercussions on the very way in which interventions are made by the analyst" ("Function and Field," 230).

17. Writes Lacan (1958), "Desire is what manifests itself in the interval demand excavates just shy of itself, insofar as the subject, articulating the signifying chain, brings to light his lack of being . . . with his call to receive the complement of this lack from the Other—assuming that the Other, the locus of speech, is also the locus of this lack. . . . Ultimately, by refusing to satisfy the mother's demand, isn't the child requiring the mother to have a desire outside of him, because that is the pathway toward desire that he lacks?" ("Direction of the Treatment," 524–5).

18. Lacan writes in 1957 that signifiers are "subjected to the double condition of being reducible to ultimate differential elements and of combining the latter according to the laws of a closed order" ("Instance," 418).

19. See especially Lacan, *Seminar II, The Ego.* Writes Lacan, "the symbolic relation is constituted as early as possible, even prior to the fixation of the self-image of the subject, prior to the structuring image of the ego, introducing the dimension of the subject into the world, a dimension capable of creating a reality other than that experienced as brute reality, as the encounter of two masses, the collision of two balls. . . . Everything that happens in the order of the object relation is structured as a function

of the particular history of the subject, and that is why analysis, and transference, are possible" (257).

20. Though English translators of Lacan usually render the mother's representation of alterity as (m)Other, I write (m)other because, as I suggest, the other that H.D. and Barnes engage with may be more imaginary than symbolic, thus in Lacanian theory would be represented in the lower case.

21. Lacan writes, "Thus it is, rather, the assumption [*assomption*] of castration that creates the lack on the basis of which desire is instituted. Desire is desire for desire, the Other's desire . . . subjected to the Law" ("On Freud's '*Trieb*,'" 723).

22. See Lacan's 1954 discussion of foreclosure (here called *excision*) in "Introduction," 308–17, and "Response," 318–33. Writes Lacan, "[Excision's] effect is a symbolic abolition. For, when Freud says, '*Er verwarf sie*,' 'he excises' castration . . . he continues: 'thereby one cannot say that any judgment regarding [castration's] existence was properly made, but it was as if it had never existed. *Verwerfung* thus cut short any manifestation of the symbolic order—that is, it cut short the *Bejahung* that Freud posits as the primary procedure in which the judgment of attribution finds its root, and which is no other than the primordial condition for something from the real to come to offer itself up to the revelation of being, or, to employ Heidegger's language, to be let-be. . . . Freud told us right away that what the subject has thus excised *(verworfen)* . . . from the opening toward being will not be refound in his history, assuming we designate by the latter term the locus in which the repressed manages to reappear. . . . Note how striking the formulation is since there is not the slightest ambiguity in it: the subject *will not want 'to know anything about it in the sense of repression.'* For, in order for him to be able to know something about it in this sense, it would have had to come in some way to light in the primordial symbolization" ("Response," 322–4).

23. Lacan, *Seminar III, The Psychoses*, 32–3.

24. The style of denegation in language can be neurotic ("I don't mean to say that my father was an ass"), psychotic ("God is a huge ass that covers me in excrement") or perverse ("I know my father isn't really a huge ass, but still"). Writes Lacan, "[*denegation*] is the inaugural affirmation, which can no longer recur except through the veiled forms of unconscious speech, for it is only by the negation of the negation that human discourse allows us to return to [being]" ("Response," 323).

25. Lacan, *Seminar I, Freud's Papers on Technique*, 102.

26. Ibid.

27. Though Klein emphasizes the auto-genesis of the split self rather than the role of actual others in its formation, others do play a role in the "reality testing" by which the subject integrates his projections with other people's actual responses. Parent figures that respond in a balanced way to the infant's projections regarding them allow the infant to slowly mitigate its agony of paranoid fear that they will return his aggression, as well as his guilt for wishing to harm them.

28. Klein, "Study of Envy," 216. Writes Klein, "The tendency of the ego to split itself and its object is partly due to the ego lacking cohesion at birth, and partly it is a defense against the primordial anxiety [of the threat of annihilation by the internal death instinct]. I have, for many years, attributed great importance to one particular

process of splitting, the division of the breast [for Klein, the primary object] into a good and bad object. I took this to be an expression of the innate conflict between love and hate and the ensuing anxieties. However, coexisting with this division there appear to be various processes of splitting, such as fragmenting the ego and its objects, whereby a dispersal of the destructive impulses is achieved."

29. Klein, "Notes on Some Schizoid Mechanisms," 11–12. Writes Klein, "The phantasy of forcefully entering the object give rise to anxieties relating to the dangers threatening the subject from within the object. For instance, the impulses to control an object from within it stir up the fear of being controlled and persecuted inside it. . . . The accumulation of anxieties of this nature, in which the ego is . . . caught between a variety of external and internal persecution-situations, is a basic element in paranoia."

30. Ibid., 6. Writes Klein, "It is in phantasy that the infant splits the object and the self, but the effect of this phantasy is a very real one, because it leads to feelings and relations (and later on, thought processes) being in fact cut off from one another."

31. Ibid., 11. Writes Klein, "I have referred to the weakening and impoverishment of the ego resulting from excessive splitting and projective identification. This weakened ego, however, becomes also incapable of assimilating its internal objects, and this leads to the feeling that it is ruled by them. Again, such a weakened ego feels incapable of taking back into itself the parts which it projected into the external world. These various disturbances in the interplay between projection and introjection, which imply excessive splitting of the ego, have a detrimental effect on the relation to the inner and outer world and seem to be at the root of some forms of schizophrenia."

32. Ibid., 5–6. Klein writes, "The result of splitting is a dispersal of the destructive impulse which is felt as the source of danger. I suggest that the primary anxiety of being annihilated by a destructive force within, with the ego's specific response of falling to pieces or splitting itself, may be extremely important in all schizophrenic processes."

33. Ibid., 15. "If development during the paranoid-schizoid position has not proceeded normally and the infant cannot—for internal or external reasons—cope with the impact of depressive anxieties a vicious circle arises. For if persecutory fear, and correspondingly schizoid mechanisms, are too strong, the ego is not capable of working through the depressive position. This forces the ego to regress to the paranoid-schizoid position and reinforces the earlier persecutory fears and schizoid phenomena. Thus the basis is established for various forms of schizophrenia in later life; for when such a regression occurs, not only are the fixation points in the schizoid position reinforced, but there is a danger of greater stages of disintegration setting in."

34. See McMahan, "Buddhist Modernism," 168–9.

35. For instance, the fifth-century Buddhist scholar Buddhaghosa writes, "As [a meditator] cultivates in this way the contemplation of dissolution, the object of which is the cessation consisting in destruction of all formations [*sankhara*, also translated as thought patterns or programs], then formations classed according to all kinds of becoming, generation, destiny, station, or abode of beings, appear to him in the form of a great terror, as lions, tigers, leopards [etc.], appear to a timid man who wants to live in peace." (Buddhaghosa, *Visuddhimagga* (*The Path of Purification*), 673).

36. Adyashanti, *The End of Your World*. Writes Adyashanti, "In awakening, what's revealed to us is that we are not a thing, nor a person, nor even an entity. We are that which manifests as all things, as all experiences, as all personalities. We are that which dreams the whole world into existence. Spiritual awakening reveals that that which is unspeakable and unexplainable is actually what we are" (5).

37. Adyashanti calls these persistent thought patterns "Velcro thoughts." *The End of Your World*, 52–3.

38. Loy, *Nonduality*. Loy argues throughout that descriptions in Buddhist-influenced contemplative traditions of personal dissolution or nothingness (*shunyata*), and in Hindu-influenced traditions of nondifferentiatiated identity with all forms (*Brahman*), may refer to the same experiences of nonduality, described in seemingly opposite terms because of the different philosophical schools from which they emerged and because of the challenges of describing nondifferentiation with differentiated signifiers.

39. See Epstein, *Thoughts*. For an overview of modern and contemporary Buddhism's marriage to psychology, see McMahan, *The Making of Buddhist Modernism*, 52–7, and Payne, "Buddhism and the Powers of the Mind," 234–55.

40. See Epstein, *The Trauma of Everyday Life*.

41. For attachment theory see John Bowlby, *Making and Breaking*, and contemporary psychologist Sue Johnson, "Couple." For relevance realization, see John Vervaeke, Timothy Lillicrap, and Blake Richards, "Relevance Realization," and John Vervaeke and Leonardo Ferraro, "Relevance, Meaning." Indeed, cognitive scientist Vervaeke describes the spectral in popular culture as signaling a collective crisis of meaning just as a psychoanalytic theorist might, though he focuses on the contemporary proliferation of zombie spectacles (*Zombies*).

42. Schreber, *Memoirs*.

43. As Atwood notes, *Abyss*, 37–8. The subject of Freud's *The Schreber Case* (1911/2003), Schreber's *Memoirs of My Nervous Illness*, is also Lacan's primary reference in replacing Freud's theory of cast-away homosexual desire with foreclosed castration as the condition of psychotic potential. For descriptions of soul murder see especially *Memoirs*, 54–61.

44. For the culturally dominant construction of schizophrenia, see the *Diagnostic and Statistical Manual-V*, 99–102. In short, two or more of the following symptoms must be present for a significant portion of time during a one-month period for the diagnosis of schizophrenia to be made. At least one of these must be symptom 1, 2, or 3:

1. Delusions
2. Hallucinations
3. Disorganized speech (e.g. frequent derailment or incoherence)
4. Grossly disorganized or catatonic behavior
5. Negative symptoms (i.e. diminished emotional expression or avolition) (99).

Further, level of functioning must be significantly affected during a portion of this time, continuous (not necessarily acute) signs of the disturbance must persist for at least six months and other possible causes for the disturbance must be ruled out.

45. See Payne, "Buddhism and the Powers of the Mind," 247. Writes Payne, "Neo-romantic popular religious culture promotes a vision of individual personal wholeness [that is] predicated on comprehending the current human condition as pathological. This is a diagnostic prescriptive narrative—commodifying religion as a product needed to cure the pathology diagnosed by religion."

46. Tolle, *New Earth*, 109–10. Writes Tolle, "Although the word [pathological] is normally used to describe a condition of disease, it is derived from *pathos*, which means suffering."

47. Ibid., 11–12.

48. Barnes, *Nightwood* (1937), 32.

49. See Charan, *Srimadbhagavatum*, and the *Bhagavata Purana*, 1.16.20 and 1.8.6.

50. See Gottesman, *Schizophrenia Genesis*, for a case study describing a patient's belief that his psyche is in special alignment with events in the outer world and that he is needed to guide the world to healing and renewal (44–50). Writes Gottesman of David's perspective: As [he was] the Messiah, his psyche mirrored humanity's problems. . . . David's duty was to fulfill God's ultimate goal—to turn Earth into a heavenly kingdom" (48–9). For spiritual framings of such beliefs, see Farber, *The Spiritual Gift of Madness*, 268–74, 362–80; Aurobindo, *Savitri*, 45, 91–2, 197–8.

51. *Samyutta Nikaya* 56.11 (*Dhammacakkappavattana Sutta*); Thānissaro Bhikkhu, *The Shape of Suffering*, 2.

52. *Samyutta Nikaya* 56.11; Thānissaro Bhikkhu, *The Shape of Suffering*, 4.

53. In the cycle that ends in fire, writes Theravadan scholar and monk Ven. Buddhaghosa, it will stop raining, fresh water and oceans will dry up, and the earth will eventually burst into flames. *Visuddhimagga* (*The Path of Purification*), chap. xiii, and Clarke Warren, *Buddhism in Translations*, 321–6.

54. For discussions of apocalyptic and post-apocalyptic visions in modernist and modern texts, including T. S. Eliot's *The Waste Land* and *The Four Quartets* and Lawrence's *Apocalypse*, see Kermode, *The Sense of an Ending*; Tonning, Feldman, and Addyman, *Modernism, Christianity, and Apocalypse*; and Heffernan, *Post-apocalyptic Culture*.

55. See Robinson, *Astral*, *passim*.

56. See, for instance, Lacan, "Instance," 412–41.

57. Loy, *Lack and Transcendence*, 78. Writes Loy, "In my Buddhist terms, the sense of self, being mentally constituted in this way [by association with objects] can never ground itself, yet neither can I help wanting to ground myself as long as I think that I am the sense-of-self: hence my *sense-of-lack*. From this failure, Sartre later derived our need for self-expression, which sublimates the pursuit of self into symbolic expressions such as works of art. Thus for Sartre, as for Freud and Lacan, symbolism is the result of frustration."

58. Lacan, "Function and Field," 206.

59. Butler, *Bodies*, 167.

60. See, for instance, David Loy, *Lack and Transcendance*, and A. H. Almaas, *The Unfolding Now*.

61. Loy, *Lack*, 57. Writes Loy, "One does not do anything with that anguish [primordial lack-as-anguish] except develop the ability to dwell in it or rather *as* it; then

the anguish, having nowhere else to direct itself, consumes the sense-of-self. Since the sense-of-*lack* is the other pole of the sense-of-self . . . primordial *lack*-as-anguish devours not only the ego self but itself."

62. Ibid., 61.

63. Lacan writes, "You can see what becomes of it: *what did not come to light in the symbolic appears in the real.* For that is how we must understand [Freud's] '*Einbeziehung ins Ich*,' taking into the subject, and '*Ausstossung aus dem Ich*,' expelling from the subject. The latter constitutes the real insofar as it is the domain of that which subsists outside of symbolization. This is why castration—which is excised by the subject here from the very limits of what is possible, but which is also thereby withdrawn from the possibilities of speech—appears in the real, erratically" ("Response," 324).

64. For discussion of the nom du père, or phallus, as signifier of castration or lack, see Lacan "Signification" and "Subversion." For its function in psychosis see "On a Question," 481.

65. Flatley, *Affective*, 80.

66. Ibid., 62.

67. Ibid., 80–2.

68. Ibid., 82, citing Adorno, *Aesthetic Theory*, 138.

69. Flatley, *Affective*, 80.

70. Ibid., 2.

71. Ibid., 48.

72. Ibid., 32.

73. Flatley writes that because traces of past others in present others, real or literary, call up our affect, "the fear or joy or shame or whatever one might feel about some inappropriate and hence repressed object can nonetheless make its way into consciousness by attaching itself to some other object" (ibid., 62).

74. Lacan, *Seminar III, The Psychoses*, 250.

75. Writes Lacan, "Every real signifier is, as such [that is, outside of the symbolic order], a signifier that signifies nothing. . . . The more the signifier signifies nothing, the more indestructible it is" (ibid., 185).

76. "The Mindful Revolution" cover story of *Time Magazine*, February 2014, sketches the rapid growth of mindfulness and meditation practices, focusing on America.

77. For instance, Adyashanti writes in *The Way of Liberation*: "We are so busy and obsessed with our restless thinking about everything and everyone that we have mistaken our thinking *about* everything and everyone *for* everything and everyone. This tendency to take our thoughts to be real is what keeps the dream state intact and keeps us trapped within its domain of unconsciousness and strife" (29).

78. Stanislav and Christina Grof, "Spiritual." The writers distinguish between "organic psychoses" which involve "underlying anatomical, physiological, or biochemical changes in the brain or other parts of the organism" and "functional psychoses" for which no medical explanation has been found (3).

79. Ibid., 10.

80. Ibid., 3–20.

81. Ibid., 10–11.

82. Perry, "Spiritual Emergence and Renewal." Writes Perry, "Opposites become vividly constellated. Forces that strive to destroy all existence enter a cosmic conflict with the benign forces or preservation and world regeneration. One pair that is quite distressing is the contrasexual component that arouses feelings of being changed into the other sex (not to be construed as homosexual panic). These are the heavy, frightening, even nightmarish elements in the process of renewal; there are other lighter elements, such as the inflated image of oneself in an apotheosis of hero or heroine, saint, savior, messiah, or king. Here one has the experience of being brought into a *hieros gamos*, a sacred or heavenly marriage with some mythic or divine figure, with all the accompanying exhilaration of erotic emotion. In this messianic role, one also believes oneself especially elected to bring about reforms of religion or society on a world scale thus effecting a significant aspect of world regeneration. The self-image is renewed in a rebirth or sometimes a new birth brought about by the fruitful event of the sacred marriage" (70).

83. James suggests in "Final Impressions of a Psychical Researcher" that supramundane others may collude with their hosts in *personation*, where a subject appears to be "controlled" by another being. Writes James, "My own dramatic sense tends instinctively to picture the situation [of control] as an interaction between slumbering faculties in the automatist's mind and a cosmic environment of other consciousness of some sort which is able to work upon them. If there were in the universe a lot of diffuse soul-stuff, unable of itself to get into consistent personal form, or to take permanent possession of an organism . . . it might get its head in the air, parasitically, so to speak, by peopling weak spots in the armor of human minds, and slipping in and stirring up there the sleeping tendency to personate." Cited in part by Duncan in *The H.D. Book*, Appendix 1, 608. Duncan extends James's term *personation* to argue that we personate ourselves just as the medium personates an "other."

84. Lacan, *Seminar VIII*, 44.

85. Morton, *Hyperobjects*, 1–2.

86. Foucault, *History of Sexuality Volume 1,* especially part V; *Discipline and Punish.*

87. As Lacan observes, "we are constantly raising problems closely related to these notions of internal freedom and of the manifestation of something enclosed within oneself. This point of view comes to a dead end very quickly, given that every type of living reality immersed in the spirit of the modern world's cultural arena is essentially going around in circles" (*Seminar III, The Psychoses*, 134).

88. See, for instance, Sword, *Ghostwriting Modernism*; Tryphonopoulos, *The Celestial Tradition*; Surette, *The Birth of Modernism*; Moody, *Tracing T.S. Eliot's Spirit*; Materer, *Modernist Alchemy*, and Duncan, *The H.D. Book.*

89. Setz, "Trees of Heaven," 137, 145.

90. See Materer, *Modernist Alchemy*; Hobson, "Credulous Readers," in *Incredible Modernism.*

91. See Farber, *The Spiritual Gift of Madness*, on the mad pride movement; for further social and ecocriticism see Žižek, *Living in the End Times*; McPherson and

Baker, *The Extinction Dialogues*: New, *Agency, Health and Social Survival*; and Morton, *Hyperobjects*.

92. Morton, *Hyperobjects*, 27.

93. Ibid., 9.

94. Ibid., 33.

95. For an overview of Lacan's theories of fetishism see Fink, *Clinical Introduction*, 170–93. Perverse and psychotic subjects, writes Fink, engage in attempts to supplement/provide the paternal function that brings the symbolic Other into existence—the perverse subject by staging or enacting the enunciation of the law, the psychotic subject by fomenting a delusional metaphor.

96. Abraham and Torok, *Shell*, 128–32.

97. Ibid., 153.

98. Abraham and Torok write that a crypt forms when "the shameful secret is the love object's doing and when that object also functions for the subject as an ego ideal" (ibid., 131).

99. Ibid., 149–53.

100. Abraham and Torok, see cunnilingus as a fetish.

101. Ibid., 119.

102. Ibid., 133.

103. Ibid., 175.

104. Abraham and Torok use the term "incorporation" to denote the internalization of objects that are not integrated into a coherent sense of self, as Freud suggests is the case in melancholia, and "introjection" to denote the ones that are, as in Freud's concept of mourning.

105. Ibid., 153.

106. Writes Lacan, "Freud thus unveiled the imaginary function of the phallus as the pivotal point in the symbolic process that completes, *in both sexes,* the calling into question of one's sex by the castration complex" ("On a Question," 463).

107. The phrase "traces of direction" is taken from H.D., *Sword*, 130.

108. From the preface to *Magic Mirror, Compassionate Friendship, Thorn Thicket*, by Tryphonopoulos and Robinson, ix. See also Hogue and Vandivere's introduction to *Sword.*

109. Pender and Setz, *Shattered Objects*, 8.

110. Taylor, *Affective Modernism*, 9. Writes Taylor, "For Barnes, traumatic memory . . . is brought into the world through the artistic process and the reader's witnessing, its validity guaranteed by these very conditions or contingencies."

111. Potter, "*Nightwood's* Humans," 65.

112. Barnes, *The Antiphon*, 133.

113. As Herring documents in *Djuna*, 54–9, and "Zadel Barnes," 112–14.

114. From a 1932 fragment quoted in Herring's "Zadel Barnes," 111.

115. See for instance Sherbert, "Hieroglyphics," 117; and Scott, *Refiguring*, 16–17.

116. Herring, "Zadel Barnes,"114.

117. Ibid., 112.

118. Ibid., 112–15; Broe, "My Art," 41.

119. Field, *Djuna*, 43.

120. Herring, *Djuna*, 268–71.
121. Coleman, *Rough Draft*, 305–6.
122. Herring, *Djuna*, 52.
123. O'Neal, *Djuna Barnes*, 30.
124. Abraham and Torok, *Shell*, 128, 154–6, 160.
125. See for instance H.D. scholars Friedman, Chisholm, DuPlessis, Gelpi, Hogue, Vandivere, Keeling, Baccolini; and Barnes scholars Kannenstine, Caselli, Miller, Coffman, Warren, Smith, and Martins.
126. H.D., *Majic Ring*, 59, 160. "Pieces make complete pictures."
127. *Cryptophoria* is not an accepted diagnosis in contemporary institutions that define and regulate mental health; thus, my argument about Barnes may be less relevant to ongoing controversies concerning the power dynamics inherent in diagnosis. Both Barnes's and H.D.'s modes of experience are, in my view, broadly comprehensible and relevant, as I hope my study shows, but I also suggest that some of H.D.'s writing evidences what are labeled as schizophrenic symptoms in the mainstream mental health field.
128. See Lacan, "Signification," *passim*.

Chapter 1

"Now it will soon be over"

Apocalyptic Closure in The Sword Went Out to Sea

I. H.D.'S CRUCI-FICTIONS

My first two chapters focus on works that H.D. saw as culminations of her life: the fictionalized memoir *The Sword Went Out to Sea* (written in 1946–1952, first published in 2007), and the epic poem *Helen in Egypt* (written in 1952–1955, first published in 1961).[1] Both works revisit various significant episodes in H.D.'s life, but are most concerned with her experience in London during and after the Blitz. At this time, she believes that she is receiving coded spirit messages from dead Royal Air Force (RAF) pilots and from a spirit named after *Majic Ring*'s Zakenuto, a male deity H.D. identified with *Sword*'s Z. These messages, if decoded and interpreted correctly, will save the postwar world from nuclear catastrophe and enable its transition into the next world. H.D. believes that Z has already manifested in one of her *héros fatals*, Peter Rodeck, and perhaps now in Dowding. Zakenuto, she writes, is a "Master in modern dress," equivalent in the occultist mythologies that H.D. draws on to a God—even to God the creator.[2] Though Z communicates less than the RAF pilots, she believes him to be somehow involved in their messages. However, the one person H.D. believes capable of decoding and interpreting these messages, Lord Dowding, dismisses them.

H.D. thinks of *The Sword Went Out to Sea* and *Helen in Egypt* as records, framings, and (at this time) culminations of her entire life, the most important parts of which have occurred already, but have yet to be understood and integrated. She believes from 1946 to the end of her life that Lord Dowding (*Sword*'s Lord Howell) is the last and most central of her great loves. She believes this even—or especially—after whatever uncomplicated happiness she finds in this love is shattered by his rejection (in February 1946) of the spirit messages that she communicated to him in letters.

She embeds this rejection within a process she outlines in letters and journals, where she writes that her literary work, including *Sword*, *Helen*, *The Mystery* (written 1948–1951), *Bid Me to Live: A Madrigal* (1918–1948), *The White Rose and the Red* (1947–1949), and *Pilate's Wife* (1929–1934), undertakes a process of personal reintegration by means of its various protagonists' searches. Her characters, who "all are . . . the same woman," look for the scattered pieces of a male "Eternal Lover" who, since he is dismembered, appears as different men.[3] This search, H.D. claims, integrates the heroines' fractured selves and achieves a triumphant conclusion in both *Sword* and *Helen*.[4]

During and after her 1933–1934 psychoanalysis with Freud, when she feels personally responsible for humanity's survival of the Second World War and for the inauguration of a new world era, H.D. imagines a personal integration through writing and psychic vision that would have broader social effects. Her work from 1939–1945 suggests that there is war because of a general lack of social and psychic integration in the world, but that her personal reintegration in writing will stop the war. She pursues the meaning of her relationships, dreams, memories, ideas, and visions, increasingly abstracted from any specific social milieu, through free-associative writing, hoping that this will eventually yield the final answer for everything. She describes her process to Dowding in a 1945 letter as "the weaving of threads from one pattern to another, from one state of being or perception to another," and explains that "the first stage of artistic, integrative work is 'to remember our own personal past' and then to open up 'a very, very wide field' . . . built up on the dream content or the subconscious material."[5] This method of exploring and discovering connections between events, things, words, and people, she believes, has a "wider application," effecting transformation in the broader social world.[6]

In "Advent," (composed of notes taken in 1933 during her analysis with Freud) H.D. writes that "new words" will be required to describe the new psychic terrain that she is uncovering.[7] In accordance with her desire to express these "new states of being" with the free-associative method that Freud encouraged, H.D.'s letters and fiction grow free-associative and word-associative to the point that conceptual meanings and cognitive trajectories often do not coalesce, though she expects that they eventually will. A sacrificial or martyred quality appears along with her new sense of purpose. In 1934, she writes to her lifelong friend and long-term partner Bryher (Annie Winifred Ellerman, 1894–1983), "My whole life, literally, is one pure and perfect crucifiction [sic]. . . . I am not, except in certain hours of writing and in certain hours of FORGETTING writing, ever free."[8] She is begging Bryher not to nag her about her writing, and poet and biographer Barbara Guest has read this passage in terms of her growing demand for autonomy in their relationship.[9] But it is also, I think, meant literally: writing is martyrdom.

The integration of self and word that is to be accomplished in her writing is described in increasingly devastating terms and by circular logic. Her integration in writing is, she intimates, both the cause of, and the solution to, the war. In *Ion* (1937), written with the coming war in mind, she offers an explanation for this conundrum:

> [The goddess Athene] pleas for the great force of the under-mind or unconscious that so often, on the point of blazing upward into the glory of inspirational creative thought, flares, by a sudden law of compensation, down, making for tragedy, disharmony, disruption, disintegration, but in the end, O, in the end, if we have patience to wait, she says, if we have penetration and faith and the desire actually to follow all those hidden subterranean forces, how great is our reward.[10]

Integration of the "conscious" with the "unconscious" is, so often, disintegrative. H.D. must integrate—become conscious of and interpret—her memories in order to stop the war; but the war and the personal suffering associated with it is paradoxically *caused* by her integration—and, through sympathetic association, the world's integration—of unconscious material, especially the primal scene, as Robert Duncan notes.[11] H.D. believes that this devastation will surely end if she follows the subterranean social and psychic forces through their upheavals. But this end, as critics have sometimes noted, is never reached in her writing: everything proffered as a resolution, a frame or pattern that makes sense of everything preceding it, quickly gives way to new problems, new possibilities. As Matte Robinson writes of her late work, "All of H.D.'s powers of analysis, both psychoanalytical and occult, are bent on seeing the clear pattern, reaching the heart of the mystery."[12] But she continues, always, searching for this clear pattern, and attempting to fit the significant people, objects and events in her life into patterns suggested to her by psychoanalysis, myth, occultism, and various objects. Since she sees material objects as holding significant messages for her, H.D. also finds meaningful patterns in them—for example, in the "sun-star" pattern on the *Ghirlanda* tripod table with which she conducted solo séances in her London flat,[13] and the pattern on a Tarot card, the Star, designed by French Martinist author Jean Chaboseau.[14]

Freud's method of analyzing dreams by looking for condensed, displaced and transposed signs and symbols provided H.D. with new motivations and strategies for reading portent into dreams, visions and events—as did the impending war, for whose outcome she felt responsible. This portent stimulated but also burdened her. Her letters to Bryher during her 1933–1934 sessions with Freud are striking in that, for all her excitement about the sessions, the letters themselves grow gloomier and more paranoid. Though the coming war and climate of fear contributed to this unease, its main cause may have been the sessions themselves—especially Freud's pathologization of her Corfu visions, and the authority he lent to the free-associative method that they practiced together. Free association begins to eclipse all other modes of meaning in her writing during this time. Increasingly, objects and events are linked with one another, causes and effects attributed, based on similarities or contiguities that appear incidental from a rational vantage point. One example is H.D.'s recurring association in *Sword* of the spirit Z with bees and graphs, because bees go "zzzz-zzzz" and graphs have jagged lines like the letter Z.[15] This can be understood as the use of metaphor and metonymy in literary expression. Accordingly, Elizabeth Anderson argues that bees in *Sword* represent H.D.'s return "to the beehive and honey as a metaphor for resurrection."[16] However, *Sword* evidences a more literal than figurative understanding of the associations between bees and other things. Anderson cites one reference to bees: the other references in *Sword* and *Helen in Egypt* do not allude to resurrection, but to the RAF pilots,[17] to graphs, maps or lines,[18] to pleated time,[19] and to Z,[20] in ways that suggest that there is something literal and universally relevant yet to be understood in their association. Associative clustering is a part of the creative process for many artists, but usually without the wish to fix these correspondences into an objectively true system of relationships, or to find out what they mean objectively apart from what they evoke subjectively. H.D.'s writing suggests an increasingly painful struggle to fix and close an ever expanding nebula of free association, and the growing idea that literal destruction, of herself or others, may accomplish this closure.

Along with this loosening of distinction and precision after her analysis, H.D. sees victimization and death—that is, loss of self—everywhere. She is preoccupied with the cult of occultist Aleister Crowley (1875–1947), whom she had never met or communicated with, and his troubling role in the lives of her former lover, Frances Gregg, and another acquaintance, the writer Mary Butts. The possibility of her own blackmail by Crowley or someone associated with him looms large in her imagination. The symptoms that appear in H.D.'s journals and creative writing as well as in records of her life might suggest to clinicians the slow onset of paranoid schizophrenic symptoms starting in 1934, leading to an "active phase" during her breakdown in 1946–1947, followed by remission.[21] The symptoms that must be present for this diagnosis, including persistent delusional beliefs and disorganized speech and writing, continue to appear in work and journals written after 1946, such as *Sword* and *Helen*.[22] For H.D., these beliefs are messianic: she believed in the paramount importance of her own personal integration to the world's salvation, and feared at times that this process might be personally lethal. H.D.'s written elaborations of unlikely seeming explanations of others' intentions and actions, and her inclusion of many unclearly related elements as relevant to a mysterious cosmic plan, suggest a confusion of inner and outer worlds.

Increasingly elaborated theories regarding others' intentions, and proliferations of unclear associations, are read as possible symptoms of psychosis not only by Lacan but also within the field of conventional mental health practice.[23] Linguistic clarity, precision, and organization of cause and effect may be the result, psychologist Norman Cameron suggests, of a limit to possibility, a limit that is lacking in *Sword* and *Helen*.[24] Likewise, Relevance Realization theorists John Vervaeke and Leonardo Ferraro describe mental health as the (usually preconscious) capacity to frame what is relevant to our functioning and well-being at any given time and limit our attention to what is not; they describe mental illness, or "parasitic processing," as beginning with a misrecognition of the irrelevant as relevant, followed by the development of maladaptive feedback loops of thought and attention that interfere with, or take over, our capacity to frame what is relevant and exclude from consideration what is irrelevant.[25]

After 1946, H.D. tends to imagine the personal and world integration she seeks not as a solo endeavor but as involving a return to the primal scene: a sexualized attack, perhaps martyrdom, perpetrated by God, or a fatal hero, or both. She came to believe during exploration of her "primal scenes" with Freud that to be a woman is, at an unconscious level, to be killed by a man—since for Freud a proper woman was, or wanted to be, the consort of a man. For H.D., to have and/or to be a child is first to die: "My child is a golden Christ-child off the Xmas tree, all very clear at the age of seven. But child meant primal scene, meant being 'killed' by a man, the father."[26] Sex with the father kills, though the offspring is messianic. The "child" is Christ, the mother destroyed; H.D. is both. "Eros and Death," which she describes in *Tribute* as "the only subjects of [Freud's] eternal preoccupation" emerge ever more as her own themes, and are associated respectively with the mother and the father, whose violent lovemaking suggests Freud's conceptual conflation of the two drives.[27]

H.D. writes that because of the early "loss" (as she sees it) of both of her parents, she also contains the male principle, and her love life is, thus, built on mixed together love and violence: "I did LOOSE [sic] both parents at the age of 3 or 4 and built up my whole love life on that love and terror mixed, and violence as of war etc."[28] During her sessions with Freud, at least, H.D. believed that this loss was the source of her bisexuality: "it was simply the loss of both parents, and a sort of perfect bi-sexual attitude arises. . . . I have tried to be the man, or woman, but I have to be both. But it will work out, papa [Freud] says and I said, now in writing."[29] Through writing, the parents will on some level be regained, the mixture of love and terror on which her love life is founded will stabilize: "So in me, two distinct racial or biological or psychological entities tend to grow nearer or to blend, even as time heals old breaks in consciousness."[30]

In *The Gift* (written 1941–1943) and *Tribute to Freud* H.D. presumably contained the male principle within herself, and at any rate did not need a particular relationship to integrate with it. However, in the work following her encounter with Dowding, this "distinct racial or biological or psychological entity" is found in him. The forces of *Eros, Eris* that are supposed to become integrated seem, if anything, more polarized, and the method by which H.D. seeks this integration seems itself disintegrative. Its lack of success is also suggested by H.D.'s long (though not continuous) residency in Klinik Brunner after her 1946 breakdown, and her move after its closure in 1961 to the Klinik Hirslanden, in Zürich, where she resided until her death. Although her later time in these facilities was voluntary, and she saw herself more as a colleague to her doctors than as a patient, her doctors continued to treat her as a patient: monitoring her, screening her correspondence, administering medication, and even restricting her social interactions.[31]

H.D.'s search for the eternal lover attempts to integrate inadequate scientific father figures, mysterious psychic mother figures, Oedipal-complexed sons, and unrecognized, messianic daughters. These figures represent her attempts to work through in writing her responses to her family. She identifies with the daughter's confusion over her maddeningly unforthcoming mother as well as the father's and the son's sexual aggression toward the mother. She seeks, most of all, to identify with the mother, for to do so would be to understand her silence.[32] These figures are all ultimately part of H.D. and thus require psychic reintegration through her writing, memories, and relationships with others. Her typology of primal, Oedipal fathers and sons and psychic, desirable mother and daughters is marshaled to explain the behavior of the men who mattered to her—especially Dowding, who is identified in *Sword* and *Helen* with both son and father, just as H.D., herself, is identified with both mother and daughter.

Toward the end of the Second World War, H.D. feels unsatisfied with writing and introspection as responses to it, and she comes to believe that her special destiny requires something more socially active. Many Londoners at this time attend séances or consult automatic writers, hoping to connect with loved ones lost in the war or with hope itself; many fear greater world devastation to come and seek guidance from friendly spirits.[33] Though not quite mainstream, this "psychical research" is viewed as worthy of serious consideration by arbiters of culture such as William James, Freud, Yeats, and Carl Jung (1875–1961), among many others. In the period 1944–1946, H.D. comes to believe that her destiny, undisclosed by mundane events, involves the agenda of the spirits, Z, and deceased RAF pilots who had been under Dowding's command during the war, and whose messages she believes she is receiving during séances that she first attends in 1943, and then conducts alone during 1945–1946. H.D. believes that these spirit messages concern a globally crucial defense operation involving psychic research, which she and Dowding must work on together.

The Sword Went Out to Sea is a "spiritual autobiography" arising from H.D.'s experiences of the First and especially the Second World War during her time in London.[34] Though it was written under H.D.'s spiritual and pen name Delia Alton and is largely narrated in the first person by its chief protagonist Delia Alton, I will be distinguishing the author as H.D. and the protagonist-narrator as Delia to the extent that this is possible. *Sword*'s principal characters and events are taken from H.D.'s life, as she writes to Norman Holmes Pearson in 1948:

> I have been so very happy with this "novel." I am writing it under a real *nom de plume* [i.e., Delia Alton], I mean, one that fits me and fits the book, so it is not actually H.D. writing it. Not that it really matters. It started—the *nom de guerre* (literally), as I wrote a volume about the experience in this war and last war, myself and friends in London, and it is too near and too intimate for H.D.; anyhow, I could not have written it as H.D. All this in time, I call the first volume *The Sword Went Out to Sea* (Synthesis of a Dream), a quote from W[illiam] Morris, the Sword, I mean . . . the main guy in the book is a certain Lord Howell and in "life," he was and still is an active acting real person.[35]

H.D. states in letters and journals, and research confirms, that *Sword* renders her most charged psychic experiences and relationships, mirroring her actual spirit messages and communications with Dowding, and her thoughts regarding their meaning and her destiny. She calls *Sword* "my first record or recording of the War II story,"[36] and ascribes her use of the pen name, Delia Alton, to its content being so "near and intimate" that she "could not have written it as H.D."[37] *Sword*'s Delia "is" H.D., especially in her capacity as psychic and visionary.

Sword is derived in part from notes taken during her 1943–1946 séances, notes she destroyed in 1947, probably after finishing *Sword*'s first draft.[38] Though these original notes, which she transmitted to Dowding in letters, are lost, and only one original letter from her to Dowding is extant, the lost letters are transcribed in her edited collection of letters and notes, *Majic Ring*. H.D. introduces *Majic Ring* as "Carbon copies of letters to Lord D.—1943—& notes with A.B. [H.D.'s medium for a time, Arthur Bhaduri]—1944."[39] These copies are very similar to the letters that Delia Alton struggles to convey to Lord Howell in *Sword*.

The events that *Sword* is chiefly concerned with, and which lead up to its composition, are as follows. In 1943–1944, H.D. lives in war-torn London and regularly holds a séance circle led by medium Arthur Bhaduri, whom she meets through a "psychic-research society." The circle also includes Bryher and Bhaduri's mother. They receive messages from a "K" and a "Z."[40] In 1943, H.D. attends a lecture given by Dowding. She has, before the lecture, already read several of his spiritualist articles and one book, *Many Mansions*.[41] Dowding speaks on his continuing séance communications with the RAF pilots he commanded, who died in the Battle of Britain. Afterward, H.D. sends him a note asking if she may join his séance circle, and he cordially responds that they are not taking new members but that this might change in the future. She initiates an occasional correspondence through "little notes," as Bhaduri recommends.[42]

H.D.'s séance journals show that she is romantically taken with Dowding at this time, and that Bhaduri affirms to her that they have some special connection and might be united in "the fire of divine love" in the future; however, Dowding and H.D. do nothing more than exchange notes until 1945.[43] In late 1944, H.D. comes to believe that she herself, in the lone séances that she begins conducting, is receiving coded spirit messages intended for Dowding from these same RAF pilots. She cannot decipher them, but is quite sure (if *Sword* renders this correctly, as it very likely does) that they concern an impending nuclear war and a crucial defense operation involving psychic radio communication. Action must be taken to prepare humanity for the coming cataclysm and world transition, which in *Sword* is called *Thermopylae*. To her it is critical that Dowding decipher her messages, since she cannot, and somehow implement their coded instructions. During 1945–1946, Dowding visits her several times for tea, and they discuss spiritualism and the messages, which she also communicates to him in letters.[44] Dowding's response to H.D.'s letters is at first one of reserved interest, but the reservations increasingly outweigh the interest. Eventually, in February 1946, Dowding writes a letter rejecting her messages, suggesting concern for her emotional balance, and denying knowledge of the RAF pilots named by H.D. He writes,

> Dear Mrs. Aldington,
>
> No. I am sorry, but I am not coming to join you in the reception of this sort of message.
>
> I don't know who Charles is, or Roland, or John, or anyone, but the whole tone is trivial and uninspiring. I know it is none of my business, but I hope you are not communicating by yourself, that you are availing yourself of the balancing presence of your friend Bryher.
>
> Solitary communication is liable to be very dangerous except upon the highest wave lengths. I am sorry that I cannot meet your wishes, but I hope that you will take my advice.

Yours sincerely,

Dowding.[45]

This letter is slightly less terse than, but similar to, the one that *Sword*'s Howell writes Delia: "No. I can not be expected to receive messages of this sort. They are both frivolous and uninspiring. Of course, it is none of my business, but it would be better if you gave up this work" (37).

Dowding himself thought that he was receiving messages from the RAF pilots who died under his command in the Battle of Britain, as H.D. knew from the 1943 lecture of his that she attended, as well as from his published accounts, before she began receiving her own RAF messages.[46] Dowding had apparently been very fond of his pilots, calling them "my boys" and "my chicks."[47] He also believed that his séance circle was receiving messages from a spirit identified as "Z." It is not hard to imagine that cryptic and sometimes loving messages, ostensibly from these same spirits, coming from a woman who, although she barely knew him, seemed to hope for a great deal, might have provoked him. Perhaps, by mirroring his "authentic" RAF messages in what appeared to him an inauthentic register, or by their undercurrent of neediness, H.D.'s communications challenged Dowding's faith in the authenticity of his own spirit messages or reflected emotional needs of his own that they may have helped him to meet, and so prompted him to validate his messages by invalidating hers.

From a psychoanalytic perspective, it is significant that Dowding assumes the role of tyrannical and absent father, claiming a position of spiritual authority that he refuses to share with H.D., and pursuing a psychic-research agenda that does not include her. Dowding makes clear that H.D.'s own spirit messages do not carry authority for him because significant messages would come from his own circle. "You see," he writes after she first mentions the spirit guide Z, "we are in touch with Z in our own circle, & so it is only natural that we should devote our principal attention to what he tells us there."[48] He even suggests—again, if *Sword* renders it accurately—that H.D.'s RAF messages were coming from "beings of a lower order" (32, 33, 97) that could "upset the balance of the world" (32). Dowding reproduces the delegitimizing response that H.D. had already perceived in Freud, Peter Rodeck, her mother, and Havelock Ellis, and that so preoccupies her. He claims access to symbolic authority—spiritual beings who help regulate the balance of the world—and attributes to H.D. the "lower" beings who might "upset" this balance. As Delia puts in in *Sword*, "not only did he repudiate the messages themselves and me, as the bearer of the messages, but he repudiated the fact of the messages and their whole content, as not being 'of any importance'" (33). Later that February, 1946, H.D. suffers psychological collapse and is moved by Bryher to Klinik Brunner, where her recovery is intermittent: in September of that year she receives electroshock treatment.[49]

In "Wintersleep," the first book of *Sword*, Dowding is chiefly represented by Lord Howell, a person "peculiarly fitted to judge and assess the findings of psychic-research workers" that others can only "approach . . . subjectively" (68). Delia, H.D.'s chief representative in this section, receives coded psychic communications, consisting of "numbers and letters" (35), and/or "dots and dashes" (105), from dead RAF pilots once under Howell's command. She cannot decipher this code, but believes he must decipher it because the messages are crucial to the impending transition from this era to the next. The pilots, writes Delia, "said that I would 'hear' [the code] but that he could understand it. They wanted Lord Howell and myself to work together" (139). This union of her perception and his understanding is necessary for the anticipated advent of world destruction and the correlative transition to the next world, which she calls *Thermopylae*:

> I was looking for the perfect image in time, superimposed on a dramatic personification or a character in a book, out of time, or in the world of imagination, poetry, or drama. When, after hearing Lord Howell lecture . . . I began to wonder how it was that he and a handful of RAF pilots had saved . . . civilization, I realized the possibility of an outstanding contemporary figure acting, as it were, or re-living a story already told. I spoke of this story as an actual historical event; I called it *Thermopylae* (100).

II. WAKING DREAMS OF CATACLYSM

Delia Alton interprets the war, and Lord Howell's and other men's dismissals of her visionary experiences by placing the men and their actions within constantly expanding interpretive frameworks. *Sword*'s form, style, and narrative(s) are very fragmented and difficult to follow: as Guest writes, "nearly impossible to decipher."[50] The connection of its parts—one sentence, paragraph, chapter to the others—is often unclear: it teems with events, objects and human, supernatural and legendary beings that are often only nominally rendered and that have no clear part in any narrative. Whether they appear as actual characters, objects, or scenes, or are referenced by a character, most of these beings, objects, places, and events appear only briefly, at least in each of their particular nominal forms, and though they may reappear elsewhere as superficially different, they remain mysteriously identical. Delia literally *is* the book's other heroines who flicker by in "Summerdream": Artemis, Hippolyta, the Painted Lady, Stella, Ariadne, Day-Star, Blanchefleur, Rose

Beauvais, Queen Elizabeth, Helen of Troy. These names signal not so much distinct characters or stories as the repetition of the historically significant encounter in Delia's "past lives" (123) with male consorts. Delia is the latest incarnation in this repeating encounter, just as Lord Howell is the present incarnation of the male hero-consorts who also appear and disappear with little more than an ill-tempered remark—or not even that: Pericles, Pylades, Julius Caesar, Normandy, I-command (no other name given), Prince Lontain, Thomas Moore, Essex, Hippolytus, and Achilles. Other significant male characters include Z and Hal Birth, who appears in medium Ben Masini's séance visions and Delia's thoughts. His role is not evident, but he is identified as the Viking Eric Ericson (reference unclear), and also the craftsman and writer William Morris (1834–1896). *Sword*'s multitude of quickly appearing and disappearing characters, objects, places, and events is cognitively overwhelming, notwithstanding Hogue and Vandivere's 2007 explanatory introduction and their three-page-long key (liv-lvi) to which characters represent which real people. As Anderson writes, *Sword*'s "dreams, séances, memories and interlocking fictional vignettes from different epochs are layered together in a jumble of dialogue, imagery and reverie with little exposition to guide the reader."[51]

This lack of guidance may equally trouble the author/protagonist, Delia, who does not seem to find, in the associative nominal chains she ponders, the meaning she seeks. She finds instead flickering patterns and signs that perpetually "ghost for" this hidden meaning, which may mean for her that they signify it incompletely. In *Sword*'s dreamlike realm, everything that appears is intermediate to this final imagined meaning. The fact that many beings and things appear as names with little else attached to them, besides other names, contributes to this ghostly quality; it is as if their substance lies elsewhere. In *Tribute to Freud*, H.D. describes signification in dreams as "ghosting":

> The [unidentified] boys in the dream . . . are ghosts. They are, that is, "ghosting" for another or others; when the ghosts take form as brothers or as uncle-father, it will no doubt be seen that they again are ghosting. Or rather if we pursue the dream content, the intermediate ghosts, should they manifest, would be seen to be a step between brothers or uncle-father. We are all haunted houses.[52]

As in dreams, so in *Sword*, too, ghosts and ghostly language signal something or someone yet to appear in complete form—and since their signification is incomplete, it is not clear who or what they may be.

Sword was drafted in 1946–1947, during and after H.D.'s first, and initially involuntary, stay in Klinik Brunner following her 1946 breakdown. H.D. continued to revise it until 1952, although she unsuccessfully attempted to publish it in 1950. "Wintersleep" was composed in Klinik Brunner and Lausanne;

the second book, "Summerdream," in Lausanne and Lugano, locations where she (respectively) wintered and summered. "Wintersleep" is mainly a first-person account of Delia's experiences during and after the war. It details her group and individual séances, her betrayal by Geoffrey, her encounters with Peter Van Eck and Tom Moore and, most of all, her attempts to associate with Lord Howell, to communicate her RAF spirit messages to him, and to understand why he repudiates them. These encounters have direct autobiographical parallels, as I have discussed. Like Delia and Howell, H.D. and Dowding met and exchanged letters concerning RAF spirit messages. Dowding ended their correspondence with an only slightly gentler version of Howell's short letter (37). As in Delia's life, too, H.D. and her husband Richard Aldington (Geoffrey) separated over his affair with Dorothy Yorke (Miranda), and H.D. and acquaintance Peter Rodeck (Peter Van Eck) met on a sea voyage, only to part suddenly. While Bryher appears briefly as "Gareth" and *Sword* is dedicated to her, she does not appear as a romantic interest or as an object-cause of the thought patterns I study, and so will not be a focus in my reading.

In "Wintersleep" Delia revisits scenes with men she cared for and lost, attempting to place them in some kind of order in relation to one another and to determine the motivations of Howell and of the numerous other Dowding-based characters. Never fully satisfied with the personal motivations that she considers as possibilities, she also considers that their rejections are not personal or even fully intentional, but part of something preordained by enigmatic powers: a cosmic "plan" (124, 127, 257), "play" (266–7), "mystery-play" (106), or "story" (7, 69). "Summerdream" begins on the same track, with Delia's thoughts pertaining to Howell's motivation, but moves into a sequence of other female protagonists who are, Delia suggests, her past-life incarnations. "Summerdream" depicts the scenes of the plan, story or play to which "Wintersleep" alludes. This play consists of the past-life scenes of other rejections of Delia's various incarnations by Howell's, scenes that are by extension rejections of H.D.–based heroines by Dowding-based heroes. These heroes and heroines, and vague, often unspecified fragments of histories and legends, succeed one another from chapter to chapter. In each, the heroine-narrator has an encounter, or reflects on an encounter, with an enigmatically rejecting, betraying, obtuse, difficult, and/or absent man who (like Dowding) is a key player at that historical or legendary moment. "None of them," records an unnamed heroine, "had the absolute choice of the place and the time of their returning," but "they would be swept back together" (175). Each chapter of "Summerdream" is set in its own minimally rendered myth, legend, or historical period, though it is not always clear which one, who the narrator is, or what is going on in the broader social context. In these chapters, the hero's conscious motivations, though still sometimes considered, are also imagined as irrelevant since his actions are preordained. "Summerdream" ends with a brief return to London in 1947, where "we," (antecedent unspecified but presumably the characters who enact each of these episodes, or this recurring episode in different settings) "went on with the play" (266–7).

In "Wintersleep," Delia recognizes Howell as the latest incarnation of the heroes of history, poetry, and drama who enabled the "turn-about or turn-over" (174) of "one civilization or one era to another," in conjunction with her own past incarnations. *Thermopylae*, the world transition that repeats in the cosmic play, once again requires their union. The assault on this vision that Howell's response to Delia's messages entails causes her breakdown: The "slow poison" that his "doubt and repudiation had dripped . . . into [Delia's] brain" took effect "after his last letter, dismissing my communications as 'frivolous and uninspiring.'. . . It was then that I visualized the streets of gibbets. It was then that I walked, eyes wide open, into hell" (95). One of "Summerdream's" unnamed heroines suggests, however, that each couple maintains their function of enabling world transition in spite of their seeming alienation: "The point was, to get them both together at the turn of the tide—I mean, the turn-about or turn-over of one civilization or one era to another. . . . All that mattered, was to get them both together. When the message came she would receive it, he would carry it out" (174). Indeed, this transition may be enabled *because* of the heroine's devastation by the hero: "For the supreme moment, one had to be prepared to make the sacrifice, to sacrifice in fact, everything but the message. . . . She [name not given] had sacrificed the supreme moment—or shall we say, she had been its sacrifice? . . . Her whole life had been a preparation, though she did not know it" (175).

However, "Summerdream's" unrelenting bleakness, many repetitions and large cast of incarnations, and the ambiguous "meaning" found in each betrayal implies a dissatisfaction—or at least an unusual kind of satisfaction—in Delia's interpretations. In both books, explanations of the rejections do not progress, as one might expect in an evolutionary sequence of incarnations and world eras, but rather co-exist and repeat statically, as do the rejections themselves. Delia's satisfaction in them is, by her own description, inert:

> I was not . . . completely satisfied with my explanation of his attitude to myself and the RAF messages, until I saw him as part of that world of poetry. The picture [of Howell alone on a ship] satisfied me. But my satisfaction was of something not so much dead, as frozen, final, static, and irrevocable. (155)

Howell's repudiation becomes part of something greater, the "world of poetry," and this makes her "explanation" of it satisfactory in a "frozen, final" way. The frozen irrevocability of Delia's picture appears in "Wintersleep" as irrevocable repetition and schematization, the constant return to the event of her invalidation and the attempt to schematize it into the final, fixed "pattern of my life" (104). This "pattern" is visual and spatial as well as temporal, but never stable or complete—it constantly changes. The inexpressibly meaningful visual patterns by which Delia schematizes or "explains" the repudiation become, in "Summerdream," inexpressibly meaningful behavior patterns, enacted by ever new incarnations of couples, who nevertheless do "not change much" (175)—particularly the man. This fixed relationship pattern of Howell's and Delia's past incarnations at transitional historical and legendary periods is the "mystery-play":

> It was a mystery-play, it would explain everything. Death would appear, in his familiar trappings. Plague, War, and Famine would be his Apocryphal companions. . . . I, myself, might be asked to walk on, in a crowd scene. . . . There was a stage-clap of thunder. There was a mechanical flight of winged devils. . . . Then the curtain dropped and there was a brief interlude. We heard the roll of drums, the blare of silver trumpets. At last, I had a place in the vast pageant and a place that was near the altar. (106)

Delia trumps the destructive force of Howell's dismissal by placing it in the repeating epochal drama suggested by her psychic insights and buttressed by occultist cosmologies. Their vexed relationship represents the "meaning" of the mystery-play—though not to her satisfaction. Delia is here, as Robinson shows, drawing on Gnostic, Rosicrucian, and Neo-Platonic belief systems wherein creation is an apparently meaningless play orchestrated by a demiurge.[53] However, there is more than a belief system behind the power of this recurring pattern in her later writing.

Psychic fragmentation and a wish for resolution, as well as occultism and anti-hegemonic experimentalism, shape Delia's interpretive project and her expectation of apocalypse. In *Sword*, the psychic splitting that H.D.'s language, characters, and objects give shape to is envisioned as ending with the splitting of the atom. Her syncretic apocalypticism, in which destruction is seen as the means to union, may be read as a wish to subjectively integrate the symbolic order—the order of language—with the imaginary order, the unity and boundlessness experienced (sometimes frighteningly) in the absence of language. Lacan's description of the "imaginary cataclysm" at the onset of psychosis could serve as a frame for *Sword*'s context, form, and content. For Lacan the psychotic break is triggered by

> the question of the subject's access to a signifier as such and . . . the impossibility of that access. . . . There follows a process whose first stage we have called imaginary cataclysm. . . . Then there is the separate deployment and bringing into play of the entire signifying apparatus—dissociation, fragmentation, mobilization of the signifier as speech, ejaculatory speech that is insignificant or too significant, laden with nonmeaningfulness, the decomposition of internal

> discourse, which marks the entire structure of psychosis. After the encounter, the collision with the inassimilable signifier, it [the signifier as such] has to be reconstituted, since this father cannot be simply a father.[54]

This description of imaginary cataclysm fits H.D.'s written response in *Sword* to Dowding's "*coup de grâce*," as Delia calls it there (86, 92). This perhaps placed into question her "access to a signifier as such" (which Lacan identifies with the phallus), since it both suggests that she cannot hold authority and represents a difference she cannot assimilate. In *Sword*, H.D. "reconstitutes" the inassimilable signifier, Dowding's rejection, as the return of a preordained cycle of sexualized violence and betrayal. She suggests further that this meaningful event is the solution to the drift of her words from their meanings. Nonetheless, it is also unsatisfying, so it appears that she hungers for the more final "integration" that she believes must follow.

III. PROLIFERATION AND THE COUP

Delia's messages and Howell's *coup de grâce* give rise to a disheveled transhistorical, transnational metanarrative that links the repressed content of the unconscious to the supernatural. Past lives, clairvoyant visions, unknown countries, languages, symbols, myths, Greek drama, English poetry, anagrams, cryptograms, graphs, and maps are all invoked as slippery reference points in an interpretive cataclysm that can never conclude because it excludes nothing from consideration. *Sword*'s heroines' relationships with their male counterparts appear as the point of vexed union for disparate principles: war and love, reason and intuition, masculine and feminine, social and psychic. Over and over, male war heroes and scions of the social order betray and brutally deny Delia and her other incarnations. Here, as Duncan writes of H.D.'s World War II writing, "The events of the London Blitz illustrate the wrath of the Father, and the arguments of the pro-war forces in English society . . . reappear as voices of the Protestant Ethic, the very spirit of industrial and commercial capitalism, in its attack on art, sexuality and Woman."[55] Dowding's rejection and World War II dovetail into a vision of a violence that is gendered, sexual and lethal, global and personal. Delia, who mentions "Hokusai" (perhaps the artist Katsushika Hokusai, 1760–1849) and Hiroshima only once, as with many other personages, things, and events in *Sword*, reflects,

> Hokusai, the most familiar of the Japanese masters, no doubt, by some magic of association, negated Hiroshima. I had felt the scar. The earth was furrowed with the irrational assaults that man had made upon her. She was always

> mother-earth. I felt that man was actually assaulting woman. I happened to be a woman. (54)

H.D., speaking as Delia, identifies with the earth assaulted by man. As Dowding is her last love and betrayer (as she thinks at the time), so the coming third war will be the last war, the final assault on herself and on the world before it cracks open and gives birth to a new era. Perhaps like Hokusai, she may "by some magic of association" negate the nuclear explosions to come. Yet, her vision of the end of the world is tinged with a vast relief: "Secret tunnels had been mined across Europe. I thought, 'I'm glad it has happened now, this is the third war and now it will soon be over'" (51).

Though the impact of the war on H.D.'s thinking at this time is apparent, her vision of world cataclysm after Dowding dismisses her messages also suggests what will call after Lacan the return from without of castration, normally internalized as entry into the symbolic order. In *Sword*, castration returns from without as endlessly repeating personal attacks and rejections directed at H.D. figures and at the earth by men, representatives of the symbolic order, and their wars. But this encounter with the father figure always remains imaginary; it is never internalized in the sense that it "takes hold" in the more widely agreed upon world. It is always the men, never the H.D. figures, who are limited, misguided in their views, and perhaps controlled by the divine being who choreographs the play. The failure of *Sword*'s heroes and heroines to understand and accommodate one another's perspectives parallels the alienation of words from their meanings in Delia's interpretive quest.

In his 1955–1956 seminar, Lacan describes a similar deferral of meaning in Schreber's use of language, wherein Schreber invokes meanings not evident, but presumed to exist, and emanating from a God he perceives as threatening. However, "the real" of God as the Big Other, the guarantor of law and meaning, is God as small other: lawless and seemingly ignorant of the meaning that he is supposed to guarantee. What maintains God's existence at all, Schreber's text suggests, is God's presumed knowledge of the meaning of His own enigmatic speech (directed at Schreber by means of talking rays) and strange creations, the "diversionary phenomena," that he deploys to torment Schreber. If God is "essentially language,"[56] at least in psychosis, one could speculate that the continual production of meaningless language maintains the possibility, for Schreber, of meaningful language. Such meaningful language is imaginable by maintaining the possible existence of God—who may yet prove to understand these ghost words. Writes Lacan,

> Here, both in the [psychotic] subject's relation to language and in the imaginary world, there is a danger, which he is constantly aware of, that all this

> fantasmagoria might be reduced to a unity that doesn't annihilate his existence, but God's, which is essentially language. . . . It is at all times necessary to produce diversionary phenomena so that God is not absorbed back into the central existence of the subject.[57]

God is connected to Schreber, more closely than either of them like, through "rays."[58] Without these rays' constant, nonsensical speech and multifarious other devices for reducing Schreber's power of attraction for God, there would be no God separate from Schreber, no one who might be capable of knowing the meaning of utterances that are nonsense to Schreber.[59] Speech, thought, and writing would cease to be even potentially meaningful without the constant elaboration and repetition that keeps God at a distance. They would simply be, as language already almost is, uncomfortable processes occurring in Schreber's body. Each of God's body-destroying "miracles," usually intended to weaken Schreber's attractiveness to him, is accomplished by the speaking rays: that is, through a repeated phrase that acts directly on Schreber's nerves. For instance, the diminution of his bodily stature is "always accompanied by the announcement, 'I wonder whether to make you somewhat smaller.'"[60] Most of the miracles are painful, but still better, Schreber suggests, than the endless nonsense of the rays themselves.

Lacan explains Schreber's narrative with the theory that he has foreclosed castration, experiencing it as external interference by God that transforms him into a woman and destroys his autonomy. For Lacan, the phallus gives an illusion of separateness "only when veiled"—that is, when it becomes a sign of the rift between signifier and signified, where "normal" modern subjects mistakenly imagine autonomy.[61] The foreclosed phallus/castration (for Lacan), or God (for Schreber) attacks this autonomy in the personal register.

In *Sword*, H.D. gives the male characters based on Lord Dowding a similar role to Schreber's God.[62] Such characters are the arbiters and agents of a meaning and plan that Delia and the other autobiographical characters can apprehend as only vague and elusive—though Delia has more hope than Schreber does that everything is ultimately for the best, and not merely the result of God's sexual weakness and bad judgment. However, like Schreber's God, Delia's male consorts are really quite bungling and conflicted, perhaps too interested in maintaining the dysfunctional present order and not sufficiently aware of reality to manage the world's renewal on their own. Schreber and Delia must think the thoughts, and surrender to the cruelty, that will enable them, probably through martyrdom, eventually to bring about such renewal.

Contemporary historian and theorist Eric Santner (b. 1955), building on Žižek's adaption of Lacan's work to political theory, reads the return of foreclosed social content in Schreber's identifications with marginalized others and martyrdom to God. Schreber writes in his *Memoirs* that his feminine "voluptuousness" attracts God's injuring, castrating "rays" and causes God to draw too near the earth, but the skewed world order perpetuated by this proximity will be healed at the time of his death "at the latest."[63] For Santner, Schreber's delusions represent a "crisis of symbolic investiture," where what is excluded from Schreber's society of late nineteenth-century Wilhelmine Germany returns in his physical experience and preoccupations. This socially foreclosed content includes the feminine, the sexual, and the Jewish. It includes also the understanding, enacted in Schreber's molestation by God, that the symbolic order, which establishes the difference between one person and another, is itself set in place by invasive and regulatory manipulations of the subject's mind and body, beginning with his father and continuing through other figures and institutions invested with symbolic authority: the understanding that, as Lacan might put it, the law is also the destruction of the law.[64] H.D.'s vision of possession by God, ghosts, and spirits is similar to Schreber's in that both evidence the impingement of something unassimilable into psychic life. They evidence, too, the knowledge that the social order is unable to protect them from the awful shadow of its unseen power.

As well as noting the vision of sexualized infringement by gods, or by beings controlled by gods, that Schreber shares with some of H.D.'s protagonists, I also draw on the *Memoirs* to highlight what critics have understood as Schreber's unintentional social commentary. While Schreber's delusions, as Eric Santner has argued, give form (Schreber's own body) to the others of late nineteenth-century German ideology, Santner does not argue that Schreber consciously intends this. He argues, on the contrary, that Schreber embodies the German ideological other without intending to; rather, he constructs his otherness in terms of the literal relations between his own body and God, his sometime doctor Professor Flechsig, and the skewed Order of the World.[65] Like the *Memoirs*, H.D.'s later prose, generally understood as intentionally counter-hegemonic, may also evidence a lack or a different kind of intentionality. Critics have already, with terminology different from Santner's, drawn attention to H.D.'s marginal identifications and her reinscriptions of the violence of oppression, but Schreber's embodied, inadvertently symbolic way of registering social violence might also be found in H.D.'s rendering of the recurring, history-making attack of heroes and gods on heroines identified with herself. Both may give body to an experience of patriarchal violence that, for most of us, remains unconscious.

In *Sword*'s hyperbolic formalism, meaning never stabilizes in words, but is imagined as perpetually beyond them. Language "ghosts for" the meaning it never fully expresses. The union of heroine and hero, the communion of his orderly understanding with her depth perception represents a return to the safer shores of a stable language—a return of meaning, identified with the next world that will soon, Delia is sure, replace the nearly defunct present one. In the meantime, Delia's constantly expanding frame of reference maintains the possibility of meaning. The meaning of Howell's repudiation, within this unlimited frame, becomes unlimited and unlimiting, but also inundating and burdensome, because Delia must endlessly consider new objects and possibilities associated with it.[66]

Howell's repudiation does limit Delia's freedom of association in a sense, by being the thing with which everything must be associated. It creates an imaginary difference, a distant man who is not really distant since he and Delia keep getting reborn as one another's consorts, and a world that becomes different—but not really—as an effect of their harrowing separation-union. *Sword*'s heroine(s) struggle to assimilate difference but fail: in each case the different perspective represented by the man is trumped by the heroine's "expanded" perspective. The repudiation, H.D. suggests in *Sword*, happens (and repeats) because the heroine's significance and deeper understanding triggers male aggression. She is what men have repressed, what their warring, divided world lacks and must regain though violent and sundering measures and perhaps her sacrifice. World destruction is associated with the hidden meaning that Delia seeks, and that violent men repress and long for. H.D.'s religious and political views appear here as apocalyptic and sometimes assimilative, not heterogeneous and pacifist, as they have been described for instance in Jane Augustine's introduction to *The Gift* by H.D. and in Susan Stanford Friedman's *Psyche Reborn*.[67] The other's perspective is subsumed by a cosmic play; his attacks give rise to new, presumably more integrated eras, yet more always remains to be violently integrated, the play continues to repeat itself in era after era, and the question of the other's motivation continues to wound.

H.D.'s later prose, her correspondence, memoirs and literary work, return in a pattern of free-associative interpretation to men's denials of the special knowledge, insight, vision, or gift that she believed gave her a unique role in the transformation and healing of the social world. Concerns emerge about others' motivations for invalidating her visionary experiences and insights. In *The Gift*, H.D. portrays her mother's dismissiveness of a "gift" that allows "Hilda" to heal the war-torn world through personal integration. *Tribute* shows continued disappointment at friend, physician, and sexologist Havelock Ellis's (1859–1939) lack of response to H.D.'s *Notes on Thought and Vision* (written 1919, first published 1982), a manifesto for the transformation of human consciousness that she believes will be spearheaded by a few special individuals.[68] In *Tribute* she takes issue also with Freud's response to visions she had while travelling with Bryher on the Greek island of Corfu in 1920. H.D. saw a series of pictures—including a chalice, a tripod, and the goddess Nike—appear on their hotel room wall. Though she acknowledges that these visions can be interpreted as "'megalomania' they call it—a hidden desire to 'found a new religion,'"[69] she nevertheless takes them to mean that there will be "another war" after which she will "go on in another, a winged dimension."[70] However, she struggles in *Tribute* with Freud's suggestion that her visions are "a dangerous tendency or symptom."[71]

After her analysis by Freud, H.D. equates the end of interpretation with the end of spectral life. Freud's own tendency to trope repressed material in spectral terms was not lost on H.D., who recalls Freud telling her that those who finish analysis are "dead . . . as dead as your father."[72] In *Sword*, however, interpretation becomes maddeningly fleeting and ambiguous, a sliding of signification with no anchoring points, "nothing to hold on to" (141). Delia's constantly expanding and dissolving interpretive frameworks suggest a thought disorder in which what cannot be apprehended generates legions of rapidly coalescing and disintegrating ghosts that sabotage the structure of what can be. *Sword* articulates not a "final rational unity," as Augustine has argued, but a constant approach to the "hidden" meaning that it continually posits, but which continually retreats from its formulations.[73]

Sword's language is always already the language of the unconscious, "ghosting for" absent meaning. As in dreams, objects *are* other objects rather than (to borrow Freud's terms) the condensed, displaced or transposed signs of them that most of us discern upon waking.[74] Delia's interpretive endeavors witness the unconscious from a place inside of it, but she is alienated from the social "conscious," linguistic relationships with others based on collective agreements regarding the meanings of words, which can be used to express differing opinions and points of view. Her difficulty in determining the appropriate responses to supernatural messages in terms of social action may be a function of her trouble finding significance that is social and not just personal, since the pattern of her thought forecloses the symbolic dimension in which the social is experienced as other than personalized. Though she can view social phenomena—like the Second World War—as having to do with her personally, for her response to be implemented as social action she requires Howell, who represents social authority. Her own interpretive process, when applied to the purely personal significance she finds, retains meaning only as an unsignified remainder that makes further interpretation and articulation necessary. Accordingly, the RAF messages that she receives in encrypted form require his translation. Though Robert Duncan rightly argues that "[H.D.'s] genius is fictive and dramatic, not philosophic," in *Sword*, the lack of philosophic structure that Duncan describes intensifies into a lack of a semiotic structure that can abstract sense data into generalizable significations, and into a creative structure within which the parts of *Sword* can cohere and resonate.[75] *Sword*'s specters do not communicate hidden but socially significant meaning, as Delia hopes, but instead signal an absence of differentiation between the social world and her own psyche. Since all things merge in Delia's thought processes, ever new thoughts, things, possibilities, characters, and events are rapidly generated and absorbed into an ever incomplete nebula of associations. These ever new terms preserve the possibility that there is something else, not yet apprehended, that may grant clarity. However, their very proliferation precludes the possibility of stable difference, of structure.

IV. SEXUAL RELATIONSHIP PATTERNS

H.D.'s struggles to establish a meaningful relation between her heroines and heroes suggest a desire to reunite the imaginary and symbolic orders via the sexual relationship. But though the sexual relationship appears as the point where cold, clinical difference and boundless unity must surely be reconciled, there is no sexual relationship.[76] Actual symbolic otherness, the "no" of the Dowding figure, is trumped by what Lacan might call the "symbolic unreal," a fantasized nebula of references associated with the maternal, the divine "plan," and the H.D. figure.[77] This fantasy replaces Dowding's differing perspective with the supreme significance of their encounter.[78] While its status as "delusional" is open to question, H.D.'s thought process at this time seems to follow the movement from the particularity of the symbolic interpersonal relationship to the self-universalizing perspective that Lacan, Perry, and Ram Dass associate with delusion. The common factor that all of these possibilities share is that the Dowding figure never has a perspective that is capable of calling the H.D. figure, or the universally significant plan, into question. Whether genuinely felt or calculated, his actions are always predetermined by the mysterious forces arbitrating the plan. Supernatural visions and messages assure H.D.'s later protagonists that their male consorts may be motivated by fear, ignorance, and despair, or may be captured by a formula established in their past lives together, or else may be adhering to "the plan" or "play" without acknowledging it. The protagonists vacillate between possibilities. The Dowding figures may doubt the truth (often unspecified) that the protagonists represent. They may be shrinking from the plan to save the world whose particulars remain unclear. Alternatively, they may be on track with the plan but deny the protagonists' roles in it as part of the plan's very strategy—which they may know while the heroines do not—or as a test for the protagonist. As H.D. writes in *Sword*,

> I must say that this apparent or real repudiation of Beauvais was part of the plan. I must argue that it was a further test of the quality and strength of Beauvais. If

> Ladies Guard must meet the war, then Ladies Guard must be tested and tried, and all weakness uncovered. My weakness was my strength. (257)

The Dowding figures' mother issues combine with these factors. They can be cruel because the heroines remind them of their mothers, or they can be, as Freudian primordial father figures, stuck on a primal scene that H.D. envisions as brutal—but these latter possibilities are also envisioned as part of the plan. The heroes may have no agency in the plan, but be helplessly under the control of the divine being, perhaps Z, who orchestrates it.

The perpetual return of the question of Howell's motivation throughout *Sword*, and the boggling procession of past-life betrayals in "Summerdream," suggest, however, that the problem of the other (meaning) subsists on a structural level. *Sword*'s messianic and sacrificial content, flattened affect, and Delia's claims that she was "dead" after Howell's repudiation suggest the annihilation of personal feeling and even of selfhood that occurs in splitting and in the drives, which take over, as Klein writes, when the desiring part of the ego is annihilated, and when access to the signifier is lost.[79]

Delia's description of the effects of Howell's repudiation suggests stimulation as well as annihilation. Though she claims "[t]he shock of his volte-face had left me, not so much frozen as inanimate and lost. I simply wasn't there, any more" (33), she later adds, "his sudden volte-face served to drive in the impressions deeper, to heighten my perception and to act as a sort of flint or whet-stone to sharpen my mind" (126). Delia's apocalyptic vision of world transition both mirrors a stimulating psychic "death" with spectacular social destruction and suggests that this destruction enables psychic and social "integration." Her desire for union with Howell, for the next world, for certainty regarding the meaning of multifarious signs, and her "integrative" discovery of these "meanings" in herself, all suggest an endeavor to mend a shattered psyche, but the cure may be the poison. The process of "integration," always reaching to encompass new objects and possibilities, itself appears to enact the cognitive and emotional shattering.

In *Sword*, at any rate, these objects and identifications do not integrate with one another into the whole vision that Delia longs for, but seem to hold great significance that never clarifies, and then quite quickly give way to something else. For Delia, the means by which final integration is to be accomplished, though suggested by dreams, visions and spirit messages, remains unclear, though aligned with the final union of the fated heroes and heroines, who represent the "conscious or scientific mind and the unconscious or dream-mind":

> Lord Howell seemed peculiarly fitted to judge and assess the findings of psychic-research workers. I had thought myself above the usual type of sensational or hysterical seeker. I still think so. But my valiant . . . effort to make a

> bridge between the conscious or scientific mind and the unconscious or dream-mind, met with but scant recognition. (68)

Delia does not think herself the type who would hallucinate spirit messages, as Howell's words imply. However, despite her self-perception, she feels that his *coup de grâce* still prevents her from bridging the scientific and dream minds, since the former is his domain. Their vexed union could be read as an allegory for the separation of personal/imaginary (the woman) from social/symbolic significance (the man), and the ensuing breakdown of signification that takes place, Lacan argues, in psychosis.

Sword represents the radical separation between its signifiers and signifieds, then, using themes of spectrality and of man's invalidation of woman. In a sense, these push back against the construction of signifier and signified by suggesting that there is something more to meaning than the mere concepts fastened to words. As Friedman and others have suggested, this may have to do with women's knowledge and agency, which has been under attack—as *Sword* witnesses—throughout history and pre-history. Though H.D. senses that this meaning, which in *Sword* and *Helen* wells up through the cracks in the symbolic order, is more than mere delusion, it is also true of *Sword* that H.D. does not deliberately thematize the indeterminacy of language or the evacuation of the concept as such—intentions that are sometimes ascribed to her when her writing appears vague and enigmatic. The spectral ambiguity of *Sword*'s language is only partly literary device, as Helen Sword maintained was true of other works in her reading of H.D.'s "cryptopoetics."[80] In *Sword*, H.D.'s language is less meant to explore the indeterminacy of signifiers than to discover once and for all what they "ghost for."[81] Delia's RAF pilots precisely desire straightforward translation, and they want it from Howell: "All [the RAF pilots] wanted was someone who would understand the numbers and letters" (35). If *Sword*'s specters thematize an uncanny, ungraspable influence on reality, and the maddening insubstantiality of language, they do so not so much intentionally as inadvertently, and to Delia's torment. These specters have literal existence and urgent social agendas that can be positively determined, she and they believe, given the right interpretive strategies. While the RAF pilots say that they "speak the same language" as Delia and Howell, they "wanted to establish a means of communication that could be shared by other people" (140). This requires that Howell translate the "infinite varieties of flash and pause, of double-flash, half-pause, and so on. It only needed a translator to put their dots and dashes into words" (150). Delia receives and records a meaningful code that awaits Howell to render it into a universally relevant system of signs. While Anderson has argued that Delia acts as a translator of spirit messages in *Sword* and, therefore, "aligns artistic and spiritualist practice, representing the medium as an artist in her own right," the evidence in *Sword* is overwhelming that Delia's messages await Howell's translation, and that she sees herself as a receiver, not an interpreter.[82] Her interpretations following his refusal to translate remain fragmentary, tenuous and unsatisfying to her.

The Morse code–like form of these messages recalls H.D.'s vision of communications from a statue, "the Delphic charioteer," in *Notes on Thought and Vision* (written in 1919, first published in 1982):

> If we had the right sort of brains, we would receive a definite message from that figure [the Delphic charioteer], like dots and lines ticked off by one receiving station, received and translated into definite thought by another telegraphic center. . . . We want receiving centers for dots and dashes.[83]

These "dots and dashes" become, in *Sword*, the form of the RAF pilots' communications. As a "receiving center," Delia appears as one of *Notes*' "two or three people, with healthy bodies and the right sort of receiving brains, [that] could turn the whole tide of human thought, could direct lightning flashes of electric power to slash across and destroy the world of dead, murky thought."[84] That these people must have "healthy bodies" suggests H.D.'s earlier note that "overmind without the balance of the other two [mind and body] is madness."[85]

The way that this madness develops is suggested in *Sword* by Delia's strained and uncomprehending mode of receptivity to the spirit world. It almost seems that Delia feels her life depends on Howell decoding her spirit messages: "All [the pilots] wanted was someone who would understand the numbers and the letters. I didn't know anyone in the Air Force, but Lord Howell and anyway, they wanted him to do this" (35). The RAF pilots cannot understand Howell's unwillingness to listen to them: "'You help,' they kept insisting" to Delia (35). Their messages, transmitted to Delia but not received by Howell, cause psychic tension to build up in her—reminiscent of the "pressure of ideas"—that psychiatrist Eugen Bleuler (1857–1939), a contemporary of Freud, describes in sufferers from schizophrenia—a term he coined that means "splitting of the mind."[86] Writes Delia,

> They [the RAF pilots] stayed as long as I could keep concentrated and didn't give way under the strain . . . it was no good my explaining that we had come to a sort of blind-alley. . . . I felt like a battery . . . that had to be completed by another battery. Or I felt like a wire, across which a voice was speaking and if the message were not received at the other end, in some way or other, the wire would break. (31)

Delia is filled, excruciatingly, with coded information that cannot be "shared by other people" because of Howell's resistance, yet this rejection somewhat relieves the incomprehensible messages' pressure by replacing them as the object of her interpretive focus. Howell's repudiation is likewise incomprehensible: Delia is perpetually dissatisfied with her explanations of it and constantly discovers new pertinent signifiers, considering their various possible significances without choosing between them, following in all directions a branching and rebranching cognitive labyrinth. Correlatively, Delia's ghosts and spirits are hopelessly ambiguous creatures whose communications are vague and platitudinous, coded or cryptic, but never determinate, as she would wish. Delia comments wryly on the volumes of spirit messages collected by the Stanford House Library:

> Being in daily peril of imminent destruction by the high-explosives, perhaps I found the letters from the dead, too vague and elusive. At such a time, we needed a surer certainty of heaven. I do not mean the fact of there being a heaven, but the facts of heaven. . . . But their [the spirits in heaven's] spiritual life seemed to be . . . without any apparent "traces of direction." (130)

Even when Delia finds "traces of direction," by which she means similarities between words or objects that allow her to identify them with one another, meaning always remains detached from the signs that "ghost for" it. Delia, unable to eliminate possibilities or associations, speaks from "inside" the social unconscious and according to its dream logic, a condition that is troped in Delia and Howell's own spectrality: "Lord Howell looked like a ghost. We were ghosts together. We were ghosts together. We were out of the same play" (84). Possibilities, since they cannot be separated, are not really possibilities at all but unclearly meaningful aspects of the same inevitability, "the same play." Ghosts, with their legendary proclivity to return repetitively with unclear agendas and again disappear, signal this simultaneous vagueness and repetition. Ghostliness suggests the incessant dissolution of a world in which others are always projections of oneself, the disjuncture of personal from symbolic meaning, which contributes to the highly personalized language of *Sword*.

V. SPATIAL AND TEMPORAL PATTERNS: GRAPHS, MAPS, CHARTS, CYCLES

The proliferating memories and associations that elusive meaning requires Delia to elaborate accrue as a spectral palimpsest within her person. Her avatars hence exist simultaneously in her present identity, allowing her to recognize others—like Howell—who are "out of the same play," who have been with her in "past lives" that are not really past but instead part of an eternal present. The palimpsestic composition of her identity is reflected by this quality in her writing. "Summerdream's" stories do not progress temporally through causes and effects but lie over one another like transparencies or "pleats" (214) as she calls them, different layers of an inchoate picture. As Helen Sword writes,

> Paradoxically, in [H.D.'s] wartime writings, she "mend[s] a break in time" not by reinstating but rather by shattering conventional notions of linear temporality, confounding history by collapsing past, present, and future into a single "spectral moment," a temporal unit, in Jacques Derrida's definition, "that no longer belongs to time . . . that is not docile to time."[87]

If chronological time, as Lacan argues (1945), can only be measured through the duration of objects—their tendency to exist for a while and then to cease existing—then the identity of avatar objects with one another annihilates time.[88] Or conversely, the collapse of chronological time annihilates difference. In *Sword*, each encounter reflects, and in a sense is, each other one, and all happen in the "event," *Thermopylae*, that causes history to "turn-about or turn-over" (174). Though they seem to take place at different periods in history, what H.D. in *Helen in Egypt* calls "time-in-time (personal time)" this history is in *Sword* "pleated," or in *Helen* circular or spiraling. Each "event" (100) or "ever-recurring 'eternal moment'" (277) represents a return to a temporal unity, and, perhaps, an opportunity for resolution of the whole through personal and world integration. This vision of a personal temporality that loops back toward eternity may call us to a less bounded experience of time and subjectivity—yet, these pleats, circles and spirals continue to proliferate and become increasingly complex. As Delia puts it,

> We followed the Z or the bee-line in its zig-zag track or path across time. Time was conveniently pleated and the pleats lay flat under the chart or map that took us from London to Lausanne, to Lugano, to Knossos, to Athens, to Delphi. . . back to London, to Venice . . . there are to-and-fro journeys and return flights, but this briefly is our path or our zig-zag in space. Time is another matter. But this bee-line or Z-line has this advantage over time, time is neatly folded. (214)

Delia cannot combat the nonmeaning with which Howell threatens her by making it part of a story, since this would require linear time with its causes and effects, beginnings and endings. Instead, she combats this nonmeaning with a saturation of associations and instances of time, always personal, within her person. Her frames of reference, outside the laws of space and time, appear unlimited. The transhistorical and regional, even universal, relevance of Delia and other H.D. based protagonists, is the "answer" that was already emerging in H.D.'s earlier work, such as *The Gift* (written

1941–1943). *Sword* re-establishes tentatively and *Helen in Egypt* asserts more confidently, that not language but rather Delia and Helen themselves are universally significant. Their personal experiences, memories, and their integration of these directly cause social upheaval, war, or peace in the world through sympathetic resonance. The task of the protagonist is thus to accomplish world integration by means of these repeating encounters, and by recognizing and cataloging everyone and everything that they contain inside themselves.

Seeking meaning in herself, Delia finds expanding, overlapping, and related social discourses that share inexhaustibly fertile signifiers: psychoanalysis, religion, history, legend and myth, all endlessly suggestive of one another and of her personal associations. Since everything gains its significance in relation to her, and to Howell's invalidation of her and her messages, her search for meaning must then become the articulation of everything.[89]

Sword repeatedly attempts to find meaning in a dreamlike or spectral explosion of *Logos*, the word as creation. To this end, it generates new characters, things and places to which meaning is unattached except through the "physical and vital realities," as Duncan puts it, of Delia's person.[90] *Sword* suggests that, through Delia's containment of everything within herself, castration can be reversed. Correlatively, the tyrannical, murky, dead order that the system of language imposes can be miraculously subverted. For Schreber and Delia, as perhaps for formalist literary critics in a less physical and vital register, writing that is also being may be the means by which the reversal of castration—the elimination of signification and return to pure *Logos*—can be accomplished. However, though *Sword* begins to work toward this imaginary containment of all things within Delia, primarily it traces an "imaginary cataclysm," a natural disaster of cognition in response to an inassimilable signifier. Perhaps because the establishment of a fairly stable delusional metaphor is far from accomplished, other ways of organizing things are attempted as well.

Delia, for instance, tries to substitute patterns and objects for symbolism as such. She senses immanent meaning behind language and other signs that "ghost for" it, and tries to apprehend it nonlinguistically through graphs, charts, maps, circles, and other patterns of various sorts, as well as through material objects and their attributes. She attempts to organize her impressions according to these visual, nonsymbolic systems, which she hopes will tell her something about her mission. But she never succeeds in abstracting meaning from momentary phenomena, just as the dreamer cannot find the "final rational unity" of her dream until she wakes to the thought structures of the day, where a symbolic meaning crystallizes.[91] Unassimilated terms proliferate during each attempted schematization. In her preoccupation with the question of the plan and the means to achieve it, "uncertainty of the outcome wins out," although the "certainty of the undertaking, the project, eludes . . . doubt."[92] This uncertainty is deferred repeatedly through ever new characters, narrative threads, associations, images, and syntheses that then branch into new dualisms.

For instance, Delia surmises that her RAF messages could be transcribed graphically if she knew, as she believes Howell does, the right way to do so. At times, she attempts to picture these transcriptions herself; but her imagined maps, graphs, and charts have no abstract significance; they do not represent something else (e.g., changes, categories, or parts of the world), as graphs, maps, and charts usually do, though she asserts that collectively they represent a zig-zag movement though time and space. They can be understood as attempts to substitute another system for symbolic language:

> [The bee] whispers or drones. He buzzes or hums. Words are not necessary. They [the RAF pilots] could have dictated a graph or a map. Without words and our sometimes clumsy spelling, they could have zzz-ed a detailed line-drawing. I could easily have transcribed the rhythm, the up-and-down, the pause and beat on ruled music paper. But they wanted Lord Howell to translate the music—or the weather-chart. . . . Now, it seems almost too easy. They had only to indicate to me the type of ruled, numbered and lettered paper that they wanted. . . . At first, they would tap out N or S or E or W or Ne or Sw, or variations of these, as I saw them in the compass sun-pattern on the *Ghirlanda* table [the table in her London flat at which she held her solo séances]. These would indicate direction or simply the side of the sheet of map-paper on which the graph began. There would be numbers, latitude and longitude. . . . They had only to indicate what sort of graph or map-paper they wanted and Howell would find it for them.
>
> "Wave-work," they had said. The hieroglyph or graph of Z or Nenu's own name is [a double zig-zag], the wave-symbol. It is W, twice repeated in one graph . . . it would be a zzz-zzz way of talking. But it might have been too easy. (140)

This fragment is representative of Delia's interest in graphic representation, her difficulty in representing anything with it, and her belief that Lord Howell would be able to make things clear. It exhibits several characteristics that have been identified with schizophrenic language, such as overinclusion (the inability to limit the boundaries of a problem), vacillation, and asyndetic or paralogical thinking. The map, graph or chart that the RAF pilots might have dictated would not have represented anything in particular, except perhaps the hieroglyph of Z's name or the shape of pleated time. Moreover, Delia's awareness of the asymbolism of her graphs as unusual—as a problem—does not seem clear. Objects, patterns, and words as objects are called on to synthesize and anchor the sliding signifiers of her thought and memory:

> There was nothing to hold on to. I tried to visualize the swallow-graph, the dart and flight, so different from the eagle's.
>
> I kept on wondering about the flight or graph of the eagle or falcon.
>
> "He has a nest somewhere," Ben Masini [Delia's medium] had said. The nest was the little tripod table. (141)

The *Ghirlanda* tripod table, the séance table whose pattern Delia describes in great detail, exemplifies an object and pattern that temporarily substitutes for the symbolic order. This substitution extends to her association of the table with "science," her father, world destruction, and personal reintegration. This table was once owned by writer, craftsman, social activist, and friend to the Pre-Raphaelites, William Morris. The title of *The Sword Went Out to Sea* is taken from Morris's poem, "Sailing of the Sword," and Morris is mentioned in *Sword* as one of the many fleeting, mysteriously relevant figures on whose identity or difference from Lord Howell, Delia speculates.[93] With the *Ghirlanda* table, the extremely violent character of stabilizing synthesis, for her, can again be noted. The messages that Howell refuses to decode have the function, Delia tells us, of arranging her past into patterns that resemble those on her *Ghirlanda* table. Delia reflects, "We do not need 'messages' to assure us of eternity. But without the 'messages' the other squares would have remained dispersed, unshaped and unassembled" (110). Though she may be certain that eternity exists, the *Ghirlanda* table's four-square pattern, organizing the messages alongside other memories, allows her to give "the other squares" some shape:

> There were four later infatuations or emotional experiences, but until I found the original foundation, they were dispersed and disproportionate. It was only after I had left London that the sequence became clear and with it, the experience with Lord Howell. This third square is related to the first square, four-square in all particulars. The last square is more difficult to define, it is the sort of crown or affirmation of the others. (109)

Through the table's pattern, Delia visually articulates and attempts to resolve the eternal rebranching and revolving of her thoughts, a cycle of thought that expands on all fronts. She compares thoughts to ripples around a stone thrown in water. The table's "circles on the sea" describe, inadvertently, her outward-rippling thought processes, where linear cause and effect have given way to simultaneity, while the "sun-star" at the center of the circles is associated with the table's "stabilizing" quality. To Delia's satisfaction the sun-star, rather viciously, captures "unwary and unpredictable motes of memory" like an "eight-legged spider" or a "Venus fly-trap":

> I said that the table was like a stone which sent out circle on concentric circle to the horizon. The sun-star of the four superimposed squares on this little table, seems on the other hand, a sort of mesh or net. The inner stars diminish until they reach a circle of about six inches in diameter, in the center of the table.
>
> In this innermost circle, there is a conventional, geometric pattern. This flower-pattern has eight petals. It is the living heart of the circle, the eight-legged spider at the center of the web, the Venus fly-trap if you will, pulsing to trap unwary and unpredictable motes of memory. (113)

Unlike the outward-rippling circles, the sun-star spider pattern gives her a sense of "completion, of finality" (111). Here, in the realm of objects that materialize her thought processes, Delia's speculations become very problematic socially, for these objects help to affirm her sense of the rightness of mass annihilations of human life. Delia reflects that "this star-circle [on the table] with its angles and diminishing flat perspective, might decorate the altar of a pyramid-temple in South America, Mexico or Yucatan" (113). This pattern is taken as a message concerning the "final outcome" of world annihilation, because these "angular motives of the gate-ways and fortifications of Yucatan" are "repeated endlessly in the weapons of modern warfare" (127). Her association of the table, Yucatan, and "the weapons of modern warfare" suggest to Delia that destruction and sacrifice "might by some miracle be justified" (127)—a comment that fits ill with the feminist pacifistic position most critics have attributed to H.D. The associative identity of these objects, conferred by the sun-star, is taken to reveal a socially significant message:

> I said the Viking ship was the table. Perhaps, we may conclude that the Viking ship was England. England is the inheritor of the tradition of the sea-kings. But all the physical or material horizons have been explored. But other horizons have lately been opened up, by new and terrible weapons of destruction. I have said that the angular motives of the gate-ways and fortifications of Yucatan are repeated endlessly in the weapons of modern warfare. If the motive of slaughter and blood-sacrifice, which I had associated with the pyramid-temples of Yucatan, had or could have any "plan," then the recent unparalleled destruction of the peoples of the world, would by some miracle and only by some miracle, be justified. Then Yucatan, meaning blood-sacrifice, had or might have a "plan" or a "part in plan." (127)

The *Ghirlanda* table is "the legitimate reward of my devotion to the 'work,' the intense, broken sessions when I concentrated so feverishly on the messages from the RAF," says Delia, because its sun-star pattern tells her that sacrificial mass destruction is part of the plan (113), since it enables "other horizons" to be explored—again, a socially problematic "reward." Since the *Ghirlanda* table "was like, or was" (123) "the Viking ship" of Hal Brith

(127), England, with its war-nourished enthusiasm for the paranormal and otherworldly—will in "the tradition of the sea-kings" explore the nonmaterial "horizons" opened up by the annihilation of most human life by atom bombs.

However, the association between the table, Yucatan, and "new and terrible weapons" may be based on more than a visual "motive" that they have in common. The sun-star also enables the psychic "integration" necessary for world salvation: "The points of the sun or star, directed outward, have in fact, like so many magnets, attracted the various memories, scattered in time and space, and drawn them all together" (120). Therefore, the spatial arrangement of the *Ghirlanda* table's pattern that Delia substitutes for symbolic language is aligned with both psychic integration—the drawing in of "various memories scattered in time and space"—and world destruction. Here, free-associative identifications and distinctions appear to replace symbolic language as a means of communication, revealing the asymbolic forms of desire.

Delia sometimes articulates differences as well as identities between things, but these are differences that would otherwise not have been in question for most readers. Often a distinction is followed by identification, as if difference, itself, might be threatening: "Campione [a region in Italy] . . . is not Persia, it is India" (138); "Lord Howell was not Hal Brith, but William Morris was. And Hal Brith was Eric Ericson. . . . But Hal Brith did not sponsor the [RAF] messages, though I said that the table was like, or was the ship. The messages were sponsored by Z" (123). The continuity that reincarnation confers to the characters in Delia's universe creates a sense of a purpose and reinforces her sense of the intention held by Z, which has yet to become clear.

Delphi's Painted Lady in "Summerdream," an alter ego of Delia's, suggests that a transition of her "pictures" from the symbolic to asymbolic realms occurred after her "dismissal" by Pericles:

> I knew the pictures would never leave me . . . but it was only after I was (as I then thought) dismissed from the golden house, that I began to see them clearly, that is, to see them as pictures, *things actual, tangible, and eternal. There is that hair-line between imagination and vision*—and that night, on the Acropolis, I crossed it. (175, emphasis added)

After this "dismissal," which echoes Howell's dismissal of Delia and Dowding's dismissal of H.D., what was once "imagination" becomes "vision" of things that are "actual, tangible, and eternal." Accordingly, identifications in *Sword*, whether between graphics, characters, objects, signs, or attributes, are literal rather than symbolic. Maps, charts, and patterns are not *of* anything: they are the things themselves. Beings and things *are* other beings and things. Past identities, however, are also present ones. They are indistinct in Delia's "spectral moment" of pleated time.

Delia substitutes for the symbolic order an imagined system in which cause and effect give way to simultaneity, a cognitive big bang of outward-moving "concentric circles" that must encompass everything. Her thoughts seemingly entertain as many possibilities and identities as possible, but the circles that she is "driven to circumscribe" ripple outward with more sense data, which she is therefore never able to abstract into a coherent system. She claims that these "circles on circles" find a cohesive force in the *Ghirlanda* table:

> The circles on circles . . . may not have merged but they must have moved. Later, I said that the circles seemed concentric and the table like the proverbial pebble, thrown on the surface of a pond. But again, there was movement, though this time, from within, as each circle grew larger, spreading from the small center out, toward the horizon. But the pattern on this table gives me a sense of completion, of finality. My mind may follow any one of the sixteen "traces of direction" in memory or in retrospect, but I myself remain where I am, unconcerned with the future, reconciled with the past. (111)

This unconcern and reconciliation, however, is followed rapidly by new "traces of direction," new paralogical synapses. Ineffable meanings in "Wintersleep" and casts of characters in "Summerdream" slip away, give way to the new, as quickly as they appear. Delia claims, "our pictures sometimes seem to be made up of unrelated segments, yet they spell something. They are the clue to the final answer, they are, among the million paving-stones of the labyrinth, the ones with the little cross marked on them" (215). However, these "clue[s]," the new, seemingly relevant associations, are the very substance of the branching labyrinth.

What Lacan calls delusional intuition and delusional formula are, in *Sword*, the forms in which signifiers are presented, whereby they refer not to signifieds but to the unsignifiable, to "meaning as such."[94] Howell's dismissal is "repeated, reiterated, drummed in with a stereotyped insistence"[95] as the formula of his past lives with Delia, and also described as a unique, ineffable encounter whose essence, which gives meaning to other events, like "the scent of lilac" cannot be described but only felt (110). In "Wintersleep" Delia relates the fourth square of her *Ghirlanda* table, which represents Howell, to the scent of lilac. Neither can be labeled, contained, or described, but each can penetrate the rest of the pattern:

> The scent of the lilac, under the gold-framed mirror, can only be felt, be sensed, be perceived. It is like that with the fourth square of the star-pattern, its dimension penetrates the senses. It can be felt, this fourth of the four squares. It can be apprehended but perhaps it can not be understood. . . . We can relate or compare this fragrance to others. It evokes emotions and we can accept or dismiss the scenes, the places, the rooms, the people that we associate with this flower. So

> we can relate scenes and emotions to the fourth square, but it is the very essence of the fourth square that eludes description. But without the "traces of direction" of the other three squares, the fourth would have remained unrealized . . . the fourth square or the qualities that I attribute to it can of course, penetrate the others, as the fragrance of lilac fills this room. We do not need a geometric analysis of our life, in order to appreciate or recognize the fragrance of a flower. But the perfume of a flower can be distilled, adulterated and preserved, though no labeled, crystal bottle can ever contain the spirit or the ghost of the flower. (109–10)

Howell's "meaning" for Delia cannot be labeled or contained. Likewise, the formulaic repetitions of "Summerdream," though seeming to take a different approach to meaning, share the sense of it as unsignifiable. While in "Wintersleep" the meaning of Howell's rejection is ineffable, in "Summerdream" its formulaic repetition takes precedence as its meaning; indeed, this repetition constitutes its meaning. The ineffable, but penetrating, meaningless "patterns" that appear visually in "Wintersleep" are dramatized as unclearly meaningful repetitive behavior in "Summerdream." However, these formulas have an overburdened quality, as if they are sinking fast into a sea of nondifferentiation:

> I had said that my star-pattern on the table in the *Ghirlanda* drawing-room was like a magic ring. I had said that I had my traces of direction. This [similarity between her star-pattern and magic ring] was one of them.
>
> But magic ring is *Zauberring*. You see what I mean. The word "magic" for us has lost its meaning. But we, he [possibly Norman Holmes Pearson or Lord Howell] and I (German and English speaking), are not only affiliated but are one in the word, ring. It was Z who first indicated to me this sort of divination. He began it with *nénufar*, but the dictionary spells it *nenuphar*; in English, it is a specialized word, though the French, *nénufar*, is the name for water-lily. But that was not enough. Z balanced, simplified or coded it, by spelling water-lis. That suggested *fleur-de-lis* and Z, I think, meant us to understand by water-lis that English-French was indicated. One can perhaps become too deeply involved with this sort of decoding, but I don't think so. Z spelt nenufar instead of nenuphar. I looked at the word for a long time. Then I got out Garry's hieroglyphs. There was a little picture of Nenu, the Egyptian sky-god. His name is found in the zodiac. His picture or his name is [a double zig-zag] which is the sign of the eleventh house of the Zodiac, Aquarius. And *far* was all right, too, *phar* would have spoiled it. So we had ancient Egypt and the present, and *far* spelt backward, is RAF. (138–9)

Delia's appeal to the reader, "You see what I mean," provokes a careful scrutiny of this passage, a concentrated effort to see what it does mean. If her oneness with Pearson (or perhaps Howell) in the word ring and her multifaceted account of the word *nénufar* is correct—that is, intended by Z—what then? Simply, that this is what *Zauberring* and *nénufar* are associated with for her. How these associations might relate to the social context to which she relates them remains unclear, but their proliferation delays indefinitely the conclusion that they don't. Writes Lacan,

> Beware those who say to you—*You understand* . . . this means that she herself isn't very sure of the meaning, and that the latter refers not so much to a system of continuous and reconcilable meaning as to meaning as ineffable, to the meaning of her own reality, to her own personal fragmentation.[96]

Just as Dowding figures in *Sword* associate H.D. figures with their mothers, H.D. figures and H.D. herself associate Dowding figures and Dowding himself with fathers, with her father.[97] Lacan writes that the function of the father in the Oedipal phase is "the introduction of an order, a mathematical order, whose structure is different from the natural order."[98] Delia looks for an order of some kind in Howell, who can "feel things . . . in a rational way" (34) and who can "understand the numbers and the letters" (35) that she receives from the RAF pilots. After his dismissal, she attempts to order her experiences through the *Ghirlanda* table's and other patterns:

> We have proved conclusively at last, that two plus two makes four. Not only has each square its four sides but there are four squares to our final pattern. The last square, although I have said it eludes definition by its very essence, yet relates the material to the spiritual, as the fragrance of the lilac recalls old scenes and events. The scenes and events can be described in . . . detail, though the fragrance of the flower eludes description. (118)

The description of the "old scenes and events" that the indescribable fragrance of lilac recalls can, she implies, indicate this fragrance in the "material" register. Likewise, the fourth square—though it "eludes definition by its very essence"—recalls, assembles, and penetrates the other three and can thus be indicated by describing them. The organization of the first three squares that the fourth square provides turns out to consist in detailed descriptions of the first three squares, or more precisely of things and events that she associates with the love interests that the squares "are" (110). Endlessly, the organization that things and patterns promise turns out to be more description, more association. Objects and patterns do not provide an anchoring point to hold the slide of the signifier.

VI. SOCIOPOLITICAL PATTERNS

Like the "provisional-improvised" men and birds that give rise to "compulsive thinking" in Schreber, fleeting characters and things in *Sword* ghost for truths that Delia must incessantly unravel, following traces of direction that split, sometimes by means of the word "or." Even Howell's "last letter had *or* had not precipitated my illness." Delia's splitting of possibilities with "or" suggests a perhaps too wide frame of reference, which has been linked to the problem-solving troubles experienced by sufferers from schizophrenia.[99] Delia maintains possibilities in a simultaneity that suggests less distinct possibilities than indistinct inevitability. Words are heavy with unclear, but certain, meaning, which awaits someone's understanding. *Sword*, intended to be, and interpreted by Cynthia Hogue, Julie Vandivere, and Augustine as H.D.'s means of recovery from her 1946 breakdown, figures instead as a binding chain of empty signifiers whose links had begun to harden some time earlier.[100] H.D.'s persistence was perhaps, in part, a response to Freud's analysis of her Corfu visions. As she writes afterward, "But symptom *or* inspiration, the writing continues to write itself *or* be written."[101] Whether verbal or visual, the spirit messages fall short of their literal meanings, but Delia is sure that they pertain to herself and to *Thermopylae* in some way. Indeed, the very opacity of these spirit messages may allow the "plan" to which they refer to remain "inaccessible, inert, and stagnant with respect to any dialectic," as Lacan writes of delusional formations.[102] Delia's conviction that the plan concerns her person in some unique way is characteristic of delusional belief as Lacan describes it:

> The subject admits . . . that these [hallucinatory] phenomena are of another order than the real. He is well aware that their reality is uncertain . . . but . . . he is certain of something, which is that *what is at issue—ranging from hallucination to interpretation—regards him*. . . . The very nature of what he is certain of can remain completely ambiguous . . . but it means something unshakable for him.[103]

As with all things and events, H.D. renders the war—and the visions and nightmares of atom bombs, scaffolds, and underground tunnels for survivors that it suggests to her—meaningful in relation to what Robert Duncan calls the "depths and heights of [her] personal reality."[104] For H.D., the Blitz is an attack on *her* that, as she sees it, breaks down her psychological barriers. Her sense of the salvific function of this attack on herself and the world is perfectly literal in *Sword*. Social destruction correlates to the need that Delia expresses to sort out and limit the proliferating multitude of things, thoughts, and possibilities that present themselves to her.

There is even an imagined necessity to sort people according to their worthiness to live. Delia imagines a recognizable demarcation between "who was and was not worth saving" from the global annihilation of the "third war" (52). Her past incarnation, Julius Caesar's first wife, Stella, laments:

> There are too many people. Something has to be done with all these people. And I was younger and I loved you and those roads and charts and maps took you away from me. *Vae Victis*. I thought of the conquered peoples, but there were so many of them and after you left I began to imagine horrible, horrible things, primitive, unutterable—I had mad fantasies. . . . I have said the house is haunted but I love it. . . . Villa Trevi is full of ghosts but this isn't a matter of the knockings and rappings I heard last winter. I had perhaps foolishly tried to help them in the village. . . . I wanted to die then. If you go, there will be no one to stand between me and the new exodus from the city. . . . I am afraid of all these people. I thought I loved them, but I don't love them. I am afraid of them. (227)

Hogue and Vandivere argue that in this chapter, "Stella seems . . . to be turning from her own illness to a restored vision of plenitude and peace, to which the vision of Caesar's actual or symbolic journey to King Arthur's blessed isle has opened her."[105] However, Stella claims not to be at peace, but rather to be afraid of people, and to feel that something must be done with them. Her claim to happiness would seem to support Hogue and Vandivere's argument, but it is strikingly unpersuasive: "Well, I'll sit down—I'm light-headed, Julius. I don't think I can stand any more of the Trevi [wine]. But, Julius, I'm so happy. You see, last winter was worse than other winters. . . . It's the Trevi—I'll rest here under the fleeces, while Nina clears the table. I am so happy, Julius" (234). Here the word "happy" seems to mean "drunk," and suggests the medications administered at Klinik Brunner, for which Villa Trevi stands. "Happy," at least, means something different than usual, something more uneasy. For Stella, this is the fear that "if you [Julius Caesar] go, there will be no one to stand between me and the new exodus from the city" (227).

In keeping with the dizzying succession of characters and frequent evidence of projection and introjection in *Sword*, "too many people" suggests both "the masses" and the unchecked splitting of H.D.'s inner life into the multitude of characters that *Sword* tosses out. The hordes that frighten Stella and the necessity that Delia imagines in discriminating between those worthy and unworthy of life, together, thus suggest the necessity of sorting, arranging, and limiting thoughts, visions, and identities. Howell articulates this need for a limit even to spirit messages in a way that Delia, who "loved" her exhausting RAF pilots "very dearly," never would (121): "There were too many of these messages. There were too many altogether. They had to stop somewhere" (152). Howell, the Air Chief Marshall, is assigned the ruthless, discriminatory qualities stereotypically associated with his role. Moreover, Delia's feminine receptivity and imaginative fecundity catalyze this aggression.

While Christine Coffman and others have suggested that the projection in H.D.'s work is an aesthetic choice that asserts a feminist and lesbian erotics and aesthetics against patriarchal visions of love and language, *Sword*'s projections do not always challenge modernism's stereotypes, but sometimes rather suggest their uncritical adoption. Delia's psychic colonization of "Ben Masini" (Arthur Bhaduri, her medium for a time) is another example of such stereotyping. Masini is, like Delia, a "strange, sensitive creature," tormented, she surmises, by his mixed parentage, who "out of the whirlwind . . . brought his pictures and his naïve, oriental fantasies" (63). However, Delia cuts off all relations with Masini because of his coming marriage:

> Masini said, "But what will you do and Gareth do if I marry Doris?"
>
> I had answered, "I don't know what Gareth will do, but I won't see you any more." He didn't understand, and I became perhaps over-effusive and motherly.
>
> "You see, Masini, we are both so terribly fond of you. . . . I have loved our work together and I can't mix it up with—with other things." (22)

This statement, in light of Delia's own mix-up between her work and her obsession with Lord Howell, suggests what Klein calls "projective identification"—the projection of her unacceptable feelings onto another person (Masini) who is then rejected. She subsequently adopts his role as medium, table-tipping in "the best Masini manner" (23). After losing touch with him she speculates on his fate in the identical terms that she uses to describe her own:

> But mal-nutrition and constant fear of the law, in connection with a recrudescence of intolerance that found legal support in the obsolete Witchcraft Act, proved too much. He took the easy way, or perhaps it was the hard way. I don't know, for by this time, I have completely lost touch with him. (63)

This closely mirrors her own breakdown: "I was terribly afraid. I thought I had broken some law. I thought that I was damned. I was damned. I didn't eat anything. I remembered our discussions of the Witchcraft Act. I wondered what had become of Ben Masini" (49). Indeed, there is no evidence in *Sword* that Masini had a breakdown, or that his marriage to Doris was a response to the overwhelming internal pressures that Delia expected from his mixed Indian and English parentage. Masini's choice seems free. The nakedness of the projection and its lack of credit to Delia suggest that its portrayal is unintentional. Here, Delia—a rich white woman—projects her conflicts, fears and desires onto an Indo-English man, who seems to depend on her and Gareth (Bryher, the heiress) for financial support, and whom she rejects when he chooses whom to marry. Delia does not yet know what the complete picture may be, but this does not necessarily imply a radical openness to possibility. She can be emphatic that events, such as Masini's engagement, which do not pertain to her in a special way, are "not in the picture."

There is, in Delia's engagements with others, an uneasy shuttling back and forth between her own perspective and the other's *imagined* one, followed by a running together of inside and outside, of the personal and the universally true perspective. Everything is fused into a single, but indistinct, perspective or picture. Nevertheless, Delia preserves a rhetorical distinction between inside and outside—for instance, in the question she frequently returns to of whether her various visionary and psychic experiences are authentic, and so have some degree of universally relevant truth, or whether they are simply the projections of her subconscious mind. However, her thought processes often suggest a conflation of both possibilities into the belief that her experiences grant universally relevant, albeit often unclear, insights. For instance, Delia speculates in "Albatross," a chapter of "Summerdream," that Howell's fear of madness caused him to repudiate her visions—just as H.D. had speculated years before that Ellis "may have thought [that *Notes on Thought and Vision*] was a danger signal."[106] In this process of assimilating the other's perspective, Delia first reopens, in "Summerdream," the question of Howell's motivation for rejecting her, which she claims she had incompletely resolved by writing "Wintersleep." Delia writes: "I thought I had settled the question of Lord Howell's motive, but Randolph [a fleeting and unspecified character not listed in Hogue and Vandivere's key] made me feel that "Wintersleep" still left the problem unsolved" (151).

Howell is in this chapter Coleridge's Ancient Mariner while the albatross is Delia and perhaps her ghostly RAF pilots. His thoughts concerning the albatross suggest Delia's own vacillation between narratives of projection and real psychic insight:

> He saw them die of hunger and thirst. They all died. There were only ghosts left, and two of them, madness and death, threw dice for his soul . . . the bird swayed, circling the dead mast . . . but this was finally, irrevocably impossible . . . it wasn't *them*, of course. . . . It [the albatross] was a phantom, another ghost. It was not an albatross. (152)

Howell tells himself that Delia, or her RAF messages, are phantasmatic and therefore inauthentic. However, Delia knows that what appears as spectral may be real. Correlatively, what appears as madness or "life in death" may be "true"; madness can be "authentic" (101). "I have at last," she writes, "traced my own madness to its source, the source of all western poetry, the source of philosophy and mythology, the Greek drama" (101). If her madness has the same source as all this greatness, can it be truly idiosyncratic—would it not partake also of universal, socially relevant truth? However, she immediately returns to the problem of the other perspective: "But I have no means of assessing the madness of Lord Howell or tracing it to its source. I can only judge him by my own standards, and his may be very different" (101).

Delia is burdened by ambivalence between internal and outside perspectives, and haunted by Freud's and Dowding's suggestions that what appears to her as meaningful external phenomena may actually have no objective validity. Though her visionary perspective trumps that of the other in her writing, this other invalidating perspective remains a source of uneasiness. Perhaps in response, she claims that it does not matter whether an (unspecified) dream is a projection or a psychic insight. In either case, it follows "the pattern of [her] life," and is thus significant:

> This desolation, once re-established [by Howell's repudiation] became a waltz, a circling within the orbit of another time-dimension. The orbit of the dance belonged, by association, to the hieratic circling of the Maidens in a Greek play. I was a maiden in a Greek play, therefore in line with the source of inspiration of all dance and music. . . . Whether the dream had or had not the quality of a so-called psychic materialization, or was projected by the submerged content of the subconscious mind, is beside the point. The dream, neatly and deftly, followed the pattern of my life. (104)

Delia's dream, she claims, has the same significance whether it is subconscious projection or clairvoyant vision. This significance comes from its circling pattern that places her "in line with the source of inspiration of all dance and music."

The rejection of Howell (Tom Moore/Pylades/*Prince Lontain*) "re-establishes" a "desolation" that becomes this dream of circling Greek maidens, "all blessed by the gift of Love." In this dream, the goddesses of Love, War, and the Moon (associated with madness) are all awarded "the apple or the apples . . . without discrimination" by Paris (105). The dream tells Delia that "Love had tempered the arrows of madness and the sword-thrust of the victor, and Love had adjusted the quivering balance till finally it stood level and at rest." Love tempers and adjusts the Moon-madness and the War-rejection, the man and the woman, and restores balance—and this is true whether the dream that tells her so is clairvoyant—that is, referring to something outside herself—or whether it is only a "subconscious projection." If it is projection, it can nevertheless tell her something true about what is outside of herself—and in that sense is not mere projection at all. In this reading of her dream, H.D. re-establishes a figurative dimension in which Love can effect reconciliation between War—the cold, oppositional reason that, untempered, destroys—and the wandering, mad Moon that is its first target. She here resolves, for a time, the battle that unfolds in *Sword* to establish her inner knowledge as external and objective in the face of the Other's no.

VII. H.D.'S "FORECLOSURES"

The slippage between *Sword*'s words and concepts parallels Delia's difficulty discovering the meaning of her interpersonal relationships and symbolizing this meaning in shared language. Language's "central signal of a possible mediation" is introduced in an asymbolic or unintentionally symbolic fashion as the vexed unions of its many heroes and heroines. Read through Lacan, *Sword*'s proliferating past-life repudiations and apocalyptic fantasies, and the imaginary relation of these to Dowding's actual repudiation, represent a "mode of mediation" that both figures and substitutes for the symbolic dimension whose absence is revealed by H.D.'s encounter with the "no" coming from a father figure.

It is interesting to note, without giving it too much weight, that H.D.'s actual father appears flimsy in her fiction, memoirs, and correspondence. For instance, in *The Gift*, *Tribute to Freud*, and *HERmione*, the mother figures are truly formidable, while the father is experienced by the child, Hilda, as "not altogether negligible."[107] Though highly respected by others, he seems unequal to the power that he represents. In *The Gift* (as well as in H.D.'s correspondence) much is made of her father's head wound, a real incident exaggerated to macabre proportions. A family friend's record of his wounding states that Dr. Doolittle had not been hit by a car (as H.D. claimed) but instead had stepped off a bus while it was moving. He was "dazed," his beard "dark with blood," but "luckily he wasn't badly hurt."[108] H.D., however, describes this incident in dire terms in *The Gift* and in a letter to Havelock Ellis. She tells Ellis that her father's "life was despaired for some time" and ascribes her great need for Ellis—presumably a less vulnerable father figure—to this event.[109] In *The Gift*, the incident becomes "concussion of the brain and his collar-bone is broken."[110] In both documents, she returns several times to the fact that her mother did not give her credit for finding her father and washing his face: "Mama did not look at us, she was looking at Papa. She did not say, "O, children, children, who was it found your father?"'[111] Hilda and her father reverse roles, she becoming the responsible and he the helpless one, but this reversal goes unacknowledged. In *The Gift*, Hilda's giftedness, her courage in washing the blood from her wounded father's face, in effect, her power, remains unacknowledged by her mother, Helen. Indeed, Hilda and Helen Doolittle's representatives rarely address each other directly in H.D."s work.

In *Tribute*, it is her unforthcoming mother that Hilda desires, though she attempts to desire her father:

> It is *she* who matters for she is laughing, not so much at us as with us and over us and around us. . . . About *her*, there is no question. The trouble is, she knows so many people and they come and interrupt. And besides that, she likes my brother better. If I stay with my brother, become part almost of my brother, perhaps I can get nearer to *her*. . . . *If* one could stay near her always, there would be no break in consciousness—but half a loaf is better than no bread and there are things, not altogether negligible, to be said for *him* [her father]."[112]

H.D. seems to be trying here, perhaps at Freud's direct prompting or simply by suggestion, to transfer her desire from her mother to her father. After all, it is "his daughter to whom [her father] later entrusts his paper-knife; he leaves the uncut magazines and periodicals for her"—to cut, presumably.[113] This attempted transference includes symbols of "castration," which are also associated with Freud. A picture in her father's study of a doctor slicing a patient's arm is accordingly transposed onto her relationship with Freud:

> The half-naked man on the table [in a picture in her father's study] was dead so it did not hurt him when the doctors sliced his arm with a knife or a pair of scissors. Is the picture called *A Lesson in Anatomy*?
>
> It does not really matter what the picture is called. It is about doctors. There is a doctor seated at the back of the couch on which I am lying. He is a very famous doctor. He is called Sigmund Freud.[114]

Freud, perhaps, confronted H.D. with the "necessity" of this libidinal transfer to her father and corresponding "acceptance" of her castration. Told that she must prefer her father, as Freud thought that normal, healthy women did, H.D. tried to talk (or write) her past and present selves into it. Dr. Doolittle apparently thought the world of his daughter, claiming that this "one girl is worth all of her brothers."[115] The mother's affirmation, however, remained at issue.

In *Sword*, Delia's father (or his ghost) "made only one pronouncement—*Stop this war*" (68). Such a pronouncement suggests the unlimited power that the father gave her. This is a power that she does not choose, yet cannot reject: "But though . . . I would have exchanged Troy and *Thermopylae* for a basket of apples, I couldn't do it" (54). Lacan writes that when the "No" of the father fails to enter the subject's psychic economy initially, language as a differential, abstract system is never acquired. Subsequent encounters with something like this "No," which may simply take the form of other people's interpretations or judgments of the subject's speech, trigger the onset of psychosis, as Lacan discusses in detail: "For psychosis to be triggered, the Name-of-the-Father—*Verworfen*, foreclosed, that is, never having come to the place of the other—must be summoned to that place in symbolic opposition to the subject."[116] When psychosis is thus triggered, "the subject moves into another mode of mediation . . . and substitutes for symbolic mediation a profusion, an imaginary proliferation, into which the central signal of a possible mediation is introduced in a deformed and profoundly asymbolic fashion."[117]

In *Sword* and *Helen*, Dowding's suggestion of a limit to H.D.'s knowledge is introduced in an asymbolic fashion as cataclysmic, erotic, eternally recurring, and productive of a claim to certainty whose object remains mysterious. Delia "would be driven, haunted until I circumscribed the circle, I mean, until I was sure of the circumference" (146). H.D.'s recurring failure to reconcile and integrate the feminine, psychic, and "unconscious" forces that her person represents with the masculine, scientific, ostensibly civilized social order (represented variously in her life by her father, Freud, Ellis, Dowding and others) gives structure in the real to the foreclosure of what Lacan calls the Name-of-the-Father or the phallus, the signifier as such that is necessary for signification. H.D. seeks to fill the gap of castration with a meaning that can never be articulated in her malfunctioning language, but is always personal. Therefore, it is Delia's person, not language, that must be meaningful, that must close this gap by containing everything.

VIII. FLESH, SPIRIT, GHOSTS

H.D. adapts—tentatively in *Sword* and more decisively in *Helen*—Freud's argument from *Civilization and its Discontents* that civilization, although built on repression, would be better off with slightly less of it. H.D. suggests rather that a good deal less of it is in order. She often associates her works' female protagonists with the mothers of their male love objects, and portrays the violence of these love objects toward her protagonists as a result of their repressed memories of their mothers, and concurrently of a universal mother. There is war because male aggression is triggered by the repressed feminine/maternal principle, identified with the works' protagonists. Civilization, since it is built on repression, must be demolished for the next world to emerge. Correlatively, the blocks in the hero's psyche must shatter to admit the memory and love of the divine feminine, the mother/protagonist. This is the repeating story that Friedman and others have rightly argued affirms feminine power and wisdom—but it affirms violence by the same logic.

In *Sword*, Delia associates herself with Artemis and Howell with Hippolytus. In *Hippolytus Temporizes* (1927), H.D.'s English adaptation of Euripides's play, Hippolytus is obsessed with Artemis because he associates her with his mother, Artemis's former maiden. A lost mother of whom Delia reminds him, correlatively, haunts Howell. Likewise, before Delia met Howell, she was "haunted, obsessed" (84) by a specter of him, her identity split into Iseult Blanchemain, wife of Geoffrey, and Iseult Blanchefleur, the future partner of Howell:

> I had seen a ghost, a specter, *chère belle fantôme*, Geoffrey had once called me, and he was right to say I didn't love him. Iseult Blanchemain loved him well enough and I protested. But Geoffrey knew enough to know there was another. He knew there was another, but I didn't know it. He sensed in me the *belle fantôme* but he could not know what I did not know. He shouted, as he called it, Hippolytus and that was a play by a Greek poet, called Euripides. He "shouted" it in Greek and I stood frozen while I listened. I was the statue that the poet prayed to. . . . I saw Hippolytus. (83)

This association of Delia with Hippolytus (intended either as Howell's literal past incarnation or as an archetype of the mother-complexed hero) suggests that her relationship with Howell is Oedipal. In H.D.'s play (unlike in Euripides's surviving version) poor Hippolytus mistakenly sleeps with his stepmother thinking that she is Artemis, realizes his mistake, commits suicide, is resurrected in a state of insanity, and dies again—a fate that Howell may wish to avoid. Howell, too, is already Achilles, Dowding's incarnation in *Helen in Egypt*: "a wisp of steel—a sword of the Spirit, if you will, and a sword that had worked God's will before, as we all know. *Troy town's down*" (46). Delia is already Helen: "I remember the walls and the pale ghost, called Helen. *Troy town's down* but the beauty they recaptured, is no longer living" (54). *Helen in Egypt*'s Helen and Achilles are explicitly one another's (and their own) mother and father: they engender themselves by having sex (288). Thus, in the overall picture that these works attempt to piece together, the cruelty and wars of men result from repressed desire—or at least, the repudiations of Achilles/Howell/Dowding, and the Trojan and Second World War result from their Oedipal issues as sons and primal ferociousness as fathers and consorts. Family traumas charge these father/consort/sons' responses to H.D. figures with *Eros, Eris*. H.D.'s sexualized attack by father/sons is repeated, these works suggest, throughout history and legend.

However, though it is true that in some of *Sword*'s versions of reality Howell's reason malfunctions because Delia is his mother or mother-substitute or daughter, the "expanded world view" that gives rise to this vision in *Sword* is less fixed than it is in *Helen.*[118] *Sword* does not provide, as *Helen* does, a coherent explanation of its hero's behavior. It does not unify her experience so much as elaborate it to forestall the nonmeaning that threatens it.

Her protagonists, H.D. seeks to establish, contain the significance that they seek. Her approach in later work to reclaiming agency in relation to authority is to place the authority figure, the man who assumes the place of the Other, in a broader context that remains incompletely articulated, but within which the heroine's unlimited, ever unfolding (self)-knowledge reveals the man's perspective and behavior as limited. H.D.'s vision of the turning over of civilization into the next world mirrors this denouement of worldly authority. Just as the difference represented by these men is subsumed by her psychic insights, so rationalistic, male-dominated civilization—aligned with the conscious mind—will re-integrate with the primitive, unconscious and maternal. For H.D., as for Lacanian scholar Anika Lemaire's "Wolf Man," "castration is lived . . . as a precondition for being cured [though] the role of the persecutor, here the castrator, is successively filled by different men."[119] The movement of meaning from language into the protagonist herself is the goal.

The figure of Helen of Troy, whom H.D. identified with both her mother and herself, sounds a messianic note in *Sword* and *Helen*. Both works suggest that H.D. experienced her anger toward the warlike and utilitarian ethos of modern Europe, and Dowding, its emblem, as *their* aggression toward her. "Troy fell because it had sheltered" her alter ego Helen, inadvertent catalyst of male violence (116). However, Helen's "frail ghost bequeathed her priceless inheritance not only to the victor but to the vanquished. The rule of war did not preclude the rule of Beauty." Helen of Troy has in *Sword* the role that H.D. sets for herself in *Ion*; both represent beauty, which H.D. defines there as the kinship of "the conscious mind of man" with subtle "unconscious forces."[120] This beauty is bequeathed to the coming civilization. The violent reconciliation that Helen catalyzes is, as *Sword* and *Helen* suggest, the union of conscious and unconscious, the source of artistic, and consequently, cultural perfection.

In *Sword*, "Day-Star" says of Athens that there are "few ghosts, few . . . emanations. That is why I love it. It is all spirit" (198). "Spirit" stands here as in *Ion* for the "integrated" artistic perfection that H.D. believed the Ionians had achieved, and that now, at this turning point, must be achieved again:

> Today, again at a turning-point in the history of the world, the mind stands, to plead, to condone, to explain, to clarify, to illuminate; and, in the name of our magnificent heritage of that Hellenic past, each one of us is responsible to that abstract reality . . . that *spirit* again stands holding the balance between the past and the future. What now will we make of it?[121]

On the other hand, the Roman "Villa Trevi" (Klinik Brunner) is "haunted," but "would be all right if they didn't interpret everything, in that morbid way they have" (224). "Haunting" is again figured in terms of perpetual interpretation, the necessity of further integration of conscious and unconscious. The absence of ghosts, the "integrated" saturation of pure spirit, pure "aesthetic drive and concentrated spiritual force," expresses itself as a perfect beauty—especially in art—that makes interpretation unnecessary.

This integrated perfection stands for the renewed language for which H.D.'s own writing searches. Like Schreber's person and the God(s) and "provisional-improvised" beings of *Memoirs*, *Sword*'s female victims, male aggressors, and ghosts express malfunctioning language, suggesting, but not articulating, a hidden meaning imagined beyond the confines of the crumbling social order. Delia's cognitive "labyrinth" and Schreber's "compulsive thinking" compel their pursuit of this meaning and result in a knowledge of the Cosmic Order in which, for both, "everything that happens is in reference to me."[122]

Like Schreber, Delia follows spectral signifiers, "traces of direction" that locate meaning in her person, in her memories, associations and writing—asymbolic though these are—and in her traumatic participation in the eternally recurring "Sacred Drama." Agency, for her, becomes a question not of behavior regarding others, but, instead, of articulating to herself what is always already contained within her. The written revisitation of her past becomes itself a political project. Perhaps, for H.D., *Sword* and *Helen*, as integrated literary works, are necessary to the coming civilization, if it is to be perfect. At any rate, H.D.'s and Schreber's work implies that their encounters with, and perhaps, as I will discuss, reversals of castration will enable the new, integrated world to rise from the ruins of the old.

Delia's task of integration and correlative world salvation, linked to the attainment of certain knowledge, raises the difficult question of how to bring together these two clusters of associations. On the one hand, there is "civilization," the "conscious mind," and the white, male, secular, intellectual tradition, which I have associated with the linguistic signifier and the symbolic order. On the other hand, there is the "primitive," "psychic," "unconscious," supernatural, nonwhite, and/or feminine, which stands for the signified and the imaginary order. In *Sword*, the integration of these terms involves the need to put psychic phenomena on a more "scientific" basis, a task to which Delia imagines Howell (with whom she associates the former set of characteristics) and herself (with whom she associates the latter) as uniquely suited. Morris writes of H.D.'s determination to integrate "science" into her conceptual framework in terms of a desire to heal the modern breach between science and the mystical or animistic. Referencing French literary theorist Roland Barthes, Morris describes "science" as one of H.D.'s "Mana-Words." According to Morris such "Mana-Words" are words a writer uses "that are [as Barthes puts it] 'neither eccentric [n]or central' yet nonetheless impart 'the illusion that by this word one might answer for everything.'"[123] Morris distinguishes three approaches with which H.D. attempted to integrate science into her writing: imitation, supplementation, and assimilation:

> Where supplementation makes science and poetry into adjacent and complementary disciplines, assimilation, H.D.'s third strategy, like imitation, her first, overlaps the two enterprises . . . in assimilation, the poet takes up a position as a practitioner who contributes to knowledge in his or her own right. The claim of this strategy is not that poetry is *like* science but that in some fashion it *is* science.[124]

Sword takes this "assimilative" strategy. In it, Delia's psychic experiences and associative process are meant to uncover empirical truth. This truth is "scientific" and should be recognized as such: "If 'We are not ready' to place psychic communication on a scientific, practical basis now, at this very moment, when will we be?" (128). The power of science to save the world is contingent on its being applied to psychic phenomena. But science is never—here or anywhere in H.D.'s writing—fully united with psychic phenomena, with art or with the unconscious realms. It always remains the term with which, try as she might, she does not identify: "Clairvoyants, as a rule, are sensitive but not scientific" (125). In suggesting a systematizing and discriminatory capacity that she does not feel herself to possess, "science" implies the possibility of answering for everything while it remains beyond her reach. Delia reflects,

> One was afraid of the end of the world. It was the end of the world, anyway. There must be another world, but where was it? It was there, somewhere. I had never doubted that. But I had made no real emotional connection with it, as my work with Masini had been for the most part, either impersonal or literary. *Lord Howell had stood out for some sort of extension of consciousness. I wanted anyhow to feel things in that way, in a rational way. Perhaps that was where I was wrong.* (34, emphasis added)

Delia's desire, associated with Howell and with the next world, to feel things "in a rational way" echoes all the protagonists' desires in *Sword* and in *Helen* for the union of their *héros fatals* and themselves, science and psychic research, Egypt and Greece, masculine and feminine, civilized and primitive, conscious and unconscious, in order to achieve the "next world." This desired integration, as well as the violent imagery with which it is imagined, suggests H.D.'s ambivalent longing for, and terror of, the modern (male) symbolic order, the realm where beings and objects are coldly differentiated from oneself and from one another, language is shared, and speech and writing may be true or untrue according to logic. Science, and the men that H.D. and her alter egos associate with it, represent the possibility of what Lacan calls castration—the possibility of admittance into their shared world of symbolic law and order. However, it is the men with their science who turn out to be castrated (in the sense of being limited and misguided) while H.D.'s expanding frames of reference contain (she suggests) their rationality, but are not limited by it. The invalidations that come from these men, however, trigger psychic cataclysm by representing her lack of access to the symbolic phallus, or determinative social power.

Robert Duncan understands H.D. as a psychic warrior who explored and testified to the strange truth that words shape us, and "reality," in a much more radical way than we realize. For Duncan, H.D. shows in work like *Helen in Egypt* that there is no ontological distinction between dreamer and dream, medium and "control": we dream ourselves.[125] The renewal that H.D. depicts is thus, he suggests, a true renewal. Yet for H.D. it is never quite accomplished. Notwithstanding her many claims of final understanding, and substitutions of beings, events and objects for conceptual meanings, she continues to deploy free-associative inter-referentiality in a literary search for answers to questions that are themselves often unclear. This search spins new connections and references in a "complex web of abstract values" that feels perpetually unsatisfying to H.D., as her unending quest to complete it suggests.[126]

IX. WAR, LOVE, BETRAYAL

Regardless of whether we believe that the intensity of her response to delegitimation by authority figures has to do with an early foreclosure of what Lacan calls the name of the father, so that the enactment of this denial by a father figure triggers a crisis, it is fair to surmise that H.D., having experiences that are beyond the pale of the ordinary and socially comprehensible, is vulnerable to delegitimation by authority figures to an extent that may be hard for many of us to imagine. The psychoanalytic theory that interested H.D. portrayed paranormal experiences as symptoms of mental illness. Such experiences were, as Robin Pappas notes, pre-inscribed as mad, "feminine" or "artistic," certainly unscientific; and H.D. struggled against this prevalent discourse, as many critics have discussed.[127] Some contemporary psychoanalytic theorists refute the idea of fixed psychic structures, and suggest that the very pathologization of a nonnormative experience invites the onset of severe disturbances. George Atwood would understand H.D.'s intense way of relating to male power and authority figures as an ongoing attempt to repair an unmet developmental need, and would understand her as particularly vulnerable to their invalidation when communicating to them the unusual experiences that she describes in *Notes on Thought and Vision, Sword,* and *Tribute*. Writes Atwood,

> An objectified psychiatric diagnosis is the antithesis of needed validation and mirroring. It leaves one with an attribution, offered up by a person invested with enormous authority, that can invade and usurp a person's sense of selfhood, that can operate like a nuclear tipped torpedo exploding in one's brain. . . . A spiraling effect occurs, wherein the operation of the medical model further injures the already devastated patient, whose reactions to the new injuries in turn confirm the correctness of the diagnosis.[128]

If Freud's pathologization of H.D.'s Corfu vision was destabilizing, Dowding's dismissal of her spirit communications—communications that she believed were of crucial social importance since they were intended to save humanity from destruction—was shattering, and it appears as a central concern in H.D.'s writing for the following decade or more. Likewise, the skepticism of her other analysts concerning the unique significance of her relationship with Dowding is rendered as a cause of anguish in *Helen in Egypt*.[129] These delegitimations are often followed by the appearance in her journals and creative work of paranoid, delusional, and disorganized feelings and thoughts. Such responses followed Freud's interpretation of her visions as "dangerous," Dowding's refusal to receive her spirit messages, Heydt's disbelief in the universal significance of her encounter with Dowding, and writer Lionel Durand's panning (as she believed) of her *Bid Me to Live: A Madrigal* in a *Newsweek* review.[130]

There was also, in each case, extensive literary production: a written struggle to understand the rejection, a deployment of patterns—including family triangles and occult schemas—and a proliferating of different possibilities without a selection of one, or, quite often, a sense of the logical or causal connection between the rejection and the possibility. Her work's multifarious characters, things, and events, whose causal relations to one another are not evident, but who are mysteriously encompassed by or contained in their H.D.–based characters, likewise suggest splitting, projection, and incorporation in the realm of thought. Her responses to Freud's, Dowding's, and Heydt's perceived rejections comprise whole books, and share the same pattern: Why, why must they be so limited and blind? Nevertheless, if they must, H.D.'s literary and spiritual alter egos will persist, go beyond their limits, encompass more knowledge with their vision, discover and integrate different parts of themselves—even though this project remains disorienting and incomplete.[131] As Delia in *Sword* appeals to Masini, "it's not the person, it's the story. The person went out of my life years ago. I hate to leave things unfinished. I wrote a sort of—a sort of novel. I can't finish it and I can't destroy it. What shall I do?" (7)

Earlier writing establishes the groundwork for *Sword*'s and *Helen*'s particular takes on family dynamics, the conscious mind's reintegration of unconscious memories, and the broader social significance of this. In work composed before Dowding's ascendancy, like *The Gift* (written 1941–1943, first published 1944) and *Tribute to Freud*, H.D. portrays her own psychic integration as a solo endeavor that has a sympathetic effect on broader social integration. In *The Gift*, the protagonist-author Hilda intuits that war, generally (including the Second World War, since the novel spans multiple time frames), is the result of a broken promise of peaceful co-existence made by Hilda's spiritual predecessors, the Moravians, to "the Indians." The Second World War is taking place because the Indian-Moravian brotherhood has been sundered through no fault of either party, but through the betrayals of other settlers: "There was a Promise and there was a Gift, but the Promise it seems, was broken and the Gift it seems, was lost. That is why, now at this minute, there is a roar [the Blitz] outside."[132] However, "a secret powerful community" is destined to "bring the ancient secrets of Europe and the ancient secrets of America into a single union of Power and Spirit, a united brotherhood, a *Unitas Fratrum* of the whole world."[133] This union of the ancient secrets of Europe and America takes place in the person or "subconscious being" of H.D., and has to do with remembering her identities in past lives:

> I had gone down under the wave and I was still alive, I was breathing. . . . I had gone down, been submerged by the wave of memories and terrors, repressed since the age of ten and long before, but with the terrors, I had found the joys, too. . . . I was Morning Star, or I was Anna Von Pahlen who had been a sort of Princess in Europe. So Europe and America had at last been reconciled in the very depth of my subconscious being.[134]

The Gift, which ends with a ceasefire, suggests that this reconciliation, centered in her own person, has a sympathetic effect, which heals the divisions between warring nations. The postwar era envisioned unites disparate cultures under the rubric of a shared higher knowledge that is, finally, the protagonists' self-knowledge. The imagined elect form a diasporic network, and each knows the same truth though it may be called by different names. This knowledge of the truth ends the Second World War when Hilda discovers that the figures that represent Europe and America for her, Morning Star and Anna Von Pahlen, are her past incarnations. This discovery reconciles them in her "subconscious being," and thereby reconciles the warring continents in actuality.

Ion, H.D.'s 1937 creative adaptation of Euripides's play, offers a similar vision of the sympathetic effect of personal integration on social integration. It describes the beauty of Ionian cultural achievement as the product of a fated union of God and mortal, tantamount to the union of "the conscious mind of man" and the "unconscious forces."[135] During its composition, H.D.

wrote to Bryher that "my work is creative and reconstructive, war or no war, if I can get across the Greek spirit at its highest I am helping the world, and the future. It is the highest spiritual neutrality."[136] *Ion*'s main concern is to recall the Ionian spirit of beauty and perfection, and to caution humanity to have faith in the "ultimate plan," notwithstanding social strife. Though Ion, founder of a perfect civilization, suffered when he opened the box containing his past and discovered the evidence that reunited him with his mother, Kreousa, their reward is Ionian culture itself, "the absolute achievement of physical perfection by the spirit of man," before it "sank into the darkness of late Rome and the Middle Ages."[137] Kreousa, mother of Ion, is an H.D. figure, the mother, through her art, of the civilization to come, in which art and beings are indistinct:

> [Kreousa] now wishes to be nothing but the mother of Ion, the mother, if she but knew it, of a new culture, of an aesthetic drive and concentrated spiritual force, not to be reckoned with, in terms of any then known values; hardly, even today, to be estimated at its true worth. . . . A scattered handful of these creatures or creations is enough to mark, for all time, that high-water mark of human achievement, the welding of strength and delicacy, the valiant yet totally unselfconscious withdrawal of the personality of the artist, who traced on marble, for all time . . . that thing and that thing alone that we mean, when we say, Ionian.[138]

Cultural transformation and perfection here involve the traumatic reunification of a divinely chosen individual with his lost mother. This will give rise to a new culture—in *Ion* perhaps an uncomfortably perfect one, considering that it was written in the shadow of National Socialism, also given to the rhetoric of perfection.

Like *Ion*, *Hippolytus Temporizes*, H.D.'s 1927 creative adaptation of Euripides, portrays mother and son figures in painful, muddled, hostile interactions. In *Ion*, Kreousa and Ion's conflict results in their discovery that they are mother and son. This discovery gives rise to Ion's founding of a perfect Ionian culture. However, H.D.'s Hippolytus, obsessed with the goddess Artemis because she reminds him of his dead mother, has worse luck. He sleeps with his stepmother thinking that she is Artemis, commits suicide on discovering his mistake, is resurrected by Apollo at Artemis's behest and, since he has become insane, is killed off again. These plays, then, portray both successful and unsuccessful unions of sons with mother figures. One gives rise to a "perfect" civilization, the other to madness and death.

While *Ion* and *The Gift* suggest that the integration of "Europe and America" or "God and mortal" cause, on the one hand, the beginning of a perfect civilization, and on the other, a ceasefire (at the very least), the apparent interminability of the Second World War, and the onset of the second

Blitz make H.D. think that there was more integration to be accomplished. In *Sword* and *Helen*, this integration appears, paradoxically, as the violent (dis)union of the women who represent H.D. with the men who represent Dowding, who see them as mother figures. The violence that H.D. sees in the war and in Dowding's repudiation, creatively revisited in *Sword* and in *Helen*, become her circular answer to the problem of the "integration" necessary for the arrival of the next world.

In contrast to the intensity between mothers and fathers and mothers and sons, the mothers and daughters in H.D.'s fiction have undynamic relationships. H.D.'s mother, when she is fictionally portrayed in *Tribute to Freud*, *The Gift* and *HERmione*, is shown withholding everything that Hilda wants: acknowledgment, information, validation, explanation, and indeed, her very presence. Eugenia Gart in *HERmione* retreats into silences that Hermione cannot explain. Helen in *The Gift* answers Hilda's questions but unforthcomingly. Hilda must turn to Mamalie, her grandmother, whose cognition is fading, whose hints and ramblings provide piecemeal information that must, Hilda is sure, all fit together somehow. Characteristically, Hilda tries to contain her mother's dismissal, "My children are not gifted," within a larger framework, suggested by psychic insight and by her grandmother's hints, in which this dismissal appears as repression. In *Helen* and *Sword*, H.D.'s alter ego Helen of Troy, like her mother, Helen Wolle Doolittle, contains, but does not explain, "the answer." The violence of the war is directed particularly at this Helen, though it is destructive *en masse*. It is tempting to speculate that H.D.'s aggression toward her own unforthcoming mother, and toward subsequent repudiators, appears in her writing as male aggression toward literary Helens and mother figures.

This maneuver would involve what Klein calls "splitting" and "projection," mechanisms to disperse the anger felt toward others and the anxiety it generates.[139] Duncan, who traces his poetic lineage through H.D., when discussing H.D.'s *Trilogy* (also written during and after the Second World War), considers the role of projection in H.D.'s perception of the war. Duncan suggests that the violence of war reflects H.D.'s rage and longing for vengeance, which she projects, exultantly, into her work: "The apocalyptic picture of the world that is also the heart under attack is a complex image of correspondences between what is felt as inflicted and what is felt in projection, of wishes for vengeance that are also fears of punishment seen fulfilled in actual events."[140] This rage is a response to perceived attacks and betrayals that are equated with the war, at least as much as to the war itself. H.D. experiences her fury *as* the Second World War, the violence of which is directed specifically at her and her alter egos, the objects of male desire and aggression. In her protagonists, aggression is absorbed through sexualized attack (the primal scene) and transformed through birth; the world ends and is renewed in an eternal cycle.[141] Friedman rightly reads the cycles in H.D.'s work as an adaption of cross-cultural mythic cycles of sex, death, and renewal. However, there is often something rapid, chaotic, overpopulated, unsatisfying, and gloomy in these cycles that set them somewhat apart from the mythic. Friedman has described "the pattern of H.D.'s . . . life and work" as a "profoundly dialectical" process in which she "repeatedly established clearly defined, imagistically rendered, polar oppositions so that she could ultimately move toward a transcendent synthesis." [142] However, Friedman's formulation, "ultimately move toward," itself, suggests H.D.'s vexed relation to "transcendent synthesis," which her later work figures as a will-o'-the-wisp of united personal and universal meaning: a meaning that her cycle can never have.

X. EXPANDING FRAMES OF REFERENCE, IDENTITY SORTING, THE "PSYCHOTIC PSYCHIC STRUCTURE"

> My love of the gods, as fairies and beings was alive in me, before I struck the bare cold reality of "facts" or the numeral star-symbol.
>
> – H.D., *Tribute to Freud*, 121–3.

As we see in H.D.'s letters and in *Tribute to Freud*, Freud reads her visions at Corfu as her foreclosed homosexual desire for her mother returning in the guise of hallucinations, just as he reads Schreber's symptoms in terms of his desire for his father—a phenomenon that he discusses in "The Loss of Reality in Neurosis and Psychosis."[143] "The professor," *Tribute* tells us, "translated the pictures on the wall . . . as a desire for union with my mother."[144] Though H.D. recasts her visions as psychic gifts, Freud's view of them as psychotic symptoms contributes to the ongoing ambivalence with which H.D., herself, reads them: "But symptom *or* inspiration, the writing [on the wall at Corfu] continues to write itself *or* be written."[145] H.D. maintains both possibilities in *Tribute* and other later work. However, the question of whether her visions and insights are purely subjective (symptoms) or universally relevant (psychic visions) seems itself to haunt her with proliferating, dissociative, and repetitive thought cycles.

Freud believes that H.D. had not negotiated the Oedipal phase successfully by repressing her primordial bisexuality to become properly, heterosexually "female": "The Professor said I had not made the conventional transference from mother to father, as is usual with a girl at adolescence."[146] Their sessions leading up to this time, as she recounts in letters, involved the exploration of her early triangles or failure to triangulate: "F. says mine is the absolutely FIRST layer, I got stuck in the earliest pre-OE stage, and 'back to the womb' seems to be my only solution. Hence islands, sea, Greek primitives, and so on . . . my triangle is mother-brother-self . . . diverse looking manifestations fit in somehow."[147] The project of Oedipal triangulation apparently continues in *The Gift* and *Tribute*, in which H.D. seems to be diagnosing her own lack of relationship to her "un-get-atable" and "giant-like" father and attempting, not very successfully, a libidinal transference from mother to father.[148] In a 1933 letter to Bryher, she reports that, according to Freud,

> There is some block and connecting link missing that he can't get at. I suppose it is the "father" vibration, for we can't, no matter how we idealize the mother-idea, get rid of the father. . . . I think I have made some funny pure classic transference, and that certain things, the "ball," these doves, represent "father," but do not link up with the actual personal father. . . . I think the link is the star-stuff, but as S.F. once or twice has given such a snort when I have gone into star-states, it sort of cripples me. . . . I am not, as you know, a sloppy theosophist or horoscope-ist, but you know, I do believe in these things and I think there is a whole other-science of them. And that is where, in a way, S.F. and I part company. I suppose that too, is symbolical of my leaving my own home and its surroundings and the strictly, so-called "scientific." But I think you will agree that star-fish stuff is my real world and that getting that, I am, in a way, being "in love" also with my father, but of course, again a mystical "father-in-heaven."[149]

Freud suggests that there is a block in regard to her actual, personal father. In her terminology, which may be borrowed from Martinist Robert Ambelain's *Practical Kabbalah*, the "father vibration" cannot be gotten rid of—but things that represent the father do not link up to the actual personal father.[150] However, she surmises, getting the "star-fish stuff" that is her real world is "being in love also with my father, but . . . a mystical father-in-heaven." Though H.D. accepted Freud's suggestion that her interest in astrology manifested her desire for her father, the astronomer, her star-states seem to replace her actual personal father with the father-in-heaven. Certainly, star-states, mother-ideas, and "other-sciences" share a hyphenated fuzzy unboundedness, a nondifferentiation, with the father-in-heaven, which the actual personal father with his "cold, scientific detachment" lacks. H.D. rejects her father's "strictly, so-called" science, and calls on a greater interpretive framework associated with "other-science": occultism, hyphenation, and the father-in-heaven. Both this passage and *Tribute to Freud* demonstrate her turn to a wider frame of reference or "other-science," which is unavailable to Freud. This turn to a wider but unclear frame of reference is repeated in *Sword*, when Howell (associated, like Freud, with her father and with coldness, detachment, and science) rejects Delia's appeal that he translate "the meaning of the numbers and letters" from the RAF pilots that Delia "could only record."

Analogously, H.D.'s correspondence suggests that her famously renewed sense of purpose after her analysis comes, not from father figure Freud, but from modifications to his analytical method that affirm the truth of her visions and the social relevance of her work (at that time, a creative translation of Euripides's *Ion*).[151] H.D.'s letter to Bryher suggests what Lacan calls a "recognition of the imaginary,"[152] which H.D. provides for herself following Freud's "crippling" response to her star-states. Viewed through a Lacanian lens, this affirmation may be precisely what perpetuates her disaster of signification. As Norman Holland notes,

> Gaps, spaces between, somehow these terrified her. In interpreting a dream about a mysterious, beautiful Egyptian princess coming down a flight of steps to find Moses in the bulrushes, she tells us how she dealt with them. . . . "Am I," asked H.D., "after all, in my fantasy, the baby [Moses]? Do I wish myself, in the deepest unconscious or subconscious layers of my being, to be the founder of a new religion?" Yes, she did. She had to believe in a religious transcendence, because that would close the gaps.[153]

I am far from intending to pathologize the belief in a "religious transcendence" of difference. However, I do see a repeating pattern through which H.D.'s "other-science" attempts to regain wholeness, following the dismissal of her visions by representatives of "strictly, so-called science." She makes the dismissal itself part of a larger pattern, wherein the exact causal connection between dismissal and pattern remains elusive.

H.D.'s preoccupation with distinguishing self from not-self suggests an attempt to order the chaos ensuing from her turn toward an inter-referential "other-science" following her analysis with Freud, as well as a means of "closing the gaps"[154] She remains occupied with distinguishing self and not-self and with the identity and difference of other people, things, and events throughout her life—as *Sword*, *Helen*, and other late works demonstrate. Holland speculates that this "urgent concern for boundaries and discrete units" relates to her work's formal qualities as well as to its content: "H.D.'s short, choppy stanza forms, her difficulties with the boundaries of sentences, or the indeterminacy of the verb forms in many of her lyrics."[155] Holland also suggests that it has "something to do with her insistence on treating symbols as having fixed meanings and the dream as 'a universal language,' despite Freud's cautions to the contrary."[156]

If symbols have "fixed meanings," for H.D., then her discovery of which person, object or event "is"—as she sometimes puts it—which *other* person, object or event becomes broadly relevant. For H.D. "symbols" are understood in a literal rather than symbolic way—if symbolism requires that the symbol not also *be* the thing that it represents. For H.D., things really are what they also stand for—not just subjectively but objectively, for others (though they may not know it) as well as for her. For instance, her *Ghirlanda* table really is "the Viking ship of Hal Birth" (127), and "the Viking ship was England" (123) in a broadly relevant sense, since these identities confirm England's (and Delia's) premonitions of England's future and her mission to explore new psychic horizons. Sorting out what everything else is and what it is not, and creating visual schemas of how things, events, and people relate spatially and temporally to the things, events, and people they are not, is thus a universally significant endeavor. From the mid-1940s, H.D.'s belief in reincarnation and spirit channeling, and also from the 1950s to her death, her belief in astral doubles, provide a rationale for her intent and ongoing sorting of identity and difference. This preoccupation and the need for it is evident in *Sword.* Robinson writes of H.D.'s sorting activity in reference to her engagement with Ambelain's and Chaboseau's work:

> With Ambelain's volumes at her bedside, she resumed the style of dream-journaling she had done with Freud in the 1930s; in these journals she began the work of composing an astral *who's who*, linking up figures from different periods of her life to show who replaces whom, what symbols stand for what people or constellations of people. . . . H.D. embarked on a program of "hermetic definition," finding the hidden astral identities behind the host of individuals she had encountered in her dreams, visions, and encounters in the *au-delà.*[157]

H.D.'s project, from the mid-1940s to the end of her life, of establishing who represents which previous incarnation or astral double partakes of, but cannot be fully explained by, the influence of spiritualist and occultist theories. It also suggests a wish to somehow give order to ongoing experiences of disorder that may have involved the perception of receiving spirit messages and visions of past lives. The chaotic form and content of her work from this period, and the identity-sorting preoccupations of its protagonists, speak of H.D.'s confusion regarding identity and difference at this time, and her deployment of occultist frames of reference to lend their meanings to her free-floating signifiers and looping thought patterns.

As Robinson notes, H.D. spends much time formulating and reformulating the correspondences of men she loved to astral initiators, expressing uncertainty about who is whom, really. Her uncertainty regarding correspondences among people and objects suggests that she views these correspondences as more literal than subjective. We can usually discern what people or things represent for us personally at a particular time, whereas discerning a fixed and universal system of correspondences might entail more guesswork and uncertainty. Robinson observes that "it is as though in these late years H.D.

arranges and rearranges the same set of puzzle-pieces over and over, trying to find the true pattern." However, he notes elsewhere, "the act of completing the pattern is, for H.D., also the search for the pattern; she often uses the term [pattern] to mean a work in progress, a search for parallels and connections." This search for fixed connections—for instance, by reformulating her understanding of which men represent which stars in Chaboseau's pattern—appears in H.D.'s late writing as a search for a symbolic order in Lacan's sense: a socially shared order of meanings rather than personal symbols. This search for a universalized system inside herself suggests confusion between inner and outer worlds, as well as the astral questing that Robinson explicates.[158]

Lacan warns against free-associative therapy for analysands with psychotic structures because of their difficulty with signification as such, and considers the potential misrecognition of the distinction between the symbolic and the imaginary orders as the greatest danger in their analysis:

> What in the subject calls for recognition on the appropriate level of authentic symbolic exchange [i.e. free association and dreams] . . . is replaced by a recognition of the imaginary, of fantasy. Thus to authenticate everything of the order of the imaginary in the subject is properly speaking to make analysis the anteroom of madness . . . we must attribute the well-known cases of fairly rapid onset of a more or less persistent and sometimes lasting delusion to a certain way of handling the analytic relation, which consists in authenticating the imaginary, in substituting recognition on the imaginary level for recognition on the symbolic level.[159]

Freud, primly scientific though he appears in H.D.'s letters and in *Tribute to Freud*, was credulous and expansive toward the supernatural in the 1930s,[160] despite his earlier dread of occultism's threat to the scientific integrity of psychoanalysis.[161] He was a member of the English Society for Psychical Research and in "Dreams and Occultism" (1932) urges the reader "to have kindlier thoughts on the objective possibility of thought-transference and at the same time of telepathy as well."[162] In *Totem and Taboo* he describes an affinity between magic and art based on their shared method of associating ideas through similarity and contiguity and on their common assumption of the "principle of the 'omnipotence of thoughts,'" in which "[r]elations which hold between the ideas of things are assumed to hold equally between the things themselves."[163] Obsessional neurosis, he notes, shares this assumption with magic and art. As Timothy Materer describes Freud's ideas,

> The artist draws on the primitive feelings found in animism just as the magician draws on them to demonstrate a power over spirits. But there is a second and even closer affinity between magic and art: both work through the association

> of ideas. . . . The artist is thus linked with the shaman, and magic with literary technique—just as an occultist would wish.[164]

In keeping with his theory that magic and art both assume, in different ways, that the relations they establish between representations of things extend to the relations between the things themselves, Freud to some extent validated H.D.'s visionary experiences and her idea of the literal correspondence of her inner and outer worlds, and of the things, people, and events in them. He did so by invoking her vocation as a poet: her visions could be "true" for her as a poet, although he did not think that they represented information about anything in the world outside of her. Since Freud was very much a scientist for H.D., his view of art and magic's affinity through shared associative modes, and his qualified affirmation of her supernatural experiences, lent scientific credence to her belief in the superiority of the "other-science" of free association and psychic vision over the rationalism that he himself represented for her.

Both Freud's and Dowding's perceived repudiations give rise, for H.D., to interpretive endeavors that trump the father figure's blinkered authority and reverse his attempted castration, but never bring the clarity that she seeks—except insofar as it may be found in the imaginary reenactment of the castration. H.D.'s psychic experiences—for instance, her Corfu visions and her RAF messages—are considered in *Tribute to Freud* and in *Sword* as functions of a potentially dangerous mental state, in which the eruptions of the unconscious may be overwhelming to the conscious mind—though their broad social significance is nevertheless affirmed.[165] In *Sword,* Delia doubts that she would have received spirit communications if in perfect health: "Given ideal conditions, comfort, security, peace of mind would the messages have come at all, or would we ourselves have wanted them? . . . If I with sincerity and conviction, later continue the 'work,' would my very peace of mind and comparative good health, in a sense, block the communications?" (68). Delia seems to shuttle somewhat between an affirmation of the noetic quality of her insights and an understanding of them as predicated on some degree of unhealthiness. Though ambivalence over competing frames of reference can be productive, H.D."s need to establish with certainty that her frame of reference was true, and others' false, as well as her constantly new associations and interpretations, suggest that her ambivalence results in a growing confusion and incoherence, and that it is not intended as a self-reflexive example of the never-ending quality of thought and inquiry. The degree of H.D.'s identification with her thoughts in these works makes the thoughts themselves the only means through which their resolution can be sought.

All of the objects, events and beings that appear in H.D.'s constantly expanding interpretive framework are somehow, she imagines, associated with the repudiation whose meaning she is interpreting. Though she frames this preoccupation with esoteric teachings such as Ambelain's writings on cycles of spiritual initiation, these teachings and beliefs do not explain the preoccupation itself—nor do they fully account for the enigmatic and repetitive qualities of her writing. Since, for her, beings and things actually "are" the other beings and things they represent—and more of these keep appearing—distinctness and precision of cause and effect, or historic time, slips into inundating nondifferentiation. The only "meaning" of repudiations by male love objects is found in the very cycle of their traumatic reenactment. H.D.'s journal entries in the 1950s and 1960s increasingly locate her life's meaning in these "initiations," or encounters ending in betrayals with men she has loved.

It is hard to say exactly when and why psychoanalytic descriptions of "psychotic" or "paranoid-schizoid" mechanisms are applicable to H.D.'s work: for instance, when they are applicable because she knew of them and chose to engage with them, and when they are applicable because of their accuracy in describing inadvertent thought patterns. It is mind-bending to try to distinguish these alternatives, perhaps because, due to the intensity of H.D.'s engagement in a perilous psychic exploration informed by psychoanalytic theory and methodology, they are not entirely distinct. I read her relation to psychoanalysis as an oscillation: she knew something about it, and it knew (and produced) something about (and in) her. The psychoanalytic theory available to H.D. certainly contributed to many images and narratives: the knives and crucified worms in *Tribute*, the grieving process in *Trilogy* (as Susan Edmunds suggests), among many other examples. Psychoanalysis, especially her sessions with Freud, may have also further promoted to her the free-associative mode of thought and expression that become so pronounced in *Sword* and *Helen*.[166] However, H.D. cannot be said to intentionally portray in her writing after 1946 a cataclysm of sequential, organized thought as a self-reflexive commentary about theories of psychotic language, or language as such: nor were these theories available to her.

Indeed, I find no intention in *Sword* or *Helen* to self-consciously reflect or rearticulate even the preoccupations, beliefs, and crises of H.D.'s social environment. These preoccupations and crises are seen as personally relevant, since H.D. believes that her psychic explorations have sympathetic effects on world events. However, though inner and outer worlds reflect one another for H.D., there is little evidence of a space outside of her dysfunctional thought patterns, which mirror the dysfunctional patterns of the social realm, and from which a self-conscious reflection on either of these could take place. The degree of H.D.'s identification with her thoughts in these works makes the thoughts themselves the only means through which their resolution can be sought.

H.D.'s work, like Schreber's (as psychoanalytic theorist Samuel Weber writes in his 1988 introduction to the *Memoirs*) "does not stand apart from what it describes, but . . . itself is included in it."[167] Similarly, the apocalypticism and the martyrdom of women by men in *Sword* and *Helen* are not self-consciously intended to comment on, or challenge, postwar Anglo-American modernism's "warrior ethos," as Hogue and Vandivere suggest of *Sword*.[168] The beliefs and preoccupations that *Sword* evidences—for instance, the preoccupation with the attacks and betrayals of beloved warrior figures, and the belief that there must be a Third World War before the balance of the world can be realigned—are actually held by H.D. at this time with no evidence of self-reflexive distance. Dreams, visions, and spirit messages in her lived experience seem to support them. Further, *Sword* and *Helen* do not intentionally communicate the experience of a breakdown in language in response to psychoanalytic theory, though H.D. delivers intentional and interesting responses to psychoanalytic theory elsewhere and in other ways. Here, H.D.'s agency is in witnessing her own semiotic disaster and perhaps in trying to reverse it by rendering symbolic meaning as being—as Schreber also attempts in his *Memoirs*.

Delia's written response, in *Sword*, to Howell's dismissal of her messages and his unequivocal refusal to receive them, suggests the collapse of symbolism, which triggers the ensuing necessity of ever new dualisms and terms, of wider interpretive frameworks, of new characters and chapters that maintain the possibility of meaning. In *Helen in Egypt*, H.D.'s "alter ego"[169] Helen attempts, more successfully than Delia, to imagine a cosmology (of sorts) within which this repudiation makes sense—a sense that does not contradict the sense of purpose that H.D.'s psychoanalytic sessions with Freud, and her extraordinary psychic experiences, had given her. This cosmological system includes her literal embodiment of language and a recurring cycle of sexualized violence directed at her, and preordained and perpetrated by God (or a male divine being). This violence is expected to result in transformation and rebirth, and is sometimes depicted as doing so, but not for long or with much conviction. Though this cycle is aligned in H.D.'s mind with cycles of initiation in occultist doctrine, its appearance in her work cannot be explained solely with reference to her engagement in occultism. The energy that drives her thought and writing about and through this devastating cycle comes, I would hold, from a psychic imperative too threatening to assimilate.

Though H.D. scholars such as Christine Coffman have rightly deplored the sexism and homophobia inherent in the Freudian conception of psychosis as well as its tenacious remainder in psychoanalytic theory, Coffman has read the construction of "the psychotic lesbian" in critical responses to H.D. as simply a means of marginalizing her work and maintaining patriarchal literary norms.[170] However, H.D.'s own critics have tended to reproduce the standard tendency to use "madness" as a mere negative and unexamined label. In their introduction to *Sword*, Hogue and Vandivere write that it displays "a mad grief—something that looks like madness but isn't, something that is closer to fury" (i). This argument posits a category of "actual" madness—undefined but inapplicable (for reasons undisclosed) to H.D. It also implies that actual mad people are not responding to social conditions, that their madness is not "mad grief" or "fury" but rather an a priori condition. If madness as a concept is rejected in literary criticism because of its brutality, it should be rejected categorically, and not only in the cases of writers like H.D. whose communications we consider worthwhile. While the term and definitions of it subsist, they should be applied, or not applied, equitably. They might also be usefully re-examined, since they will haunt, and their denial will have to be repeated. Though Schreber's *Memoirs* informs our very understanding of what madness is, Schreber responded with sense, ingenuity, and courage to the conditions that he was experiencing. I validate Schreber rather than invalidating H.D., in part by drawing attention to the uncertain ground for the discursive division between madman and creative visionary.

For H.D., the mother is Love, "dream/vision," the unconscious; the father and Death are science (including psychoanalysis), the conscious mind. Union is deadly to the mother. H.D.'s association of psychic powers with insanity suggests a discursive pitfall, perhaps resulting from the encounter between "science" (as Freud and its early practitioners wished psychoanalysis to be understood), paranormal experiences, and H.D.'s occultist and spiritualist beliefs. I use the terms "occultism" and "spiritualism," hoping that they will encompass various permutations of Western esoteric thought and practice including Theosophy, Hermeticism, Gnosticism, Rosicrucianism, table-tapping, and the various other sectarian beliefs and practices that H.D. used to frame and understand her own psychic explorations. Psychoanalysis aligned supernatural visions with psychotic hallucination; to see and hear things that others do not see and hear was always, for Freud and for psychoanalysis in modernity generally, a dangerous symptom. Further, the spiritual transcendence that occultism posited translated, in H.D.'s understanding of Freud's system, as either psychic integration or madness. In *Sword* and *Helen*, the male hero (aligned with science, pragmatism, war, and hegemony) attacks and delegitimizes the heroine (aligned with psychic insight, creativity, love, and counter-hegemony). This attack is devastating, but necessary to their processes of integration, which H.D. sometimes suggests will be completed at some future time. Concurrently, H.D. asserts her feminine psychic experiences in the face of delegitimation by father figures. Charles LaChance rightly notes that H.D.'s female characters "are terrorized by and yet gravitate toward omnipotent males," but rather than desiring mere sexual surrender as he suggests, these characters desire legitimation, are shattered by delegitimation, and are unceasing in their interpretive efforts to salvage it.[171]

As the imaginary order sought to assimilate the symbolic within H.D.'s psychic economy, so her epochal vision after the Second World War sought to assimilate difference—religious, cultural and personal—under the rubric of higher knowledge and integration. H.D.'s solution to the estrangement of science (the hero) from enchantment (the heroine) is to give birth to a new world order in which the scientific and the psychic are reunited. This rebirth, her later work suggests, will be accomplished through writing. As Augustine notes, H.D. "believes in [language's] substantiality because body (matter), speech, and mind (spirit) are one, not divided; therefore language, like the spirit of God, has the power to create something beyond itself."[172] In H.D.'s writing, body and language, thing and word, do reunite; however, something always remains unintegrated. H.D.'s faith during this time is that the forces of destruction she identifies with the male principle will, by uniting with her, engender a new order in which meaning is clear and difference is negated. This order will be born, *Sword* suggests, from her ruins and the ruins of the world after the "third war" (*Sword* 51).

H.D.'s thought during the 1940s and 1950s was increasingly influenced by spiritualism—though she distanced herself from it—and later by occultism. In the 1940s, she attended (and conducted solo) spiritualist séances, and in the 1950s increasingly adopted the ideas of occultist writers, "Denis De Rougemont, W.B. Crow, Jean Chaboseau, Dmitry Merejkowski, Arthur Weigall, E.M. Butler," and especially Robert Ambelain, as Robinson catalogs them.[173] Freidman also calls Ambelain "the focus of [H.D.'s] occult activities."[174]

As well as being influenced by discourses in psychoanalysis and occultism, H.D. was tremendously affected (as Sylvia Dobson and Elizabeth Willis discuss) by her direct experience of the London Blitzes and by news about the so-called fission bomb, current in the media at the end of the Second World War.[175] This influence may well be present in *Sword* and *Helen*'s recurring themes of simultaneous destruction and salvation. H.D. witnessed the end of the Second World War by means of a new weapon with an unprecedented capacity for swift obliteration—a weapon whose power was generated in the same way as the sun's life-giving power. However, this witnessing affected different people differently; the message of destruction as salvation delivered by popular news rhetoric took hold in H.D.'s work to an unusual extent.

Though the influences of psychoanalysis, occultism, spiritualism, myth, war, war rhetoric, and other external factors cast some light on the fragmented form and enigmatic content of H.D.'s later work, *Sword* and *Helen* are also shaped by what Lacan describes as the "imaginary cataclysm" and the establishment of a "delusional metaphor." This cataclysm was triggered, textual and biographical evidence suggest, by Dowding's repudiation, though the war set the stage. I read *Sword* as predominantly exemplifying the cataclysm phase and *Helen* as the formation of a delusional metaphor, although cataclysm and metaphor join in a feedback loop.

In *Sword* and *Helen*, this feedback loop appears as multitudinous characters, things, possibilities, and events, whose causal relations to one another are not evident, but are somehow all encompassed by H.D.–based characters. All beings and things in these works, whirled around in a repeating, imaginary catastrophe, seek reunification in a field of eroticized aggression: the passionate male attack on Delia/Helen that is the cause and *raison d'etre* of all beings, things, and events. This is the vision that gives these works "meaning," as their protagonists claim, though this mode of meaning remains unsatisfactory to them. These works grapple with a catastrophe of language that, in Lacan's theory, arises after the encounter with an other who assumes the missing place of the father, or One-father, for the subject with a psychotic structure. Lacan writes that this other "need but situate himself in a tertiary position in any relationship that has at its base the imaginary couple a-a'—that is, ego-object or ideal-reality—to involve the subject in the field of eroticized aggression that it induces."[176] To assume this place of the One-father, which for the psychotic subject was never there, "sets off a cascade of reworkings of the signifier," the signifier of difference that gives language its symbolic function. These works grapple with (in Lacan's terminology) this catastrophe of language that arises after this encounter.

XI. AGENCY, MAGIC, MYSTICISM, INTENTIONALITY, HEALING AND H.D. SCHOLARSHIP

Now that it has become possible to discuss religious belief and experience without the superciliousness that the genre of literary studies would have demanded ten years ago, H.D. scholars are suggesting more directly that she had mystical experiences—states of consciousness that elude representation and conceptual understanding, and which involve, as Anderson puts it, "a passion for the divine [where] imagination and affect have primacy over doctrine."[177] The suggestion that H.D. is a mystic, or someone with profound spiritual insights and experiences, usually meshes in critical readings with accounts of her social vision as pluralistic and regenerative. Writes Friedman, "*Trilogy* is profoundly antiauthoritarian and antifundamentalist, building a hope for peace out of the mystic's sense that there are multiple pathways to the divine."[178] Similarly, Lisa Rado sees H.D.'s engagement with expanded states of consciousness as conjoined to a celebration of "spiritual power—particularly the power to renounce an ideology of death, to embrace a healing affirmation of life, to renew and restore transcendent vision by challenging familiar, primarily gendered orthodoxies."[179] Anderson argues that H.D.'s "highly creative, idiosyncratic mysticism" insists on "the material, and therefore the contingent and historical" and that the divine she envisions is not a determinate entity, but "at most an ambiguous, changeable presence."[180]

As well as being traced to her pacifist, inclusive, and heterodox social vision, H.D.'s unusual (from a Western academic perspective) experiences and states of consciousness, and mystical passion, are traced, in critical accounts, to the pluralistic and open-ended approach to meaning that the majority of established scholars see in her writing. H.D.'s rebellion against "sterile logic, trivial reason"[181] in her search for meaning is understood as proceeding from mystical understanding. For Augustine, "[H.D.] understood that the path is the goal."[182] Donna Krolik Hollenberg suggests that H.D. presents a mystical vision that "reconciles contradictory experiences . . . in language that mediates between the sacred and the profane."[183] H.D.'s dissolution of the boundary between subject and object is also discussed without explicitly religious terminology by McCabe, who suggests that the fluidity of her sexual identity correlates to "the dissolution of the boundary between subject and object, lover and beloved," in her poetry—a dissolution often associated with mystical experience.[184] Anderson argues that H.D.'s mysticism is not "overly transcendent" but "contingent," and thereby refutes Madelyn Detloff's and Tony Trigilio's readings of *Trilogy* as privileging (in her words) "narrative closure," "singular authority," and "a violent vision of the end of history." She holds that H.D. instead imagines transcendence as an "immanent [. . .] rebirth."[185]

I agree that unusual experiences and states of consciousness, a longing for the unbounded, and knowledge of various mystical traditions influence the style and content of H.D.'s writing, but I find problematic commentary in which the influence is understood as wholly positive. Unusual states of consciousness, as religious and psychological studies show, do not necessarily preclude suffering and confusion, or ensure that entirely counter-hegemonic, open-ended, or life-embracing discourses will accompany them. An author's mystic states cannot guarantee that their writing will necessarily be personally restorative or socially progressive. Indeed, contemporary studies suggest that recourse to mystical states of consciousness and the beliefs they suggest are used by many religious spiritual practitioners as defense mechanisms against unresolved personal conflicts, a process popularly termed "spiritual bypassing."[186] The conflicts and behavior patterns associated with them are maintained regardless of the subject's mystical experiences of nonduality or union with the divine. An example of spiritual bypassing is magical thinking, which, writes psychotherapist Robert Augustus Masters, "relies heavily on 'signs'—apparent clues, whether internal or external—that seem to point us in a certain direction or to affirm something that we already intuit, giving us the green light to go ahead."[187] According to Masters, "magical thinking both makes us feel more significant than we actually are [since the signs are meant for us specifically, not for others] and reinforces the feeling of being part of something immeasurably vaster than us; while these may seem like positive things, they can buffer us from the impermanence and inevitably contingent nature of our existential condition."[188] Likewise, though conceptual, social, and interpersonal boundaries are indeed dissolved in H.D."s thought and writing, and this does correlate to its plurality and open-endedness, I hold that difference and lack—which parallel the impermanence and contingence Masters identifies—are not fully transcended but re-emerge in violent and threatening forms, creating new confusions, affects associated with suffering, and troubling patterns.

Though the divinity H.D. imagines is indeed ambiguous, it has designs that are determinate and, she imagines, may involve her sexualized martyrdom. As Anderson notes, H.D.'s vision of transcendence does involve rebirth as well as immolation, but the cycle of death and rebirth that she depicts retains a devastating traumatic charge. Further, there persists in this cycle a relentless pursuit of resolution. This opens the question of whether H.D. means her writing to champion open-endedness and contingency, or that it does so, at least somewhat, inadvertently and to her torment. While I agree with Anderson that the material and divine are inextricable in H.D.'s writing, I hold that, in the works I study, H.D. longs for a material and divine reality that is not contingent and open-ended but somehow final—an end to the cycle of death and rebirth that her work depicts. Her contemplation of surrender to the dominating Other at times has a curiously flat, desolate rather than ecstatic, quality that appears in quite mechanistic terms as a literal takeover of agency reminiscent of what Lacan calls imaginary capture.

H.D.'s sacrificial vision may be, as psychologist George Atwood argues of Schreber, a concretization of her feelings of annihilation at the hands of male authority figures, but it is pervasive and sustained enough to call into question readings of her work as championing life and renewal over death. Further, her tendency, at times, not so much to include, but rather to erase the points of view and agency of others calls for a nuancing of the critical near-consensus that she presents a pluralistic, heterodox vision. H.D.'s texts quite often subsume others' perspectives into a "picture" or "pattern" in which the Other who challenges her appears ordained by divine decree or driven by family-of-origin issues—but never as acting from conscious motives and in self-possession.

The question of the respective roles of the agency of either characters or author in H.D.'s later writing is unresolved. To what extent people undergoing a loosening of cognitive associations choose to communicate in a more free-associative way is still in debate, probably because the answer varies over time and for each individual. Moreover, the question of what free choice actually is remains unresolved. Certainly, with H.D., intention is initially involved in her movement into less conventional ways of associating thoughts. If, as Lacan suggests, there is in psychosis little or no illusion of stable connection between signifiers and signifieds, it would make sense to look for other ways of expressing the meaningfulness that is now experienced without reference to concepts. H.D. certainly chose to use and adapt the interpretive strategies furnished by psychoanalysis and occultism, and she defended her beliefs spiritedly, as it were, from Freud's atheism. Many "sane" people would do the same. Certainly, H.D.'s free-associative style was a choice at times—perhaps, in some sense, all of the time. But the absence of an underlying order, a pattern that does not hurtle outward in every direction for fear of excluding anything, is at least at certain points experienced as disastrous—as her constant search in *Sword* for patterns and conclusions as well as her desire for apocalypse show. Perhaps the broad leeway in occultism for free association, and the scientific validation H.D. believed that psychoanalysis gave free association, contributed to this slow eclipse of logical organization by free association in H.D's later thought and writing until, in *Sword*, she struggles to regain structure, "to feel things . . . in a rational way" (34).[189]

Many people believe that there are forces at work in the universe or in their lives that science has not accounted for. However, people experiencing schizophrenia or psychosis tend, more than others, to perceive mysterious external forces and beings imposing (often cryptic) imperatives on them, personally. H.D.'s work suggests such a perception, not only in its references to such beings, but also through its mode of meaning. Terms that usually partake of a more symbolic, subjective dimension in occultism and psychoanalysis, such as "mother," "father," and "integration" appear in her work as if their meaning was not subjective, but instead predetermined by some outside force. The task that remains for H.D. is to figure out who is who in this predetermined cast of characters and sequence of events, and perhaps to be martyred by the enigmatic being, the invisible giant who runs the show and who arbitrates meaning. For her, I suggest, the disappearance of difference is experienced not only as mystical union—at least not solely in the recuperative sense that Anderson highlights in her work on H.D. – but also as traumatic sexualized invasion and chaos.[190]

Robert Duncan writes of H.D. that her poetics brings language into the unfolding moment, both creating and renewing history through its resistance to the impersonality of conventional language. Her free-associative style is key to this renewal. But after H.D.'s 1946 breakdown, the aesthetic success of this style and its effectiveness in renewing language by giving words and phrases new meanings and valences was curtailed by her difficulty in relating to it as a semiotic system. Duncan himself, as he describes it in *The Truth and Life of Myth* (1968), locates meaning in his own poetic process of play, which also refuses linguistic stability and (as he sees it) renews language's vitality. H.D., too, imagines a "dead, old, thousand-times explored old world of over-worked emotions and thoughts,"[191] and after her analytic sessions with Freud, she envisions her destiny in terms reminiscent of Duncan's: "I must find new words as the Professor found or coined new words to explain certain as yet unrecorded states of being!"[192] "Yet," she notes, "if I become more 'human' I seem to lose my sense of direction, or my prose style."[193] Unlike Duncan, H.D. has a vision of truth as potentially beyond the reach of her words, which "ghost for" it. In *Sword*, the "re-creation" of the old world is far from a matter of aesthetic play. Meaning detaches itself from H.D."s words, and language becomes an obstructing, rather than a revitalizing, force. Apocalypse is imagined as the only means to its renewal. H.D.'s vision of salvific destruction to bring in the next world, like Schreber's, symptomizes the deterioration of her language's symbolic function and its longed-for reinstatement. As signifiers float free of meaning and accrue palimpsestically in her body, her own demise is seen as redemptive, an ending, a beginning, a real difference, which is paradoxically union. Passionately anticipated death and the coming of the next world represent the end of malfunctioning language, the hoped for advent of an order in which signifier and signified, man and woman, achieve union at last in the wondrous sign.

As I touched on in my introduction, H.D. scholarship has often taken H.D.'s own view of the effects of her writing as integrating and restorative, both for herself and for the world. Friedman notes Freud's influence on H.D.'s vision of "Eros, Eris" in later work, but sees H.D. as reinscribing repressed Eros, which Friedman associates with "the woman's world."[194] For Friedman, H.D.'s allusive, "alchemical" approach to language transforms the seemingly violent aspects of her work: "In her apocalypse, the fires of war morph into the purifying flames of alchemical transfiguration."[195] Dianne Chisholm reads H.D. as writing herself out of the fixity of melancholia and into the more dynamic process of mourning.[196] As Chisholm sees it, in *Helen in Egypt*, H.D. reformulates Freud's opposition of the life and death drives by "eroticiz[ing] the death drive"—particularly by means of Achilles's and Helen's "ecstatically therapeutic" encounter—and thereby returning repressed feminine sexuality to civilization.[197] Likewise, Hogue and Vandivere present *Sword* as a personally and socially "curative" restoration of "the lost strength of the feminine [to] the world skewed by the dominance of a warrior ethos."[198] Augustine also describes *Sword*, though without political inflection, as a "recovery document" that enabled H.D. to retain "the expanded world view which spiritualism brought to her and . . . the sense of giftedness and female empowerment that support her self-identification as a writer" by giving her traumatic interactions with Lord Dowding "a final rational unity."[199] In each of these readings, and many others, H.D.'s literary responses to patriarchal figures and institutions are seen as effecting personal and social reintegration and synthesis with a feminine principle.

Consecutively, writers on H.D. have tended to focus on "exploring the literature rather than explaining it,"[200] entering as deeply as possible into H.D.'s own frames of reference.[201] Some scholars attempt to establish, as H.D. herself sometimes did, meaningful patterns within the writing—and thus conceptual order in the "network[s] of potentially significant associations and contexts" (to borrow from James Maynard) that they describe.[202] Others suggest that students attempt to track down H.D.'s allusions as a way of entering into her work's conceptual scarcity. Such scholarly exploration often lingers in what Adalaide Morris calls the "generativity" of H.D.'s work: its shimmering webs of associations and liminal spaces between meaning and nonmeaning.[203]

At the other pole from identification with H.D., and emulation of her mental processes, are writers, outside of the circle of established H.D. scholars, who take rather dim views of H.D.'s work (for instance, see Randal Jarrell, Lawrence Rainey, or Charles LaChance), or who suggest that her writing gives evidence of maladaptive psychic processes like splitting (Norman Holland). One scholar who, with what we might call poetic license, both celebrates H.D.'s work and writes openly about the splitting, projection, and wrath that it sometimes evidences is H.D.'s friend and aficionado, the poet Robert Duncan (1919–1988) in *The H.D. Book* (written in 1960–1961, first published in full in 2011).[204] However, in general, polarized critical responses almost seem to dramatize the embattlement of masculine and feminine principles, and the need for their "integration," elements with which H.D. herself was so concerned.

Though background knowledge can indeed illuminate enigmatic material, the critical excavation, explanation, integration, and speculation on H.D.'s bottomless troves of associations must contend with the radical instability of meaning that drives her referentiality. Historical and intertextual criticism that seeks to uncover the meaning of H.D's later work through intertextual references walks in the shifting sands of her own search for meaning. H.D. herself remains unsatisfied with these open-ended networks of potentially meaningful nouns, and while such dissatisfaction has itself been read as an anti-hegemonic refusal of determinate meanings, I see rather than a refusal of determinate meaning a singular faith in it, a passionate search for it and inability to find it. It cannot be found because H.D.'s language, in her books and journals, is slipping from the order in which words take meaning through their differentiation from other words, which enables them to indicate distinct meanings. Rather, H.D.'s formulations express the absence of symbolic differentiation characteristic in psychoanalysis of unconscious and preconscious processes. H.D. seeks to encompass difference itself in her unbounded interpretive endeavors—but difference remains alien and threatening, a return from without. Correlatively, the "recovery" she documents often looks and feels like more wounding.

H.D.'s desire for a union of understanding with father figures whom she saw as scientific, such as Freud, Ellis, and Dowding, and her vulnerability to their responses when she communicated her psychic insights to them, speaks in part to her own sense that her thoughts and experiences are too far from the orderly, scientific, patriarchal realm. Her desires and vulnerabilities also imply a wish to connect with such a father figure, and to thereby unite the psychic and the scientific through her own connection to another. Though after her analysis with Freud, and especially after the Second World War, H.D. saw her writing as key to her recovery, self-knowledge and spiritual journey, from a psychoanalytic viewpoint it suggests what Lacan calls an "imaginary cataclysm" and the defensive formation of an inchoate, repeating "delusion" that may sabotage recovery—if recovery is seen as an end to suffering.

In her "Preliminary Comments on the Meaning of *The Sword Went Out to Sea*," Augustine describes *Sword* as a "recovery document," the writing of which allowed H.D. to retain "the expanded world view which spiritualism brought to her and . . . the sense of giftedness and female empowerment that support her self-identification as a writer" by giving her traumatic interactions with Dowding "a final rational unity."[205] Though Augustine is likely correct in her view that the writing of *Sword* helped H.D. to stabilize after her breakdown, no final rational unity underlying her traumatic experience becomes apparent in it. Although interpretations of Dowding's behavior are proffered, *Sword* ends as it began: with a multiplicity of interpretations and a postponed conclusion, in both senses of the word. The penultimate and final chapters end and begin with: "we went on with the play. We went on with the play" (266–7). The dedication, to "Gareth" (Bryher) reads, "It's not lost. This will go on somewhere." Hogue and Vandivere's introduction to *Sword* also reproduces this critical approach to H.D.'s later work. They argue that *Sword* describes a "curative" process that healed H.D. by restoring "the lost strength of the feminine" that balances "a world skewed by the dominance of a warrior ethos," (xxxvii) and that, "as part of a body of women's literature written around World War II," it helps scholars to "reorient and reconfigure modernism" (xvi). However, *Sword*'s status as a recovery document—both for H.D. and for modernism, as we know it—is complicated by its fixation on and eroticization of this "warrior ethos." The "[i]mages of invasion, defense, and siege [that] permeate *Sword*" (xlii) comprise, in their repetition, the only "unity" it may have. The "cure" that H.D. in *Sword* imagines and at times welcomes involves what she calls *Thermopylae*, a cataclysmic world war in which *Sword*'s heroines and fatal heroes play an unclear but crucial role. H.D. suggests in *Sword* that this war repeats itself in each historical epoch, enabling its transition into the next. Hogue and Vandivere's reading of *Sword* presents H.D.'s exultancy in the war, her "love life" of "love and terror mixed," as a protest that "*war* is mad." Though they are not necessarily wrong, *Sword* does not display a thoroughgoing rejection of war. Lara Vetter writes that *Sword*, as well as other later prose, "interrogates nationalism and imperialism by exposing the impact of the public on the private sphere."[206] I will offer a contrary account of this work, where H.D. envisions the impact of her own private sphere rippling outward into the world, where the violence that male love interests direct toward her heroines is reflected through mystical syncretism as conquest and war. While Morris argues, persuasively, "the ethical work of H.D.'s texts is to put into question the possibility of 'having done,'" this "ethical work" in *Sword* it appears inadvertent and entailed H.D. much suffering.[207] To have done, finally, is her great longing: "I thought, 'I'm glad it has happened now, this is the third war and now it will soon be over'" (51).

H.D. imagines her later writing and her recovery as synonymous, particularly in the cases of *Sword* and *Helen*. In 1951, she writes to friend and scholar Norman Holmes Pearson (1909–1975) "Yes—the Sword is important. But simply again, as a record and a record I could not have done, if I had not persisted, even at Küsnacht, on REMEMBERING. For me, it was so important, my own LEGEND. Then, to get well and re-create it."[208] However, it seems to me that this view of H.D.'s later writing, which has persisted through the decades, has over-determined critical responses to it. If this protects H.D.'s status in some sense, it does so by sacrificing engagement with her work.

Sword does not document a recovery, but rather witnesses the unconscious from a place inside it, searching unsuccessfully for a way into the functioning of consciousness—a way to knit the conscious and unconscious. H.D.'s free association of words, objects, people, and events does not synthesize what was once distinct into a new understanding. Rather, her free-associative language describes the absence of symbolic differentiation characteristic of unconscious and preconscious processes. The difference on which language is predicated enters the unconscious landscapes these works depict chiefly as eroticized, recurring attack. Correlatively, the "recovery" that they document is, I have argued, shattering. Indeed, the relationship of this endeavor of recovery and integration with actual recovery, in the sense of an alleviation of suffering, may be one of sabotage.

NOTES

1. Hogue and Vandivere, Introduction to *Sword.* Hogue and Vandivere write, "Initially writing a fictionalized memoir (a *roman vecu*, as she puts it), H.D. engaged her 'gift' to see further than individual circumstances and attempted to create Sword as a cultural 'autobiography' speaking not only of individual trauma but working through the trauma of a civilization in critical transition (in some sense from colonial Empire to postcolonial nation-states" (xviii).

2. H.D., *Majic Ring*, 37, 161.

3. H.D., "H.D. by Delia Alton," 181–2.

4. Ibid. Writes H.D., "She [two of her protagonists, who 'are, they all are, the same woman'] knows . . . that 'women are individually seeking, as one woman, fragments of the Eternal Lover.' As the Eternal Lover has been scattered or disassociated, so she, in her search for him. . . . She seeks him in fantasy, myth. She has found him, of course. But she can not yet correlate or relate the various entities that make up her own fragments, though in Egypt they were related for her; the formula was presented. . . . She knows that to keep him, she must lose him. . . . She cannot know that she knows this, until she has progressively retraced her steps, redeemed not so much the fragments of Osiris, as of his sister, twin or double, the drowned or submerged Isis" (182).

5. H.D., quoted in Hogue and Vandivere, Introduction to *Sword*, l–li.

6. Ibid., l.

7. H.D., *Tribute*, 145. "Advent" was assembled in 1948 and published as Part II of *Tribute to Freud.* Writes H.D., "I am on the fringes or in the penumbra of the light of my father's science and my mother's art—the psychology or philosophy of Sigmund Freud. . . . I must find new words as the Professor found or coined new words to explain certain as yet unrecorded states of mind or Being! . . . We retreat from the so-called sciences and go backward or go forward into alchemy."

8. Friedman, *Analyzing Freud*, 498.

9. Guest, *Herself Defined*, 218.

10. H.D., *Ion*, 254.

11. Duncan, *The H.D. Book*, 127. Writes Duncan, "In the fairy-world, the otherness or alien nearness of the dead and of hidden elements, of illusion and delusion in our daily life, the witchcraft of phantasy and the bewitched obsessions of madness, all the psychological dangers, combined as if they were the heart's wish. The specter that haunts Europe Marx had called the hidden wish of the human spirit in history; the traumatic image Freud had called the repressed wish of the psyche—the primal scene."

12. Robinson, Introduction to *Hirslanden Notebooks*, xxv.

13. H.D., *Sword*, 113. The *Ghirlanda* table, as H.D. calls it, came to H.D. after the death of her friend, writer and Pre-Raphaelite scholar Violet Hunt (1862–1942). Writes H.D. in 1945, "The 'Writing' continues but the mysterious or mystical symbol writing on the wall of the hotel bed-room, in the Ionian island of Corfu, spring 1920, is now (in 1945) in Delia Alton's apartment off Hyde Park in London, the ABC of a child's alphabet-chart. It is the tapping of one of the three feet of the tripod table that

had been brought me, during the war, after the sale of Violet Hunt's effects, soon after her death" ("H.D. by Delia Alton," 192).

14. Chaboseau is the author of *Le Tarot* (1946), a work that influenced H.D. from the 1950s onward. From it she borrows the pattern in which she places the major male love interests in her life, who H.D. considers as "initiators" into higher states of being.

15. H.D., *Sword*, 140.

16. Anderson, *H.D. and Modernist Religious Imagination*, 109.

17. H.D., *Helen*, 43, 46.

18. H.D., *Sword*, 140; *Helen*, 46.

19. H.D., *Sword*, 214.

20. Ibid., 40.

21. The *DSM-V* distinguishes two phases in the psychotic break: "Prodromal symptoms often precede the active phase, and residual symptoms may follow it, characterized by mild or subthreshold forms of hallucinations or delusions. Individuals may express a variety of unusual or odd beliefs that are not of delusional proportions (e.g., ideas of reference or magical thinking) . . . their speech may be generally understandable but vague; and their behavior may be unusual but not grossly disorganized" (101).

22. Ibid., 99.

23. The *DSM-V* describes, in some individuals suffering from schizophrenia, "deficits in the ability to infer the intentions of other people. [Thus they may] attend to and then interpret irrelevant elements or stimuli as meaningful, perhaps leading to the generation of explanatory delusions [which] frequently persist during symptomatic remission" (101).

24. Psychologist Norman Cameron, in a 1939 attempt to analyze the schizophrenic language of disorganization, writes that the cognitive links normally joining causes and effects are missing in it. "In the place of well-knit sequences," patients who were asked to finish sentences using the word *because* invoked "a cluster of more or less related elements." Cameron, "Experimental," 52. In contrast, "a normally syndetic, or linked-together, logical organization would have automatically eliminated all but one or two . . . possibilities, and in this way have restricted the solution to something more clean-cut and precise" (52–3). The associative clustering that Cameron describes appears in *Sword*, in H.D.'s endeavor to explain Dowding's repudiation. *Helen*, though it also displays associative clustering, suggests that this process results in the formation of a fixed explanatory delusion, the beginnings of which appear in *Sword*.

25. Vervaeke and Ferraro, "Relevance, Meaning."

26. Friedman, *Analyzing Freud*, 485.

27. H.D., *Tribute*, 103. See Freud, *Beyond* (throughout).

28. Friedman, *Analyzing Freud*, 507.

29. Ibid., emphasis added.

30. H.D., *Tribute*, 32, emphasis added.

31. Guest notes that "Bryher had been asked to limit her visits by Dr. Heydt, who decided that H.D.'s equilibrium was upset" (*Herself Defined*, 328). Vetter discusses H.D.'s frustration at Klinik Brunner's "suppression and surveillance" of her personal mail (*Curious Peril*, 175).

32. H.D. avowedly fixated on her mother and her mother's name, and believed that this fixation indicated "the direction of [her] soul's journey." In *Majic Ring* she writes, "But even the truth of a child's 'fixation' on a mother and a mother's name, on Helen, on Hellas, on the Hellenes (on, if you will, Helios) is only a sign-post, is only an indication of the direction of the soul's journey, which journey was already predetermined before the child Delia was born" (99).

33. See Sword, *Ghostwriting Modernism*.

34. Augustine, "Preliminary Comments," 130–2.

35. Hollenberg, *Between History and Poetry*, 76.

36. H.D., *Magic Mirror*, 137.

37. Hollenberg, *Between History and Poetry*, 76.

38. As Hogue and Vandivere surmise (Introduction to *Sword*, xxii).

39. See Tryphonopoulos's 2009 edition of *Majic Ring*. Jane Augustine has been able to match Lord Dowding's extant replies to H.D.'s letters in *Majic Ring*. Hogue and Vandivere reference Augustine's findings in their Introduction to *Sword*, xlvii. "In an e-mail note to the editors written on May 18, 2005, Augustine confirms that the letters are 'actual'—that she has been able to match Lord Dowding's extant replies to H.D.'s fictionalized letters in *Majic Ring* (there are to date no extant originals).

40. Hogue and Vandivere, Introduction to *Sword*, xxv–xxvi.

41. Ibid., xxvii.

42. Ibid., xxviii.

43. Ibid.

44. Ibid., xxxi.

45. H.D. Papers, YCAL/Beinecke.

46. Hogue and Vandivere, Introduction to *Sword*, i.

47. H.D., *Majic Ring*, 196, 206.

48. Ibid., l.

49. See Vetter, *Curious*, 10–11; Guest, *Herself*, 278-9, 283.

50. Guest, *Herself*, 278.

51. Anderson, *H.D. and Modernist Religious Imagination*, 26.

52. H.D., *Tribute*, 146.

53. Robinson, *Astral*, 76–7.

54. Lacan, *Seminar III, The Psychoses*, 321.

55. Duncan, *The H.D. Book*, 339.

56. Lacan, *Seminar III, The Psychoses*, 100.

57. Ibid.

58. Schreber, *Memoirs*, 69.

59. Ibid., 166.

60. Ibid., 132.

61. Lacan, "Signification," 581.

62. Vetter speculates that H.D. may have read Sigmund Freud's long paper on Schreber, published in 1911, between 1946 and 1948, while she was assembling "Advent" from notes taken during her analysis to publish as the second part of *Tribute to Freud*. Thus, Vetter argues, H.D. may have intentionally modeled Delia's apocalypticism and messianism after Freud's account of Schreber's (*Curious*, 75-6).

However, there is no mention of Schreber, or of reading Freud's work, in H.D.'s letters and journals from this period, which often document profound influences. Further, if the powerful overtones of apocalypticism and messianism in *Sword* are to be attributed to H.D.'s having read Freud's work on Schreber, this influence must have been so great as to extend to *Helen in Egypt* (written from 1952–1955) as well, since the latter shares these themes, and also shares Schreber's themes of invasion and control by God. Vetter writes that while Delia "had an apocalyptic vision of World War III," H.D.'s journals suggest that she "probably did not" (*Curious*, 212). I would argue rather that H.D. felt more comfortable expressing her vision as a "novel" (her quotation marks) than avowing it in journals and letters that she expected eventually to be published: she had become skilled at sheltering her beliefs from people who she knew would not take them seriously. She herself writes that "Delia Alton" is a "*nom de plume*" that she assumed because *Sword*'s content is "too near and intimate for H.D." (Hollenburg, 76). Thus, though Vetter finds my "slippage" between H.D.'s and Delia's beliefs "at times troubling," (212) I read the evidence as suggesting that H.D. herself privately drew little distinction between them, seeing "Delia Alton" as a name under which she could express her spiritual vision.

63. Ibid., 252.

64. Santner, *My Own Private Germany*, 63–99.

65. Ibid., 86. Santner argues that "the characterization of disciplinary power as counter-law secreted by and within the law exactly parallels Schreber's efforts to elucidate what he calls conditions contrary to the Order of the World, conditions under which . . . God takes an exceptional interest in and comes to have knowledge of *living human beings*. One might say, then, that the chronic state of emergency generating the bizarre array of symptoms and delusions described in the *Memoirs* was inaugurated by that partial suspension of the law effectuated by the disciplinary power to which Schreber had been exposed since early childhood and to which he was exposed again, though in a different form, in the psychiatric institutions of Flechsig and Weber. Schreber's soul murder becomes, from this perspective, a sustained traumatization induced by exposure to, as it were, fathers who knew too much about living human beings."

66. See Apollon, Bergeron, and Cantin, *After Lacan*. Cantin explains the disorganized character of delusional psychosis thus: "It is as if the elaboration of the delusion were not subjected to or governed by the laws of language, but rather by the underlying fantasy that the delusion serves to support—the fantasy, that is, of the omnipotence of the Other to which the delusion responds and which the delusion works to maintain, though all the while trying to escape from it . . . *one could almost say that delusion treats the real by attempting to subjugate the symbolic to the imaginary*" (95, emphasis added).

67. Friedman, *Psyche*, 207–96.

68. H.D.'s response to Ellis in *Tribute* resembles her later response to Dowding: "I thought he would be so interested. But he appeared unsympathetic, or else he did not understand or else he may have thought it was a danger signal" (130). Later again, "It had really been a great shock to me as I had visualized Dr. Ellis, during the time of writing my notes on thought and vision, as a saint as well as a savant" (148). The

strength of her reaction can also be seen in her letters to Bryher, which show delight in the betrayal of Ellis's urination fetish to Freud and in Freud's dismissal of his work as "immature." However, she continues to solicit Ellis's affection and approval in their personal correspondence.

69. H.D., *Tribute*, 51.

70. Ibid., 56.

71. Ibid., 41.

72. Ibid., 141.

73. Augustine, "Preliminary Comments," 130–1.

74. See Freud, *The Interpretation of Dreams* and "Dreams and Occultism."

75. Duncan, *The H.D. Book*, 586.

76. For a further discussion on the non-conjunction between the drives and the sexual relationship see Lacan, *Seminar XX, On Feminine Sexuality*, especially 111–12.

77. Lacan, *Seminar I, Freud's Papers on Technique*, 117.

78. This accords with Lacan's description of erotomania: "The erotomaniacal delusion is addressed to such a neutralized other that he is inflated to the very dimensions of the world, since the universal interest attached to the adventure is . . . an essential part of it." Lacan, *Seminar III, The Psychoses*, 43.

79. Klein, "Notes on Some Schizoid Mechanisms," 7. Writes Klein, "Omnipotent denial of the existence of the bad object and of the painful situation is in the unconscious equal to animation by the destructive impulse. It is, however, not only a situation and an object that are denied and annihilated—it is an object relation which suffers this fate, and therefore a part of the ego, from which the feelings towards the object emanate, is denied and annihilated as well."

80. Sword, *Ghostwriting Modernism*, 118. Sword argues that H.D. "deployed cryptopoetic strategies not to reveal some timeless universal truth about death—the code broken, the hieroglyph interpreted—so much as to explore the slippery borderline between death and life and, by extension, the slipperiness also of the verbal signifiers we must use to describe whatever is unknown and unknowable."

81. Lacan, "Instance," 431.

82. Anderson, *H.D. and Modernist Religious Imagination*, 38.

83. H.D., *Notes*, 26.

84. Ibid., 27.

85. Ibid., 17.

86. From Greek *skhizein*, "to split" + *phrēn*, "mind." See Bleuler, "Basic Symptoms," 613–15. "Pressure of words" would be more accurate in my view, since it is not ideas but rather words that Bleuler's patients describe.

87. Sword, *Ghostwriting Modernism*, 127.

88. Lacan, "Logical Time," 161–75.

89. Delia's attempted articulation of everything suggests what David Rappaport, writing on schizophrenic language, calls "overmeticulousness," in which "the subjective experience [is] that the central idea [here, the "plan"] has not been communicated until all of its facets have been conveyed. Thus many things that usually go without saying will be explicitly communicated." Rappaport, *Organization and Pathology of Thought*, 589.

90. Duncan, *The H.D. Book*, 586.
91. Augustine, "Preliminary Comments," 130–1.
92. Laplanche, *Hölderlin*, 91. In Hölderlin's later essays, "[t]he thinking proves to be extremely difficult to sort out . . . it often clings to formal points of emphasis, like mathematical formulas the terms of which are subsequently subjected to circular permutations in which the meaning sometimes vanishes in favor of false symmetries" (88).
93. Hogue and Vandivere, Introduction to *Sword*, xxvi.
94. Lacan, *Seminar III, The Psychoses*, 33.
95. Ibid.
96. Ibid., 55.
97. Guest, *Herself Defined*, 261. Writes H.D. (quoted in Guest): "[t]o recall my father is to recall the cold, blazing intelligence of my 'last attachment' [Dowding] of the war years in London."
98. Lacan, *Seminar III, The Psychoses*, 320.
99. See Von Domarus and Cameron, in *Language and Thought*, 59, 120–1.
100. See Augustine, "Preliminary Comments," 130–1; Hogue and Vandivere, Introduction to *Sword*, xxxvii.
101. H.D., *Tribute*, 51, emphasis added.
102. Lacan, *Seminar III, The Psychoses*, 22.
103. Ibid., 75.
104. Writes Duncan, "H.D.'s apocalyptic vision in the *War Trilogy* . . . provides an historical perspective in which the experience of London under attack in the Second World War becomes meaningful in relation to depths and heights of personal reality, depths she had come to know in her psychoanalysis with Freud and then in new terms with the study of occult and hermetic lore, heights she had known in aesthetic and erotic ideals as early as her first work" (*The H.D. Book*, 337).
105. Hogue and Vandivere, Introduction to *Sword*, xlii.
106. H.D., *Tribute*, 130.
107. Ibid., 50.
108. As recorded in Guest, *Herself Defined*, 18.
109. H.D., in Friedman, *Analyzing*, 197.
110. H.D., *Gift*, 194.
111. Ibid., 193.
112. H.D., *Tribute*, 34.
113. Ibid.
114. Ibid., 34–5.
115. Guest, *Herself Defined*, 14.
116. Lacan, "On a Question," 481.
117. Lacan, *Seminar III, The Psychoses*, 87.
118. Augustine, "Preliminary Comments," 130.
119. Lemaire, *Jacques Lacan*, 246.
120. H.D., *Ion*, 254.
121. Ibid., 255, emphasis added.
122. Ibid., 197.

123. Morris, *Live*, 8.

124. Ibid., 59–60, emphasis in original.

125. Duncan, *The H.D. Book*, 608–11.

126. Robinson, Introduction to *Hirslanden Notebooks*, ix.

127. See Pappas's 2009 article "H.D. and Havelock Ellis." Pappas argues that even scientists and pseudo-scientists who studied extraordinary states of consciousness (including those experienced in pregnancy and under the influence of psychedelic drugs) discursively distinguished their "scientific" perspectives on such experiences (even while under the influence of hallucinogens themselves) from the perspectives of women and artists. She extrapolates the discursive maneuvers by which Havelock Ellis separates the scientific from the artistic and feminine perspectives, and privileges the former, in his studies of peyote use and pregnancy. This bias, for Pappas, makes its way into Ellis's analysis of H.D.'s *Notes on Thoughts and Vision*, whereas in contrast *Notes* does not construct extraordinary psychic experiences as pathological or unobjective but seeks a perspective in which neither the scientific nor the artistic framework is privileged. I would argue on the contrary that the perspective that H.D. presents in *Notes* and elsewhere subsumes the scientific just as surely as Ellis's scientific language subsumes the artistic. I read, in Ellis's article on peyote (1902), ambivalence similar to H.D.'s. It is as if both H.D. and Ellis want to bridge the gap between the masculine-scientific and the feminine-artistic poles but are trapped within the discourse that they represent—as if these discourses cannot be brought together as equals. One inevitably subsumes the other, just as do the heroes and heroines in H.D.'s work.

128. Atwood, *Abyss*, 35.

129. H.D.'s analysts at Klinik Brunner include Erich Heydt, its owner Dr. Theodore Brunner and perhaps friend and sometime analyst Walter Schmideburg, who was also a patient there for a time.

130. H.D. and Durand met twice, briefly, in 1960: once when he visited the Klinik Brunner to interview her for a review of *Bid Me to Live* forthcoming in *Newsweek*, and once in New York where she had gone to receive the Gold Medal for Poetry from the American Academy of Arts and Letters, Foreword to *Hermetic Definition*, ii. The 1960 review is patronizing and dismissive in tone; see *Hirslanden Notebooks*, 93–4, appendix 5. According to Guest, Durand did not write this review, though H.D. believed that he did (*Herself*, 321).

131. *The Flowering of the Rod* also places the repudiation and denial of an H.D.–based character into a larger context in which it is shown as misguided and/or cowardly and/or triggered by haunting memories. Published in 1946, shortly after Dowding's invalidation, it stages it with yet another cast of characters: he as Kaspar and Simon and she as Mary Magdalene. Kaspar/Simon's behavior, as Susan Edmunds points out, is cast as a repression of a memory arising from his unconscious. Writes Edmunds, "[j]ust as Freud suggests that his patients' acts of 'negation' or disavowal are attempts to deny their own unconscious thoughts . . . Simon's denial that he knows Mary (like his subsequent attempts to 'eject' her from his house) suggests that he does in fact know her, even that she is wrapped up in his self-knowledge" (*Line*, 79).

132. H.D., *Gift*, 212.

133. Ibid., 214.
134. Ibid., 219.
135. H.D., *Ion*, 254.
136. Friedman, *Analyzing Freud*, 530.
137. H.D., *Ion*, 257.
138. Ibid., 254–5.
139. Klein, "Notes on Some Schizoid Mechanisms," 5.
140. Duncan, *The H.D. Book*, 339.
141. This is not introjection in Abraham and Torok's sense, a positive process by which new objects become integrated with the ego's existing models. Klein's usage, in which the introjected objects may remain separate within the ego, and which is closer to Abraham and Torok's "incorporation" more accurately renders the mechanisms to be found in *Helen*.
142. Friedman, *Psyche*, 152.
143. Freud suggests in "The Loss of Reality" that the ego in psychosis, instead of siding with external reality at the expense of the id, sides with the id at the expense of foreclosed ("*Verworfen*") external reality. This entails a reconstruction of reality which hallucination often abets (569–70).
144. H.D., *Tribute*, 44.
145. Ibid., 51, emphasis added.
146. Ibid., 136.
147. Friedman, *Analyzing Freud*, 143.
148. H.D., *Tribute*, 38.
149. Friedman, *Analyzing Freud*, 331–2.
150. In *The Practical Kabbalah*, Ambelain writes that the "vibrations" of sounds cause the "ideas" linked to them to appear (*Kabbalah II*, 77). These "ideas" which resemble Jungian archetypes but have their own "life" include "mother-ideas" (*Kabbalah I*, 174). Writes Ambelain, "Each sound is intimately associated with an idea, which forms the counterpart. Through this, when we evoke a particular sound in our mentality, an idea which is linked to it immediately appears. If we continually maintain a like spiritual idea in the consciousness, mentality liberates itself little by little from its impurities, its nature is refined and it then transmutes into Fire, issued forth from Malkuth, the superior fire. Ruach, the very essence of the 'MOTHER' then shines forth in its entire splendor. The mentality, composed of subtle essences, invisible substances, then sees the schema restored in full, to these constitutive elements, their original purity" (*Kabbalah II*, 77). See also Friedman *Analyzing Freud*, 331.
151. Writes Sword, "H.D. manages in her 'tribute' both to celebrate the famous psychoanalyst's memory and to skewer his most deeply held beliefs, portraying him as a 'beloved light-house keeper' . . . whose denial of the afterlife would in time be proven to be wrong. . . . She concludes her memoir by associating her self with Goethe's Mignon, leading her symbolic father and protector . . . over terrifying 'chasms or gulfs' to the promised land far beyond the grave, 'the land where the orange-tree blossoms'" (*Ghostwriting*, 109–11).
152. Lacan, *Seminar III, The Psychoses*, 15.
153. Holland, "H.D.'s Analysis," *PsyArt* (no pagination), citing H.D., *Tribute*, 37.

154. Ibid. Writes Holland, "the child H.D. evidently dealt with potential gaps, not by suffering them passively, but by actively closing them herself."

155. Ibid.

156. Ibid., citing H.D. *Tribute*, 71.

157. Robinson, *Astral*, 9.

158. Writes Robinson, "'Located' between the physical and purely intellectual realms, the astral plane has been described by twentieth-century occultists as analogous—or even identical—to the fourth dimension. The physical body has an immediate double—the radiant body—but also an astral double. The astral body is yoked to the physical body, consciousness shifting to it during dreams. Occasionally, though, one's consciousness can shift to the astral while awake, either in an unconscious or conscious exteriorization (or 'dédoublement')" (*Astral*, 52).

159. Lacan, *Seminar III, The Psychoses*, 15.

160. See Freud, "Dreams and Occultism," 54.

161. See Jung's testimony, quoted by Colin McCabe in his introduction to Freud's *The Schreber Case*. Jung records that Freud told him in 1910, "'My dear Jung promise me you will never abandon the theory of sexuality. . . .You see we must make a dogma of it, an unshakable bulwark.' . . . Somewhat astonished, I asked him: 'A bulwark, against what?' Whereupon he answered, 'Against the black muddy tide,' here he hesitated for a moment, then added, 'of occultism'" (McCabe, "Introduction," x).

162. Freud, "Dreams and Occultism," 54. See also Materer, *Modernist Alchemy*, 9–10.

163. Freud, *Totem and Taboo*, 85.

164. As Materer explains, in sympathetic magic "the destruction of a carven shape of a person will stand for the destruction of that very person [similarity], or the anointing of a knife will alleviate the pain of a wound made by the knife [contiguity]. In this association of ideas, Freud identifies two principles—similarity (as in the carving) and contiguity (as in the weapon); in literary art, the principles would be termed metaphor and metonymy. Believers in animism use magic to gain control over the spirits, thereby imposing their will on the world and even triumphing over death. Freud compares such magic to art because our civilization credits the 'omnipotence of thought' only in 'the field of art. . . . People speak with justice of the 'magic of art' and compare artists to magicians" (*Modernist Alchemy*, 11–12).

165. See H.D., *Tribute*: "For my head . . . is already warning me that this is an unusual dimension, an unusual way to think, that my brain or mind may not be equal to the occasion. . . . Here is this hieroglyph of the unconscious or subconscious of the Professor's discovery and life-study, the hieroglyph actually in operation before our very eyes. But it is no easy matter to sustain this mood, this 'symptom' or this inspiration" (47).

166. Foucault argues in *The History of Sexuality Vol.1* that psychoanalytic discourses *produced* the desire and subjectivity that they purported to free or analyze, 77–131.

167. Weber, Introduction to *Memoirs*, xli.

168. Hogue and Vandivere, Introduction to *Sword*, xxxvii.

169. H.D., *Magic Mirror*, 17.

170. Coffman, *Insane*, 147. For Coffman, H.D.'s free association and projection was an "effort to define a modernist poetics of the visionary that is inflected through female same-sex desire" (146), and a challenge to "the phallogocentric terms of the symbolic order that produces [the unrepresentability of the homosexual-maternal]" (152).

171. LaChance, "Sexual Sublime," 47.

172. Augustine, "Preliminary Comments," 132.

173. Robinson, *Astral*, 10. Robinson maps H.D.'s encounters with the ideas of the astral plane and astral body: "Likely the first time H.D. encountered the idea of the astral body was in the 'Yogi books' Pound brought her in the mid-1900s. [Hindu mystic Ramacharaka's cosmological system, which they outline] is similar to the Theosophical septenary scheme, which feeds the terminology used by spiritualists. The Hermetic/Rosicrucian scheme, espoused by the Martinists Robert Ambelain and Jean Chaboseau, use a slightly different system, influenced by the Kabbalah. . . . At times Ambelain talks of a triple scheme (physical, astral, and spirit bodies). . . . Unless one is an expert in the occult, the terminology and cosmology in the Theosophical and Hermetic branches are similar enough that they might as well be the same" (11).

174. Friedman, *Psyche*, 175.

175. See Dobson, "Shock," and Willis, "Public."

176. Lacan, "On a Question," 481.

177. Anderson, *H.D. and Modernist Religious Imagination*, 7.

178. Friedman, "Teaching Trilogy," 141.

179. Rado, "Portraits of an Artist," 52.

180. Anderson, *H.D. and Modernist Religious Imagination*, 3, 32.

181. H.D., *Trilogy*, 40.

182. Augustine, "Teaching H.D. and Spirituality," 69.

183. Hollenberg, "She Showed a Way,"147.

184. McCabe, "Teaching Sex," 97.

185. Anderson, *H.D. and Modernist Religious Imagination*, 31–2; Detloff, *Persistence*, 83–7; Trigilio, *"Strange Prophecies Anew,"* 84–7, 111.

186. See for instance Trungpa, *Cutting through Spiritual Materialism*, and Masters, *Bypassing*. Masters describes spiritual bypassing as "the use of spiritual practices/beliefs to avoid dealing with painful feelings, unresolved wounds, and developmental needs" (1).

187. Masters, *Bypassing*, 61.

188. Ibid., 63.

189. See Rust, "Schizotypal Thinking."

190. See, for instance, Anderson, *H.D. and Modernist Religious Imagination*, 37. Writes Anderson, "By foregrounding her 'mad grief' [in *Sword*] H.D. sets the stage for the rest of the narrative to develop various strategies for healing from the practical—removal from the scene of the trauma—to the visionary—Delia experiences consolatory as well as frightening hallucinations. The text becomes a 'recovery document,' as the psychoanalytic cast to the narrative highlights." However, Anderson notes that H.D.'s "recovery is affected by returning to the distressing symptoms of her illness and seeking to make sense of her breakdown by relating it first to her own

previous experiences and then to the larger pattern she traces through the historical vignettes."

191. H.D., *Notes*, 24.

192. H.D., *Tribute*, 145.

193. Ibid., 149.

194. Ibid., 264. Friedman argues that in *Helen* Achilles's "assault [of Helen] turns into love" because Helen invokes the mother-goddess whom he, like civilization, has repressed (*Psyche*, 257). However, the loving or therapeutic quality of this experience is not evident in the text. Rather, it appears violent and traumatic.

195. Friedman, "Teaching Trilogy," 140.

196. Chisholm, *H.D.'s Freudian Poetics*, 122–3.

197. Ibid., 187. Chisholm describes *The Gift* as "a recovery and a working through in writing" (124). Similarly *Helen*, instead of "presenting [Eros and death] as essentially or dialectically oppositional," presents them as "one" (184). Though "Achilles's meeting with Helen is painful it involves a shattering reunion and re-initiation into the mysteries of life and death which they experience together as ecstatically therapeutic" (212).

198. Hogue and Vandivere, "Introduction," xxxvii.

199. Augustine, "Preliminary Comments," 130–1.

200. Debo and Vetter, Introduction to *Approaches*, 6.

201. See, for instance, Rado, "Portraits," Thomas, "Creative," Pondrom, "Helen," Keeling, "British," Sword, "Digital," and Hirsh, "God," in *Approaches*, ed. Anette Debo and Lara Vetter. Rado suggests that we "invite students to consider . . . how they imagine the different modes of experience [that H.D. delineates] (physical, intellectual, artistic, or spiritual) and the relations among them. . . . What texts, sights, or experiences enable them to enter into expanded states of consciousness?" (51).

202. Maynard, "Robert Duncan's," 148. For examples see Friedman, *Psyche* (throughout) or "Teaching," and Lesley Wheeler, "Mapping."

203. Morris, "Ticking Differently," 60.

204. Writes Duncan, "The apocalyptic picture of the world that is also the heart under attack is a complex image of correspondences between what is felt as inflicted and what is felt in projection, of wishes for vengeance that are also fears of punishment seen fulfilled in actual events" (*The H.D. Book*, 339).

205. Augustine, "Preliminary Comments," 130–1.

206. Vetter, *Curious*, 22.

207. Morris, *Live*, 13.

208. Hollenberg, *Between History and Poetry*, 104–5.

Chapter 2

"How phrase or how frame the problem?"

Helen in Egypt's Formless Question

I. FORMLESS QUESTION AND SHATTERING ANSWER

Helen in Egypt is generally considered the masterpiece of H.D.'s later work. Although formally it is a poem, it is to H.D. "the final epitome of [her] novel or the novels" written in and after the war years, and "the final and complete solution of the life-long search for the answer—the companion in-time and out-of-time together."[1] She sees its protagonist, Helen, like *Sword*'s Delia, as her alter ego. "I am alive in the Helen sequence," she writes in *Compassionate Friendship* (1955), the second work in a memoir trilogy including *Magic Mirror* (1956) and *Thorn Thicket* (1960).[2] H.D. writes that Helen is "[her] alter-ego or . . . double—and that my mother's name was Helen has no doubt something to do with it. This is myself, Helen out of the body, in another world, the *eidolon* [ghost or astral double] of the legend."[3]

The poem was begun in Lausanne, where H.D. wintered between 1947 and 1953, and Lugano, where she summered, alone in beautiful hotels with occasional visits from her daughter Perdita, friend and former analyst Walter Schmideburg, and Bryher. It was completed in Klinik Brunner, where she returned in 1953, after two serious abdominal surgeries. Though she had considered it finished, she revised it there, and at Norman Holmes Pearson's suggestion, added explanatory prose introductions to each canto. It was first published in 1961.

Biographer Barbara Guest, and others, have observed that the poem recreates H.D.'s relationships with the men who were important to her. Achilles is almost entirely based on Lord Hugh Dowding, and Paris on her sometime analyst Erich Heydt with, critics have suggested, a little Ezra Pound added. Theseus has been seen as based chiefly on Freud, but I will suggest that

Walter Schmideburg and/or Klinik Brunner's owner and chief physician, Theodore Brunner, were also role models.

Helen has little narrative or setting, and what there is shifts like a dream, and perhaps indeed exists only in its protagonist Helen's thoughts. As in a dream, characters and objects appear without preamble or explanation only to disappear without a trace, to again manifest in, and as, one another. Nothing holds a stable identity or cause-effect relation to anything else—except, perhaps, Helen and Achilles. Like its setting and narrative, *Helen*'s characters are not clearly rendered: most of them appear and disappear rapidly without evident contribution to the action or narrative, as if the poem were an Ancient Greek and Egyptian theme party that its guests dressed up for, but then left immediately after putting their heads in the door. Formally the poem is composed mostly of questions, answers, and admonitions that do not have a clear relation to one another or to the scenes or actions of the poem, though relations are implied. Mystifying answers to unclear questions produce new and more mystifying questions. The either/or choices that the questions offer are often between things, characters, and possibilities whose significance in the poem is unclear, and whose appearance is very brief. Accordingly, each question and answer leaves the reader a little more confused as to what exactly is being asked and explained, what the protagonist Helen "understands," and how this relates to the rest of the poem. Apparently, the (unidentified) narrator shares our uncertainty: "And Helen understands, though we do not know exactly what it is that she understands. To her, 'It is all very simple'" (191). What Helen would like, one senses, is to find "the direct question that will tell her everything" (47). However, the question cannot be formulated because, as its totalizing phraseology suggests, there is nothing outside it. It can only be circumnavigated through a series of inchoate questions.

Friedman notes that the poem's first book, "Pallinode," places itself in the tradition of Stesichorus of Sicily—whose *Pallinode*(s), according to commentators, never placed Helen in Troy.[4] *Helen* is thus aligned with the traditional Greek epic (though Stesichorus does not appear again), of which it has been considered a feminist critique and re-articulation. Though its settings are vague, it begins with Helen in an "Amen temple" in Egypt, possibly speaking to Achilles who appears a few pages later, mysteriously transported from the killing fields of Troy. In *Helen*, as Matte Robinson discusses, Egypt stands for what H.D. believes to be the astral plane, conceived as a nonmaterial dimension parallel to our terrestrial or material plane, and adapted by branches of occultism from Indic religions. Helen and Achilles's encounter is a reworking of, and intended as the astral component of, H.D.'s relationship with Dowding.[5] When Helen mentions the name of Thetis—Achilles's mother—Achilles recognizes her as Helen of Troy and/or as his mother, and his enraged attempt to throttle her becomes, I will argue, a rape. Though

Friedman claims that in this scene Achilles's "assault turns into love," I will suggest that love, or Helen's consent to the sexual encounter, is nowhere evident.[6] Though Helen may retroactively acquiesce to it—at any rate, she wishes to remember it once it is over—depictions of the event and later references to it suggest a traumatic physical invasion rather than a consensual act. I call this encounter a rape because it looks like one to me despite Helen's retrospective and ambivalent acquiescence.

From this encounter, we are later told, Helen engenders (paradoxically, since they already existed) a multiplicity of beings including Helen and Achilles themselves. The encounter also catalyzes Helen's great need and search for answers, which is evident throughout the rest of the poem. However, the questions to which these answers are to be applied are rarely clear. They concern her identity, as well as the meaning behind the rape and other events—for instance, the meaning behind the Trojan War in which she may or may not (this is another question) have participated. Exchanges with Achilles and questions and assertions follow the rape: some are unclear, while others concern the meaning of his words and behavior. Helen imagines the meaning that she seeks in terms of Achilles's motivation for his "first boorishness" (47), in terms of the meaning of their encounter in the larger scheme of things, and also as something unspecified beyond these.

In the second book, "Leuké," Helen departs for Leuké and Paris, and later for Theseus. However, although each provides some solace and council, both former lovers dismiss the importance of Helen's relationship with Achilles. These dismissals provoke her departure from them and her return, in imagination at least, to Egypt and to Achilles—or to the "image or eidolon of Achilles" (208). In the third book, "Eidolon," the eidolons (Ancient Greek for image or ghost, and the theosophical term for the "astral body") of Achilles and Helen appear about to be reconciled, but Helen is called back to the mundane Leuké and to Paris, who is still intent on repudiating her relationship with Achilles. After this, it is hard to say where the text locates her physically, if indeed she has physical being at all. She revisits previous and new scenes in memory—and/or in her astral body—and in this way appears to be reunited with Achilles.

I will draw on H.D.'s notes and biography to argue that Helen's questions and answers trace a thought pattern that was to somewhat stabilize H.D.'s emotional and cognitive life in the frozen embrace of a repeating scenario of eroticized invasion, sacrifice, union, and (perhaps) renewal, depicted in the poem as Achilles's rape of Helen. This rape represents the "answer" to an unclear question that Helen seeks throughout. It does so by acting as the beginning and endpoint in an imaginary cycle of traumatic recurrence, which appears in H.D.'s mind as a powerful thought pattern, but also in her imagination as a recurring event of cosmic significance—though the significance itself shifts in each retelling. The answer to the question of Dowding's repudiation, which *Sword* begins to formulate and *Helen* knits together, conceives it as an annihilating, yet repeating, mother-father-son reunion that resolves (perhaps) the alienation of masculine and feminine principles in the world order. H.D. seeks integration and completion through cognitive comprehension, but failing this, through the assimilation of the signifier of difference within a system that is not personal and symbolic, but literal and universal—an all-determining cosmic pattern whose center is H.D. herself. Though this pattern remains ever shifting, ghostly and incomplete, a thought pattern is fomented in it, in which the phallus is imagined both as a penis entering her (or her alter egos) in a sexual encounter and as a birthing and re-absorption of the universe, and, therefore, the containment of everything, hence all difference, within herself. This explanation of the signifier of difference as part of the repeating pattern of her special destiny, and as motivated by erotic aggression, anchors its meaning somewhat, but also appears retraumatizing. H.D. seeks to contain and nullify the trauma of her encounter with Dowding, and the traumas of other negative or equivocal reactions from authority figures that confront her with difference, but this search, and the "answers" she finds, themselves become shattering reenactments.

In *Helen*, the cyclical encounter with the male lover coincides, for H.D., with the spiritual cycles of initiation preliminary to what occultist Robert Ambelain terms "Reintegration into the Divine."[7] *Helen*'s characters, including Helen, emanate from and are absorbed, excruciatingly, back into a many-named God, just as Schreber and his "provisional-improvised beings" come from, and return to, a God who, as Weber writes in his introduction to the *Memoirs*, "corresponds to meaning."[8] H.D. in *Helen* draws on Ambelain's vision of the union of the divine mother-father-son triad within each initiate.[9] Ambelain writes of the primary importance of personal re-integration with the mother: "The key to all success resides in the art of awakening in us the Divine spark emanating from the 'MOTHER.'[10] Likewise, the encounter in *Helen* of H.D. figures who are also divine mother figures with son and father figures is expected at some future time to fully unite mother, father, and son. However, this union is depicted bleakly in the poem, with overtones of the sacrifice and takeover of the characters involved: Helen by Achilles, and both perhaps by the God who, it appears, controls Achilles (87, 230).

Interfering, talking rays for Schreber and unclear questions and mysterious objects for Helen seem to circle the intensity of a union with God, which both envision, at least at times, as unbearable. Schreber, like Helen, believed that "the eternal cycle of things" was "the basis of the Order of the World."[11] God's roles as beginning and end point in this cosmic cycle and as "soul-murderer" are of equal interest to him:

> This exposition of the "forecourts of Heaven" may give an indication of the eternal cycle of things which is the basis of the Order of the World. In creating something, God in a sense divests Himself of part of Himself or gives different form to part of His nerves. This apparent loss is restored when after hundreds or thousands of years the nerves of departed human beings . . . return to Him as the "forecourts of Heaven."[12]

Though I hesitate to make too close a parallel, the cyclical "Order of the World" that Schreber describes in his *Memoirs* is reminiscent of the cyclical play or plan that H.D. describes in *Sword* and *Helen.* In both, a departure from God alternates with a seemingly brutal reunion with God, which is yet imagined as necessary for renewal.

Though *Helen* refers to the cosmological system provided by Ambelain's work and places its characters and events within the cosmic pattern of initiations that Ambelain describes, the poem's incorporation of occultist patterning is not the main cause of its impenetrability. On the contrary, Ambelain's frameworks, and other esoteric frameworks, are in part attempts to clarify and structure an agonizing formlessness. H.D. found in some occultist texts a resonance with her concern with the integration of science and spirituality, and other abstract values, her quest to subsume differences of perspective into a metanarrative, her interest in diagrams and schemas depicting things unclear to most people, her belief in discernible (to the elect) levels of spiritual seniority, and her anticipation of otherworldly interventions and world transformations. Occultism, like psychoanalysis, spoke to her belief in the importance of personal and social integration, and of family triangles. However, just as H.D.'s deployment of psychoanalysis does not fully account for the enigmatic qualities of her texts, neither does the influence of occultism. *Helen*—like *Sword*—is enigmatic chiefly because H.D.'s thought is spiraling in abstraction and confusion.

Likewise, though Ambelain's conceptual schema and those of psychoanalysis frame an enigmatic cycle, or wheel, of integration and departure in *Helen*, they are not, I suggest, the chief sources of its power and significance for H.D. Rather, this significance is similar to what Schreber assigns to God's approach and departure.[13] The experiences that Schreber depicts in his *Memoirs*, as Weber argues in his 1988 introduction, enact Schreber's replacement of symbolic differentiation with imaginary and embodied differentiation—which for Schreber, as for Helen, is also, paradoxically, a harrowing, invasive union.[14] There is a slippage between identity and difference that in both H.D.'s and Schreber's writing is associated with takeover or violation by another, with fragmented or proliferating identities, and with their own role, likely through martyrdom, in the renewal of the world. Though Schreber's vision is more entirely and consistently literal than H.D.'s, H.D.'s vision, as evidenced in *Helen* and other texts from this period, is more literal than has been acknowledged—though Robinson's reading of *Helen* establishes that the characters and events in it have literal (albeit sometimes astral) existence in her belief system.

H.D. in *Helen in Egypt* imaginatively creates a universe where writing and being are one and the same, and replaces the symbolic universality of shared language with Helen's and the rape's universal significance as the creation, destruction, and integrating container of the fragmented universe. Achilles's sexual invasion of Helen, and the "miraculous birth" (288) that follows it, stages this imaginative reversal of castration into nondifferentiation or incomplete differentiation. Like language, but in a more corporeal register, birth, death, and the skin usually mark the limit where identity becomes difference. In the rape and miraculous birth depicted in *Helen*, all of these limits are invoked and traversed. Achilles repudiates Helen's words and attacks her, asserting their sexual and symbolic difference, but this attack reverses into a traumatic union that is also timeless and eternal. In Lacanian terms, the lack imposed by the father figure appears as eroticized aggression, because difference as such is not fully internalized. A repudiation reverses into a literary depiction of a rape. This may be because actual negation, disinterest, or disengagement in her loved one's response is in this instance even more difficult for H.D. to assimilate than it is for most of us—perhaps impossible.[15] This event abolishes difference, yet is also the marker of difference. A symbolic order predicated on the idea of difference is precluded: oneness as singularity, and its opposite, oneness as nondifferentiation, are imagined as paradoxically identical.

Helen, like Schreber in his *Memoirs*, is invaded by God(s) and men, as well as partially identified with, or embodying, multitudes of others—who are also not entirely distinct from one another, and who also are, or may be, controlled and invaded by one another. The idea of control would have been familiar to H.D. from her séance years: in spiritualism, "controls" are the spirits that most often possess the medium, acting as interlocutors with other spirits and directing séances to some extent. Zakenuto, who H.D. believed was (a) God, was one of these "controls."

Helen's identity is threatened by the overwhelming "eternal moment" of her rape by Achilles. When contemplating this moment she must "fight for her identity, for Helena," because "the lure of his sea-eyes/endanger[s her] memory" (37). To "invoke" the letter in Egypt is, for Helen, to retain identity, to be—like the vulture—a writing-being or "living hieroglyph" (23). This invocation of identity involves remembering. Achilles's annihilating "anger" seemingly changes Helen from a "letter" to a mother herself, the thing that all letters recall:

in the dark, I must have looked
an *inked-in shadow*; but with his anger,
that ember, I became
what his accusation made me,
Isis, forever with that Child,
the Hawk Horus. (23, emphasis added)

Prior to the desire to remember, Helen voices a desire to forget associated with the initial attack. The desire to forget is a response to the throttling, while the desire to remember is a response to its transition into sex:

O Thetis, O sea-mother,
I prayed, as he clutched my throat
with his fingers' remorseless steel,
let me go out, let me forget,
let me be lost
O Thetis, O sea-mother, I prayed under his cloak,
let me remember, let me remember,
forever, this Star in the night. (16)

This procreation/remembering saves Helen at the time of the rape, when she gives birth to the "thousand sails" that "brought them together. If she forgets this, she is lost." In subsequent traumatic recollections, too, she remembers other loves and family to "temper or balance" the "suspense" (162). If forgetting/castration is the aggressive father, remembering is the mother and castration's reversal, the unity of the letter and being. Motherhood is envisioned both as corporeal and as literary production, a union of writing and being in which castration is reversed. In Achilles's attack on Helen, memory and identity (the mother) and repression and difference (the father) unite. But not entirely to Helen's satisfaction: "O God-father," she begs Theseus subsequently, "teach me to remember/teach me not to remember" (185–6). Remembering and forgetting may both be necessary to shore up an identity under attack, Helen suggests—as Ruth Leys may also suggest in her discussion of trauma resolution.[16]

The inchoate questions that Helen and *Helen*'s narrator articulate wheel around Dowding's rejection, which, as I suggest in the last chapter, places H.D.'s entry into symbolic language in question. I argue that it is this question of the desire of the Other that H.D. seeks to "phrase or . . . frame" (63) in the poem. This uncertainty, or unformed question, articulated in the poem as "What is the answer?" (46) and "How phrase or how frame the problem?" might also have taken shape as "What does the Other want?"—the question that arises, Lacan writes, in the standard process of subject formation, where the intervention of the father figure in the mother-child dyad first throws the subject into question.[17]

This mysterious want envisioned in the Other wavers in the poem between desire and demand. It has to do, at times, with an inarticulate imperative directed at Helen—like the tyrannical "You must!" that Lacan describes. The divine being manifesting in Achilles, and orchestrating "the play" (230) within which Helen and Achilles's encounter takes place, is depicted in the poem as mandating and controlling as distinct from desiring. Nevertheless, the question of the Other's desire persists in the sense of something yet to be understood—about Achilles's motivation in attacking Helen, and about "everything." Helen's musing, near the end of the poem, on Achilles's loss of, and repressed longing for, his mother, Thetis, recasts the Other as incomplete, as desiring rather than demanding, which represents the poem's most profound resolution, though the sense persists of an overwhelming divine imperative and of Helen's impending martyrdom to this demand.

Over the years that H.D. composed *Helen*, the radical groundlessness of meaning triggered by Dowding's repudiation lingered. She seeks, in the poem, to re-anchor meaning by establishing that writing and being are the same—as Lacan argues Schreber does in his *Memoirs*.[18] H.D. also suggests in *Helen* that the "meaning" of writing-being, and also that the difference between the writing-being and its "meaning," is Achilles's rape of Helen. *Helen* is, itself, intended as writing-being; it *is* the indecipherable script that it seeks to interpret. All of its events, images, and beings are the progeny of, and consequently take significance from, the rape. It represents and reverses symbolic castration in an imaginary register in which the imperative appears as a tyrannical, "You must," a rape, rather than a "No."

Whereas H.D.'s prose response to Dowding's repudiation appeared as a nebulous cognitive upheaval in *Sword*, *Helen* begins to fix the beliefs and associations pertaining to this experience into a wheel, a circling around a central emptiness that seems to call for the generation of ever new terms and associations to fill it temporarily. Accordingly, Helen's and the reader's minds are whirled around and eventually dropped by the poem. *Helen*'s words do not consistently "gel" (a favorite word of H.D.'s in later life) with concepts, occultist or otherwise, but orbit one "eternal moment" (277) whose meaning is itself. However, whereas H.D. in *Sword* seeks more anxiously to unite words and meanings, in *Helen*, she more easily allows words unclear meanings, since they gain significance in relation to Helen's rape and generativity, and to the divine being who, Helen speculates, wills this, and perhaps participates in it. Perhaps for this reason the generation of new terms slows from its hectic pace in *Sword*, though questions, answers, characters, and events in *Helen* still succeed one another in a rapid, chaotic way—as if perhaps subject to the will of an incorrigibly enigmatic and inconsistent creator, as Helen speculates.

Helen answers with circular logic the mystery that *Sword* returned to obsessively: how to integrate Dowding's repudiation of H.D. into "the plan," now imagined more as an overarching cosmic plan than a plan to accomplish impending postwar world transition, and yet maintain the heroine's key role. *Sword* proffers many possible motivations for the Dowding figures, but does not fix on anything for long. In *Helen*, H.D. uses Freudian and occultist models more confidently to make Dowding's repudiation the "Alpha and Omega,"[19] the beginning, end, and meaning of everything. Taking place chiefly on the astral plane, where words (*Helen* suggests) are embodied and castration is reversed, Achilles's rape of Helen both dramatizes and "answers" the question of the Other's desire by recasting it as demand, though desire briefly re-emerges later in the poem. It seeks also to establish that Helen contains the phallus—through which everything gains meaning. However, in spite of this claim to answers and meanings, Helen and the poem's narrator continue throughout the poem to produce unclearly formulated questions. Likewise, objects, characters, memories, and alternate identities that are imagined as significant, but whose significance is not clear, continue to appear and disappear rapidly throughout, leaving little or no trace on the poem's action.

Helen's subdivided, proliferating, telescoping characters, gods, and indistinct otherworldly beings (who are also all, mysteriously, one or two), and its redoubling, referentially unclear text suggests psychic shattering, projection, and incorporation. The proliferating shards of self-image that the work depicts appear as fleeting characters, intentions, roles, and objects that come into the picture and vanish with no apparent causes or effects, other than their genealogy in Achilles's rape—Dowding's shattering rejection. Characters and uncharacterized beings like the "swarm," difficult to distinguish and organize, gain their literal existence from the rape, since Helen conceived them by it. The ideal self, the object of the other's (indeed of everyone's) gaze, is personified as the fragmented and subdividing, but also miraculously unitary, and universally significant, Helen. However, the continued proliferation of subjects, objects, and unclear questions, as well as the desolate tone of the poem, suggest no resolution. Even the moment of "*La Mort, L'Amour*," in which difference is invoked, but transcended, has an uncertain remainder. Achilles and Helen "will always be centralized by a moment, undecided yet. Though *La Mort, L'Amour* will merge in the final illumination" (271). The final meaning is identified with the sexual encounter of Helen and Achilles, H.D."s and Dowding's alter egos and astral doubles, although this encounter, despite having already occurred on the astral plane, has (somehow) yet to reach its final version. In 1957, H.D. writes of her relationship with

Dowding, "Later, I seem to think, somewhere else—not here—there will be the consummation."[20]

II. *HELEN* IN *EGYPT* AS AFFIRMATION OF THE FEMININE

Early described by Friedman and Rachel Blau DuPlessis as a re-inscription of the lost power of the feminine, and by Albert Gelpi as a particularly feminine progress toward mystical union, *Helen* has more recently been discussed in terms of its indeterminacy, its ambivalently reactionary political import, and its immersion in occultism. Friedman describes the poem as an epic re-telling of the patriarchal Helen myth from an empowered feminine perspective, in which Helen resists various male versions of herself in her quest for the self-generated feminine identity that Friedman envisions as the poem's central concern. In Gelpi's interpretation Helen dismisses the advances of the wrong men in order to remain true to her ideal, which he describes as the feminine mystical unification of all her selves in death, represented by Achilles. Friedman notes the influence of Freud's theory of the life and death drives, *eros* and *thanatos*, on H.D.'s vision of *Eros, Eris* in *Helen*. However, she sees the poem as a reinscription of *Eros*, which for Freidman is associated in the poem with "the woman's world."[21] In *Helen*, Friedman writes, Helen's thought process "clarifies . . . the values" of this world, the "peace and harmony"[22] that must be restored to blasted civilization. Friedman argues in reference to what I read as Achilles's rape of Helen, that Helen's "appeal to Thetis [which] transforms Achilles's hatred into love"[23] encapsulates the poem's vision of the battle of love and death and the recovery of the past that allows love to triumph. However, this triumph of love Friedman claims is not evident to me in the poem. Helen is "loved of War," says Theseus, but War is still around doing the "loving"—very badly and distantly, as one would expect. In a similar vein, Gelpi argues that "with that name [Thetis] Helen and Achilles are reconciled as lovers and siblings."[24] Rather, it is the name of Thetis that instigates Achilles's rape (15, 277).

This rape is first described in a prose introduction early in the poem. Achilles, disoriented by his sudden relocation from Troy to Egypt, suddenly recognizes the identity of Helen, who he has encountered "on the beach" (13). He is further provoked when she reminds him of his mother: "Again, [Helen] thinks of [Thetis] and reminds Achilles of his divine origin, "O child of Thetis." This is quite enough. Can you throttle a phantom? He tries. The end is inevitable (15). Achilles, the poem tells us, "caught at [her] wrist," (16) and "'clutched [her] throat/with his fingers' remorseless steel" (17). Helen's immediate response to this is a wish for death or psychic departure: "Let me go out, let me forget/let me be lost" (17). Immediately afterward, however, "under his cloak," she prays: "Let me remember/forever, this Star in the night" (17).

Helen returns to this event often, with intense ambivalence, in thought and memory. Though she values and wishes to remember it, she also describes it as devastating throughout the poem. As she puts it, "As the light of the Star [her encounter with Achilles]/glows clearer, the shadow grows darker" (84). This shadow has not received critical attention—critical responses have described the encounter only in positive terms, as a transformation of aggression into love. I found these responses disturbing. The initial description and later references to it suggest a traumatic invasion, notwithstanding the more positive sounding significance it also has for Helen, who remembers it as a "Star in the night" (17, 76) and "the only answer" (86). Helen—and Achilles, who may have been under the control of a divine, and perhaps malevolent, being—are depicted as having no agency in the event. Further, its effect on Helen, and the more sinister and destructive resonances that it maintains throughout the poem despite Helen's (and literary criticisms') attempts to imagine it in positive terms, suggest a sexual invasion rather than a consensual act.

The poem's message, Friedman writes, is that "all male violence is an incomplete, culturally damaging turn from unaccepted maternal love and power and, by extension, from the life-force of the Great Goddess."[25] But Helen reflects that without the war, there would have been no rape—and this would have been a bad thing: "They [Helen and Clytemnestra] must forget the war and its consequences—but no, there is this yet, unresolved—without war, there would have been no Achilles, no 'Star in the night'" (76). The "Star in the night," as Helen calls the rape, is Helen's "only answer" (86) to her formless question.

DuPlessis has rightly noted the relation of repressed love for the mother to the violence in *Helen*: "*Helen in Egypt* seriously intends itself as an anti-war text, which uses an examination of the roots of violence in repression of love of the mother to propose an alternative."[26] But what alternative to violence does *Helen* propose? War is coupled with love—as Achilles is with Helen—but retains its violence. Helen herself describes her rape as the "ultimate experience, *La Mort, L'Amour*" (288) and as "the absolute of negation" and chooses this annihilating absolute over the gentler role of "Dendritis" that Paris offers her, with its "Love without arrows" (140). Helen's question, whether "Zeus decrees that, forever/Love should be born of War?" (32), implies that Love is indeed born of War, and that this birthing does not eliminate War. No more could Freud separate the two, as H.D. knows.[27] Swiss theorist Denis de Rougemont in his *Love in the Western World*, an important text for her, also insists that this is impossible.

As well as being read as life affirming and anti-war, *Helen* has been read as communicating a less literal understanding of occultism than H.D.'s previous work. Helen Sword has written that "only when [the RAF messages] became starkly unambiguous, requiring action rather than interpretation, did H.D. reject her wartime spirits and replace them with the metaphorical, purely literary ghosts who haunt the beaches and pages of *Helen in Egypt*."[28] Rather, as Robinson has argued, these ghosts literally represent H.D.'s and Dowding's astral selves meeting on the astral plane, a meeting that has shattering and re-integrating effects on the "terrestrial plane." H.D. sees the astral plane as a place where certain people, "who are not shadows or shades,/ but entities, living a life/unfulfilled in Greece" (*Helen* 89) can visit in their astral bodies when living. It is so considered in many branches of occultism, and various permutations of Hinduism and Buddhism, where this plane is also the place where most souls go after the death of the body. It is where, in Dowding's *Many Mansions*, the deceased RAF pilots dwell. Instead of signaling metaphor or other intent commonly recognized as literary, *Helen's* "ghosts" suggest H.D.'s belief that her astral double journeys to the astral plane, where the significance of events on the material plane is found, and words are embodied.

Robert O'Brien Hokanson has drawn attention to *Helen*'s indeterminacy, arguing that "[r]ather than simply offering a rebuttal to the legend of 'hated Helen,' *Helen in Egypt* investigates the dilemma of imposing form on experience and demonstrates the elusiveness of the 'true' story."[29] He sees in H.D."s style an intentional troubling of "conventional modes of thought and representation," a "critique" of these modes rather than a largely inadvertent drift from them. Cyrena Pondrom also observes that the poem's "fragmentary, partially contradictory narratives," rather than cohering into a narrative, radically destabilize reality and "shatter . . . the coherence of the world."[30] Susan Edmunds has linked Kleinian theory to the poem's "fantasies of maternal violence," which "continue to preoccupy H.D. in *Helen in Egypt*."[31] Britain, she argues, represents the Kleinian "bad mother" to H.D. (the bad mother and good mother are fantasies of part-objects that result from splitting). The violence to *Helen*'s accused but ultimately sympathetic mother figures thus suggests to Edmunds H.D.'s ambivalently conservative response to the 1952 Egyptian revolution aimed at ending British occupation. While this reading is possible, the evidence suggests that the Egyptian revolution did not loom large in H.D.'s mind during the poem's composition. The poem's primary importance for her, as her letters and memoirs show and the poem's content suggests, lay in its rendering of her significant relationships.

The vaguely formulated, confusing questions and answers that occur in a somewhat rising tempo throughout *Helen*'s three sections concern the identity and difference, and real or ghostly existence of Helen's various selves and of the characters, objects, and settings in the poem. They concern as well the purpose of the God who she believes orchestrates it all. These questions and answers do not "mean" anything in the usual sense: they do not take stable positions within a structure of meaning, because the poem has none. Though Helen's questions appear coherent in and of themselves, they rarely knit with the poem as a whole or with one another. Rather, they blur into one another, reappear even after they have been "answered," and are no sooner answered than another pops up. They seem to fall into the uncertainty that motivates them rather than to formulate it. The poem attempts to resolve the formlessness of its questions by presenting various signifiers (sound-images, words) that it asserts are the same, or that contain and are contained by one another, or that are redoubled through repetition in another context: signifiers that "are" other signifiers replace signifier-signified relations. Other forms of splitting of text and character also attempt to re-create the signifier-signified structure. Helen's own behavior mimics the poem itself: she contains, repeats, and recalls word-images that she briefly identifies with the "answer" to her questions, but like the poem itself she is trapped in an endless deferral in which meaning is promised anew by each new character, object, image, or term, but never closed.

The lack of lack experienced in foreclosure is implicated in the formlessness of Helen's question. Helen always already contains everything. Her question cannot take shape, except as the question of the question. Since language is enabled by lack, Helen's question, "How phrase or how frame the problem?" could be synonymous with the question, "What is language?" The problem cannot be framed in language, because there is nothing that does *not* concern it. H.D.'s incipient desire to enter the symbolic realm is stymied by her foreclosure of anything outside herself. The poem therefore offers us Helen herself—albeit rather tentatively—as the solution to the question of the question.

The exceptions to the formlessness of Helen's questions and answers are her questions and answers concerning Achilles's, Theseus's, and Paris's motivations: "the problem of why [Achilles] had, in the first instance, attacked her" (18), and why Paris and Theseus discourage her from contemplating her relationship with Achilles. These precise questions concern actual events: Dowding's repudiation of H.D.'s RAF messages and Heydt's, Brunner's, and/or Schmideburg's discouragement of her preoccupation with Dowding and her beliefs about the significance of their relationship. The clear questions and answers begin in "Pallinode," with questions of Helen's culpability in the Trojan War, and quickly refocus on the motivation for Achilles's rape. Helen also considers his general ruthlessness, and his penchant to sacrifice women—with whom she identifies—to the demands of war.

In "Leuké," Helen finds herself in the company of Paris and later Theseus. The clear questions here concern the motivation of Paris's repudiation of her relationship with Achilles, and she later considers Theseus's motivation for his dismissive attitude toward Achilles, as well as returning to the motivation of Achilles for his raping Helen and "sacrificing" women. "Eidolon" contains fewer questions and claims to understanding. It revisits and re-evaluates previous scenes, and the unclear answers found in them, suggesting equally unclear alternatives. In it, too, characters and things are sorted according to identities and differences that seem to be predicated on contiguity. But it does formulate *Helen*'s most comprehensive explanation for Achilles's rape of Helen; she reminds him of his mother. Indeed, she is his mother.

III. SEXUAL ENCOUNTERS WITH DIVINE BEINGS

I do not know how often what Lacan calls "delusional metaphors" or "delusional formations"—visions that defend against (and perhaps depict) the threat of annihilation experienced in the psychotic break—involve a fantasy of the sexual entry of divine beings into a subject who conceives and gives birth as a result.[32] In published case studies, the scenario is widespread; Schreber, for example, shared it. As philosopher Gilles Deleuze and psychoanalyst Félix Guattari point out, Schreber's preoccupation with reproduction, genealogy, and motherhood has not received as much critical attention as his preoccupation with his penetration by God since it does not illustrate Freud's theories as well.[33] I argue that like Schreber's, Helen's fertility following her rape, imaginatively reverses castration by transforming it into procreation. Language thereby becomes being. The rape and miraculous motherhood of Helen and Schreber depicted in the *Memoirs* and in *Helen in Egypt* suggest in psychoanalytic terms not only imaginary castration in the form of sexual subjugation by a powerful male figure, but the imaginary reversal of castration: the argument that Helen and Schreber physically contain the ultimate meaning of all things (the phallus, the divine life of God) and that they give birth to a more alive, meaningful world than the rote, invasive, and senseless one that they experience. Transpersonal psychology, too, suggests that such "fantasies" or "delusions" actually represent, as mystical visions are understood to in some circles, an insight into a fundamental truth about internal transformation or about the unfolding of human history.[34]

Charles LaChance attributes H.D.'s vision of sexual immolation in part to her upbringing, writing that the "paragon of sexuality in H.D.'s early work [is] a willful god or man who devastates yet fulfills women's bodies and minds" and that this "sexual sublimity," may proceed from "Christian masochism . . . as she was 'reared' in Moravianism, a sect celebrating 'Wounds' of 'the sacrificial victim' Christ in hymns bloody-minded and sexual."[35] Miranda Hickman, though disagreeing with LaChance's description of H.D."s work as "phallocentric," also finds in it "a current of masochistic desire for surrender to a power that might obliterate,"[36] and calls for a nuancing of critical readings that have H.D.'s work unequivocally opposing violence or domination.[37] LaChance goes further, suggesting that contrary to critical orthodoxy, H.D. "in her spiritual life and art . . . bows to a brutalizing conservatism: a patriarchy of salvational male sadism and female idolization of pain."[38] James Gifford reads H.D.'s journal references to Lawrence Durrell to argue persuasively that H.D. saw herself, and that Bryher also saw her, as masochistic, or at least powerfully and multivalently affected by images of male brutality and female vulnerability.[39]

I agree that the sexualized immolation of the feminine by the masculine appears throughout H.D.'s work, and disturbingly so in *Helen*; however, I don't agree with LaChance that this is mere sexual masochism. For one thing, H.D.'s work shows a genuine puzzlement with this vision—a disappointed expectation that it will fulfill. Though the idea is proffered that Helen's sexual attack by a God-possessed hero is "the only answer" (86), *Helen* retains a floundering quality that undermines these assertions. Though like LaChance I see rape in *Helen*, I do not see there the glorification of rape that he finds in her early poetry. LaChance reads the sexual resonances in mystical texts and in H.D.'s poems as referring only to conventionally sexual acts, particularly to heterosexual rape. He makes no distinction, for instance, between St. Teresa of Avila's visions of being pierced by a flaming spear and any other sexual fantasy of "debasement."[40] To me, H.D.'s and Saint Teresa's texts do not exclude or even sublimate sexuality, but include it among their ways of longing for, and experiencing, the dissolution of boundaries and encounters with something beyond them.

Helen claims she understands (though it is not clear what) without needing to decipher the signifier. Thus she can find meaningful the "one finite moment" that has "no before and no after" (301), no dialectical meaning. The meaning that the rape enables, she finds, is the rape. The event that provoked the formless question is itself the only answer. *Helen* likewise *is* its own meaning. Like Schreber's *Memoirs*, it reverses castration by casting itself as the very system of signifiers, and as the very meaning of the encounter, that is in question.

IV. NEGATIVE MEN

As critics have observed, the explanations tendered by *Helen*'s male authority figures, based on Dowding, Heydt, Freud, Brunner and/or Schmideburg, are resisted. Paris is dismissed as a bitter Trojan with an Oedipal complex who knows little of the sea. Achilles, too, is seen as warped by the High Command and as reacting to his mother issues. Even Theseus, Helen believes, is unfairly partial to Greece at the expense of Egypt, and to Paris over Achilles.

Helen's various answers to the questions of Helen's consorts' motivations are comprehensible, albeit inter-referential and not governed by the known laws of time and space. These answers represent in Lacan's terms the growth of the "delusional metaphor," which stands in for the paternal metaphor. By questioning H.D.'s version of reality and offering their own in contrast to it, the men on whom Theseus, Paris and Achilles are based placed themselves in the position of Lacan's "name of the father," the place where symbolic meaning is determined, as I discussed in my introduction and first chapter. A subject with what Lacan calls a "psychotic structure" has no precedent, he writes, for this is a call to the order where language is shared and meaning is open to contestation.[41] Such a call, for Lacan, addresses the subject-position that he cannot fully assume—that of the castrated subject. It can therefore catalyze psychotic breaks in persons with "psychotic structures"—structures where castration, as entry into the symbolic order of shared and stable language predicated on repression, has been foreclosed. If we follow Lacan, the men who dismiss her vision may assume a place that, for H.D., was never fully there—a tertiary place alien to her internal structure of object relations, which in Lacanian theory might be described as the dyad of the subject and her ideal reality.[42] Though I question Lacan's claim that this cataclysm proceeds from an inability to relate to another outside of a narcissistic dyad, I agree that the responses of these men opened cracks in a meaning-making enterprise that was incredibly important to H.D.—one on which her sense of self relied—and that these cracks fill with mysterious and proliferating literary objects (beings, things, and words) whose meanings and place in a larger whole are unclear. Alternatively, what fills the cracks that open in meaning for H.D. may be objects—perhaps hyperobjects—or others whose magnitudes and intensities most of us miss because of the boundaries within which meaning unfolds for us.

The hole that opens up in response to invalidation fills up for H.D. with a multiplicity of others in perhaps narcissistic, certainly referential, sometimes malign, relations to herself. We see these others in the many fleeting characters and things that populate *Helen*. The insistence and repetitiveness with which Achilles's rape is invoked as the "meaning" of these beings places it, in Lacan's theory, as a delusional metaphor—an "imaginary phallus" rather than the "symbolic phallus" that normally structures language. This phallus, rather than functioning as the unconscious internalization of difference that allows clearly distinguished words and concepts, appears in a nonsymbolic modality in *Helen* as an attack and union on which the meaning of everything else is fastened. Its nonsymbolic modality correlates to the segmentation and vagueness in *Helen*'s language, as well as to the confusion of its protagonist.

The rape, the sacrifices of other female characters (who also represent Helen and therefore H.D.), and Helen's disagreements with Paris and Theseus are all modeled on H.D.'s real encounters with men. However, as the poem progresses it becomes less clear to which textual or extra-textual stuff the poem's action and Helen's questions refer.[43] What is suggested, however, is that Achilles's rape answers Helen's questions in some as yet to be determined way. This encounter, "the only answer," is "the series or circle of the ever recurring "eternal moment" (277). It *is* the eternal moment, the circuit's simultaneous beginning and ending, cause and effect. As such, it retroactively gives meaning to each of H.D."s "cycles" or "sequences," as she describes the phases in her life as distinguished according to her predominant love interests. The narrator tells us that "the mind can not answer the 'numberless questions' but [her] heart 'encompasses the whole of the undecipherable script,' when it recalls the miracle, 'Achilles's anger' and 'this Star in the night'" (85). Yet paradoxically the question that Helen asks herself most often concerns finding the reason for Achilles's rape. Her several conceptual explanations mesh somewhat: she reminds him of his mother, she is his mother, he is controlled by a divine being, and they are part of a play ordained by this being that eternally reenacts their encounter. However, none of these explanations of it is satisfactory to Helen. Her beliefs that it is itself the "answer" to the question of why it happened, and the answer to the unformed question that she seeks to formulate, also leave her unsatisfied, as her many subsequent questions show. The rape's shortcomings as an anchor for meaning can be observed in the drift of *Helen*'s text, particularly its multifarious, mysteriously overlapping characters and unclear expressions, questions, answers, settings, and meanings. At times, H.D. uses alliteration and rhythm, patterning, counting and sorting, and the materiality of imagery, memories, and objects as replacements for a structure that does not settle in her thought. She also tries to sort things out by identifying characters as identical or different, containing or contained.

Formal and imagistic renderings of splitting, such as dividing and telescoping identities, proliferating words and objects, and words encapsulated in quotation marks for no apparent reason, occur in *Helen* as responses to male characters' attacks on Helen. These attacks are modeled on H.D.'s real encounters with men who challenged or dismissed her beliefs regarding her special role in the world and her relationship with Dowding. Images of splitting suggest that H.D. experienced therapeutic interventions advising her to stop revisiting her memory of Dowding as harmful. Hence Helen's emphasis on resisting male advice and "never [forgetting] Achilles" (170) and their "Star in the night":

but I would not go yet,
I must have time to remember
Dis, Hades, Achilles. (199)

Helen's reminiscences are challenged. Before the imminent return to Achilles to which Thetis has summoned her, Helen subsists in her "small room" and ambivalently receives the attentions of Paris. For Paris, modeled on her doctor and analyst at Klinik Brunner, Erich Heydt, Helen "died, died, died/when the Walls fell" (131) and Achilles "never loved [her]" (143). Paris tells Helen that there was no meaning in the Trojan War and her encounter with Achilles was fulfilled on another plane of existence: "She died, he says, that is all there is about it" (131). Erich Heydt's response to H.D.'s belief in the supernatural significance of her encounter with Dowding is not hard to glean from this.[44] In *Compassionate Friendship* H.D. writes of Heydt,

> He had scant sympathy with my War II story of the RAF and communications as for Lord Howell. I felt his attitude was un-professional and destructive, especially as he had urged me to tell him about the War II novels, the first of which, *The Sword Went Out to Sea*, was a reconstruction of my contact with Lord Howell, through and because of the messages we had received, as narrated in the *Magic Ring*. Though much of the material is re-worked in *The Sword*, I had actually put aside *The Ring*, after I finished the first rough copy, winter 1944, and never saw it again until Bryher brought it to me from London, last winter, 1954. . . . Anyhow, we are back in late summer, 1953, when Erich went off, leaving a question un-answered and a possible compassionate friendship un-resolved. This break in time, in continuity was more than compensated for, by my beginning the new Helen sequence, Leuké. I didn't much care then, what he did, thought, or was. He had acted as a dynamic liberator or inspiration for my Greek epic.[45]

In *Helen in Egypt*, Helen ascribes Paris's dismissal of her encounter with Achilles to the rage of the defeated. By extrapolation Heydt, who is German, is both the defeated Oedipal son and a German nationalist. He desires the mother who belongs to the father, Dowding, the British victor in war over the Germans. Paris/Erich is the son-lover in the Oedipal triangle, jealous of the father-lover:

they the many, the One [RAF pilots]
were born of myself and Achilles,
our Son; but there is another,
single, alone, proud and aloof,
no Greek but a Trojan;
he hated Achilles; Achilles
was not his father

nor was I, Hecuba, his mother;
did he hate Hecuba?
she exposed him on Ida

H.D. is gripped by suspicion in parts of *Compassionate Friendship* that Heydt, who acts "as if one personality over-shadowed or over-lapped another," is a Nazi spy, controlled by a mysterious being or beings. Heydt's controllers might include "Tiresias," "X," "Bally" (Gustav Bally was a German psychoanalyst and contemporary of Heydt), or "Boss" (Heydt's analyst was Dr. Medard Boss).[46] Indeed, she fears Heydt might be working in Klinik Brunner ("Küsnacht") simply to get at her in some way as part of a secret psychic experiment in the interest of German political sabotage: "Zurich was always notorious for its spy-ring, its counter-espionage and espionage circles. If the pseudo-Boss is the head of a spy-ring and Erich one of his chief minions, then what? Do they think I can be of use to them?"[47] While she calls these fears "sheer melodrama on my part," she is nonetheless genuinely afraid. She hesitates to tell Bryher, who "would have feigned indifference or called it paranoia,"[48] and to whom she "will not mention X,"[49] but she considers leaving Klinik Brunner to avoid Heydt's secret agenda involving her.[50] However, she is reassured by confiding some of her concerns to Bryher, and by Bryher's establishing through her contacts that Boss and Bally are indeed analysts and thus hopefully not leaders of a spy-ring. Writes H.D., "There may be an X but we have established that Medard Boss and Dr. Bally are not altogether a screen."[51]

In a literary reflection of H.D.'s speculations about Heydt, Helen's Paris hates the Greeks because they defeated the Trojans in the war and because, though Paris kills Achilles on the plains of Troy, he cannot defeat Achilles's significance to Helen. Heydt/Paris and his people are castrated, inadequate to challenge the power of Achilles/Dowding, victorious English war hero, law-making father figure: "What could Paris know of the sea, la mer, la mère, the mother?" (304) Only Achilles could know her. Helen appreciates Theseus's "power and tenderness," to which she temporarily ascribes the completion of her (unknown) task: "What was Helena's task?" She cannot altogether say, only that through the power and tenderness of Theseus, "it was finished" (206). However, it is Achilles's attack to which Helen consistently returns to anchor meaning (206). Only Achilles, the "invincible, unchallenged Sire" (5) who had "saved . . . civilization" (*Sword*, 100) "could break his heart/and the world for a *token*,/a memory forgotten" (304, emphasis added). Only the victorious father, not the former lover or defeated son, can castrate the world for a token, a sign, an entry into language and into the writing-being. However, with their Oedipal and primal complexes, Paris and Achilles can hardly be blamed for being a bit negative sometimes. Consequently,

Heydt's and Dowding's refutations of H.D.'s viewpoint, on which Paris's and Achilles's grumpiness is based, cannot place her viewpoint into question because it proceeds from these complexes, not from considered, authoritative perspectives. Such refutations can only evidence the repressions and complexes of the refuters.

The dizzying cognitive repercussions of the psychic splitting caused by her male consorts' advice are suggested by Helen's convoluted responses to the challenges of Paris and Theseus. Here, as elsewhere, splitting, initially a defense, increases confusion. Paris's advice, though inadequate to come between Helen and Achilles, produces more signs of splitting: the "rent veil," the "attributes of" Aphrodite (145), phases with unclear meanings that are placed within quotation marks, and Helen's departure for Athens and Theseus. As a prose introduction enigmatically explains,

> [Paris] has asked, "why remember Achilles?" and apparently, Helen has turned on him with the accusation that it is he who has "recalled the past." There is despair and envy in him, "hatred, fear of the Greeks." There is that shadow, that prescience, even now in "this haven, this peace, this return." He is "defeated even upon Leuké." For her, there was "healing . . . death or awakening . . . the love of Achilles." The final retort of Paris is, "I say he never loved you." (143)

The advice from Paris and Theseus to "remember other loves"(165), and their unwelcome reminders of Achilles's womanizing, create further identities and questions in Helen. Immediately after Paris's "final retort" of "I say he never loved you," Helen "appears [to Paris] 'in rent veil'" like Aphrodite's, and suggests that Paris "has accepted and must accept 'a tattered garment' or an incomplete or partial manifestation of the [unidentified] vision." Paris does not know any better, though what it is that he does not know is unclear. Heydt, perhaps, was not initiated into knowledge of the astral plane, where H.D. and Dowding, she believed, encountered one another in a more meaningful way than was evident in their encounter on the terrestrial plane. The prose introduction states that Helen, presumably in Paris's vision, "was suave and elegant, her 'garment sheathed' her, as she 'stepped from the painted prow'. . . but now, she has taken on the attributes of another" (145). This other is Aphrodite, and Helen's assumption of her attributes angers Paris, who asks, "Do you dare impersonate her?" (145). Helen departs from him in response and "finds her way to another lover" (147), Theseus, "baffled and buffeted and very tired" (151). But Theseus, in this capacity perhaps based on Dr. Brunner and/or on Schmideburg, also advises Helen to let go of her concern with Achilles. He tells her to "leave [Achilles] with the asphodels" and brings up, inappropriately, Helen feels, Achilles's other lovers:

> He seems deliberately to have stepped out of the stream of our and of Helen's consciousness. Why? He has told her that she was safe with him. He reminds her that she "found life here with Paris." His Achilles lingering with Polyxena ("leave him with the asphodels") is not Helen's Achilles "on the desolate beach." (172)

Theseus's counsel, too, is followed by images of splitting and disintegration. His reminders of Achilles's other loves produce the "voice within" Helen (174) and her return to "Egypt but in a Greek mode" (178). The voice within Helen is the voice of another Helen whose consciousness the preceding Helen does not share: "There is a voice within me, listen, let it speak for me" (174). This new Helen speaks authoritatively to, as well as through, her host Helen on the subject of other characters' identities with one another:

> if Thetis was Cypris, Cypria,
> (you say) who could not Achilles be?
> in the temple, in the dark,
> in the fragrance of the incense,
> without touch, without word,
> by a thought, Amen begot Amor. (180)

The new Helen is an intense one, with "passionate devotion and dedication to "the rage of the sea, the thunder of battle, shouting and the Walls" (176). She represents the answer to the first Helen's question, does the ember glow in the heart of the snow? (174) This question, though unclear, suggests that the absolutes of heat and cold are one, or at least containing and contained, united in extremity. Helen's splitting, perhaps an attempt to avoid the pain that Theseus's words evoke, is accompanied by the extreme thinking in which wellness and death become one: "Is it Death," asks Helen subsequently, "to know/this immaculate purity,/security?" (194) The new Helen tells Theseus that Achilles's other loves did not matter to either of them and immediately remarks on the "beauty of arrows,/each bringing surcease, release (177). This unjealous, death-loving Helen within Helen then begins to identify gods and goddesses as identical with one another:

> Again, the "voice" seems to speak for Helen. . . . It takes us back to Egypt but this time in a Greek mode. Isis is Cypris (Cytherea) and Isis is Thetis. Amen-Zeus is the father of Isis-Thetis-Aphrodite (Cypris). We cannot altogether understand this evocation, the rhythms must speak for themselves and their alliterations, Cypris, Thetis, Nephthys, Isis, Paris. Proteus, the legendary King of Egypt, as we have learned before, takes many shapes. (178)

Whatever the rhythms and alliterations of her speech may have to say for themselves, Helen of Sparta soon bewilders and overwhelms the previous Helen—though the former may manifest in the latter to protect her from Theseus's words. After Helen of Sparta's cluster of questions and assertions concerning the identity and difference of the poem's deities, the first Helen cries, "Stop—O voice prompting my strophies/stop—how could that be?" (180) How could all of these beings be one another?

V. SELF-QUOTATIONS AND ENCAPSULATIONS

Self-quotations with no clear significance are another way that the poem splits and takes its (other) self as its meaning/being. Words that appear in the verses reappear within quotes in the prose sections, which were written later at Norman Holmes Pearson's suggestion to "explain" the verses. Generally, the prose simply repeats the verse in declarative form with parts of it in quotation marks. However, instead of explaining the content they surround, the quotation marks suggest that the prose means something else. But what? Words that were once part of a question now have mysterious meanings, proffered as answers to unclear questions that have somewhere been posed, or as parts of new questions. Someone is being quoted, usually Helen, but her own expressions, with their rapidly appearing, nonconsecutive terms, seem to refer to a source that we do not have. We do not know what Helen means. However, by repeating the words and placing them within quotation marks, the prose introductions suggest that someone understands—or will in the future. An extremely high proportion of the words and phrases that compose *Helen*'s prose introductions are encapsulated in these mysterious quotation marks. Sometimes the text within these quotation marks also appears in verse sections, which usually render Helen's thoughts—for instance, "Achilles's anger" and "this Star in the night" appear in verse. However, "numberless questions" and many other words and phrases enclosed in quotation marks appear in the poem only once: they are not repetitions of words that appeared first in verse. In either case, it is not clear what the quotation marks are intended to convey. Do the words mean something other than, or as well as, what they say—and if so, what? If they repeat or prefigure Helen's thoughts in the verse sections, how are their meanings altered or extended when they appear within quotation marks and explanatory prose sentences? If they are not repetitions of Helen's thoughts or speech, does someone else speak them? And if so, who—and what does this someone mean?

Schreber tells us that he uses quotation marks to indicate that an expression has been "suggested . . . from outside" by voices.[52] For instance,

> I did not invent the expression "forecourts of heaven," but like all other expressions that are in inverted commas in this essay (for instance "fleeting-improvised men," "dream life," etc.), it only repeats the words which the voices that speak to me always applied to the processes concerned. These are expressions *which would never have occurred to me*, which I have never heard from human beings.[53]

"The processes concerned" are the bodily transformations that accompany these expressions. They are, Schreber eventually discovers, intended by God to torture him into losing his reason, which would enable God to withdraw from him. God, an ambivalent lover, pursues this plan intermittently; his approaches alternate with withdrawals, especially as Schreber learns how to withstand the torment of the phrases by simply repeating them without thinking about them, which echoes how the voices themselves represent senseless repetition.

Helen contains a similar phenomenon, but with the suggestion that the strange and seemingly meaningless phrases indicate something more positive than the mind games of a cruel and ignorant God. God's intentions are hopefully not compromised by his own misunderstanding and ambivalence, as with Schreber's God, but are part of a benevolent plan that will—that surely must, Helen seems to expect—render the relations between its component parts perfectly clear in the end. Redoubling and repetition therefore safeguard "meaning" by encapsulating words in quotation marks, to await the coming of the Other who knows what they mean. The prose does not clarify what it quotes, but stores it. Meaningless words are not simply intended to drive Helen crazy. The revelation of their meaning must await the final answer that she anticipates. In the meantime it is enough for Helen to reinscribe them so that they will remain part of the complete picture to come.

The encapsulating of words in scare quotes in anticipation of an interpreter to come, especially in the prose introductions, is another way in which the poem splits. This becomes evident when, for instance, Helen asks, "What is this 'simple magic' of a 'ring of no worth, a broken oar' that finds more favor in the eyes of the 'Regent of Heaven' than the priceless treasure 'from the uttermost seas?'" (280) The ring and the oar have no obvious referent in the poem, nor does the Regent of Heaven. They do not appear elsewhere. Their magic is the subject of a question whose answer, Helen perhaps finds, cannot be defined, but which nevertheless exists: "Perhaps it can not be defined. It is a 'secret treasure' but Helen implies, as she counts 'the seven and seven slats of the ladder or the bars of light on the wall,' that it could only be judged or assessed if 'God would let me lie here forever'" (282). The actual meaning of the words in quotation marks, Helen finds in this dissociative-sounding passage, could only be determined in the synchronic dimension of eternity.

They do not refer to diachronic meaning. The answer to their question could be ascertained only through the quantification of something apparently unrelated, such as by counting "the seven and seven slats of the ladder or the bars of light on the wall." Words have meanings that cannot be thought about, addressed in time or by other words, nor measured by their use in speech and writing. Their significance is elsewhere: endless and indefinable.

Helen's language in such passages is at a remove from interpersonal speech, thought, and feeling, and while it can still create beautiful atmospheric effects, at times it plunges—surely inadvertently—into bathos. For instance Achilles's re-dedication to "a new Command"—that of Formalhaut, the "Royal Sacred High Priest of Love Rites"—suggests, by Formalhaut's encumbered title, the absence of narrative introduction of him, and his rapid appearance and disappearance, not living language, but gratuitous and lifelessly ornate words and beings (210). Most of the characters in *Helen* are similarly glorified and fleeting. These multiplying and telescoping characters, both human and divine, suggest what Lacan calls "a proliferation of imaginary modes of being" as the poem's response to the "interpellation to which the subject is unable to respond."[54]

Helen's multiple and telescoping identities, repeated scenarios, enigmatic quotations, unclear questions, and short-lived patterns appear in response to the formless question of the other's desire, but give rise to more failures of signification. The delusion elaborated in the text rests on a nonreferential language that requires new characters, objects, and associations to be generated constantly in lieu of meaning. As Delia does in *Sword*, Helen tries to figure out "the answer" by following a trail of signifiers, hoping that the "picture" will become clear retrospectively when all are chain-linked together. However, the many dualisms that she tries to bring together, such as Egypt and Greece, Egypt and Troy, "personal time" and "eternal time," Eros and Eris, Paris and Achilles, Troy-Helen and Egypt-Helen, the child and the mother, and the father and the mother are no sooner imaginatively brought together than another distinct term appears. Something always remains "unintegrated" with the "complete picture," and marks the contours of a hole that opens up in her language. Achilles's attack, though it appears as the completion and apotheosis of the cycle, perhaps only keeps the wheel spinning.

Helen's encounter with Achilles seems as though it should function as what Lacan calls a *point de capiton*, an anchoring or quilting point for the poem's meaning.[55] The *point de capiton* is the place on a chain of signification where as Lacan describes it "the signifier stops the otherwise endless movement of the signification" by seeming to connect to a signified, thereby enabling a false sense of stable meaning.[56] Yet the many causes, effects, and objects associated with it continue to divide and multiply, perhaps because their causal relations to it are never clear. The same words refer to many different things; things are or refer to many other things; many explanations are proffered for the same thing; many names and characters are actually the same being in some unclear manner or unclearly related. *Helen* does not organize its characters and action into a single frame of reference or a network of causes and effects, but clusters them around the single cause and effect of Achilles and Helen's encounter. Like Schreber's *Memoirs*, it seeks to resolve the foreclosed symbolic wound of difference through the fecundity of its protagonist. In Egypt, understood by H.D. as the astral plane, beings *are* "letters" and "writing"; to write is to give birth. Thus, Helen is the mother of herself and everyone else—of the poem itself. Still, in the end, the narrator calls on an unidentified Other to answer Helen's inchoate questions: "One greater than Helen must answer, though perhaps we do not wholly understand the significance of the message" (303). Helen may be, produce, and understand the writing that is the epic poem *Helen in Egypt*, as the poem asserts; however, the poem also suggests that some knowledge pertaining to what this is all about remains elsewhere.

The idea of events or "pictures" only becoming intelligible once the "ultimate plan" is revealed appears often in H.D.'s later work. It may have been popular in séance circles during the Second World War; Arthur Bhaduri and Dowding both admonished H.D. to view her paranormal experiences as containing meanings that would become clear over time. *Majic Ring* suggests that Bhaduri encouraged H.D. in the practice of piecing together different visionary images and words. He would give her "pictures" that came to him during his séances, and tell her that they would form a whole, piece by piece, with patience: "Pieces make complete pictures."[57] Writes H.D.,

> We have had so many references to "plan" and "pieces." On December 10 for instance, here with [Bhaduri's séance] table, we had *each piece goes with time*. And I find that I wrote to Lord Howell on December 11, "*Each piece goes with time* seems to indicate the 'plan' as a picture-puzzle with the separate bits scattered about, to be fitted together later in the *eternal plan*."[58]

Correspondingly, *Helen*'s narrator tells us that Helen wishes to read progressively, "picture by picture," the way Achilles reads:

> "Picture by picture," Helen would read the star-script, as Achilles had done. Paris will come back, he "will reflect the past" and Helen as she was "before the ultimate Mystery." But Helen in her mind, or "in my crystal" as she calls it, "would see further." She would relate the pictures in time to the pictures in eternity, as she "strove in the precinct, to decipher the Amen-script." (204)

Each "picture," each signifier, may have a meaning that is not evident in the present, but that will become clear at some future time, or perhaps "in eternity." In this time or dimension outside of time, the swirling, ghostly world will become clear retroactively.

Bhaduri's spirit-channeled responses to H.D.'s questions at their séances as transcribed in *Majic Ring* are sprinkled with such admonitions: "One part at a time. Patience" and "P-e-a-c-e. We have an eternal plan—hurry not—each piece goes with time."[59] These messages, as well as Helen's frequent admonitions to herself to be patient, to "take her time about it," I speculate, may be responses to H.D.'s urgent struggle to fix the meaning of her experiences and her difficulty in doing so. This was perhaps not well addressed by Bhaduri. By the circular logic that their séances seemed to encourage, the ultimate revelation to come would provide her with the meaning of everything preceding it. Confusing and disempowering events would be understood as contributing to the greater whole of her life's purpose. For a time, this purpose was envisioned as her crucial role in bringing about the next era of the world, and she had hoped that Dowding would do his part in it by interpreting her spirit messages. The concrete, action-oriented agenda she envisioned as their purpose was replaced instead with his repudiation, which she imagined as somehow having a purpose. In *Helen*, the meaning that Helen is sure exists, but which does not refer to anything specific—the answer, perhaps, that has no question—is fastened on the imaginative re-working of Dowding's repudiation, Achilles's attack on Helen. Just as this encounter serves Helen to anchor a meaning that otherwise seems inchoate and formless, H.D.'s encounter with Dowding serves her for years as a transcendentally meaningful event, though new significant elements enter the picture in H.D.'s later life, and other love interests and memories suggest the need for expanded organizational models.

VI. WRITING-BEINGS, SWARMS, THE ASTRAL PLANE

> When [H.D.] speaks of "*where thought dwells,/and beyond thought and idea,/their begetter,/Dream, Vision,*" these—*thought, idea, dream, vision*—are not concepts or terms of a phenomenology but entities, *dramatis personae* of her universe. "Sword" and "Word" are poetic counterparts of daimonic beings in Neo-Platonic hierarchies, having their creative necessity here in the plasticity of the immediate reality of the poem rather than in the requirements of a philosophic structure.
>
> Robert Duncan, *The H.D. Book*, 586.

If God, the Other, is as Lacan tells us "essentially language," the question that haunts *Helen*, the "agony/the question that has no answer" (276) might, consecutively to "What does the Other want," be formulated as "What does language mean?" Lacan writes,

> The syndrome of action from without, as naïve as it appears, does underlie the essential dimension of the phenomenon, the psychotic's exteriority in relation to the entire apparatus of language. Hence the question arises whether the psychotic has really entered language.[60]

Instead of answering this question by referring to the relationship of signifiers to signifieds and envisioning language as a symbolic apparatus, H.D. seeks to bring signifiers to life. In the poem, H.D. envisions the astral plane/Egypt as the land of the living signifier. The living beings in it, like Helen and the bird that "hooted past" *are* writing or letters (13):

> but when the bird swooped past,
> that first evening,
> I seemed to know the writing,
> as if God made the picture
> and matched it
> with a living hieroglyph (23)

These beings constitute one of H.D.'s attempts, in *Helen*, to make words *be* so that there will be no need for them to *mean*. She can then be literally "alive in [her] Helen sequence." The narrator and Helen, thus, need not interpret the events and images that they describe, which Helen sometimes acknowledges: "It is not necessary to read the riddle. The pattern itself is sufficient and it is beautiful" (32). H.D. seeks in *Helen* to render meaning as being by identifying its characters with signifiers, or "writing."

The actual writing that composes the poem, Helen also suggests, contains meaning that may not be apparent, but which someone, surely, understands. Though H.D. was increasingly framing the significant events in her life with her understanding of Ambelain's ideas, as Robinson discusses and as her journals during this time show, she does so indirectly in work written for publication.[61] Though occultism's influence on her work from *Helen in Egypt* onward is great, as Robinson shows, H.D. shies away from occultist terminology and separates herself discursively from the "banal" spiritualists for most of the period of her interest and involvement.[62] However, she gradually adopts esoteric ideas and visual schemas; for instance, she places the significant men in her life in the schema derived from Chaboseau's visual rendering of the Tarot card of the Star.[63] In Chaboseau's picture, lesser stars surround a large star and, for H.D., each star represents an "initiator" into higher states of being, as described in Ambelain and Chaboseau's "Hermetic/Rosicrucian scheme" of spiritual reintegration.[64] Martinism, which Robinson describes as "a Masonic offshoot of Rosicrucianism," appealed to H.D., he writes, because it "emphasized levels of initiation that opened deeper, more authentic access to the traditions once the adept grades were achieved."[65] This major initiator is identified in the period of *Helen*'s composition as Dowding, and even though later in H.D.'s life the initiator becomes a composite of characters, Dowding always remained important to her.[66]

H.D. at the time of *Helen*'s composition was using Ambelain's conceptual models to frame her relationships with different men in terms of cycles of major and minor initiation, including initiation into astral realms.[67] She imagines these initiators as forming a pattern, a pattern with Dowding at its center. "Eidolon" (also the title of the poem's third book) means "astral double" for Ambelain, and "ghost" and "image" in ancient Greek. Though in theosophy "astral double" refers to the astral body as opposed to the material body, H.D. expanded the term's meaning and claimed Hugh Dowding (as well as *Helen in Egypt*'s Helen) as her astral double, a status bestowed, at least in part, by their identical initials.[68]

One possible reason that the astral plane and astral projection are not fully explicit in *Helen* may be H.D.'s knowledge that her readership was comprised not of fellow initiates but rather literati who would lack a frame of reference for such things and perhaps have difficulty taking them seriously. However, these references, as Robinson discusses, are clear enough to readers with background knowledge of Western esoteric thought—or, I would add, of Eastern traditions in which the astral plane, and astral bodies, figure prominently. H.D. distinguished her terrestrial, astral, and celestial selves according to Ambelain's model.[69] As she writes in *Thorn Thicket*,

> There are three phases, "*militante* (terestre [sic]), *souffrante* (astrale), *triumphante* (céleste)." There is "un *corps*, un *double*, une *âme*." This is the circle, in which the *Madrigal* War I marriage is the corps, the Lord D. contact in War II, the double, and the inspiration, the poetry running through this, before it and after, the âme.[70]

On the astral plane Helen and Achilles, H.D.'s and Dowding's "eidolons," meet and part in "the second long-playing disk," as H.D. calls the astral phase, of her "cycle" of initiations into truth. The first phase was her marriage to and parting from Richard Aldington: "The meeting with the *double* in War II is superimposed on the *corps*, the marriage or love-affair of War I."[71] H.D. and Aldington met on the terrestrial plane, and H.D. and Dowding's meeting in the astral world is "superimposed" on this corporeal meeting. Describing *Helen*, H.D. writes,

> This is myself, Helen out of the body, in another world, the *eidolon* of the legend. But she is not alone. There, she meets the legendary Achilles, a phantom but a reality. There I, there Helen lives out her war—her wars. There, in the second long-playing disc [the astral phase of her cyclical spiritual journey] is Helen with Achilles on one side, on the other, Helen with Paris. There is the

> conflict solved—as The Woman Within [a book] asks, "Is it true, I wonder, that the only way to escape war is to be in it?"[72]

H.D. suggests that this second "cercle" is completed in Egypt, with Dowding:

> We repeat *Madrigal* or *Marriage*, 20 years later, with another war. But this is what Robert Duncan calls the "astral H.D."[73] Lord D. as I have said, was H.D. too and was an "astral H.D." We met on that plane. There was the *choc en retour* [magical backlash][74] as the Cabalists call it, the 1946 coming back. I was very ill.[75]

H.D. attempts to resolve the trauma that her corporeal relationship, or nonrelationship, with Dowding triggered by imagining it as the fated astral cycle of a series of initiatory encounters. This initiation takes place in the timeless, looking-glass world of the astral plane, Egypt. Here, Dowding's and H.D.'s astral doubles, unlike their corporeal selves, have consummated their relationship. The poem, *Helen*, plays an active role in this astral encounter, perhaps literally (if an astral event can be literal) creating it.

Egypt, the astral plane, is the world in which writing *is* being, the eternal dimension beyond the bar of Lethe, river of repression or forgetfulness. In "Pallinode," which is set there, Helen, who "does not wish to forget," therefore, "achieves the difficult task of translating a symbol in time, into timeless time or hieroglyph or ancient Egyptian time" (13). This "symbol in time" is a bird that "hooted past." Helen tells Achilles, about to shoot it, that "the shape of this bird is a letter" and that it is "dedicated to the goddess here":

> I am instructed, I know the script,
> the shape of this bird is a letter
> they call it the hieroglyph,
> strive not, it is dedicated
> to the goddess here, she is Isis. (13–14)

This bird-letter that triggers Achilles is a reference to the *letters* H.D. sent Dowding that he repudiated. She calls them, in *Sword*, "*winged word*[s]" (30). These letters contained the coded messages delivered to H.D. by the RAF pilots. She was convinced that Dowding could interpret this code though she herself could not. These letters, with their messages from astral beings, become actual "winged words" (bird-letters) on the astral plane. H.D. suggests that here, on the astral plane, beings such as Helen and the bird-letter *are* manifestations of what, on the "terrestrial plane," is writing. Terrestrial writing manifests as astral beings.

Although it does not appear in her initial description, Helen later claims that a "swarm" had surrounded her during Achilles's attack. She refers to the swarm with many terms whose relevance is not always clear. She calls it, among other things, a spread of wings, a thousand sails, an unnumbered host, a galaxy, a cloud of snow, a veil and a Holocaust, and also gives it proper names associated with mythic son-figures: Euphorion, Eros ("the Hawk Horus" as she calls him), and Paris—since "Paris" is "the one name for the thousand lost" (41). The multiplicity of this swarm is emphasized by the large number of terms by which Helen refers to it as well as by the terms themselves, but it is also, she tells us, one. Notwithstanding its identity as the progeny of Helen and Achilles, which is instantaneously engendered by the rape, the swarm also caused the rape: "It is "the 'thousand sails' that brought them together. If [Helen] forgets that, she is lost" (37). This "thousand sails" refers to the RAF pilots, Dowding's "boys" and "chicks," whose communications H.D. sought to convey to him. Helen claims that it/they shelter her from the intensity of Achilles's anger:

> it was they, the Holocaust,
> a host, a cloud or a veil
> who encircled me, who sheltered me
> when his fingers closed on my throat. (38)
> there was never such a spread of wings
> such a play of golden feathers,
> though I did not see them,
> I heard them, as I heard myself say,
> O Thetis, O Sea-Mother. (42)

The swarm that Helen gives birth to protects her in two ways. First, referring to the RAF pilots, it suggests that the letters containing coded messages that H.D. sent Dowding were legitimate communications from these ghostly others. Secondly, as a signifier, the swarm undercuts difference by its claim to simultaneous unity and multiplicity. Though they are singular nouns, "swarm," "host," "cluster," and "galaxy" refer to gatherings of distinct entities or things. They "seem one but are many" (43), and conversely are an "infinite number," but "yet one whole":

> the Child,
> Aphrodite sent,
> Love begotten of War
> and the sea-enchantment together;
> the veil of Cytheraea?
> a cloud or a swirl of snow,
> a swarm, an infinite number,
> yet one whole, one cluster of bees,
> as a trail or a Galaxy

of numberless stars,
that seem one but are many (43)
it was they, the veil
that concealed yet revealed,
that reconciled him to me (44)

As well as protecting Helen, the swarm also aids somehow in her attempt to reclaim the dark side of Achilles, who has split into Osiris and Typhon: "As Isis seeks to reclaim Osiris with the help of their Child, the sun-god Horus, so Helen, with the aid of 'the unnumbered host' would gain spiritual recognition and ascendancy over 'Typhon, the Destroyer'" (28). This swarm, then, allows difference to also be/come unity, both in itself and for "other" characters. It reconciles Helen (temporarily) to the problem of difference that Achilles's attack represents.

Achilles's rage and jealousy that the "unnumbered host" are Helen's and not his suggests one of H.D.'s explanations for Dowding's repudiation: he was angry because the RAF pilots chose to communicate with her and not him. In *Helen*, Achilles the father is jealous of the mother:

O Child, must you seek your mother
while your father forever
attacks her in jealousy?
"I begot them in death, they are mine";
must death rule life?
must the lily fade in the dark? (28)

But Achilles's wrathful attack and penetration of her fertilizes Helen, and, in another temporal paradox, causes her to give birth to the very swarm whose preference for her provokes him. Helen reflects that

with his anger,
that ember, I became
what his accusation made me,
Isis, forever with that Child,
the Hawk Horus. (23)

In another two-directional movement of time, Helen and Achilles also engender themselves, although they are also subtly identified with the swarm/Paris/the Hawk Horus: "The promised Euphorion is not one child but two. It is 'the child in Chiron's cave' [Achilles] and the 'frail maiden,' [Helen] stolen by Theseus from Sparta" (288). Achilles, as well as Paris, is Helen's son, and Helen is her own mother and daughter. There is no unidirectional time to make this impossible.

VII. THE ONE AND THE MANY, MEANING AS SUCH

Helen's many different words and identities are part of a "complete picture" that is never understood cognitively, but which is instead literally contained within Helen, as incarnation, mother, writer, and writing:

> She seems to have identified herself with her own daughter, Hermione, with her sister's daughter, Iphigenia, and with Clytemnestra, her twin-sister, "one branch, one root in the dark." Now she seems to equate Orestes, her sister's son, with Achilles. She has said of Achilles, "let me love him, as Thetis his mother." Now of Orestes, "has he found his mother? will he ever find her? can I take her place?" She would recreate the whole of the tragic scene. Helen is the Greek drama. Again, *she herself is the writing.* (91, emphasis in the original)

Helen identifies with Iphigenia, Clytemnestra, Polyxena, and Hermione as well as being, the poem suggests, all of *Helen*'s many goddesses, notably Thetis, Isis, Cytherea/Aphrodite, Artemis, and Persephone. She is also several Helens: Helen of Troy, Helen of Egypt, Dendritis or "Helena of the trees," and Helen of Sparta. Achilles is also Osiris, Typhon, Orestes, Heracles, and Hades/Dis. Paris is also Adonis, Eros, Orestes, Euphorion, the "swarm" or "galaxy," and Horus, as well as being "incarnate Helen-Achilles" (185). Achilles and Theseus, the poem tells us, are the light and dark aspects of the same being (190), which makes them Castor and Pollux. Though polarized, they "meet finally in 'Helen in Egypt' and 'Helen in Hellas forever'" (190). Helen and Clytemnestra are their twin sisters, "half, part of the tale of Troy, half, bound to the Dioscuri, 'twin-sisters of twin-brothers'" (71). Everyone, indeed, is ultimately either Helen or her male counterpart, the son-father-lover-God.

The portentous introductions and rapid disappearances of seemingly powerful, fantastic and mysteriously significant beings, as well as the simultaneously single and multiple identities of the text's characters, suggest psychic splitting and a sort of mental "fast forward" that saps these beings of their aesthetic power, as if the poem were music played at triple speed. Multiple beings "manifest" in single bodies or in the text itself, and the vast majority of them appear with a bang and disappear unceremoniously within a page or two. The "delusional metaphor" does not organize them into a sequence of cause and effect, but simply absorbs them. Delia in *Sword*, in fact, compares her thoughts to "unwary flies" that are "caught" and "collected," to her relief, by a "sun-star" that behaves like a "Venus fly-trap" (113).

In *Helen* multiplicity, whether birthed or recollected, is imagined as a preserving force. Helen and the narrator both suggest that profusions of beings (who are also one or two) "temper or moderate" Helen's overwhelming experience with Achilles. In order to "progress in life" (117), Helen must "balance" this experience by recalling and identifying her "other loves" (165) and her family: "It is as if Helen wanted to recall her immediate 'family,' as protection or balance against the overwhelming fact of her Fate or Destiny, her meeting with Achilles" (68). During the meeting, she was "protected" by a "swarm" of pure multiplicity that she had instantaneously conceived and delivered. To help her deal with its intensity, she afterward remembers her "immediate family"; later with Theseus, she remembers her other lovers. However, since these other beings are not clearly separate from Helen herself or from one another, more uncertainty and tension is generated around questions of their identity and difference. The simultaneous unity and multiplicity of beings troubles the usual one-to-one relation of word to meaning. The splitting and introjection of *Helen*'s characters, and the alienation of the work's words from its meanings, reflect the same process of psychic splitting.

Melanie Klein writes that apropos of the splitting of the ego, some split-off identities are endowed with positive imaginary qualities, some with negative. Such distinctions are drawn in *Helen*, where Helen represents the initiated, reborn, "astral" H.D., the principle of pure Love (or Beauty in *Sword*), while Clytemnestra, betrayed by her husband, Agamemnon, and slain by her son Orestes, is a figure for the earthly, angry H.D., betrayed by Aldington and Dowding (with their other women) and refuted by Heydt. Clytemnestra's daughter, Iphigenia, also represents H.D. betrayed, "summoned to Aulis, on the pretext of a marriage to Achilles," (72) she is "pledge[d] to death" so that the Greek armies might sail to Troy. Achilles facilitates this "sacrifice" of Iphigenia by playing the role of groom. He also demands the sacrifice of Polyxena, as well as having his way with "Chryseus, Deidamia, Briseius" (172)—and God knows whom else, as Theseus upsettingly points out to Helen. These women were betrayed by Achilles, but their names, the narrator reflects, "seem unrelated to our Achilles concept" (172). Helen's Achilles "on the desolate beach" is not Theseus's "Achilles lingering with Polyxena" (172). Achilles, too, splits into different identities seemingly predicated on his relationships with different women.

> Why does Helen recall Iphigenia? Does she identify herself with her sister's child? Does she feel that she, like Iphigenia, was "a pledge to death" and that like Iphigenia, she had been rescued at the last moment? She reminds us that Iphigenia was summoned to Aulis, on the pretext of a marriage to Achilles. (72)

The poem evokes a multitude of sacrifices of women by men, one pair following another: "But Achilles ('I tell and re-tell the story') has been an accomplice. He, as well as her own father, would have sacrificed Iphigenia.

Helen returns constantly to this theme of sacrifice" (84, emphasis added) and populates it with different "players" who are also herself (230).

Schreber also asserts the eternal nature of the answer. It is eternity in which the wound or rent in the order of the world could be healed: "the Order of the World carries its own remedies for healing the wound that has been inflicted on it: the remedy is *Eternity*."[76] Schreber writes, "The concept of *eternity* is beyond man's grasp. Man cannot really understand that something can exist which has neither beginning nor end, that there can be a cause which cannot itself be traced to a previous cause. And yet eternity is one of God's attributes."[77] However, Schreber hopes to "prove . . . by means of definite examples" that "divine creation is a creation out of the *void*."[78]

Schreber's examples are definite, though stated in a roundabout way out of a concern not to expose God to blame and ridicule. The example that he immediately offers to prove that "divine creation is a creation out of the *void*" is God's earthly fathering of Jesus by Mary. His *Memoirs* begins by asserting that "things exist which are true though [humanity] cannot understand them."[79] For instance, "nobody would maintain that God, as a Being endowed with human sexual organs, had intercourse with the woman from whose womb Jesus Christ came forth."[80] Given, however, the actual changes to Schreber's reproductive organs (apparently so enjoyable to God) and his sexual encounter with Ariman (the "lower god"), the rest of the *Memoirs* suggests that, in fact, this is precisely what had happened to Mary and that this is also what is now happening to Schreber. It is in the nature of rays to penetrate Schreber. That God created man "in his image," Schreber discreetly admits, "has to be understood literally, which no human being has so far dared to do."[81] Schreber has replaced Mary as God's female consort.

Sexual penetration by God, for Helen and Schreber, takes place in what they describe as the dimension of eternity. Schreber tells us that "a human being who in a certain sense can say *that eternity is in his service*, can afford to ignore all nonsense in the certain knowledge that ultimately a time must come when nonsense exhausts itself and a sensible state of affairs returns."[82] God's attribute of "eternity" allows him to create things out of a "void"; the "rent" in the order of the world will be filled by the offspring that will "issue from [Schreber's] lap."[83] God's creations in the meantime are the "fleeting-improvised" beings with their nonsensical speech that He conjures up to interfere with Schreber. This state of affairs is contrary to the proper order of the world, in which creation takes place through the reproduction of species.

Schreber and Helen both suggest that their meetings with God in eternity fertilize them and allow them to give birth to a new order. Since it is only in the temporal dimension that a hole in meaning opens up for Schreber and H.D., they build up systems of causality in which the meanings endowed to words and events by their sequential relations to one another are completely replaced by the repetition of an "eternity," or an "eternal moment" that freezes time's movement and the disordered sliding of the signifier. Eternity is the only reference point, the beginning from which everything issues and the ending to which it returns. In eternity, which is outside of cause, effect, and sequentiality, creation and sense simultaneously emerge from, and return to, the bodies of Helen and Schreber.

If critical responses to *Helen* have often referred sparingly to the poem's actual text, preferring to summarize its meaning as they understand it, this may be because the poem requires "eternity" to mean anything. The verses run on with new associations, and Helen herself asserts that she could only determine "the answer" to a formless question through an act of quantification that would take forever. In fact, that is exactly what she is doing in *Helen*, though the reader may not realize it. The poem has no temporal dimension, "no before and no after," but "only the ever-recurring 'eternal moment,'" the moment of the rape (277). All of its characters, associations, images, and things are laid out in the dimension of eternity, where "the wheel is still" (202). Their meaning awaits the reader who can enter this dimension.

VIII. THE WHEEL OF TIME

In *Helen*, the experience of difference in time, of the difference of one time from another, reverses into timelessness. Helen's encounter with Achilles "out-of-time" (i.e., on the astral plane) is established in the poem as the beginning, end, birth, death, and purpose of everything. In place of forward-moving time, *Helen*'s cycles of castration-union, imagined with circular logic, embody cause and effect, birth and death. However, this eternity has a threatening side for Helen. Timelessness, as experienced in the astral rape, is "too great a suspense to endure" (162), a formulation reminiscent of Caruth's theory that "what causes trauma . . . is a shock that appears to work very much like a bodily threat but is in fact a break in the mind's experience of time . . . the *missing* of the experience, the fact that, not being experienced *in time*, it has not yet been fully known."[84] For Helen this timeless bodily shock must be "balanced" by movement in time, however illusory. Thus Helen "must be re-born, that is, her soul must return wholly to her body." Within this body, "the memory of breath-taking encounters with those half-seen must balance and compensate for the too intense primary experience" (162). Though the rape is the only moment that exists "in eternity," Helen must depart from, and return to, it by remembering and forgetting, which creates "[t]ime-in-time (personal time)" (202). This forgetting and remembering promote the departure from, and return to, the "Absolute" (199), "the 'eternal moment' of [Helen's] constant preoccupation, *La Mort*" (301). Her remembrance of other loves and family "re-vitalize and re-awaken Helen" (160). This remembrance of others, which alternates with the remembrance of the eternal moment, generates a multitude of associations that moderates the traumatic "suspense" of timeless union.

> She will encompass infinity by intense concentration on the moment. She has finished her cycle in time. But out-of-time or beyond moon-time, are the "widening star-circles." But she will not attempt to escape "the moment" by a flight to infinity with "wild wings." She will bring the moment and infinity together "in time, in the crystal, in my thought here." (200)

Helen's wish to "bring the moment and infinity together" in her thought suggests a desire to unite this recollected multiplicity with the "one finite moment" that has "no before and no after" (301). However, the multiple terms (time, crystal, thought) proffered for the location of this synthesis and the use of unclear quotation marks obscure what exactly is being brought together with what, and where this union might be happening.

These loops and wheels "in-time" perhaps represent departures from, and returns to, the "eternal moments" (277). Because of the identity of "eternal moments" with one another, "time-in-time," where one moment is distinct from another, forms circles or spirals that begin and end in eternity. In *Sword*, H.D. describes this eternal moment in terms of a repeating encounter that causes the "turn-around or turn-over of history." In *Helen*, she suggests that the annihilation of Helen, which is also unification with Achilles, paradoxically *results in* the very sequence of events that bring it about: the birth of Helen, Achilles and Paris—who is himself also identified mysteriously as the "unnumbered host" who fought the Trojan War. The host that fought in the war is Paris and the war was caused by Paris's seduction of Helen. The war itself resulted in the death and transportation of Paris to Leuké, and the transportation of Helen and Achilles to Egypt, the "astral plane," the timeless dimension where he rapes her and it all begins again. Achilles and Helen engender themselves, grow up, fight, are perhaps killed, re-enter Egypt, copulate and are reborn. Characters, places, objects, substances, and words exist not in linear time but within the "wheel" (258), a procession of terms that return to the "ever-recurring eternal moment." This "Zodiac hieroglyph, comes to life with the magnetic intensity of these two" (271), Helen and Achilles. Though Helen's "mind goes on, spinning the infinite thread" (297), the enigma that fastens it remains the same, the fixed point where the wheel is "still" (202).

Achilles's rape of Helen, though occurring in a timeless cycle of return, is paradoxically where this cycle begins and ends. The prose tells us that

"Time-in-time (personal time) . . . as well as star-time (the eternal) seem alike incalculable to Helen, without Achilles" (202). Without the "eternal moment," neither "personal time" nor "the eternal" can be calculated, since the rape fastens all temporal events to the eternal. In Egypt, Helen and Achilles are out of time: "Time values have altered, present is past, past is future. The whole heroic sequence is over, forgotten, re-lived, forgotten again" (57). Meeting where "present is past and past is future," they beget the selves who act in past and future "personal time," and thus return to the moment of "eternal time" (202). Everything else in the poem, "in-time" on the material plane, is aligned with Helen's other companions.

Achilles's attack on Helen not only engenders their lives, but is also the combined cause, effect, and purpose of the war: "Is it possible that it all happened, the ruin—it would seem not only of Troy, but of the 'Holocaust of the Greeks' . . . in order that two souls or soul-mates should come together? It almost seems so" (5). Troy was breached and fell "in memory" of Achilles's sexual attack:

> why did I invoke the mother?
> why was he seized with terror?
> for that was Victory
> and Troy-gates broken
> in memory of the Body (7)

In H.D.'s *Helen*, war and rape mirror one another endlessly. Troy falls in memory of the rape, but the war also causes—occurs for the sake of—the rape, the integration of the principles of War and Love that are ultimately contained in Helen. The rape of Helen causes the war and is necessary to end the war. This encounter, further, is first cause and final destination not only of Helen and Achilles, not only of the war, but of their catalytic action on the world, of history itself: "Achilles seems grudgingly to apologize for his first boorishness, 'I was afraid.' Who indeed would not be, at sudden encounter with the admitted first-cause 'of all-time, of all-history.' Fate, Death, Reintegration, Resurrection?" (47)

Since H.D puts Egypt outside of time, Helen can return in memory or in astral form, after the rape, to the earlier time of her relationship with Paris: "In the light of her inheritance as a neophyte or initiate, she would re-assess that first experience" (112). The cycle beginning in Egypt plays itself out in "personal time," earlier times on the "material planes" of Leuké, Sparta, Athens, Mount Ida, Chiron's cave, and Troy:

> and War came; Hecuba like Jocasta
> was overthrown (by Paris, by Oedipus,

> the son); O the web is sure
> . . .
> he of the House of the Enemy,
> Troy's last king (this is no easy thing
> to explain, this subtle genealogy)
> is Achilles's son, he is incarnate
> Helen-Achilles; he, my first lover,
> was created by my last;
> . . .
> how could I know, the fire-brand, the ember,
> the Star would return—but other (185)

Paris, the "fire-brand," is here the return of Achilles, the "ember" (185). Paris is Achilles's son, his slayer and himself, and Helen is the mother of both. When Helen mentions the name of Thetis, she both represents and *is* (*Helen* wishes to establish that these are the same) Achilles's "careless, unspeakable mother" (253), responsible for his death in Troy:

> the invincible armour
> melted him quite away,
> till he knew his mother;
> but he challenged her, beat her back,
> *are you Hecate? are you a witch?*
> *a vulture, a hieroglyph?* (261)

Achilles's unflattering questions perhaps recall the "beings of a lower order" (the sorts of beings with whom witches communicate) from whom, Dowding suggested, H.D.'s spirit messages came.

All the things and events that begin and end in the rape partake of pasts and futures that they inhabit in great numbers with no fixed organization. They can be taken apart, mixed around, and changed. "Personal things" can be "re-assembled in different order as thoughts and emotions." Before and after the "eternal moment" is the teeming, chaotic multiplicity that delights Deleuze and Guattari: disorganized, incompletely rendered "things"[85]:

> it was Love, it was Death,
> but what followed before, what after?
> a thousand-thousand days,
> as many mysterious nights,
> and multiplied to infinity
> the million personal things,
> things remembered, forgotten,
> remembered again, assembled
> and re-assembled in different order

as thoughts and emotions. (288–9)

Helen's cosmos develops a sense of sequential time not by having a temporally continuous unfolding of events, but from the splitting of the eternal moment in which all is one in Helen. Helen lingers in and savors the multiplicity engendered by that splitting, and returns to the moment of oneness, experienced as the flip side, perhaps, of the multiplicity. As Deleuze writes, "eternal return . . . does not express an order as opposed to the chaos engulfing it [but] is nothing other than chaos itself. . . . To the coherence of representation, the eternal return substitutes . . . its own chaodessy."[86]

This chaodessy for Helen, however, is imagined as the alternative, not the correlate, to her shattering "eternal moment." She therefore anticipates with both gloom and a shade of relief the return of a sacrificial event such as Achilles's attack on her at the beginning of the poem, and the fates of Iphigenia and Polyxena. Achilles, near the poem's end, has "promised/ Another white throat to a goddess," his mother Thetis, whose name provoked his attack on Helen at the beginning of the poem. The prose introduction tells us that "Helen herself seems almost ready for this sacrifice or, at least, for the immolation of herself before this greatest love of Achilles, his dedication to 'his own ship' and the figurehead, 'an idol or eidolon . . . a mermaid, Thetis upon the prow'" (245).

In Schreber's time, too, chaos holds sway and God looms threateningly near. The cycle of departures and returns of souls or "nerves" to God is thus very rapid. God, writes Schreber, is supposed to leave divested nerves alone until the death of the bodies that house them, rather than forming nerve-attachments with them as in Schreber's case.[87] The proper order of the world requires time as well as eternity. When the proper interval is maintained, the individual soul's return to God as "rays" is blissful; however, when the interval between departures from, and returns to, God is shortened or eliminated, the result is violent and grotesque.

This havoc results initially from a plot by Professor Flechsig (Schreber's doctor for a time) to form a nerve-connection with God, but it subsists because of God's continued attraction to Schreber. God, normally at a great distance from Earth, "was forced [first by Flechsig, now by his attraction to Schreber's nerves] to draw nearer the earth again and remain relatively close to it. [Thus] the earth has once again become the permanent scene of divine miracles."[88] God seeks (intermittently) to annihilate Schreber, or at least Schreber's mental powers, with his "miracles" so that he can sever their nerve-connection and withdraw to the proper distance. God's miracles, accordingly, always pertain to Schreber and are usually accomplished by the miraculous "fleeting-improvised" men, birds, and insects temporarily given shape to torment him.

IX. THE GOD OF DEATH

The rapid cyclical movement and dereliction of personal autonomy in H.D.'s and Schreber's cosmic visions perhaps suggest what Lacan calls the death drive, and describes as a circuit of departure and return in relation to a lost object that is actually a part of oneself. Lacan cites Freud's description of his grandson's *fort/da* game, a constantly repeated cycle of loss and recovery, as an example of this drive. Whereas for Freud, *fort/da* represented a working through of traumatic loss, for Lacan the motive for the repetition involves the symbolic order. The pleasure, and sense of stability and consistency, that repetition itself maintains replaces the desire to work through the loss.[89]

In psychosis, however, there is no original lost object, real or imagined: loss has been foreclosed. It returns in the real in threatening forms, whose cycles of departure and invasive return are perceived as originating outside of the subject, as with Schreber's God and Helen's divinely controlled Achilles. The return of the terrible lover alternates with abandonment by him, an intensity that approaches and then withdraws. Lacan writes that sufferers from psychosis, rather than "entering" language, are "inhabited, possessed, by language."[90] Helen's and Schreber's Gods, both rapists, take them over prematurely, taking an agency that neither Helen nor Schreber have had the time or opportunity to give freely. This alternates with a withdrawal that, though moderating for Helen, leaves her both forsaken and vulnerable to the attacks of inferior beings. What Schreber and Helen's experiences suggest is a sense of an annihilating force for which they do not feel ready. To return completely to this force is to be sacrificed. Even Helen only seems "*almost* ready for this sacrifice—at least, for the immolation of herself" to Achilles's great love. For all Helen and Schreber's emphasis on the importance of surrender to this looming martyrdom, their anticipation of union with the divine lacks the rapturous, or at least heightened, affect that can usually be seen in mystical writings. But the alternatives to martyrdom, Helen's endless ruminations and Schreber's "terrible, monotonous" persecution by talking rays that repeat "ever recurring phrases," are not much better.[91]

If God's existence in psychosis, as Lacan tells us, is "essentially language,"[92] perhaps it is language that is envisioned as the threatening shadow of God. Language can express differences and opinions that wound, and which have wounded H.D. Or perhaps by "essentially language," Lacan means that God is the unconscious symbolic system predicated on difference and lack, which renders us subjects or, in psychosis, more overtly persecutes and subjugates us. At any rate, for Schreber and Helen multiplicity, nondifferentiation, and meaningless rote speech appear to circumvent this threat. Even the rote repetitions of Helen's "players" and Schreber's mechanical birds, while they may be meaningless, at least do not express genuine difference, incredulity, or animosity, but simply mechanical repetitiveness. Instead of the return to God/language, a shaky stability is derived for Helen from the repetition that Theseus advises, of "always another and another and another" memory, "lest you return to that other/and flame out, incandescent" (187). This remembering, proliferation, and repetition "balance and compensate for" the "incandescent" encounter, perhaps with the symbolic order of language and lack, whose threat generates new unclear questions, new memories (162).

The alternative to this deferral of union, Helen suggests, is actual death. If motherhood and conception involve endless remembrances of things that pertain to the cycle of death and rebirth, the alternative is annihilation alone: to forget, to be lost (17). At one point Helen surmises that "I am only a daughter;/no, no, I am not a mother,/let Cypris have Amor" (191). The daughter's consort is not Amor, but his negative opposite. It appears that her destiny, like childless Persephone's, lies with an "absolute of negation," Hades/Dis:

> So there must be no rivalry with either the earth or the heaven mother. Helen says, "I am only a daughter." She will not compete with Demeter for union with her Absolute or with Leda for this same Zeus. There is another Absolute, that of "the crystal, the center, the ice-star." It is the Absolute of negation, if you will, or of completion, "this immaculate purity," and hence in a sense, of Death. Helen has said, "my heart had been frozen, melted."—So she compares herself to Persephone and recalls Theseus' question, "Did you too seek Persephone's drear icy way to Death?" Helen's answer is yes, "I found or was found by Dis." (195)

God is completely annihilating to the daughter who is "not a mother," who cannot conceive (of) herself. The Helen who is "only a daughter" with no capacity to remember, give birth, or (re)create multiplicity experiences love with longing as death without birth:

> O flame-tipped, O searing,
> destroying arrow of Eros,
> O bliss of the end,
> Lethe, Death and forgetfulness,
> O bliss of the final
> unquestioned nuptial kiss. (183)

Though there is longing, there is icy fear. The "bliss," too, seems equivocal, since it is identified with "Persephone's drear icy way to death," the dismal "Hyperborean dwellings," where "Achilles waits" (195–6).

X. TELESCOPING IDENTITIES AND SOUL MURDER

Many identities and names manifest in Helen, enacting and responding to H.D.'s unusual perspective on identity and difference on the levels of both language and being. Lacan, who envisions language as including the social universe that surrounds and permeates the normal subject, accounts for the experience in psychosis of inhabitation or invasion (and feminization) from without by arguing that it represents language's entry into, or invasion of, the organism. For Lacan, the foreclosure of difference in psychosis results in attempts to assimilate language in a bodily and imaginary (rather than symbolic) register by assuming the feminine position in a sexual relationship to language. Helen and Schreber's passive, feminine position in relation to aggressively sexual male divinities (and multitudes of other smaller entities) symptomize this bodily and imaginary reversal of "castration" or entry into language represented by the invasion of the body/mind by language. As Lacan discusses, we find in Schreber's writing,

> the notion that the imaginary identity of the other has a profound relation to the possibility of fragmentation and segmentation. That the other is structurally multipliable and divisible. . . . There is also the telescoping of these images inside one another. On the one hand one finds multiple identities of the one same character, on the other there are these little enigmatic identities. . . . These identities, which in relation to his own identity have the value of an *instance* . . . penetrate, inhabit, and divide Schreber himself.[93]

Helen's imaginary others, like Schreber's, are inside her or part of her, and also inside and part of one another. Helen's experience of control by an omniscient other resembles Schreber's fantasies of "soul murder" by what he calls "nerve language," the language that acts on him from without and that feminizes him.[94] Like Helen's, Schreber's feminine identity contains language and beings. But they divide him into parts rather grotesquely, while in *Helen in Egypt* Helen is divided poetically into several Helens, as well as other named characters such as Thetis. For instance, Schreber writes that certain "fleeting-improvised-men . . . unloaded into my body a part of their bodies in the form of a foul mass. . . . M. repeatedly placed himself into my arm as a so-called 'large nerve' (a jelly-like mass about the size of a cherry) through which in a certain sense he participated in my thinking and my sensations like the other rays or nerves."[95] Although Helen does not describe anything so nasty, she is not always certain whether her thoughts are her own "or the thoughts of another," even when she appears to be thinking them. She contains distinct identities that speak, think, multiply, and divide. Indeed, other than their division along gender lines, their "distinctness" seems comprised mainly in one identity's ability to "manifest as" another, and think, speak and act in ways that seem foreign and involuntary to the other identity (178).

Identities, though they "come together" in Helen, are otherwise divided along the gender line. Questions of identity and difference are infinitely subtle and gradated within each gender category. The way that beings are one another cannot be described, only suggested by phrases like "Amen begot Amor" (180). The poem suggests that Thetis, Aphrodite, and Helen of Sparta are distinct from the initial Helen, although not very, or always. Male gods are likewise not entirely distinct from one another or from Helen's male counterparts, but the indistinction of male gods often regards their "control" of other characters. The omniscient being—variously referred to as Amen, Zeus, Proteus, Thoth, Formalhaut[96] ("the Royal Sacred High Priest of Love Rites"), and the-Nameless-of-Many-Names—controls and/or manifests in Achilles, and arguably in all the characters in the poem.[97] In this capacity, this being may also have a darker side as "Calchas" (87) and "the Command," who also control Achilles.

Helen, brooding on Achilles's culpability in female sacrifice, reflects, "As the light of the Star glows clearer/the shadow grows darker" (84). As the rape increasingly illuminates the other events that she recollects, making it clear that they are all part of a predetermined endless cycle, the fearful aspect of this cycle becomes more apparent. Splitting takes the potentially sinister form of telescoping, in which one being is occupied and controlled by another. Achilles, for instance, was "under compulsion, and at the command of the Greek soothsayer, Calchas" (87) when he participated in the attempted sacrifice of Iphigenia. His general cruelty is the result of control by "the Command," and/or by "a spirit master," a godlike astral being in Ambelain's work who is identified, in different works of H.D.'s later period such as *Majic Ring* and *Hermetic Definition*, with (Z)akenuto and Amen. Again, the immanence or personation of God, or of beings who are not *not* God, is rendered in terms of coercion or invasion.

Helen's own understanding of Achilles's involuntary behavior comes from a "Message" from the outside, she is fairly certain. She experiences her thought as the whisper of a Presence:

> How does the Message reach me?
> do thoughts fly like the Word
> of the goddess? a whisper—
> (my own thought or the thought of another?) (87)
> Helen is not sure, but suggests that the voice comes from outside:
> I swerve about to surprise
> this Presence, this Voice,
> but the long arcade is empty;

has Nephthys stepped from her pillar
or from her frame upon the Wall?
is it Nemesis? is it Astarte? (88)

The voice tells her that Achilles's life would have been forfeit if he had not co-operated with the plan to sacrifice Iphigenia (87). This argument, Helen decides, "on the material plane, justifies Achilles, and Helen would call him back" (87); however, it may not, she suggests, justify "his first boorishness" (47) on the astral plane, since the astral plane is beyond physical life and death. However, Achilles's subsequent improved behavior also appears as the result of control by Theseus, Formalhaut, or Amen-Zeus. Achilles is made to crawl by many: even Theseus commands him to say, "Theseus commands me" (208).

The distinction of container and contained correlates somewhat to the gender division since God, the ultimate male, always "manifests as" lesser males, and Helen, the ultimate female, ultimately contains all. The omniscient God, Theseus, and Achilles "meet finally in 'Helen'" (190). Helen/Thetis, the sea-mother, "mer, mère, mere, mater, Maia, Mary,/Star of the Sea,/Mother"[98] is where all boundaries and distinctions melt. But however capacious Helen becomes, the question of identity and difference subsists.[99]

Weber surmises that Schreber's conviction that the human race can be renewed through his transformation into a woman[100] expresses an attempt to *reverse* this castration by making it visible, material, the subject of his own speech. Writes Weber,

> What Schreber would like to see established is the fact that *he holds God within his body*, that the *Wunde* of castration—which *is* not, and yet which is *not* nothing, insofar as it allows gender difference to articulate itself—has corporeal existence as a *Wunder* (wonder). Schreber's text attempts to control this difference, which structures both language and the subject (as a sexual being), by making the difference *visible*, so as to repeat and reverse the moment—the "apparition," as the voices say—when castration was discovered.[101]

Accordingly, Schreber's wounds and "unmanning" are seen by God, talked about by the rays, and by Schreber himself; this is, indeed, what draws them to Schreber. God's occupation of him is physical. In Lacan's terminology, Schreber has the phallus—God's—in his body.

Like Schreber's "unmanning," Helen's sexual ravishment and "sacrifice" by an out-of-control divine, or divinely possessed, masculine being is potentially globally salvific, an act of divine violence that may replace the disintegrating world order. Her fertility transforms castration into procreation, language into being. Schreber imagines himself as fertilized by a tormenting, lustful God (who also wishes to "forsake" him) so that the "rent"[102] in the

"Order of the World" can be healed and the "human race can be renewed."[103] Helen, like Schreber, is "stricken, forsaken," raped, and left alone (5). Like Schreber she is consort to the phallic Other: Achilles, the "unchallenged Sire," and the omniscient God manifesting in him during the rape. On being entered, she reverses castration by giving birth to the "swarm" that is both "One" and "many," and also to herself, Achilles, Paris and Euphorion—who are all mysteriously one with one another and with the swarm. Helen and Achilles's autogenesis asserts that identity and difference are the same. The separation imposed by the father figure is replaced by the physical differentiation of organisms, which yet "come together," begin and end, in an "eternal moment" inside of Helen. In Helen, difference is identity, identity difference.

If multiplicity is preserving, Helen suggests, oneness is annihilating. The splitting of God makes him bearable. His Oneness is

> what few may acknowledge and live
> what many acknowledge and die
> he is One, yet the many
> manifest separately (78–9)

God's Oneness, like Achilles's rape, is overwhelming, and is tempered by multiplicity both birthed and imagined. "Without the souls or 'the sails of the thousand ships,' [Helen's] encounter with Achilles would have 'burnt out in a flash' or burnt her out, like Semele, when Zeus at her request 'revealed himself'" (45). God's annihilating oneness is shattered into multiplicity, and re-unified in Helen.

Helen's fecundity and recollection and patterning of multiplicity "temper or moderate" the "signifier One," as Lacan terms it, that is foreclosed in the psychotic structure. One is not one: the "swarm," "galaxy," "cloud" of little entities that appear in the "eternal moment" is nominally singular yet divisible—like everyone in the poem. The many names the poem offers are not attached to distinct beings, but overlap. The splitting, mixing, matching, and telescoping of characters' singular identities and names in *Helen* all reflect the same process at the level of the sign: the destabilization of one-to-one correspondences between signifiers and signifieds, between names and beings, the impossibility of words meaning anything singular and distinct.

XI. THE NAME AND THE REPEATING PLAY

Helen does not see her identity in the terms of agency or an ongoing narrative based on her choices. Her story is not really a story but rather, she tells us, a play, one that is not really hers but God's—a God with inscrutable motives, who controls the characters' actions from behind the scenes, who perpetually calls this play, as well as her identity, into being. *Helen*'s characters do not respond to one another, Helen speculates, any more than actors in a play would respond to one another's lines with personal reactions. What appears personal in their interactions is in fact "scripted" by God and learned "by rote" by Helen and by "the players" whom God "lured" (234). As the narrator asserts, "It is a play, a drama—'who set the scene? who lured the players?' The players have no choice in the matter of the already-written drama or script. They are supremely aware of the honor that 'all song forever' has conferred upon them" (230). Similarly Schreber, because of the disruption of the "normal . . . Order of the World," is forced "from without" to use the repetitive, meaningless "nerve language," a language in which words are repeated by rote, without the intention to express an inwardly generated meaning.[104] The one exception to this externally generated, eternally repeated, unspontaneous script is, Helen suggests, her "unrecorded" sexual encounter with Achilles—though Achilles too, she suggests elsewhere, may have been under another's control during his rape of Helen. With this possible exception, *Helen*'s "players" must surrender to the action of God's play rather than framing narratives of their own, and the identities conferred on them thereby are, of course, roles rather than "real" selves. Whereas subjects using symbolic language usually identify (for better or worse) their "real selves" with their stories, and correlatively, meaning with language, here "the story" belongs to a controlling God.

This all-powerful God's "decree" also involves "a question asked/to which there was no answer" (230). Helen asks,

> was it [antecedent unclear] a question asked
> to which there was no answer?
> was it Paris? Was it Apollo?
> was it a game played over and over,
> with numbers or counters?
> who set the scene?
> who lured the players from home
> or imprisoned them in the Walls,
> to inspire us with endless,
> intricate questioning?
> why did they fight at all?
> . . .
> how will the story end? (230 – 1)

These questions—whose subject, "it," is unspecified, but may possibly refer to the loss of Troy—pertain to the "decree" that Helen must "accept without question." Helen poses several possible nouns for the unclear "it," which may refer to either proper names (Paris, Apollo) or more probably to the cycle of eternal recurrence, "a game played over and over," like the fort/da game. To have a name, an identity, that is both single and multiple, "one name inseparable/from the names of the Dioscuri/who are not two but many," Helen must fully accept the incomprehensibility of God's "decree," the cause of everything. She must accept that there is no sense to be made of the other's demand, no words for it. The inscrutability of this God, who "is the word," and his fondness for the repetition of the same cosmic drama is, as in *Sword*, probably derived from Gnostic and Neo-Platonic mythos where creation is senseless, a play that will only end happily in a nonmaterial realm. However, God's inscrutability also mirrors the senselessness of the words themselves. The poem's repetition of them in a "play" and in quotation marks may represent an attempt to hold the empty place of their missing meanings, which as Robinson's research also suggests may become clearer in the astral dimension of Egypt.[105]

It is the players', maybe the poem's own, unquestioning repetition of "the already-written drama or script" (230) that guarantees Helen's name, a name that is perhaps writ on water and must, therefore, be reinscribed. Helen tells us that her name, both single and inseparable, one and many, subsists on condition of her surrender to God's "decree":

> I have talked with Proteus—or—
> another (whoever he be,
> he manifests variously);
> Nameless-of-many-Names he decrees
> that *Helena* shall remain
> one name, inseparable
> from the names of the Dioscuri,
> who are not two but many,
> as you read the writing, the script,
> the thousand-petaled lily. (104)

Every name and object in this passage seems to simultaneously meld and divide, erasing difference as such. Further, Helen's name will "remain/one name, inseparable" from the many names that are offered in the poem, only on condition that "she accepts, without reservation and without question, the decree of God (who, as I have argued, takes the place of signifying language), whom she names as the Absolute, the King of Egypt, Proteus or Amen, the "Nameless-of-many-Names" (105). This decree, though presumably the one in the verse above, is now unspecified, and may also (as Albert Gelpi reads it) refer to God's will that "Helena/be joined to Achilles" (102). At any rate, surrender to an imperative, probably to sexual union, is necessary to secure her name, and this name is both singularly one and inseparable from the multitude.

Though the occultist texts that H.D. read provide conceptual groundwork here, the parallels of Helen's understanding with Schreber's (as described in his *Memoirs*) are also striking. Schreber, like Helen, anticipated "that great fame will be attached to my name surpassing that of thousands of other people much better mentally endowed."[106] This possibility is mentioned consecutively with the "alternative," that "by divine fertilization offspring will issue from my lap."[107] Schreber's emasculation and sexual ravishment by God is, he writes, "connected to the basic plan on which the Cosmic Order seems to rest, that in the case of world catastrophes which necessitate the destruction of mankind on any star . . . the human race can be renewed."[108] Schreber's surrender to "unmanning," "imperiously demanded" by the order of the world, enables his motherhood of a new race, since "nothing could of course be envisaged as a further consequence of unmanning but fertilization by divine rays for the purpose of creating new human beings."[109] Helen, likewise, is fertilized and has her name immortalized by surrender to an imperious God and presumed acceptance of his enigmatic "decree," though the poem does not tell us that this acceptance actually occurs.

Likewise, Schreber's God and Helen's are both enamored of repetition. His miraculous "fleeting-improvised" beings do nothing but repeat the same phrases, which they, like *Helen*'s characters, have "learnt by rote."[110] These beings, for instance, repeat the phrases "do not forget that rays must speak" and "don't forget that all representing is nonsense."[111] The loathing that Schreber frequently expresses for these "predetermined concoctions of thoughts spoken into my head by senseless voices in tiresome, monotonous repetition" exceeds even the bleakness of his references to the "miracles" that destroy his bodily organs.[112] Schreber's cultivation of "feminine voluptuousness," the enjoyment of intercourse as a heterosexual woman, mitigates both voices and miracles. It is intended to make the rays stop their hated "nonsense," and hence to return the order of the world to a normal state. Both Helen and Schreber, then, understand their direct encounters with an aggressively sexual God as exceptions to the rule of predetermined, unspontaneous language. Helen, after acknowledging that "the players have no choice in the matter of the already-written drama or script" (230) and that she herself "seems almost to speak by rote," then "breaks off, as it were, from the recorded drama to remind us of the unrecorded . . . her first meeting with Achilles, 'on the ledge of a desolate beach.'" (234). Likewise, Schreber's direct encounter with the "posterior" God, Ariman, is "intense, so that anybody not hardened to terrifying miraculous impressions as I was would have been shaken to the core." Although Schreber writes that "*what* was spoken . . . seemed calculated to instill fright and terror into me," he instead felt "largely . . . admiration for the magnificent and the sublime."[113] The reason for Schreber's admiration is this: "everything that was spoken was *genuine*, not phrases learnt by rote as they later were, but the immediate expression of true feeling."[114] There is in Helen's "unrecorded" and Schreber's "genuine" sexual encounters with God a spontaneity that, though violent, is treasured because it is otherwise completely lacking from their experience. Schreber *infers* that the phrases that the rays repeat may mean something to God, but the rays themselves, like the players in *Helen*, "reel them off without knowing the sense of the words" any more than Schreber does.[115] These fleeting-improvised beings have no autonomy at all: "They must reel off the crammed-in phrases without any regard of time and circumstance and irrespective of whether they want to or not."[116] They are not only without autonomy, but their function is to annihilate Schreber's autonomy by injuring his body and forcing him to think continuously on the sense, or lack thereof, of their words. Alternately, God may accomplish his "interference" with Schreber by stimulating the nerves of a nearby human being, causing him to begin "talking to [Schreber] or making some other noise."[117] The horror of the divine miracles resulting from God's increased proximity seems to consist in their destruction of autonomy. Miracles are accomplished by beings that have no—or suspended—autonomy, and seek to destroy Schreber's autonomy. He calls this destruction "soul murder."

Schreber writes that the forming of "nerve attachments," where God through these attachments draws closer to humans and to the earth, is contrary to the Order of the World, for one thing because it endangers God's existence, and for another because humans "should have autonomy over their own thoughts," as Schreber repeatedly maintains: "I also ought to have the right of being master in my own head against the intrusion of strangers. But this is not possible as regards the rays, because I am not in a position to prevent their influence on my nerves; this rests on God's power of miracles."[118] Schreber asserts, "Under normal (in consonance with the Order of the World) conditions, use of this nerve-language [words repeated in a definite order as when a person under normal circumstances wishes to learn them by heart] depends only on the will of the person whose nerves are concerned."[119] However, because of a skewed order of the world resulting from the nearness of God, Schreber is victim to the "tendency innate in the Order of the World, to *unman* [that is, to divest of autonomy] a human being who has entered into permanent contact with the rays."[120] For Schreber this loss of autonomy has to do with the contemptible, droning "automatons" whose rote phrases destroy Schreber's power of free thought. Only his cultivation of the "feminine voluptuousness" that resembles divine bliss allow him to mitigate God's and other rays' malignity toward him, which is not autonomy, but rather sacrifice.[121]

Just as Helen and Schreber remain somehow alienated from signification, language/God remains external, yet invasive, and the meaning his "play" provides is unsatisfactory. Lacan argues that when a narcissistic relation to an imaginary other replaces the relation to the symbolic Other as bearer of meaning, this other appears not only as invasive and controlling rather than separate, but also as holding the initiative that the "normal" subject imagines himself to hold:

> At the heart of the psychoses there's a dead end, perplexity concerning the signifier. . . . I suppose that the subject reacts to the signifier's absence by all the more emphatically affirming another one that as such is essentially enigmatic. I told you that the Other with a big O, qua bearer of the signifier, is excluded. The Other is thereby all the more powerfully affirmed between it and the subject, at the level of the little other, of the imaginary. . . . This is where all the between-I phenomena that make up what is apparent in the symptomatology of psychosis take place—at the level of the other subject, of the one who holds the initiative in the delusion—in the case of Schreber, Prof. Flechsig or God.[122]

In *Helen* we may read, through Lacan, a replacement of the symbolic "big Other," the Other as structure and locus of meaning, with an imaginary big Other—who, since he is in Lacanian terms imaginary and not symbolic is actually "the little other," a narcissistic reflection, perhaps, of her own anxiety or aggression. This seemingly big, but actually small, other has the initiative, directs an enigmatic demand at Helen, and directs the world within which she finds herself. Though she may not understand it, or even know what it is exactly that she doesn't understand, there is no doubt that the demand is somehow concerned with her. Her surrender to it guarantees her name, but as during the rape, this demand also threatens the memories through which she rediscovers herself. This other offers an abyss, a meltdown of thought and dissolution of identity, a lack too terrible to encounter directly.

Likewise, Schreber's surrender to God's sexual enjoyment involves the cessation of genuine thinking, or the replacement of meaningful words with ghost words. He calculates his mental workings to resemble thoughts without actually being thoughts. Rather, the "not thinking of anything thought" mentally repeats the rays' empty words without engaging with them.[123] This prevents God's rays from withdrawing from his body while allowing him to cultivate "feminine voluptuousness," which does not mix with actual thought. He believes that his surrender of independent thought to rote phrases, like Helen's, guarantees his immortal name, and perhaps his motherhood to a new race.[124]

XII. FORGETTING AND REMEMBERING, SIGNIFYING AND BEING

Helen imagines both remembering and forgetting as integral to her uncertain quest. The father-son figure's attack and rape is aligned in the poem with forgetting and with writing as signification. This attack, however, is subverted into an act of procreation, aligned with remembering and with the transformation of symbol into being. Here, being substitutes for clear, stable correspondences between signifiers and signifieds. Through embodiment and procreation *Helen* "matche[s]" "the picture" made by God, identified with writing, with its own "living hieroglyphs" (23), which I have called writing-beings. *Helen* suggests that memories *of* the mother, themselves, actually *are* the mother, and that writing actually *is* the thing the writing depicts. The poem suggests its own auto-signification with its writing-beings, "letter[s] who recall" the goddess, who is mother to them all. Though they can be "recalled" or "invoked," they are not merely memories, but also the actual thing remembered. The "letter" is alive in this realm of the unconscious, where memories, which like signifiers, are representations of something not present and also real, bodily presences. Words and thoughts are more real and embodied than we know, albeit perhaps in an astral realm. Hence, they are in some sense external to ourselves.

H.D. saw herself and Dowding as building bridges to the other realms of existence. To be, like Helen, "both phantom and reality," both word and flesh, is to enter Egypt, the astral plane, but not to "forget," as the dead souls who dwell there generally do (3). In much modern occultism (as well as the religions it borrowed from) the astral plane(s) are temporary dwelling places for souls, who usually forget their previous forms. They can also be visited by divine beings, and by spiritually advanced humans, who project their astral bodies there, but do not (usually) forget and become unmoored from their corporeal ones in the human realm. H.D. believed in a special category of humans, those whom her writings refer to as "initiates," "neophytes," or "twice-born." In *Helen,* these initiates visit, or belong in, Egypt. Achilles is mostly absent from Helen because he is at work building a "light-house" in Egypt for "others like ourselves,/who are not shadows or shades,/but entities, living a life/unfulfilled in Greece" (89). As Dowding wished to reassure England's uninitiated that their loved ones were alive and well in the beyond, so Achilles wishes to take "the wisdom of Amen and Thoth/back to the islands" (90).

Helen, too, is concerned with bringing one plane of existence nearer to the next. She does this mainly through the cultivation of her memories. These seem to be endangered in Egypt, the astral plane where memory is wiped clean for most people, who enter only after death. In Greek myth, Lethe, the river of forgetfulness, bars the land of the dead from the land of the living. In the poem, Lethe must be crossed to enter Egypt. The river suggests the bar between the conscious mind and unconscious memories: "Lethe, as we all know, is the river of forgetfulness, passing from life to death. *But Helen, mysteriously transposed to Egypt, does not want to forget. She is both phantom and reality* (3, emphasis added). Helen remembers through "invoking" a "letter": "From the depths of her racial inheritance, she invokes (as the perceptive visitor to Egypt must always do) the symbol or the 'letter' that represents or recalls the protective mother-goddess" (13).

The bird-letter that Helen invokes because she "does not want to forget" (3) is "dedicated" to Isis, the mother-goddess. In the poem's associational realm, memory is the "mother," as H.D. also states in *Notes on Thought and Vision*: "Memory is the mother, the begetter of all Drama, idea, music, science or song" (23). By cultivating her memories, the poem suggests, Helen protects herself and both invokes and becomes the mother.

As the mother figure, Helen is unforgettable: "Who will forget Helen?" the poem asks again and again, as it describes the destruction of Troy (121–4, 127). Who will forget "the admitted first cause of all-time, all-history?" (47) Helen is the object of eternal preoccupation in both senses, literally occupied by multitudes of others, and the object of attention and memory for multitudes of others. As "writing" without specific meaning, she is occupied by infinite possible meanings and identities. Simultaneously, as a corporeal being, she gives birth to everything and remains the thing that everything regards.

For Achilles, Helen is the mark of the thing lost (his mother) and also, in some mysterious way, she *is* his mother. Achilles, who seeks to control and interpret what is represented, is angered by the slippage of representation into being embodied by Helen. Representations associated with the mother are many: wooden doll, bird, octopus, flying fish, grasshopper, mermaid, Helen herself. The narrator calls them "symbols of a Greek sea-Goddess" (107). However, they do not have a narrative framework within which to take meaning; they appear and disappear quickly, with no obvious relevance to the rest of *Helen*. To Achilles, with his story of loss and recovery, at least some of these representations have symbolic meaning. They stand for what he has lost. After the young Achilles loses his mother, Thetis, he constructs a representation of her:

> a sorcery even more potent,
> a wooden doll
> that Thetis' child hid away;
> O mysterious treasure,
> O idol, O eidolon,

with wings folded about her (291)

On the plains of Troy, Achilles literally reads Helen. He interprets her movements on the Walls as signs for Yes/No, and predicts the future by watching her movements and counting her steps: "Achilles looks to Helen as 'a new oracle': if she pauses here or there—yes. If she goes on here or there—no" (53). Helen is the oracle for Achilles that H.D., herself, wished to be for Dowding.

In Egypt, Achilles sees Helen as a sign for Thetis, the sea-goddess, la mer/la mère. Helen is "Thetis-eidolon" (284) and "hieroglyph," the mark of the "meaning," which Achilles reads and remembers. She is "[t]he symbolic veil to which Achilles had enigmatically referred," which "resolves itself into the memory of a woman's scarf, blowing in the winter wind" (55). The memory of Thetis is "the power/that swayed Achilles" (56) during the Trojan War, causing his death and transport to Egypt. It is because Helen recalls to Achilles a memory of having lost "the scene of his boyhood and his childhood's secret idol, the first Thetis-eidolon" (284), that Achilles attacks then rapes her. Achilles thus "break[s] his heart/and the world for a *token*/a memory forgotten" (304, emphasis added). Achilles reads/attacks the writing that *is* Helen. The father rapes the mother; the lawmaker rapes, reads, splits apart the writing-being. But why? Why can not my *letters*, my winged words, my children simply be the truth? Why should writing not be being? What is this "language?":

> O Child, must it be forever,
> that your father destroys you,
> that you may find your father?
> . . .
> O Child, must you seek your mother
> while your father forever
> attacks her in jealousy?
> "I begot them in death, they are mine" (28)

I have the phallus, says Achilles. I raped the writing-being so that writing and being might be alienated, and I might control the meaning of writing. Dowding said, more or less, your messages, ostensibly dictated by the RAF pilots, are false. I am the arbiter of what *my* RAF pilots have to say. But what is symbolized soon breaks out of the deadening encasement of the symbol, in a swarm, a galaxy, a multiplicity whose name is in the singular. Is not every singularity split from everything else, from primordial nondifferentiation, only by the name hung on it? But a name cannot make something a singularity, as swarms and galaxies show us.

Helen's search for "the answer," however, hinges on the question of identity, and seems to require Achilles's co-operation:

> But still Helen wants "some simple answer." She feels that Achilles can give it to her. But she delays asking *the direct question that will tell her everything.* When she introduces it, it is in a roundabout way. She knows that her name was Helen, in Sparta, in Greece. But she wants to know of that other, "walking upon the ramparts." She does not directly ask Achilles if he recognizes in her the Helen of his first accusation, "I have seen you upon the ramparts." Is this Helen actually that Helen? (47, emphasis added)

The question of identity and the question of the question are placed persistently in close relation to one another. Questions and assertions of identity and language shadow one another throughout the poem. Achilles asks Helen a very similar question to the one she asks him: another question of Helen's identity followed by a question of language:

> How are Helen in Egypt
> and Helen upon the ramparts,
> together yet separate? (63)
> how have the paths met?
> how have the circles crossed?
> *how phrase or how frame the problem*? (63, emphasis added)

XIII. OBJECTS, NAMES, AND RHYTHMS AS ANSWERS

Helen's circumnavigation of the formless question pertaining to identity and language proceeds by means of unclear questions and answers, claims that she need not find the answer, that she already understands it, and/or that she contains it. Such claims are followed by more unclear questions and answers and the rapid-fire invocation and disappearance of objects and beings. We can see this circular process in the wake of Achilles's initial formless question to Helen, "Which was the dream, which was the veil, of Cytherea" (36), a question full of signifiers and free from signifieds. The referent(s), the "which-es," of the sentence are unidentified: Achilles may be asking Helen whether it is Troy or Egypt that is illusory, but "which" may not refer to either of them. Likewise the nouns, "dream" and "veil," may refer either to two distinct modes of unreality, dream *or* veil, or to the same one, dream/veil, as opposed to something else. Achilles, then, is asking Helen to apply two nouns that designate either one or two unspecified unrealities to either one or two unspecified subjects, possibly Egypt and/or Troy.

Though "the dream" and "the veil" are later associated in Helen's mind with Troy and Egypt—"was the dream, Helen upon the ramparts?/was the veil, Helen in Egypt?" (85)—Achilles's question never becomes clear. Helen is certain only that it pertains to her in some way. Initially, she, understandably, does not understand his question: "What does he mean? She does not know. We do not know" (37). What she finds significant, however, is that "for the second time, he has spoken her name. That is sufficient" (37). Achilles has posed a formless question, a question whose referents are unclear, but he has said her name. That is "sufficient," perhaps, to guarantee her identity, notwithstanding the challenge to her position as a subject of language that his question, because of its formlessness, poses. Helen takes identity as a name.

H.D. responds to Achilles's question, finally, by taking two nouns in the verse section and citing them in the prose section, where they appear to be the answer to the formless question: "Achilles' early question, 'Helena, which was the dream,/which was the veil of Cytheraea?' is answered, and Helen herself has answered it, 'they were one.' They are 'the ships assembled at Aulis,' and—a mermaid" (238). Here, Helen answers the question of difference and identity that attaches itself to "the dream" and "the veil" by claiming their identity with two more objects that suddenly appear and disappear, one in quotation marks. The formless question is "answered" by the contiguity of these terms. The logic may be that one of the ships that sailed to Troy has a mermaid on the prow, the mermaid stands for/is Egypt and therefore Troy and Egypt are one. Contiguity is identity. Theseus reminds Helen that

> we have only guessed
> or half-guessed
> . . .
> whose was the ensign (painted on the prow)
> of one whose name, even, will be
> an eternal enigma (163)

To guard herself, Theseus had advised Helen to remember "small reliques" (164) instead of recapitulating to "her own apotheosis" with Achilles. But these small relics, themselves, are evidence of the apotheosis; they are compared to debris on a beach "after a wreck" (164). Again multiplicity, meant to guard Helen against the "emotional experience" (162) with Achilles, is also a product of, and recalls, it.

The events in time that inspire her questions, Helen says, cannot be abstracted: "There is no other sign or picture/no compromise with the past" (86). Specific memories cannot become an abstract conceptual system that enables symbolic language and clear questions. Helen wishes instead to "encompass" the memories themselves in her heart without having to understand what they mean:

> the heart does not wonder?
> the heart does not ask?
> the heart accepts,
> encompasses the whole
> of the undecipherable script;
> take, take as you took
> Achilles' anger, as you flamed
> to his Star,
> *this is the only answer*. (86, emphasis added)

This passage suggests the resolution of thoughts and feelings into images. The question of Achilles's motivation is answered by a visual memory of his behavior. Helen asserts a kind of formalist reading of her memories: they do not *mean*, but *are.* Helen wishes, it seems, to resolve the events into a whole, visual "undecipherable script," and to "encompass" this "script." *Helen* itself is perhaps the fullest expression of her attempt to do so. In "Pallinode," the bird-letter, a symbol "in-time," perhaps accomplishes this. Though a letter, it is alive, a "shape" that "parallels" the "timeless, hieratic symbols," inanimate marks not subject to birth and death:

> The dream? The veil? Obviously, Helen has walked through time into another dimension. But the timeless, hieratic symbols can be paralleled with symbols in-time. Helen herself had realized this, on her first meeting with Achilles, "the shape of this bird is a letter, they call it the hieroglyph." There are other hieroglyphs, Thetis has reminded her, a grasshopper, a flying fish, an octopus—these are Greek symbols of a Greek sea-goddess—"Helen, come home." (107)

Beings in Egypt appear as parallels "in-time" for "timeless," abstract symbols. Egypt itself is reduced to a mark, a "'delicate sea-shell'" (114). They are, the text wants to establish, hieroglyphs that "parallel" symbolic language. Helen claims acceptance of the indecipherability of visual objects: "Let the temple walls flower with 'the indecipherable Amen-script.' It is not necessary to 'read' the riddle. The pattern itself is sufficient and it is beautiful" (32).

Though for Lacan a "psychotic structure" implies an asymbolic relation to language from the beginning, it seems to me that words once functioned symbolically for H.D.—or at least, more than they did during the time she wrote *Helen.* Helen's many protests, in the poem, suggest an awareness of what it is that she cannot understand, the "indecipherable Amen-script," that is too accurate, and the longing for understanding too strong, for this understanding never to have existed. No sooner does Helen claim contentment with the indecipherable signifier or memory as "the only meaning," than she is beset by another question crying for an answer, often concerning Achilles or God:

> Achilles, Achilles come back,
> you alone have the answer;
> the dream? the veil?
> is it all a story? (88)

Is there nothing but a story, a tale told by an idiot? "The harpers" may describe Helen and Achilles's meeting, over and over, "forever." But will they ever tell Helen its meaning?

> "How have the paths met?" This is indeed the lesser personal mystery. "The harpers will sing forever of how Achilles met Helen among the shades," but perhaps they can not tell us *why* they met, for exactly what reason "the circles crossed." This is part of the Greater Mystery. Helen will not force an answer from the oracle. She will take her time about it. (64)

While she waits patiently for the meaning of the meeting that is so much in question, Helen, like Achilles, "counts the tread of her feet," finding signification perhaps only in this numerical quantification: "No, I will not challenge/the ancient Mystery/I will count the tread of my feet" (64). Indeed, we can perhaps discern in this rhythmic, counted tread, "faster or slower, but never changing the beat, the rhythm," the very meter of *Helen* itself, counted by H.D.[125] "The rhythms," the narrator tells us, "must speak for themselves, and the alliterations" (178), since the words are not providing a layer of sense. The poem offers images, rhythm, and meter in place of signification. Helen's continuing efforts at quantification and schematization as alternate structures of meaning, however, create more associations—sometimes bizarre ones:

> I place my hand on a pillar
> and run my hand as the blind,
> along the invisible curve
> or thc line of chick or bee;
> where are we?
> and what is the answer? (46)

This reference to the RAF pilots who Dowding referred to as "my boys" and "my chicks"[126] suggests the desire of Delia in *Sword* to graph their communications into a line, which—she expects—will zigzag. She associates this with bees, since the zigzag "would be a zzz-zzz way of talking" (*Sword*, 140). In *Helen in Egypt*, Helen's idea that a pillar is a "line of chick or bee" represents an attempt, like Delia's imagined graph, to resolve something incomprehensible into a pure shape, and to attach this to an unclear question. The indecipherable code dictated to Delia by the RAF pilots comes to typify the elusiveness of meaning of all signifiers.

H.D. attempts to redress the failure of meaning by loading words into Helen, who "brings together" terms that lack a place in the symbolic structure by connecting them all to herself. As Robert Duncan puts it, in *Helen in Egypt* "the sense increases that as the artist works to achieve form he finds himself the creature of the form he thought first to achieve."[127] Consistent with the poem's attempted rendering of signification into pure visual image or graphic, Helen herself is the object of everyone's gaze. She encompasses all undeciphered memories, associations, and identities that enter the field of this gaze. Schreber tells us more directly than Helen that "everything that happens is in reference to me." This is not vanity, he explains. It is simply that "since God entered into nerve-contact with me exclusively, I became in a way for God the only human being, or simply the human being around whom everything turns, to whom everything that happens must be related, and who therefore, from his own point of view, must also relate all things to himself."[128]

This belief grows in H.D. following her analysis with Freud. Subsequent work repeatedly seeks to "reconcile" different principles contained in herself and her alter egos, in order to end the social strife (particularly the Second World War) caused by their division. Whether or not these principles are also identified with another person, such as Dowding, does not change that fact that they must be reconciled not interpersonally, but within herself only. Blending psychoanalytic and occultist paradigms, H.D. envisioned this inner work of following "traces of direction" as enabling not only psychic integration, but also a personal and social movement into higher realms of existence. I acknowledge the wisdom of exploring and reconciling our inner conflicts rather than—or at least before—taking them up with the others with whom we associate them, and I share H.D.'s belief in a relation between inner growth and positive social change, and her belief in eternity as well as in time. These insights seem to me to support the arguments of Grof, Ram Dass, and many others that so-called mystics and so-called psychotics are exploring similar psychic, or supramundane, terrain. Here perhaps not only H.D. and Schreber, but even some visionaries of occultist movements, are languaging similar premonitions. However, there is something more here for H.D.—a belief that she alone redeems everyone and everything else, which distinguishes her view from mystical teachings and from psychoanalysis.

XIV. HELEN AS ANSWER

Though the Amen-script, the word of God, is indecipherable, H.D. asserts that Helen *is* it, and therefore understands it on an intuitive level. She "understands" by *being* "the writing" that the other reads. Helen attempts to substitute for the missing place of what is signified with the pure signifier (in Lacan's terminology) that she herself embodies. Recurrently, Helen asks Achilles to explain to her the link between her identity in Troy (London during the Second World War) and in Egypt (the astral plane). "What was she then, if she was there, at all, in Troy. His answer is unequivocal and final, 'a fountain of water in that desert . . . we died of thirst'" (47). Achilles's answer, though it does not seem "unequivocal" since it is an analogy, tells us that the Greek armies perished for lack of Helen—as well as because of Helen.

The figure of Helen of Troy heralds a new world order. Helen's power, greater than the "Iron ring" of "the Command," seduces Achilles away from "the Command" and causes him to die and become a "new mortal" in Egypt. Her universal desirability catalyzes the Trojan War. She is unforgettable and irresistible: Achilles dies because of a glance that they exchange; Paris dies because he cannot forget her.

The capital letters consistently given in *Helen* and other later writing to terms like Love, Beauty, and War, as well as their consistent identification with H.D. and Dowding, suggest a belief that she and Dowding were divine principles or incarnations. Perhaps, as Robinson suggests, they are "egregores," beings who are formed, according to Robert Ambelain, from the beliefs, ideals, and rituals of a particular group, and who also belong to particular texts. Writes Ambelain, "Religions and magicians have always used immutable texts . . . which, by reason of their immutability and common repetition, are "living" texts, composed of "living" words, with real egregores in their turn."[129] War is one of the egregores that Ambelain mentions, and "Helena," H.D. tells us, is "the name of Love" (95). Helen also "takes on the attributes" of Aphrodite, goddess of love, in response to Paris's refutation of her encounter with Achilles.

The encounters of divinized mother, father, and son figures are now drawn from Ambelain's as well as Freud's visions of family dynamics. The union of Helen and Achilles (who is also Paris, the son) represents the union of the egregores, Love and War, and also the union of mother, father and son. It is by this union that Love and War, Helen and Achilles-Paris, give birth to themselves. The "integration" that produces Beauty and Love is both the cause and the effect of the violence that attacks Beauty and Love. The cosmic cycle catalyzed by Achilles's rape is, thus, "the only answer" (86) to the question of its cause. Achilles raped Helen so that the world could be recreated, so that

Achilles could rape Helen. In H.D.'s *Ion*, the union of Ion and Kreousa gives rise to a perfect Ionian civilization, which H.D.—who gauges a culture's perfection by the beauty of its art—describes as the "greatest aesthetic miracle of all-time."[130] In *Helen in Egypt*, Helen is the "eidolon" and "egregore" of Love, the divine mother who must integrate with War, the father-son, to give birth to another (artistically) perfect civilization or perhaps to a perfect epic poem like *Helen*. The poem suggests that the product of Helen's "integrative" rape by Achilles, the "ultimate experience, *La Mort, L'Amour*," is literally the poem itself, the perfectly beautiful offspring of these physical embodiments of "War" and "Love" or "Beauty" (288). H.D.'s protagonists attract the male violence necessary for renewed, perfect, beautiful civilization, which is also perfect artistic production.

The unidentified prose commentator tells us that because Helen "herself is the writing" she does not need to interpret it: "Helen herself denies actual intellectual knowledge of the temple-symbols. But she is nearer to them than the instructed scribe; for her, the secret of the stone-writing is repeated in natural or human symbols. *She herself is the writing*" (22, emphasis in the original). Instead of understanding the symbol "intellectually," she *is* it, like God in the Gospel of John.[131] She is God's, Amen's, "opposite number for just that flash in time," as she puts in *Majic Ring*:[132]

> Proteus, the legendary King of Egypt, as we have learned before, takes many shapes. Could he "manifest as Achilles?" If so, (the question is not asked but implied), could he manifest as Paris? Then, could the two opposites (the slayer and the slain) merge into one, and that One, the Absolute? This last question is implicit but not formulated in the final phrase or strophe, "Amen begot Amor." (178)

Helen, appearing as Delia in *Sword* and as the "opposite number" of God, is also, like God, the word.[133] Her search for the meaning of other people's behavior is therefore a self-referential search. The "clues" in her memories provide "the only answer." Helen is the meaning of *Helen in Egypt*.

Although H.D. probably has the Gospel of John in mind when she asserts that Helen "is the writing," her assertion is not meant to signal only that Helen is God incarnate, though it is meant to do that. Her wish to establish this lives alongside a wish to return through writing to a state of nondifference between signifying and being. H.D. notes, and ruminates over, John's claim that God is the Word: "He is the Word, the word is made up of letters. He is all the intermediate letters and he is the infinite combination of the letters in English and in every language. If he is the Word, he is essentially part of the language."[134] God, perhaps, presents nondifference. What he says *is*, and this is how creation occurs. So Schreber also notes with interest, "God *wills* that something should be, and by dispatching rays with this will, *what he wills immediately comes into existence*. The Bible expresses this significantly with the words "God said, let there be light, and there *was* light."[135]

For Schreber, rays, which "must speak as soon as they are in motion," are the words of God.[136] However, Schreber notes that "divine creative power" seems dependent on "drawing nearer to [the] body," celestial or corporeal, "on which creation was to take place."[137] This is also true in *Helen.* Hence perhaps, the necessity that Schreber and Helen take the divine into their flesh. If God is the Word of the original Law, then the Incarnation, the Word made flesh, can reverse that Law. The moment of castration can be, as Weber puts it, "reversed." The order of things that language put into place can be renewed, perhaps through living language. The idea of simultaneously material/corporeal and scriptural production is repeated in H.D.'s later writing, for instance, in the *Hirslanden Notebooks* (journals written in 1957–1960) and in her last long poem *Hermetic Definition* (1960). These works weave into her psychic and mythic tapestry her 1960 encounter with another man she thought was rejecting her, Lionel Durand.[138]

Helen's questions of identity mirror the question of the relation of word to meaning in the poem itself. Since everything that happens in the outer world is "about" her, the truth about herself is the articulation of everything. Her difficulty formulating questions and theories results from the limitlessness of the objects that are somehow relevant and related to her. The sense of a "real" truth beyond whatever answers she may have found persists, though it is disavowed. H.D. sometimes expresses a concern that the "threads" on the loom of her memories and associations were woven together "too loosely," an image that may suggest the drift of her thoughts from clear to enigmatic relevance.

Violent destruction that is also synthesis and rebirth remains a constant throughout H.D.'s later writing, though new players step in and others recede or merge into one another. The "next world" becomes less material than it appears in *Sword* or *Trilogy*, more of an alternate dimension (an astral or celestial plane) that co-exists with the "material plane." Although subsequent work shows that H.D. is still looking for the ends of her thoughts, *Helen* is a triumph in that it arranges them into a circular thought pattern that somewhat stabilizes its sense of meaning. The temporal dimension signified by the birth/death prevents meaning from collapsing in on itself because death and birth, which signal difference, suggest that difference, time, oneness, and eternity are all still possible.

H.D.'s troubled relation to the symbolic order perhaps correlates to her responses to other people's differing views, where the other view is swallowed by her "expanded" vision. However, the frequent return of the question of the other's perspective suggests that this problem is only incompletely resolved by these foreclosures. Though the delusional metaphor substitutes the imaginary difference of the rape's birth and death for the difference between signifying and being, Helen's search for the truth still circles the question of what is signified. H.D., like Helen, continues to appeal to others for answers and then appropriates their offerings with her characteristic turn to an unclear frame of reference and ghostly terms whose meaning she is sure they cannot comprehend, as she herself cannot. The question that the encounters with Freud, Dowding, and Heydt gave rise to (i.e., the question of language itself) persists. The "next world," "answer," or "ultimate plan" that H.D. longed for so desperately is the symbolic order, which she repeatedly foreclosed. This longing was persistent. H.D., like *Helen in Egypt*'s Helen, Kreousa in *Ion*, Delia in *Sword* and *Majic Ring*, and Hilda in *The Gift*, continued to doubt and interpret, and to crave reassurance that the "ultimate plan" was still operative and that she still had an important place in it.

NOTES

1. H.D., *Magic Mirror*, 98.
2. Ibid., 119. This trilogy mainly details her relationship with Erich Heydt during her stay at Klinik Brunner and further considers the meaning of her encounter with Dowding. My chapter title is taken from *Helen in Egypt* (63), hereafter cited in the text as *Helen*.
3. H.D., *Magic Mirror*, 92.
4. Friedman, *Psyche*, 60. Stesichorus of Sicily's *Pallinode*(s) are not extant, but are discussed in other ancient Greek texts and in contemporary summaries.
5. Robinson, *Astral*, 93. Robinson argues that *Helen in Egypt* represents "an astral initiation, a peek behind 'the Veil' into 'the Dream' (*Helen*, 107). . . . Like H.D.'s other historical accounts of initiations, *Helen in Egypt* takes place in an imagined space that is at one remove from reality or 'in-time'; she is at the Amen temple but it is not the Amen that H.D. meets in her present, for this is another age, appropriate to a different avatar."
6. Friedman, *Psyche*, 257.
7. Ambelain, *Kabbalah II*, 75.
8. Weber, Introduction to *Memoirs*, xxviii.
9. Writes Ambelain: "If we recapitulate the steps of our Reintegration into the Divine, we can state the process as follows:

1. Man is a reduction of the Universe, an image of God. We carry in us a spark emanated from the 'MOTHER' (Malkuth). If we bring this spark to life, we allow the Divine essence of the 'MOTHER' to penetrate us, and we assimilate it. When the 'MOTHER' is within us, we are, by the channel of analogical correspondence, in the 'MOTHER.'

2. If the 'MOTHER' is one with the Son (or Father), being in the 'MOTHER' we are in the Son, and the 'MOTHER' being in us, the SON is also there . . .

3. If the SON (or Father) is one with the FATHER (or Ancient of Days), then the SON is within us, and the FATHER is also within us. And if we are in the SON, we are in the FATHER too. . . .

These three postulates flow from the very concept of the Divine TRI-UNITY." (*Kabbalah II*, 75).

10. Ibid., 75.

11. Schreber, *Memoirs*, 53.

12. Ibid.

13. In his introduction to Schreber's *Memoirs of My Nervous Illness*, Samuel Weber writes, "Schreber's most significant fantasies concern the body on one hand, and language on the other; that body and language stand in the closest possible relation to each other . . . we are dealing with a text which does not stand apart from what it describes, but which itself is included in it" (xli).

14. Ibid., vii–liv.

15. This is true in Lacan's theory of psychosis in which the big Other (described variously over time as language, the unconscious, the symbolic order, radical alterity and the other sex) is foreclosed and substituted for by the small other of the imaginary order. The imaginary other is a narcissistic projection whose interest and attention are always trained on the subject—though this interest, in psychosis, is often malignant.

16. Leys, *Trauma*, 2–3, 146–52, 300–7, and throughout.

17. Writes Lacan, "We must also add that man's desire is the Other's desire [*le désir de l'homme est le désir de l'Autre*] in which the *de* provides what grammarians call a 'subjective determination'—namely, that it is qua Other that man desires. . . . This is why the Other's question [*la question de l'Autre*]—that comes back to the subject from the place from which he expects an oracular reply—which takes some such form as *'Che vuoi?,'* 'What do you want?,' is the question that best leads the subject to the path of his own desire, assuming that . . . he takes up that question, even without knowing it, in the following form: 'What does he want from me?'" ("Subversion," 690).

18. Writes Lacan, "these nerves [part-entities that torment Schreber through nonsensical speech and physical invasion] just like the divine rays *(Gottesstrahlen)* with which they are homogeneous, are nothing but the entification of the spoken words they hear (S. 130, which the voices formulate as: 'Do not forget that the nature of the rays is that they must speak')" ("On a Question," 450).

19. H.D., *Majic Ring*, 46.

20. H.D., *Hirslanden Notebooks*, 34.

21. Friedman, *Psyche*, 257.

22. Ibid., 261.

23. Ibid., 256.

24. Gelpi, "H.D.," 129.

25. Friedman, *Psyche*, 257.

26. DuPlessis, *Struggle*, 114.

27. Writes H.D., "Eros and Death; those two were the chief subjects—in fact, the only subjects—of the Professor's eternal preoccupation" (*Tribute*, 103). *Helen*'s theme of the union of *La Mort, L'Amour* or *Eros, Eris* suggests Freud's conceptual merging of the life and death drives into a single aggressive drive in his later work.

28. Sword, *Ghostwriting Modernism*, 131.

29. Hokanson, "Is It All a Story," 331.

30. Pondrom, "Approaches to Teaching *Helen in Egypt*."

31. Edmunds, *Line*, 6.

32. Writes Lacan, "It is the lack of the Name-of-the-Father in that place which, by the hole that it opens up in the signified, sets off a cascade of reworkings of the signifier from which the growing disaster of the imaginary proceeds, until the level is reached where signifier and signified stabilize in a *delusional metaphor*" ("On a Question," 481).

33. Deleuze and Guattari, *Anti-Oedipus*, 89. Write Deleuze and Guattari, "It should be noted that Judge Schreber's destiny was not merely that of being sodomized, while still alive, by the rays from heaven, but also that of being posthumously oedipalized by Freud. From the enormous political, social, and historical content of Schreber's delirium, not one word is retained, as though the libido did not bother itself with such things" (57).

34. See Perry, "Spiritual Emergence and Renewal" and *Trials of the Visionary Mind*.

35. LaChance, "Sexual Sublime," 33, 39.

36. Hickman, "Uncanonically," 18.

37. Ibid.

38. LaChance, "Sexual Sublime," 44.

39. Gifford, "H.D.'s Hirslanden Notebooks," 3–4.

40. LaChance, "Sexual Sublime," 35.

41. Writes Lacan, "I teach that the Other is the locus of the kind of memory he discovered by the name 'unconscious,' memory that he regards as the object of a question that has remained unanswered, insofar as it conditions the indestructibility of certain desires. I will answer this question with the conception of the signifying chain, inasmuch as—once this chain has been inaugurated by primordial symbolization (made manifest in the *Fort!Da!* game, which Freud elucidated as lying at the origin of repetition automatism)—it develops in accordance with logical connections whose hold on that which is to be signified, namely, the being of entities, is exerted through the signifying effects I describe as metaphor and metonymy. It is an accident in this register and in what occurs in it—namely, the foreclosure of the Name-of-the-Father in the place of the Other—and the failure of the paternal metaphor that I designate as the defect that gives psychosis its essential condition, along with the structure that separates it from neurosis" ("On a Question," 497).

42. Writes Lacan, "this One-father must . . . come to that place to which the subject could not summon him before. For this, the One-father need but situate himself in a tertiary position in any relationship that has as its base the imaginary couple *a-a'*—that is, ego-object or ideal-reality—involving the subject in the field of eroticized aggression that it induces" ("On a Question," 481).

43. See, for instance, White's discussion of paranoid schizophrenic illness. Writes White, "[i]n the early stages of the illness it is generally possible to see a connection between the patient's misinterpretations of reality and his personal wishes, needs, and fears. As time goes on, however, the delusions tend to spread out in a disorganized fashion. Magical forces and mystical powers come into the picture" (*Abnormal Personality*, 547).

44. H.D., *Magic Mirror*, 125–6.

45. Ibid.

46. For instance, H.D. in *Compassionate Friendship* writes, "I think the story [*The Mystery*, which she leant to Heydt] was read by Tiresias—what can I call him?—and that the note that Erich wrote about it was dictated by him. . . . I think I have gained, rather than lost, in visualizing Heydt as almost 'controlled' by this 'Boss' or 'Bally.' . . . Heydt would not have had time to find these references and books, even if he had had the intelligence to build up for me, this series of associations—if we can "build' associations and I think we can" (ibid., 146–7). Her interest for Erich's possible "spyring"she believes, may involve her association with Ezra Pound (143, 147). Though Lara Vetter has noted several passages in *Compassionate Friendship* and *Thorn Thicket* that cast doubt on H.D.'s belief in this story (*Curious*, 179-80), I read the affective charge this story carries as overriding her nonbelief, to impact her thoughts and responses. Vetter reads H.D.'s fear of Heydt at this time as "a fiction that embeds a critique of the Freudian process," where the analyst's surveillance and decoding of their subject's speech, and their mimicry (as Vetter reads it) of genuine identification with their subject, reflects a spy's work of gathering information and betraying trust. I agree with Vetter that H.D.'s vision of male authority figures receiving and decoding (her) information, and betraying her, likely has roots in her sessions with Freud. Indeed, many such "delusions," as George Atwood argues, may be literalized renderings of analytic subjects' felt experiences of betrayal, violation, and unresponsiveness from their analysts or doctors (*Abyss*, 14 and throughout).

47. Ibid., 147.

48. Ibid., 146.

49. Ibid., 148.

50. Ibid., 147.

51. Ibid., 149.

52. Schreber, *Memoirs*, 54.

53. Ibid., 49, emphasis in original.

54. Lacan, *Seminar III, The Psychoses*, 255.

55. See for instance, ibid., 268–9.

56. Lacan, "On a Purpose," *Écrits*, 303.

57. H.D., *Majic Ring*, 59, 160.

58. Ibid., 121.

59. Ibid., 31, 53.

60. Lacan, *Seminar III, The Psychoses*, 250.

61. Robinson, *Astral*, 12.

62. Writes Robinson, "*Helen in Egypt* introduces [occultist] ideas that will be reworked in all the subsequent poems . . . with *Helen* acting as an introduction to the puzzle or pattern that must be solved" (*Astral*, 107).

63. See ibid., 40. "In *Compassionate Friendship* H.D. discusses 'seven brothers or minor initiators. Ezra [Pound] was the first of these'; Erich Heydt does not represent an eighth, but instead acts as what Freud would call a 'determinative' of the set of 'minor initiators.' She illustrates the group of initiators as a constellation, borrowing language from Chaboseau: '*Dans le ciel brillent sept étoiles, inégalement disposées auteur d'une bien plus grande*' ('Seven stars shine in the sky, unevenly distributed around a much larger one'). Dowding, she concludes, is 'the large Star, *étoile sacerdotale et royale* . . . the final initiation, the integration, the final father-image,' (*Friendship*, 122). The minor initiators are the individual smaller stars, Heydt is the constellation that surrounds the large star, and Dowding is the star in the middle."

64. Robinson, *Astral*, 11.

65. Ibid., 14.

66. Ibid., 40. "The completion of the Delia Alton novels, time, and distance were doubtless all factors in H.D.'s re-evaluation of Dowding's role in her narrative, as was the introduction of new people and a new phase of life. But Dowding remained an important figure in her writing (and her dreams) until the end, and she wanted to make sense of his never-waning presence in her psyche."

67. Robinson, *Astral*, 9.

68. H.D., *Magic Mirror*, 176. Writes H.D., "Is this the *Consecration du Cercle*? (sic). . . . Does the Circle dictate the material as well as the spiritual aspects of life? There is Heydt-Heydt . . . but this is balanced by the H.D.–H.D. of the War II contact, and by the earlier, almost perfected formula of the War I Madrigal. The H.D. of D.H. Lawrence almost does the trick, D.H.–H.D., but not quite" (*Magic Mirror*, 191).

69. Writes Ambelain, "The soul of the text is that which is expressed thereby, the general idea which emanates from it. The material body is the word which expresses it. The double, the plastic intermediary, is the human thought which accompanies the word" (*Kabbalah I*, 45).

70. H.D., *Magic Mirror*, 176.

71. Ibid., 181.

72. H.D., *Magic Mirror*, 92.

73. H.D. understood as a significant slip her misreading of a phrase in a letter from Duncan—"the *actual* poet H.D." as "the *astral* poet H.D." (*Magic Mirror*, 174, my italics).

74. "*Choc en retour*" in Robert Ambelain's description is the "psychic backlash" that inevitably comes from the practice of magic. Tryphonopoulos and Robinson, preface, *Magic Mirror*, xvi. H.D. sees Dowding's repudiation as the effect of this *choc en retour* brought about by her solo séances, though she also explains it in other ways.

75. H.D., *Magic Mirror*, 173.

76. Schreber, *Memoirs*, 60.

77. Ibid., 42.

78. Ibid., emphasis added.

79. Ibid., 41.

80. Ibid., 42.
81. Ibid.,194.
82. Ibid., 237.
83. Ibid., 214.
84. Caruth, *Experience*, 61–2.
85. Deleuze and Guattari, *Anti-Oedipus*, 309. Deleuze and Guattari write that Lacan discovers the "reverse side" of the oedipal structure mother-father-son, the realm of part-objects: "This reverse side is the 'real inorganization' of the molecular elements: partial objects that enter into indirect syntheses or interactions . . . pure positive multiplicities where everything is possible, without exclusiveness or negation . . . signs of desire that compose a signifying chain but that are not themselves signifying, and do not answer to the rules of a linguistic game of chess, but instead to the lottery drawings that sometimes cause a word to be chosen, sometimes a design, sometimes a thing or a piece of a thing, depending on one another only by the order of the random drawings, and holding together only by the absence of a link (nonlocalizable connections), having no other statutory condition than that of being dispersed elements of desiring-machines that are themselves dispersed! It is this entire reverse side of the structure that Lacan discovers, with the 'o' as machine, and the 'O' as nonhuman sex: schizophrenizing the analytic field, instead of oedipalizing the psychotic field."
86. Deleuze, *Sense*, 264.
87. Schreber writes of God's proximity, resulting from his attraction to Schreber, disrupting the order of the world: "By and large God left the world which He had created and the organic life upon it (plants, animals, human beings) to their own devices and only provided continuous warmth of the sun to enable them to maintain themselves and reproduce, etc. As a rule God did not interfere directly in the fate of peoples or individuals—I call this the state of affairs in accordance with the Order of the World. [However, in exceptional cases] the nerves of *living* human beings particularly when in a state of high-grade excitation, have such power of attraction for the nerves of God that He would not be able to free Himself from them again, and would thus endanger his own existence" (*Memoirs*, 48).
88. Ibid., 196.
89. See Lacan, *Seminar II, The Ego*, 90, 221–35, and Ragland, *Pleasures*, chap. 5.
90. Lacan, *Seminar III, The Psychoses*, 250.
91. Schreber, *Memoirs*, 72.
92. Lacan, *Seminar III, The Psychoses*, 100.
93. Ibid., 98.
94. As Weber argues, Schreber describes his emasculation as possession by a language that acts on him from without. Writes Weber, "Because of its very structure, nerve language is anything but an expression of 'genuine feeling': it is much less an expression than an impression, something remembered, not the expression of something inward but the emergence in the interior of something outwards, something 'learned by rote' . . . as a nerve the subject does not speak, it is spoken. Although Schreber does not say this in so many words, he writes it; or, perhaps more precisely, it writes him" (Introduction to *Memoirs*, xxxvii).
95. Schreber, *Memoirs*, 115.

96. As Robinson notes in *Astral*, the name Formalhaut is taken from Chaboseau: "Fomalhaut, another aspect of the 'Large Star' from Chaboseau, becomes 'Formalhaut' in *Helen in Egypt*, who stands for 'the Nameless-of-Many-Names' or Proteus, echoing the Protean figure of the dreams in the *Hirslanden Notebooks*. This protean figure can ultimately be traced back to the entity she has called 'Amen' and 'Aquarius' and even 'Santa Claus,' and is thus closer to her Amen than is Amen: '[Formalhaut's temple] is the same Amen-temple, at all times, in all places, on all planes of existence.' This temple is thus the astral form of the temple, proper to the dimension in which she finds herself, the Platonic form of the temple behind all the other temples" (93).

97. Ibid., 93. "Achilles, the Dowding double, is 'commanded by Formalhaut,/the Initiator,'" (*Helen*, 208). Recalling that Dowding is identified as *étoile sacerdotale et royale*, which is Chaboseau's description of the Fomalhaut aspect of the Large Star, and equally recalling that he is the major initiator, it is strange here to see the two associated and yet separated, especially when considering that Dowding and the many-named Protean figure later become two distinct entities in the Eden Retrouvé dream and subsequent *Hermetic Definition.*

98. H.D., *Trilogy*, 17.

99. Thetis, both sea goddess and (Achilles's) mother, who manifests in Helen, brings maternity and non-differentiation together in a single name. In H.D.'s associative network, the sea is the mother, the "word bitterer still, *mar*,/sea, brine, breaker, seducer,/giver of life, giver of tears . . . mer, mère, mere, mater, Maia, Mary,/Star of the Sea,/Mother" (*Triogy*, 17).

100. Schreber, *Memoirs*, 72–3.

101. Weber, Introduction to *Memoirs*, xlix.

102. Schreber, *Memoirs*, 50.

103. Ibid., 72.

104. Ibid., 69.

105. See Robinson, *Astral*, 71–5.

106. Ibid., 214.

107. Ibid., 214.

108. Ibid., 72.

109. Ibid., 148.

110. Ibid., 72.

111. Ibid., 121, 152.

112. Ibid., 151.

113. Ibid., 124–5.

114. Ibid., 124.

115. Ibid.,166.

116. Ibid., 170.

117. Ibid., 199.

118. Ibid., 175.

119. Ibid., 69.

120. Ibid., 72.

121. Schreber, *Memoirs*, 151–2. As Weber describes Schreber's logic, "the cosmological system worked out by Schreber's 'compulsive thinking' sets him up as

the object of God's gaze and the vanishing point into which pour the effects of the wounded cosmic order" (xlix).

122. Lacan, *Seminar III, The Psychoses*, 194.

123. Schreber, *Memoirs*, 226.

124. Lacan, "On a Question," 469.

125. Lacan writes that "in structural analysis, as in the analysis of the relationship between signifier and signified, we discover relations between groups founded on sets that, whether open or closed, essentially comprise reciprocal references" (*Seminar III, The Psychoses*, 184).

126. See Tryphonopoulos's endnotes to *Majic Ring*, 196, 206.

127. Duncan, *H.D. Book*, 52.

128. Schreber, *Memoirs*, 197.

129. Ambelain, *Kabbalah II*, 48–63, *Kaballah I*, 41–5. *Thorn Thicket* and *Compassionate Friendship* also testify to the influence of Robert Ambelain's *The Practical Kabbalah*—in which the mother-father-son triangle and the necessity for their integration also appears—on *Helen in Egypt*, *Kabbalah*, 33. The mother-father-son triangle also appears in *Sword*, where Delia associates Howell with her father and son, as well as herself with Artemis and Howell with Hippolytus, *Sword*, 83. In *Hippolytus Temporizes*, H.D.'s creative 1927 adaptation of Euripides's play, Hippolytus substitutes Artemis for his mother as the object of his insistent and disastrous Oedipal complex. In *Helen in Egypt*, Klinik Brunner Doctor Erich Heydt shares the position of son (and father) with Dowding/Howell.

130. H.D., *Ion*, 257.

131. In *Majic Ring*, H.D. writes that "if [Zakenuto, 46] [or God, 34, or Amen, 48] is the Word, he is essentially part of language" (46). The Word that was God, she reflects, said, "I bring not peace but a sword" (34). Helen, too, is essentially part of language, *Helen in Egypt* tells us, and Helen is "loved of War" (178). H.D. writes in *Thorn Thicket*, "The war was my husband" (170).

132. In *Majic Ring*, H.D. writes, "I was [Amen's] opposite—well, his opposite number for just that single flash in time. A picture was projected, we were in the picture, I did not see the picture, I was in the picture, the *tableau*, if you will, the cinema 'still.' . . . We [Delia and Masini] had got behind the scene, as it were, or had come on the stage with the Manager or Director, before the play began" (34).

133. Ibid., 24–5.

134. Ibid., 34.

135. Schreber, *Memoirs*, 184, emphasis in the original.

136. Ibid., 121.

137. Ibid., 184.

138. See *Hermetic Definition*, 49–50. Here, in H.D.'s poetic response to Durand's death, "Star of the Day," Durand's death is equated with her maternal delivery of him through writing.

Chapter 3

"Which is the holier?"

Ryder's (W)holes

I. RESISTANCE, CAPTURE

In the next two chapters, I will read Djuna Barnes's *Ryder* and *Nightwood* as suggesting, like H.D.'s work, an unusual openness to unbounded states, and powerful thought and language patterns that may serve in part to stave off or mediate the more devastating experiences described in them, of singularity or individuation reversing into invasive unity or shattering dissolution. These patterns may recur because their end, the sense of oneness that comes with the hiatus of referentiality, appears too foreboding. Barnes's work, also like H.D.'s, I will argue, represents this threatening oneness in dramatic events, and in patterned, circular thoughts and expressions where signifiers and signifieds are unusually disconnected. The power with which these patterns appear, within minimalistic contexts and narrative structures, conveys to readers the sense of dynamic nonconceptuality for which both writers are known.

For Lacan, as I note in my introduction, so-called perverse and psychotic subjects, in contrast to neurotic subjects, lack lack. The felt sense of something lacking and of subjugation to an order is partial (disavowed) or missing (foreclosed), and thus diminished or prevented altogether. Psychotic subjects do not experience separation from the mother, or desire predicated on lack, and do not enter the symbolic realm in which conscious and unconscious mind are barred (reliably separated) from one another. Perverse subjects enter the symbolic order incompletely, experiencing the mother as distinct from themselves, but not as limited by, or desiring, anything outside the mother-child dyad.[1] Writes Lacan in 1956,

> Let's suppose that [a subject's childhood] situation entails for the subject the impossibility of assuming the realization of the signifier father at the symbolic level. . . . He's left with the image the paternal function is reduced to. It's an image which isn't inscribed in any triangular dialectic, but whose function as

> model, as specular alienation, nevertheless gives the subject a fastening point and enables him to apprehend himself on the imaginary plane. . . . Insofar as the relationship remains on the imaginary, dual, and unlimited plane, it doesn't possess the meaning of reciprocal exclusion that is included in specular confrontation, but possesses instead the other function, that of imaginary capture.[2]

Perverse and psychotic subjects experience, at least at times, an other whose ferocious imperative is directed toward only them. They hence engage in attempts to supplement or provide the paternal boundary that brings the symbolic Other into existence. The perverse subject seeks to establish this boundary by staging or enacting the enunciation of the law, and the psychotic subject by fomenting a delusional metaphor in which the enunciation of the law is rendered in imaginary terms.

Lacanian psychoanalyst Bruce Fink ascribes the appearance of the perverse structure almost exclusively (as he sees it) in men to the greater and more genitally localized erotic charge that exists between the male child and the mother figure.[3] However, the young Djuna Barnes's relationship to her grandmother, Zadel Barnes, may constitute an exception; Zadel's letters to her granddaughter, at least, take their erogenous zones as sites of their love.[4] Barnes felt lasting loyalty to her grandmother; however, although she never said so outright, she may also have experienced their love as sexual, as I discussed in the introduction. She writes of their relationship in ways that are usually reserved for sexual love. For instance, to Coleman in 1935, referring to her family's disapproval of her affair with the married artist Peter Neagoe (1881–1960), she writes, "I think suffering for love is how I have learned practically everything I know, love of grandmother up and on—and because, just because, I don't and won't regret it, I get hell from mother and Saxon [her brother]."[5] At any rate, whatever the particulars, Zadel's (and Wald's) treatment of sexual boundaries as oppressive and unhealthy had widely noted effects on Barnes's sense of self, and on her self-presentation.

Read in this light, Barnes's characters and language cite a childhood in which psychic differentiation was recast as cryptophoria and subjectivity constituted by haunting. It is tempting to theorize that as ghosts in Barnes's work seem to abandon, yet control, its characters, so her early exposure to her father's and grandmother's abusive practices might have caused her to perceive others as simultaneously abandoning and controlling her. From these beginnings Barnes, as author, repudiates yet remains haunted by familial power figures, a relation that extends, finally, to an overarching power-inflected vision of the human species and its politics. Contrary to many critical accounts, I suggest that what agency may appear in Barnes's work does not constitute a refusal or revision of social or parental imperatives. Agency appears instead as a haunted, nearly predetermined volition, which retains a trace of difference. In this manner, Barnes's work may be read to invoke not only its own secrets, but also the author's own history. Barnes's cryptic style establishes a difference between knowing and not knowing that acts as a boundary for the "impending and inaccessible" mother figure (*Nightwood* 2–3). However, this boundary also binds the characters, whose actions become increasingly bound by their words.

Scholars have noted that, in Barnes's oeuvre, ambiguously referential language, juxtaposed and shattered narratives, cryptic, fragmentary imagery, and weird character behavior confound the reader seeking clarity, and have little obvious causal relation to one another or to the story taken as a whole. Though it is understood in more thoughtful ways in recent scholarship, in her time this lack of plot and clear import is generally taken as a flaw by editors and contemporaries, and to some extent by herself because, unlike H.D., she relies at times on her literary reception for income: contracts, royalties, and support by patrons, which are somewhat contingent on her perceived success. To Emily Coleman she writes,

> I can't, I never have been able to plot or plan a book or give it, apparently any structure. I don't really think I know what structure is in the accepted manner, or is it that I don't believe in it, for me? . . . It has always been my failure, people from the beginning have cried for plot, I can't think one up.[6]

Neagoe, Barnes's friend and lover at the time when she first offered a draft of *Nightwood* (1936) to friends and editors, responds to the text, to Barnes's torment, by observing "*Nightwood* is a soliloquy. . . . There is nowhere, in all I have so far read, a trace of imparting. . . . It remains a soul talking to itself in the heart of the night."[7] Editor after editor rejects the manuscript on the grounds that it is somehow not meant for other people. Even T.S. Eliot, who eventually championed it though editing it extensively, writes all too famously that *Nightwood* would "appeal primarily to readers of poetry,"[8] and adds later, in an unpublished preface to *The Antiphon*, that *Nightwood* would appear "tedious and incomprehensible" to "people of conventional taste." Eliot correlates this narrow appeal to Barnes's style, which "shatters the normal structure of the English (or of the American) language."[9] Her early critics go further, portraying her work as altogether meaningless. Biographer Andrew Field writes rather patronizingly in 1983 that "philosophizing was not native to Miss Barnes; some intellectual digestive process converts thought into peculiar and rather charming, but meaningless, stylization."[10] Field sees the "tableau vivant" or "artistic unit . . . sufficient unto itself," and claims it, rather than meaning, as the Barnes reader's source of satisfaction.[11] Louis Kannenstine, though an early champion of her work, locates its value almost exclusively in its imagery. He reads her strategy for managing "flux" in her writing's "arrest of . . . experience" and "capture [of the] image."[12] In his reading, Barnes's characters' lives are "struggles to become one unqualified whole, either one thing or the other, but they are blocked by the recognition of their duality, their inescapably fractured being."[13] He sees Barnes's images as substituting for coherent meanings and for the narrative structures that normally enable them.

Barnes's alleged nonmeaning is challenged in early and recent feminist scholarship, where *Nightwood*, primarily, has been described as feminist and queer, as deliberately confounding clarity, patriarchy, and univocity and invoking alternative modes of agency and articulation, even alternative social realms and modes of identification, that inform its character behavior and imbue its silence.[14] Similarly, critics of *Ryder* (1928) have generally seen it as offering alternatives to patriarchy. Sheryl Stevenson has described in its imagery an opposition of "female versions of cultural ideology" to dominant ones, where "outlaw women" undercut hegemony through "parody and revision of dominant Western texts and myths."[15] Daniela Caselli argues that Barnes's work stages its own unnaturalness in order to expose "[t]he erosion of patriarchy and of genre [that] takes place . . . through linguistic proliferation, mimicry, and indecency."[16] Though Barnes sometimes admits to intentionally combating patriarchal discourses, she also tends to align her work with a universal ideal of modernist "high art" as exemplified for postwar critics by celebrated male writers like James Joyce and T.S. Eliot (a dear friend in later life) and to repudiate those who associated her oeuvre with marginal, especially queer, subjectivity.[17] *Nightwood* and *Ryder* obviously do depict marginalized modes of sociality: circus people, queer and transgendered people, night people, Jews in Europe between the world wars, polygamous, matriarchal, and alternative households and lifestyles. However, her works' strange images and enigmatic character behaviors not only suggest marginal and alternative realms and subjectivities, or the failure or refusal of narrative meaning and identity, but also have personal, circular trajectories. They invoke (and dispel) particular determinate content that surfaces among their fragments.

II. CREATIVITY, UNKNOWABILITY

As Kannenstine and Catherine Setz have discussed, a theist-and spiritualist-inflected sensibility underlies Barnes's hard-bitten, irreverent persona and oeuvre.[18] Her letters to Coleman contain an ongoing, Biblical-toned discussion of right and wrong, good and evil, which renders Coleman's dualistic religious vision in the language of possession.[19] Haunting and possession are understood literally in Barnes's early family circle, which itself came to haunt her work. Her grandmother and chief parent figure, Zadel, is an enthusiastic spiritualist and medium, "visited" in séances held throughout Barnes's formative years by the spirits of famous men including Ludwig van Beethoven, Franz Liszt, Lord Kitchener, and Jack London.[20] After Zadel's death, Barnes's stepmother Fanny inherits her talent for "stepping aside" for the entry of spirits, including Zadel herself.[21] The Barnes family's spirits are understood to speak and act through their hosts' bodies for the duration of their visits. Though Barnes positions herself as incredulous toward spiritualism and mocks ghostly visitations, for instance in *Ryder*, nevertheless, the vocabulary of haunting and possession appears in her work and letters. Her 1934–1935 letters to Coleman apply this vocabulary to normally exalted states, describing love as a debased possession and creativity as a sublime one. Barnes writes, for instance, that God, or the "true good," can possess subjects and that this possession is the source of creative genius:

> An evil person is always <u>too</u> near, no matter how far his evil reaches it is also always in your hands, you even feel that you are dealing it out . . . with true good you do not feel this (unless you are Jesus which we are not as humans, so we cannot go into that part of it) in fact when you do feel you are dealing out good, as I did with Robin [Thelma Wood, Barnes's long-term partner and great love], that is a sin—it has to be impersonal and untouchable—only in art does one deal it out, and then as you know, it is not dealt out by you or me, but is put into our hands by some sort of magic or miracle—just for a brief hour or so, it is as tiring as the work of mediums."[22]

Artistic creation is for Barnes a channeling of a "true good" which otherwise only Jesus channels. She maintains this vision throughout her life. Author and photographer Hank O'Neal recounts that "she once said to me, 'When you're creating it's just you and God—then it's only God. The greatest ecstasy is when you're possessed and don't know why.'"[23] Barnes's God is good, and she imagines that this creative possession may be contingent on her ethical choices: "I always thought that if I did anything wrong, if I took a pencil that didn't belong to me, if I was dishonorable in any way . . . then I would be unable to write a word."[24] Barnes relates in a way that she, herself, sees as largely unconscious to an incomprehensible, impersonally good other, surrender to whom may enable creative genius.

Barnes's remarks suggest a divinity whose unknowability makes it inaccessible, except during creative possession. O'Neal recalls her frequent emphasis on her own unknowing in relation to divinity and the "mystery" of life and death.[25] Decades earlier, in *Ryder*, Barnes depicts a God and a Jesus that, the narrator claims, the reader should not presume to know (5). Mockingly she writes of Kate Careless's (Fanny's) mediumistic trances: "She alone who is too ignorant for beauty alone may see beauty; she who is too vulgar for religion may be vouchsafed the word" (223). Yet, this position of unknowing receptivity is what she envisions in her own creative process, and by the same token in her relation to "true good." If God is unknowable, divine possession may result in art whose meaning is unknowable, perhaps in part because it is not mediated by the authorial plotting and structuring that results in narrative coherence. Barnes's channeling of the true good, though she distinguishes it in her letter from channeling "an evil person," may yet resonate with the possessions that she depicts in *Nightwood*. Barnes by her own account is moved by unknown forces in her art.

The unknowability exemplified by God is, according to O'Neal's description, a state to which Barnes herself aspires near the end of her life, when she lives in near total isolation in a Greenwich Village flat.[26] O'Neal, one of her last contacts, writes,

> The mystery she had so consciously cultivated for so many years ruled out [the possibility of help from fans]. Even if there had been no such mystery her pride would have prevented any outside assistance . . . pride, independence, solitude, and anger at a world she neither understood nor wished to be a part of were all that kept her going at the end of her life. She stated this eloquently time and time again.[27]

This cultivation of unknowability may correlate to Barnes's sense of vulnerability in relation to other people. Though she early achieves financial independence and renown as a journalist, a number of factors combine in her later life to throw into stark relief the power of others over her fortunes, her social standing as an artist, and her personal boundaries. One factor contributing to her felt disempowerment is the enigmatic form and style of what she considers her best work: *Nightwood* and *The Antiphon*. At a time when editors insist that *Nightwood* and *The Antiphon* are incomprehensible to the general public, Barnes relies for their reception on the mediation of few sensitive readers with the clout to legitimize them in literary circles. T.S. Eliot, poet Edwin Muir, and United Nations Secretary-General Dag Hammerskjold all mediate Barnes's relationship to her public, and though her regard for them, and their loyalty to her, weather the complications inherent in this role, many real and potential intermediaries are alienated by Barnes's fierce struggles to regain power. As well as relying on others to promote her art, Barnes in thin times relies on the financial support of her brother Saxon, and of heiress Peggy Guggenheim, yet refuses any conditions they attempt to place on her in return. To help her is to have some power over her, and this power must be held very gently.

O'Neal, called to Barnes's side by their mutual friend, the photographer Berenice Abbot (1898–1991), found her virtually alone and took up management of her financial and literary affairs. Yet Barnes comes to perceive O'Neal as both controlling and abandoning her and, after three years, dismisses him. He comments that Barnes "hated [her] dependence" on him, yet that her revocation of his status as her manager occurred just after he spent a week away (to her devastation) on a business trip. O'Neal records that she "kept repeating, 'You had control over me and I can't stand it!'"[28]

Besides his perceived control over her life, Barnes's anger at O'Neal involves his foreword to a 1979 reissue of *Ryder*, which she felt publicly exposed her. She had approved it for publication, but by 1981, maintains that O'Neal's "totally acceptable foreword," as he calls it, had "ruined her reputation."[29] In it, he states with careful modifiers that *Ryder* is "somewhat Rabelaisian," that passages of it were deleted by American censors, and that it is "slightly autobiographical, at least to the extent that various characters in the narrative are easily traced to Miss Barnes's immediate family." He discloses, too, that a dispute between Barnes and *Ryder*'s first publisher, Horace Liveright, prevented its reissue for nearly fifty years.

Though Barnes told critic James Scott and other contemporaries that *Ryder* was entirely autobiographical, it is understandable that she might later prefer to shore up her boundaries by leaving this and her disputes with publishers private.[30] As a woman of colorful reputation living alone, her work received as lurid, grotesque, marginal, *and* autobiographical, Barnes is vulnerable to stigmatization. Age, illness, sexism, heteronormativity, the death of friends, and a rapidly changing world contribute to her vulnerability. But adding force to these factors, I think, is her psychic vulnerability in situations where her boundaries are not entirely hers to control. Seven decades or more after her sexual boundaries are ripped away by Wald, Zadel, and Faulkner, she struggles to protect her felt sense of autonomy against perceived predatory and voyeuristic others. This struggle may take the form of refusals and battles over various terms, arrangements, promotional endeavors and public representations, all proffered variously by O'Neal, publishers, would-be biographers, journalists, filmmakers wishing to produce *Nightwood*, libraries wishing to hold her letters and manuscripts, enthusiasts wishing to quote her work, and even banks offering terms of investment.[31] Barnes's worst fear is that a relative will render her entirely helpless and exposed by consigning her to a nursing home. This is a fear that anyone might share, but it may also evoke earlier betrayals by relatives that resulted in boundary violation.[32]

O'Neal describes Barnes's cultivation of "mystery" as self-directed, yet notes that it was "crucial to her existence."[33] It proceeds, her work suggests, from a childhood where parental demand preyed on psychic differentiation, entailing behavior and speech that locked away the truth of her experience, and finally herself, from the untrustworthy world.

III. EMBEDDED WORDS

For Abraham and Torok, fetishism symptomizes cryptophoria,[34] where subjects know that the fetishized object, phrase or practice is not identical to the unspeakable lost object and scene, yet somehow persist in the paradoxical belief that it is. This has, of course, a correlative effect on the relationship between language and the subject, and in the case of Barnes's work, the relationships among author, character, and language. At first glance, it seems that Abraham and Torok understand fetishism differently than does Lacan: namely, as an oblique way of calling on the lost love object and forbidden secret, so that the libidinal charge associated with them is generated. However, their account of fetishism is not as different from Lacan's as it first appears. In Lacan's model, the fetish supplements the father figure's bar on the demand of the mother, but also represents the mother's demand—just as Abraham and Torok's fetish both invokes and contains the shameful secret. Like Abraham and Torok's fetish-word, the Lacanian fetish represents both the paternal prohibition and the *jouissance* associated with what is prohibited.

However useful these theories may be in describing psychic mechanisms, discursive attempts to categorize subjects as "fetishists" and "perverts," ironically, have difficulty establishing their boundaries. For one thing, since it is not difficult to see "normal" heterosexual sex as itself a staging of castration, psychoanalytic theorists have found it difficult to demarcate perverse sexual behavior from whatever other kinds of sexual behavior may exist. It may be that in perversion, limits are unusually emphatic and central: for instance, in sadomasochism, one person imposes highly dramatized "limits" (immobilization, cuts, whip-lash marks, and/or other visual representatives of castration) on another person, often setting consensual limits on these limits ahead of time, and both identify with the one who is being limited. Further, the mechanisms of perversion and fetishism in theory, both clinical and speculative, appear in various social arenas. Various psychoanalytic theorists see all sexual behavior (Tim Dean and, arguably, the later Freud), all creative writing (Julia Kristeva, Shoshanna Felman), and/or all ideology (Žižek) as constitutively fetishistic, since they all, in different ways, stage and undo castration. In some clinical theory, perversion is seen as a borderline condition that is no longer neurosis but not yet psychosis. As well as seeing perverse subjects as somewhere *between* psychotic and neurotic/normal, there have also been suggestions that they are *both* psychotic and not psychotic, or perhaps have multiple personalities (Goldberg), one or more in each category, as Abraham and Torok's theory might also suggest. Goldberg describes, instead of the usual "horizontal" split between conscious and unconscious knowledge, "vertical" splits that divide consciousness.[35] To add to this inundation of the theoretical boundaries of perversion, it is often difficult to distinguish between neurosis and psychosis when they are discussed in clinical case studies; hence, the interminability of discussions that attempt to determine into which of these categories Freud's patients Little Hans, the Wolf Man, Dora, and other famous "cases" belong. These discursive convolutions seem at times to almost dramatize fetishism, itself, in their encapsulation and preservation of the categories, "pervert" and "fetishist," whose vague meanings yet draw power from the loved shadows of Freud and Lacan.

Notwithstanding this trajectory toward the universal, fetishistic disavowal as a mechanism can be seen to varying degrees in writing, and in behavior. As I discuss in my introduction, the repetition, embedding, and resistance to interpretation that characterize Barnes's writing also characterize fetishism, as I render it through the theories of Lacan, and Abraham and Torok. Her images, stories, and character behaviors present a history of relations, a history that is not meant to be viewed or read, but rather missed: her strangely sexualized relationship with Zadel, and perhaps with her father. Like the fetish, the Barnesian tableau praised by Field and Kannenstine distorts a particular history in signs that are filled with another signification, which thereby bars it from the reader.

IV. LIVING PICTURES, MOTIONLESS MOVEMENTS

The suspended image that Kannenstine sees as Barnes's answer to oscillation between extremes, and Caselli sees as confounding clear meaning, I read as marking the divisions, that Esther Sanchez-Pardo also discusses, in Barnes's narratives and characters.[36] The image elides something that is yet present in them.

Lacan traces the split in the subject to the apprehension of the image as such.[37] Unlike the real world, which is always shifting temporally and spatially, the image is immobile and timeless, perfectly accessible to the gaze. In Barnes's work, it both presents and abjects a trace of a "particular," a real-world bodily history. The word *particular*, for Barnes, indicates what is not signified, what has not been abstracted into a "general" sign. The particular has a variety of signals in her work: silence, movement, departure, spectrality, ambiguity, gaps and holes, dirt, and, as Catherine Whitley has also noted, excrement.[38] It is what her writing seeks to approach, but the approach is always also a departure, the departure an approach. The particular haunts the word and the image.

Kannenstine's and Field's decisions to "reach not beyond the image" (*Ryder*, 3) may have contributed to an early critical tendency to overlook the rich and complex meaningfulness of Barnes's prose. Barnes's allusiveness got her first "book" (*The Book of Repulsive Women*) past American censors, who failed to notice the references to lesbian sex that are obvious to contemporary readers. *Ryder* and *Nightwood* too, have frequencies that have only begun to emerge in critical responses. Barnes's prose, as her skill developed, comes closer to saying nothing direct while remaining meaningful.

Lacan writes—perhaps justifying his own rebuslike style—that "full speech" is fuller the more fragmentary, indeterminate, and seemingly pointless it is.[39] Full speech is "identical to what it speaks about."[40] In other words, full speech is identical to psychotic speech in that both are the speech of the unconscious; however, full speech appears in fragmentary, vanishing form in nonpsychotics, where it is often "a tiny scrap, surrounded by an aura of uncertainty."[41] It appears fleetingly in *Ryder*'s and *Nightwood*'s images and *tableaux* as holes, voids, and ghosts, and also in pairs of things, often with a hole in between. The picturesque image is fetishistically frozen, "mythic" in Roland Barthes's sense, but has a hole with a vanishing, excremental, memory trail that, Barnes suggests, should not be too eagerly washed away.[42] As in Freudian dream analysis, the forms and ostensible meanings of Barnes's images and scenes must be seen as separate, and sometimes very incongruent, for the full speech hidden in them to emerge.[43]

Barnes's writing perhaps acts as a "second event" that, as she theorizes it, "gives. . .body" to preceding ones by calling both her love and its prohibition into being: representing an other that is somehow too near, yet also inaccessible.[44] *Ryder* (1928) and *Nightwood* (1936) both represent this other in the registers of form, imagery, word choice and character behavior. Precise and often repulsive, their images startle with a sudden, fleeting luridness. They often have no obvious causal relation to one another, or to the story taken as a whole, but embed fetishistic fantasy in their very structure and syntax. Rather than suggesting that Barnes herself was bound to it, however, her ability to describe fetishistic mechanisms suggests, if anything, that she had distance from them, although freedom, in Barnes's writing, is always haunted.

In *Ryder* and *Nightwood* disavowed content is depicted as simultaneously fixed and moving. In these works Barnes, perhaps trying to externalize her ghosts or thought patterns, reports on the movements of objects: their genuflections, falling and fixity, departures and returns, perambulations and trails, introjections and evacuations, their merging, splitting, going down. Cathy Caruth has drawn attention to the invocations (by Freud, Lacan, and Paul de Man) of falling and departure as transmitting the break in consciousness that defines trauma; repeating images of falling and departing in Barnes's work may be read in this sense.[45] But these images also, in being invoked and enacted by characters, transmit something of the content associated with the trauma. Barnes's objects and characters' movements, so repetitively departing, falling, and descending, yet motionless, hold the complexities of her meanings, and point, as Tyrus Miller puts it, "to the place and conditions of meaning's decline and fall."[46] Perhaps this is why when one meets *Nightwood*'s Nora, the Barnes character, "at the opera, at a play, sitting alone and apart," Nora's eyes "report not so much the object as the movement of the object" (52). In *Ryder*, disavowed content likewise appears syntactical, incidental and/or as merely passing through. Its ghosts are "in the picture" permanently yet fleetingly, in the act of departing or falling out of it. The ghosts are always already in the past, or the future—perhaps in what Miller describes in a sociohistorical register as "a *posthumous* future in which stories told of selves are already extinguished in advance"—but the ghosts are always present in their departure from the present.[47] Mechanisms of disavowal are also suggested by this unending exodus and fall. Since disavowal knows as well as not knowing, it requires ongoing spoken and behavioral acts of negation that do not so much erase its object-cause, as pose it fleetingly. The departure of these objects suggests the immanent return to (and re-emergence from) the unconsciousness that characterizes their disavowed status.

V. ORIFICES AND ISSUES

Ryder (1928) describes, in a variety of literary styles, the lives and times of the Ryder family and those associated with them by blood or sex. The chapters rapidly skim the lives of a Ryder great-grandmother and grandmother before coming into intermittent focus on the three-generation household of the grandmother, her son, his wife, his mistress and their eight children. This household is modeled on Barnes's own. *Ryder*'s fifty chapters are a series of vignettes, monologues and (a few) poems that pertain loosely to the Ryder homestead, its environs, lineages, neighbors, sociohistorical context, stories, ideologies, and characters. Its central characters appear in most of these. On first publication, *Ryder* was immediately censored by the American Post Office, to Barnes's great indignation. The expurgated passages had to do with bodily fluids, as Paul West tells us in his afterword to the 1990 Dalkey edition. Although to everyone's surprise *Ryder* quickly became a bestseller, it has not shared *Nightwood*'s high critical acclaim. Although some later criticism has taken its socially subversive and biographical elements seriously, it has only recently (for instance, by Taylor, Miller, and Caselli) been recognized for its aesthetic and theoretical complexity.

While I agree with Taylor and Caselli's theses about the literary work of Barnes's textual proliferations, multivalent affects, and polyphony, I maintain that Barnes also depicts *Ryder*'s characters' psychic negations, and the correlative gaps in its ideological universe, as the nightmare aspect of this multitudinousness. Barnes problematizes the idea that proliferation and polyphony are wholly positive strategies, chiefly by associating them with Wendell's unbridled sexual reproduction. Wendell, an advocate and exemplar of proliferation, is unable to maintain and support his two families and in *Ryder*'s last chapter sends his wife and her children away to fend for themselves, as Barnes's father did to her mother, herself and her two brothers.

The gaps and holes that appear among pluralities in *Ryder* are consistently associated with the disavowals, betrayals, and boundary violations of characters by other characters. Wendell's excision of part of his family from the whole is one of many examples of the exclusion of characters that often appear alongside images of ghosts, gaps, holes, cracks, and dualisms. Taylor writes that "'gaps' are not necessarily loci of meaning in *Ryder*" because "for Barnes the issue of hiddenness or textual lack is connected to the problem of censorship"; she argues that rather than being represented by textual gaps, "the complexities of 'sexuality and sexual abuse' are present at the very surface of Barnes's playful text."[48] The complexities of sexual abuse do appear at the surface of the text, in the book's structure, imagery, and narrative. But the way they appear points to something that is elided, distorted or violated by the power operations that determine the surface of the text and for which the censored substitution of asterisks for explicit words may have been an apt metaphor for Barnes. To suggest this elided content, Barnes relies especially on images of holes and dualities, doubled formal structures, and fragmented narratives. These gaps and redoublings, she further suggests, are effects of all speech and writing. They depict what is abjected by the forcible transmutation in speech and writing of the body into symbol, the particular into the general, the unnatural into the false natural or, in Barthes's sense, mythic.

The personalities of *Ryder*'s characters correlate to the ways that they relate to these textual gaps and negations, whether they fixate on them, intent on filling them, are split or swallowed by them, or gesture self-reflexively toward them. The characters thus function as exemplars of different modes of denegation, defined, as Miller puts it, "by their relation to the absence left behind by the evacuation of sense from language, gestures, and action."[49] However, my intent is less to draw psychoanalytic profiles of *Ryder*'s characters than to introduce the curious ubiquity, variety, and effects of gaps and dualisms in *Ryder*, and to suggest the ways in which they might represent Barnes's own concern with establishing and problematizing psychic boundaries. I read *Ryder*'s widely noted commentary on the specific political conditions of the time as proceeding from a more central preoccupation with articulating gaps in language and consciousness, the modes by which people negate them, and the personal and social effects of these negations. Read in this way, *Ryder* is a psychoanalytic *tour de force*, an archaeology and typology of personal and social fragmentation. The ghosts that populate its ruins are themselves articulations that are imbricated in the splitting process.

The kind of subversion that held Barnes's lasting interest, and that *Ryder* does not undermine even as it offers it up, is a language that gestures at the disjunctures that alienate it from particularity and materiality, or synonymously, as Miller argues, from the possibility of framing narratives of present self-identity. The styles of *Ryder*'s narrator(s) and voices of its characters are scintillating and evocative, multivalent (signs seem to simultaneously denote two or more things and evoke many more), ambiguous (images, relations between objects and events, descriptions and plots, signs and significations are all unclear) and idiosyncratic (pictures and signs are disarranged, removed from their usual contexts and placed in alien ones or do not refer to a clear meaning). This is language that draws attention to its own unreliable and polyvalent signification, what Miller calls its "erosion of distinction across a range of formal, stylistic, and thematic registers."[50] Through parodies of literary genres and anachronistic texts, ambiguous and multivalent language, and framing and juxtaposition of narratives, Barnes exposes—story by story—the fantasies of fetishistic universality that, she implies, is invoked by her snippets of narrative. Her devices open gaps in these fantasies, and within these gaps lie the particular physical realities that language secretes, in the sense both of expelling and of making secret. These gaps and secretions are often associated with images of the anatomical parts that they suggest to her: anuses and vaginas, and the excrement and infants that issue from them, tend to signal full speech, as Lacan describes it.[51] Though I doubt that Barnes intended this precise typology, I would suggest that infants are predominantly aligned with melancholic or hysterical language, and excrement with sadistic and cynical language.[52] Melancholically incorporated others, preserved within the subject by silence or enigmatic speech, reappear in childbirth or in spectral form; digested (discursively appropriated) others return as excretion.

Barnes suggests that this abjected matter somehow constitutes the nourishment of the discourse that abjects it. *Ryder*'s narratives and images are haunted by the particular body or thing eaten and digested by language. Representation itself entails the digestion of the particular by the sign. Language thus feeds on the body or the particular, "that which thou art," and transmutes it into picturesque "shit," "a sign against thy body" (5).[53] In *Ryder*, the "whole" is the "hole" filled with someone's narrative (or actual) shit. The particular, the hole that appears in full speech, passes into the general, the whole. Speech is unmoored from particular meanings, except when it buries these meanings in indirect articulations. The ghost of the eaten body, the particular, appears in and moves through *Ryder*'s images of enclosed spaces:

rooms, pairs, pictures, orifices and other holes and framed spaces, as well as structural and narrative and, as Miller argues, epochal gaps.[54]

Barnes, here, self-reflexively rearticulates personal negations and abjections and their effects, both on her relationships to other people and on the social world in general. This rearticulation may have served to strengthen her sense of autonomy in a world where, as her work suggests, personal autonomy is robbed by power figures and hegemonic discourses. However, the problem with this rearticulation as a means of shoring up boundaries is that there is no stable difference between what is defended against, the disavowed content, and the rearticulation itself. While the particular hole and the general whole could be said to be one more binary opposition in *Ryder*, their difference is a matter of perspective, like figure and background in the pictorial illusion in which you see either a goblet or two profiles facing one another. The form that the gaze fixes on is real: the other is ghostly. This constantly reversing opposition between particular and general, spoken and unspoken, being and haunting is the frame within which *Ryder's* other shaky oppositions (for example, hegemony and counter-hegemony) emerge and pass away. The discursive conflation between the ideological wholes that the narrator(s) and characters like Wendell articulate and the holes in these wholes that swallow up characters like Julie, other violated girls, and ghosts suggest the instability of the negation that structures this opposition. The gaps in *Ryder* depict not repression, not the unknown, but rather disavowal. *Ryder*'s narratives do not repress, but rather "disarrange" themselves by disjunction of their parts. Narrative fragmentation, ambiguous language, and images of gaps and dualities might be read as Barnes's rendering of a literary unconscious in an experiential world that recognizes only consciousness.

Besides anatomical splits, childbirth, and excrement, another way that *Ryder* reveals the splitting and redoubling effects of languaging is through its stories within stories and its fragmentary vignettes. Like the archways that *Ryder*'s "stiltsman" compares to the open legs of a woman, "the natural heritage erected to man's achievements," stories and vignettes within and alongside one another frame each other and reveal wholeness as a lie (20). In its structure as well as content, *Ryder* foregrounds the frames of narrative and genre by which "the picture" is necessarily constituted. Since each story and vignette is both picture and frame (for other stories), there can be no consistent choice of foreground and background. Each gives way, re-emerging only perhaps at the edges of another one. Like a body in a perverse fantasy, these parts seemingly function independently of one another in "conglomerate juxtaposition."[55] The stories they tell are "nothing erased but much submerged" as a result (13). As the pictures that lie inches thick on Sophia's walls present more resonant images underneath sensationalistic and trashy newspaper clippings pasted on top, so *Ryder*'s palimpsestic form buries the depth-meanings it presents:

> At forty [Sophia's] pictures were an inch deep, at sixty, a good two inches from the wall; the originals were, as she herself was, nothing erased but much submerged. . . . Even Alex had gone, he, who had for so long held sway, slowly ebbed, and in his stead rose that last tide, clippings from newspapers. For in the end this was her court—false prophet, false general, the pretty girl untimely raped, some woman aptly killed, some captain who claimed discovery of the North Pole, some Jack who had climbed a steeple top; all in a conglomerate juxtaposition, and under all, smiling in forlorn inevitability, Beatrice Cenci, Shakespeare and the Divine Dante. (13–14)

As well as the novel's conglomerate structure and imagery, the *Ryder* family dynamics could be imagined to mimic Sophia's newspaper "court": the "false prophet" (Wendell) and "false general" (Sophia herself), "the pretty girl untimely raped" (Julie), "some woman aptly killed" (Wendell's first infidelity), "some Jack who had climbed a steeple top" (Wendell or Timothy), and underneath all this, forlorn and inevitable family ghosts.

Like Sophia's clippings *Ryder*'s characters and chapters, too, obscure or gainsay rather than support one another. The voices of its characters and unidentified narrator(s) deliver a cacophony of stories that serve their speakers' particular interests and desires with naturalized arrangements of signs.[56] The stories proliferate with figures and images of duality surrounding a question or an opening, often associated with an anus or vagina. The one who believes these stories within stories or who swallows them whole, *Ryder* suggests, is swallowed up by them.

VI. PREDATORY IMAGES

The image, not the thing, is what *Ryder* proscribes in chapter one, "Jesus Mundane," whose narrator mandates fetishism in King James biblical language, instructing the reader to "[r]each not beyond the image" (3), and to follow convention. While Taylor reads this instruction as "Barnes's maxim" and "the theory of reading that *Ryder* proposes," I don't see reason to take this instruction more at face value than any other narrative instruction in *Ryder*.[57] Ryder has many voices, which, like the narrator of "Rape and Repining," who states for instance that a girl, because she has been raped, "should be Scourged! Flayed! Whipped! Stocked! Cried against! (28), are not meant to present Barnes's views. I read "Jesus Mundane" rather as framing the world in which *Ryder* unfolds and suggesting the way in which most of its own characters do relate to it. Indeed, I read in certain passages and chapters the downfall of the mandate that "Jesus Mundane" offers.

> Go not with fanatics who see beyond thee and thine. . . . Go thou, then, to lesser men. . . . Thy rendezvous is not with the Last Station, but with small comforts, like apples in the hand, and small cups quenching, and words that go neither here nor there, but traffic with the outer ear, and gossip at the gates of thy insufficient agony. Reach not beyond the image. For these idols and these lambrequins [etc.] are not for thee in the spirit, but for thee only in the outward manifestation; nor are the Beasts for thee. (3)

In this dystopic manifesto, speech and knowledge are static, "go[ing] neither here nor there," and spectacular, barred from the "Thing" that lurks behind them. This split between image and thing causes a logorrheic, potentially infinite redoubling: the attempt to fix a sublime object "beyond," which keeps dividing and retreating from representation. "Neither shalt thou have gossip with martyrs and saints and cherubim. . . . For some is the image, and for some the Thing, and for others that Thing that even the Thing knows naught of, and for one only the meaning of That beyond That" (4). Because the reader's desire, his "wound" and "need" for the speaker (presumably Jesus Mundane) are unknown by him, his behavior must consist in the mimicry of other people. His identity and his language are copies of "outward manifestations." He is limited to surface effects: "And speak not of Me, for thou knowest not of what thou speakest. . . . Nay, thou knowest not the extent of thy wound, nor the matter I have with it, neither knowest thou how far thy soul comes toward me, nor yet how far I lean outward to catch it by the hand" (5). In the universe proscribed by *Ryder*'s scripture, identity and speech should be mimicry. *Ryder*'s text gives form to this mandated mimicry with its many and celebrated parodies, and the strange slippage of identity between its characters and the characters in the stories they tell. All, *Ryder* suggests, are images of "Things" which are somehow more real.

Ryder's characters relate to this unreal state of affairs by being, like its structure and its stories, variously fractured. Sophia, the grandmother, who through her secret begging is the Ryder family's sole source of financial support, and Wendell, son and father, an infantile, promiscuous patriarch intent on fathering children, both exemplify perverse disavowal and identification with power. Sophia and Wendell's sadistic language use attempts to fix social relations with themselves as (quite literally) inside the other, as the thing that splits the other. Sophia, a "cynical" pervert, tells lies that she knows are lies, hoping that others will believe them. Wendell, who fully identifies with the Other, tells lies that he believes are true by virtue of his having told them. He literally "knows not what he does," as Kate remarks (159).[58] Amelia,

Wendell's martyred and miserably fertile wife, could be described as masochistically or melancholically perverse (the two are synonymous for *Ryder*'s purposes). Amelia criticizes but swallows the lies and family arrangements Wendell proffers; although she knows very well that he is a fraud, she nevertheless imagines him sublime until the end. Anne, her sister and correspondent, is phobic, perpetually appalled by smut and grotesquerie, her fixation on it identical to that of the fetishist, Horace Chubble, except in the tenor of her enjoyment. Kate Careless, Wendell's more contented mistress, knows that Wendell is perverse and their relationship "disgusting," but has developed a taste for "the flavor of motherhood" (170 – 1). Julie and Timothy are Amelia's older children, and Elisha is Kate's older son. Julie, *Ryder*'s Barnes character, is silent in an attempt to refuse the splitting between knowing and not knowing imposed on her by her family and their language use. This attempt is not wholly successful in *Ryder* or, if we read it as an extension, in *Nightwood.* Both Julie and *Nightwood*'s Barnes character, Nora, are cryptophores, split and haunted by the ghosts of their loved ones. Wendell's lovers, Molly Dance and Lady Terrence Bridesleep, are depicted, on the contrary, as humorous, idiosyncratically perverse women who refuse *Ryder*'s symbolic equivalent of feminine melancholia by refusing to conceive Wendell's children. Molly Dance, an exuberantly sloppy counter-mythographer whose stories are crafted to "suit" her, is self-reflexively ideological and, in that sense, responsible.[59] Timothy, logorrheic, pours forth proliferating, free-associative lists and dualisms. Like Wendell's unbridled procreation and subsequent disowning of part of his family, Timothy's "issueless repetition," filled with images of holes and dualisms, suggests that the counterpart to the multiplying impulse that *Ryder* seems to celebrate may be a tendency to pointlessly fracture wholes into parts.[60] Dr. O'Connor, who delivers the Ryder children and could therefore, by *Ryder*'s logic be anti-melancholic, is an exemplar of a perhaps more useful self-awareness than that available to the Ryder family. O'Connor favors palimpsestic imagery, unclear referentiality, wide-ranging parody, double entendres, and narratives in which what first appears to be a story progresses in such an unclear and absurd manner that it opens "storyness," or narrative, itself, to uncertainty, as Miller also notes.[61] O'Connor's language does not pose distinct possibilities, but suggests vacillations in signification itself, words that straddle multiple meanings, which are separated by silences. The idiosyncratic narratives, double entendres, and palimpsestic particulars deployed by O'Connor, some (unnamed) narrators, and other characters (such as Molly Dance) gesture persistently toward aporias, as if opening holes in a too-full language. Nevertheless, meanings seem to fill these holes almost as quickly as they open; nonmeaning is apprehended only as fleeting.

The first exemplar *Ryder* offers of the perverse relation to language that "Jesus Mundane" proscribes is Sophia Grieves Ryder. Though partially undone by her loyalty to Wendell and her grief over her second husband, Sophia is what Žižek calls a "cynical" perverse character: she does not believe her own lies, but hopes that others will. Sophia is the authority of the family because she is willing to deceive everyone and believe no one, including herself. Her very nickname, "the general," suggests both military authority and the opposite of the "particular"—that is, it represents language itself, always split in Barnes's universe from the particulars of its referents. Accordingly, though, "where the race in general enters a man's head . . . there, in the end, you'll find many persons in particular," the general Sophia's lies cover these particulars (45). Knowing "the way into the heart of man," (15) which is "an insulting shape" (238), perhaps split in two, Sophia buries herself there with "the simple magic of the word 'mother'" (12), the first word spoken in whatever language by most infants, evoking their first heartbreak.[62] Sophia's early years suggest the formation of this relation to the Other:

> In that house of thin partitions and sounding existence, she had hatched on every side and, coming forth, noted with approbation the moment when sympathy in the father for the new-born, newly come, took him at four in the morning in dangling nightshirt, to the "Floating Bowl" (or night vase), for as she later wrote to her friend Tollop, of the Gazette, "It did please me to see in my father consternation and its accompaniment." (9)

This "accompaniment," given Barnes's love of wordplay and elliptical presentation of the abject, is constipation. Thus, having constipated her father,

> In after life . . . proved a step in the mastering of her métier. When Sophia came of age and set up house for herself (as her humorous stock would have done before her), she rendered tribute to this memory by making something both rounded and excellent to enshrine it, for she ordered and saw executed, five fine chamber pots of a lustrous finish with one line upon their bellies' surface (just under the lip, lettered in flourished gold, and garnished with devices in bows and cupids) of the axiom,
>
> "Needs there are many
> Comforts are few
> Do what you will
> 'Tis no more than I do." (11)

Sophia's gaze, then, freezes her father in mid-dump, and she commemorates this vision with a series of inscribed chamber pots. These give her bygone father permission to finish the job, and tell him that, nonetheless, his dump is no greater than hers. The final chamber pot, "dedicated to her own use" and reading "Amen," suggests that the preceding verse is also addressed to the heavenly father, whose excrement is thereby declared no greater than her own (11), just as the anal-sadistic infant of Kleinian theory would wish. Sophia's ability to produce shit on par with God's is vouchsafed by the immaculately (or spectrally) conceived Wendell, the product of an "infusion" of Beethoven's ghost, with an "aroma . . . ripe to the nose of justice" (169).

Klein writes that in the anal-sadistic phase (which for some lasts a lifetime), excrement is seen as a harmful substance and its release as an attack on the parents or parent substitutes. Retaliatory excremental projectiles from the parents are then feared. If the subject is able to progress beyond this "paranoid-schizoid" apprehension of battling part-objects into an apprehension of the parents as "whole objects," the sadistic urge to destroy their "bad parts" will oscillate with depressive guilt and the anxious desire to make amends. This depressive vision of whole objects is what, in Sanchez-Pardo's reading, *Ryder* demonstrates the failure to achieve. Taking her cue, we can read Sophia's chamber pots as an anal-sadistic challenge to the paternal "symbolic order" (to impose Lacanian on Kleinian theory) that allows us to judge and generalize. Indeed, later we learn that Sophia "was the Law" to her family. She sets herself in the place of power as "the general," "greater than" those who devour her, and equal to the father in the manipulative power of her shit. She becomes this Law by being devoured and sublimated into testimony. Her devourers say, "She is greater than we":

> She was the law. She gave herself to be devoured, but in the devouring they must acclaim her, saying, "This is the body of Sophia, and she is greater than we." Devour her they did, and said, "This is the body of Sophia, and she is greater than we"; all but Julie, who loved her most. It was Julie who gave this queen her mortal hurt, for that she loved her best. Sophia offering her heart for food, Julie spewed it out on a time, and said, "I taste a lie!" And Sophia hearing, cried in agony, but Julie went apart. (16)

Julie's discovery of Sophia's lies splits her apart from her family and from herself. Sophia knows that her lies weigh in against the truth for the hearer regardless of whether they are believed. "Know the truth as she may," she said to herself, "the thing I've seemed will balance the account" (15). And indeed, Julie "held" Sophia's lies in "after life . . . as the best part of a capacious soul," a formulation that suggests disavowal and the cryptophoric "incorporation" of Sophia's lies in Julie's psychically fragmented "after life." Abraham and Torok describe "incorporation" in terms reminiscent of Julie's unsatisfying consumption and internalization of Sophia's lies: "The Fantasy of incorporation is the first lie, the effect of the first rudimentary form of language. It is also the first instrument of deception. Satisfying need by offering food does not sate the actual and persistently active hunger for introjection. The offer of food only serves to deceive it."[63] This unsatisfying food comes out as shit: "of the banquet doeth the turde tell" (65). But for *Ryder*'s characters, there is no "real" food, no experience that broadens and nourishes the ego, as Abraham and Torok imagine that there can be.[64] We are told that Sophia lies to her family, but *Ryder* provides little in the way of examples, perhaps because examples of lies would have to be contrasted with examples of truths. Sophia hides her begging; her "Do not strike her" (109) may redirect attention from Wendell's sexual abuse of Julie; and the stories she reads to Julie fetishize dying little girls—yet these lies are the very fabric of the Ryder family's existence.

Ryder does allude to a divine excrement that Sophia might challenge with her own, but of this, "Jesus Mundane's" narrator tells us, nothing is known. The loosening and tightening of the human heart, he tells us, is nothing akin to the same action in God's bowels:

> When thy heart loosens to hear the Miracles, and of the dead arisen and the damned that were and are not, and yet are, when thy heart tightens to the direction and the way to Holy Places, that have been found and lost again forever, think not that it is a tithe of the loosening and the tightening that was among the bowels of Him who gave them birth and who gave them death in the selfsame dream. For thou knowest nothing of the mighty rains of Heaven that come down of Him and that return to Him, *that even thou might be included and yet made nothing, for thou wast only one within the way*. (4, emphasis added)

God's excrement "includes" the hearer and "yet [makes him] nothing," "only one within the way," another turd in the divine chute. It is such an unknown God that Sophia (re)incarnates. Her transubstantiation, the offering of her body to her family for food, demonstrates the work of language, the passage of the particular body (hers) to the general "claim," the excremental narrative. Secret-ed and excreted, Sophia's body becomes a smaller scale rendition of the "heavenly rains" in which the subject is "included and yet made nothing." At least, this is Julie's experience of her place in Sophia's stories. Accordingly, the picture, on page 11, of Sophia excreting into her chamber pot as Alex arrives on the scene, is identical to the picture, on page 90, of the "heavenly rains" in the marks that indicate the sources of the effluence and the effluent itself: one or two rounded part-shapes (representing distended posteriors) from which a deluge of dotted lines issues from a single point, as excrement does and rain does not.

Ryder's characters acknowledge the transmutation of the body into excremental language. Man, Amelia tells Kate Careless, has intercepted the shit that should have gone to earth with floors, and then replaced it with words.

"What can prevail now that we put floors and pots beneath [shit] . . . but only man going head foremost, offering a word. And what is there in a word that is magnificent or of help to the land?" (115) By man's "vision," laments Amelia, the droppings that sustained nature's cycles of consumption and excretion now fall short (114). Unlike Sophia, who commemorates prematurely arrested shit (her father's constipation) in verse, Amelia sees arrested shit as something she must clean: "you can't expect but that we'll have the dunging when [Wendell] has such faulty fancies" (116).

This cleaning of the turds on civilization's platforms is what O'Connor warns against in *Nightwood*. Since excrement is the only remaining testimony to the digested particular, washing it away erases history and alienates, says O'Connor, "the American" from himself. Amelia's "dunging" (Kate, as usual, is too lazy to participate) corresponds to her melancholically perverse attitude toward Wendell's mythology. Though she knows that he "nests with vermin, [and] beneath the shadow of his wings, corruption breeds" (150), she nevertheless grants him the place of the Law, seeing him as "nature in its other shape" and "a deed that must be committed" (241). Though criticizing the "faulty fancies," Amelia cleans the ensuing shit and swallows the shittiness of his other domestic arrangements, imagining him sublime until the end.[65] Her cleaning of his pigeons' shit mirrors her internalization of his lies and her eventual effacement of herself from the family.

Amelia's dream of an "Ox of a Black Beauty," who asks her for "a place in your God, or I go to acquaint him that I am, and he will damn himself in me, for there is need of that also" suggests the disavowal involved in her deification of Wendell (99). In the dream, she peeps through the keyhole into a room where she also lies on the bed, dreaming. The walls are lined with pictures of "women going from nowhere to nothing, with snood and long leaning throats and hands held loose for lack of sorrow" and a tapestry of "Friars going from nowhere to nowhere, holily." Split into past and future, one place and another place, this "nowhere to nowhere" and "nowhere to nothing" render the placelessness, the constant receding movement into the future, the past, the elsewhere, with which Barnes portrays disavowed content. These friars and women, though fixed in picture frames, go from "nowhere to nowhere" and "nowhere to nothing" as if the depicted act of going creates a doubled nowhere: one to come from and one to go to, both outside of the picture. The dream-self of the doubled Amelia denies the ox, telling him he "must labor." This denial represents her characteristic barring of uncertainty, which returns, as I will show, in her "labor" of childbirth. Instead of giving the ox "a place in [her] God," Amelia "turned and turned about in the chamber, taking things up and laying them down" (99). The effects of Amelia's melancholia also appear in *Ryder*'s stories within stories, told by Wendell and Amelia, of redoubled women and death in childbirth. Splitting and redoubling is the natural state of women, Amelia and Wendell suggest, although it generally results in death, since splitting copulation with a man is followed by deadly childbirth.

The chief man to create and fill the gap that narratives make in "woman," Wendell's stories assert, is Wendell. He is the father whose injunction, thick with innuendo, is to "enjoy!"—and it is he that must be enjoyed. A textbook pervert, he imagines himself as completing his mother, Sophia, calling himself the "life" of her "suffering" and "note" of her "instrument" (169). Her own wish to be buried with his cock ring, "the ring of bone given to me by the hand of my second son, Wendell, first intended, and carved with painstaking lust, that the utmost aboriginal satisfaction, due the women of his house, might be rendered," suggests that his perverse position does originate from her desire (80). A weird intimacy is also suggested by Wendell's description of Sophia's breast as the "preliminary basting" in a series of (otherwise sexual) encounters that "cooked" him (168).

Wendell, the "Father of All Things," divides women from themselves and from one another (210). He is *Ryder*'s chief mythologist, the father of its fragmented and distortedly rearranged universe. In his stories, his self-interest is not distinct from the stories' meaning. Wendell believes in the determining power of speech and identifies fully with his enunciations: "What I would be, that I say I am, and thus, eventually, I become" (165). He assumes the place of the Lacanian big Other to whom all language is addressed: "I sport a changing countenance. I am all things to all men, and all women's woman" (164). Wendell's stories—not lies, but perversions—signify what Barthes might call "Wendellness." Nothing is erased, but all is arranged in the service of Wendellness.

Wendell's story of the Beast Thingumbob, in chapter 27, is an instance of this arrangement in the service of Wendellness. Here Thingumbob's love, "the Cheerful," asks Thingumbob to prove that he loves her by promising to bury her, and describes language as deception: "Tell them [her coming children] thenceforth nothing of me, nor picture me to them in any way . . . for I am, and soon shall be as I am not, and they must know no deception" (121). While the Cheerful may be "right," consonant with Barnes's own view in denouncing language and the "picture," the Wendellness signified is that mothers need not be spoken of since they, too lofty for the deceptions of language, prefer no commemoration. The male need only impregnate and bury the female to prove that he loves her. Wendell, one of whose affairs has already resulted in death in childbirth, becomes the ideal lover by implication.[66]

Unlike Sophia, who impersonates "everyone's mother" but knows better, Wendell really thinks he can be everyone's father (176–7). Thus, when Lady Terrence provides him with "No Child also," he is silenced and perforated: "Wendell opened his mouth, but no sound came" (211). For Wendell, women's vision "corrupts" them by threatening his universal status. "There are no good women," he tells Elisha. They "see too much from the start" and do not "take sides" (his side, of course) as he thinks they ought. "Confinement would, in fact, only make the matter worse, for alone, they act before God. That is religion" (225–6). Even if a woman were isolated, it would be God, not Wendell, who was her object. Wendell, who believes in justice, defines woman as the "spectator" of injustice, who watches "one man betraying another" from the audience. Wendell fears that woman, not "tak[ing] sides," preserves the anamorphosis contained in the gaze, the gap where specters haunt his narratives (224).

Both Wendell, in particular, and *Ryder*, as a whole, suggest that women find in the inexplicit, unclear and inevident the parts of themselves that were left there. Wendell contrasts his own liking for certainty with the likings of women, who, "with some unknown dexterity, take comfort from anything that has no evidence" (203). O'Connor ascribes this to "God in them," and claims, "It accounts . . . for the peculiar difference in the suicides of man and woman" (203). Whereas women rarely theorize their actions, he suggests, man must have theoretical "platforms" that elevate him to himself. He must identify his corpse with an absolute in order to make of suicide an "absolute" act in philosophical terms. Says O'Connor,

> A man may commit suicide for any number of the same reasons that a woman commits suicide, but he never lets the effect seal the cause, he reasons it out, he leaves notes, he says it was this, or that, or the other, in an endeavor to place himself on an equal footing with God. It is to him death of God and the father. . . . He goes to his mirror . . . he looked into that mirror as a lad, and understood that face. What must it be, when he looks and sees a face he does not understand? Troubled—why? Because he cannot kill himself without including his will in that action. He knows that if he kills himself, he is a slave of that action, so with the soul of a slave he bargains, and makes great argument about a thing that has not only no base for argument but no way but the way including his will. He says to himself, "I must abandon you. How shall I abandon you?" Thus, he makes for himself a pact. "If I kill me, my corpse shall be, in my terms absolute, and by myself, myself made not myself—voilà!" (203)

Here, man identifies his corpse with his own ideal ego, which he wishes to preserve intact even in death. The circular logic by which he clings to autonomy in death by splitting himself and having one part do away with the other results, says O'Connor, from his knowledge that there is duality: "God and the father" (204). Women, on the other hand, "one and all commit, in that act, their body to death's custom, neither making bargain nor asking for precepts and points of departure, nor platforms for philosophy, because women know that there is God only" (204). "Woman," O'Connor suggests, surrenders wholly in death to something not herself. The difference between woman's "God only" and man's "God and the father" is in reason's "great argument," which allows man to imagine himself in dialectical terms in death as in life, "by myself, made not myself."

Man is split and incontinent God splits man, and preys on man through woman. Woman is what man tries to fill himself by filling: "for man there is nothing that on him preys but God, and He upon him preys night and day, dreaming of greatness, threaded on the human agony, as man sets his game spinning on the helix of a vixen's whim" (206). God tops man through woman. Man, trying to fill her, instead finds himself in the reverse position, "threaded" by God. Like a "shadow jackal," *Ryder* tells us, "woman" preys on male civilization and the reason that has accomplished it, transforming it when it "enters" her by some peculiar bodily alchemy. Man is therefore prompted to ask,

> What is woman? Wherein comes that of her which we are not? What destroys our reason in her, when we see it enter her as we would, and come forth as she will? What in her, like a shadow jackal, preys upon the mound of our accomplishment, dragging off that of it we thought most rotten with defeat, to make of it a halter and a noose? For man rides the monster civilization, but to woman goes the shoe cast of it, in which is the exact record of the journey. (206)

What is buried by civilization returns via woman to hang it. Thus women, who keep this "exact record" of civilization's journey, unman men. Wendell's encounters with the Lady Terrence Bridesleep and Molly Dance can deflate his fantasy of universal fatherhood not only with particulars and desires that he cannot contain, but also by bringing the "past" (creation stories, things that they've eaten, shit) into the present. It is God, these passages assert, who "threads" or feminizes Wendell through his contact with women, who defeat his dialectics with their atemporal, aspatial messes. His encounters with them subject him to a present that (unlike the "monster civilization") cannot be straddled and ridden because it includes the past and future.

A "child" himself, Wendell identifies as each child he begets (204). Like himself, his children shall be "All Things" (210). He re-enacts a fantasy of polymorphous becoming with himself as his own Protean product. However, his dump of Amelia finally forces him to relinquish the positions of father and child: "I have no children. I have unfathered myself" (239). This auto-unfathering is followed by his first subjection to the gaze of the "creeping things" of the world:

> the creeping things that he had not numbered or known, looked at him from a million eyes, and his eyes were there also . . . and he spoke not. . . . And everything and its shape became clear in the dark . . . and lifted their lids and looked at him; in the air and in the trees and on the earth and under the earth, and regarded

> him long, and he forbore to hide his face . . . they lifted their lids and regarded him, and spoke not in their many tongues. . . . Closing in about him nearer, and swinging out wide and from him far, and came in near and near, and as a wave, closed over him, and he drowned, and arose while he might yet go. (242)

Wendell finally imagines himself from the other's perspective: "his eyes were there also," watching himself. Perhaps for the first time, he sees where he is not. The gaze of the other "came in near and near, and . . . closed over him." Wendell, *Ryder*'s last picture, both drowns and arises to go. He splits into two and, ghostly, passes away.[67]

While Wendell's relation to language's duality and gap is perverse, Timothy seems to envision it in an even more literal, embodied way. His diction and concerns persistently articulate dualities and gaps that he tries to fill, it seems, by saying everything.[68] However, his method of pairing and listing things itself illustrates the difference that separates one word from another, the difference that structures language, but cannot be put into language. Timothy, "who was God and the Father," is a geyser of lists and dualisms, his compulsive collecting and pairing of words suggesting his alienation from them:

> Quoth Timothy: I hate and I loathe and I love and I mourn thy body and soul. The old and the new, the dying and living, the sign and the symbol, the follies and foibles, thy good and thy bad, thy sick and thy well, thy ups and thy downs, thy riches and wants. Thy thickness and thinness, thy roundness and flatness, thy wet and thy dry. [Etcetera, etcetera]. Exclaiming and saying, quoting and sighing, they stood far asunder and clove to each other. Saying and sighing, exclaiming and talking, over and over, forever a little. (134)

Perhaps because of his need to speak in dualisms, Timothy is keen to place "holiness" between the eyes of others, particularly those of an unnamed whore. He claims that

> all beasts have the holy look who have their eyes on either side, for they are apart and contrive not together, and the one sees not what is seen by the other, and mix not their roots—the ox and the goat, the lamb and the deer. . . . "And I would," he added, "that your own eyes were not so dumbfounded acquainted, for it's a terrible time I'm having setting holiness between them; and there, I fear me, it will meet its death of tight strangulation." (197)

Timothy would split the whore's gaze so that one eye did not see what the other saw, like his own schizoid vision that can see only pairs of things. If her gaze was split he could "set . . . holiness between" her eyes. For Timothy, "God and the father," "holiness" describes the psychic fragmentation that motivates his compulsive arrangement of things into pairs and lists. These eyes, between which he is unable to set a gap, unhallow Timothy by focusing together on him.

Molly Dance has a similar effect on Wendell as the whore's on Timothy. Liking "all things, of all kinds, all at once, in the same place" (193), she establishes a space that Wendell is unable to split with himself. He instead finds a multitude of others in it, most notably God, the father of Molly's last-born, whom Wendell had hoped to father. Molly and the whore refuse to provide a discursive or physical space, beyond the sexual encounter, for Wendell and Timothy to fill.

Other characters in *Ryder*, rather than being eager to fill the space, neutrally acknowledge it as something that exists in itself. It appears to them as habitat for things that both are and are not. Sophia's mode of possessing Julie, "I had no daughter ever, and she is that daughter," suggests that Julie both does and does not exist. Similarly, Lady Terrence's "You need No Child also, my good man, all fathers have one" (211), suggests Wendell's simultaneous fatherhood and childlessness. Elisha's determination to remain "uncrammed of learning as a gooseberry . . . with a saddle as empty as it is possible for nothing to make it" suggests both occupation and nonoccupation of the Ryderly "saddle," the place where the gap between the legs is filled (236). Likewise, O'Connor's "two in front" and "two behind" who all sigh "Holy! Holy! Holy!" suggest a nether space where what is not lingers (138).

VII. UNENDING DEPARTURE: JULIE

This nether space is traversed by phantoms "without cease":

> Through the twilight of the capacious room went the cohort of those gone, forgotten and remembered and forgotten again. Trailing regal garments, dust colored and death worn, and threadbare of the grave—a lamb and a phantom, and the phantom's lamb, and the lamb of the lamb, and foremost, a prince in point-lace, with touching sweet honey-colored curls, holding in the curve of a cradling velvet arm, the supine form of a girl-child with the blood of the rape flowing in a thin, fine, ever-widening stream, the slotted insertion of her communal dress, petal by petal, falling, the bride's bouquet in her betrayed hands, and passed out through the wall without cease. (159)

These ghosts are not explained, do not linger in the "capacious room," but pass away continuously as if their very nature is to be constantly leaving, but never gone. The operations of disavowal and cryptophoria appear here as synonymous. Both render the known as not known by imagining it as continuously in the process of vanishing, leaving or falling. The ghost words forever depart from scenes that seem to be about something else. As Caruth puts it, "in a world of falling, reference could not adequately describe the world."[69] *Ryder*'s characters relate to these holes in its scenes variously. They attempt to fill them with words, or with themselves or others, or else they fixate on them, gesture ambiguously toward them, or fall into them, becoming ghosts themselves.

Julie, the Barnes character, falls into language's aporias. She denounces family lies but does not replace them with anything, since she doesn't have anything. Sophia's remark that Julie *is* Wendell, but "unhung, and you are slung like a man; it will make the difference" suggests that Wendell, denouncing social law, replaces it with the law of his own organ, whereas Julie, not having one, denounces "Wendellness" but replaces it with nothing (170). Of all the characters in *Ryder*, only Julie makes no claims except indirectly through her dreams. Her dreams are full of falling: "The cat jumped up on the fence, and from there into the bough, and the birds stood away from him and he leapt, and mystery took away the ledges and places of the world utterly, and the cat fell, down falling, surprised, falling surprised forever, and no one to tell it to" (122). Unlike the trajectory of shit in patriarchal civilization (according to Amelia), the cat's downward movement is never arrested by the platform of "faulty fancies." Like the specters that "passed through the wall without cease," the cat "falling surprised forever" figures the continuous traumatic disavowal of Julie's experience, of Julie herself. Julie herself falls through the cracks of the unspoken in *Ryder*'s stories, having no place in its myth-world.

Nightwood's Nora is also always falling: "There is a gap in 'world pain' through which the singular falls continually and forever; a body falling in observable space, deprived of the privacy of disappearance; as if privacy, moving relentlessly away, by the very sustaining power of its withdrawal kept the body eternally moving downward, but in one place, and perpetually before the eye" (51). This passage visually renders the fall of the trauma victim through the "gap" of what is not included in "world pain." This is perhaps the incommunicable pain of incestuous love and loss, which renders its victim "singular" but unprivate, both "known" and elided by every act of speech, both still and falling. Nora, this passage suggests, is prey to a simultaneous visibility and abandonment, and like Julie, she is also subject to a constant, vertiginous groundlessness and departure. The "platforms" on which man erects his "faulty fancies" are not for them; their position in relation to the gap in language is to fall through it, or be buried in it.

The stories that Julie reads and hears are, as Taylor discusses, about beautiful little girls who are dying picturesquely according to the conventions of the Victorian sentimental novel. The effects of these stories on Julie involve splitting and falling. Barnes implicitly associates the splitting by which Julie identifies with storybook characters with the splitting effects of sexual abuse. Julie, being read to, "is many children, suffering the tortures of the damned, kneeling at the parent knee, in all ages, all times, and all bindings, becoming what books make of a child" (106). After hearing the story of Little Emily's relinquishment of "the needle" and death, Julie is "tor[n] away" from her beloved Sophia by "darkness . . . while she yet lay upon [Sophia's] breast."[70] The needle elsewhere in *Ryder* is a trope for the vagina: "[h]as not Science proved that . . . the Thread makes no Conquest of the Needle, and the Needle has not a leaning to the Thread?" (26) Emily's relinquishment of the needle suggests the violation of her dying body, as well as probably parodying Louisa May Alcott's sentimental novel *Little Women* in which the dying Beth March cannot lift her needle to sew, as Taylor notes.[71] This death scene is followed by Julie's dream of the cat with no foothold in the "ledges and places of the world." Taylor argues that such scenes draw attention to the sensual detail with which the deaths of children are described in Victorian sentimental novels and, by extension, the sexually pleasurable, as well as painful, affect that these scenes evoke. But further, images and tropes, like the needle, which stands for the unspeakably violated hole of the child's vagina, also suggest the aporias of the Victorian sentimental genre as well as of Ryderly discourse. Rape and incest constitute a hole in "world pain," through which its victims fall "forever . . . and no one to tell it to."[72] Because Julie and Nora are constantly falling and vanishing out of their own stories, their "secrets" belong not to them but to the texts in which they appear. Julie and Nora are elided by their own open secrets, *Ryder* and *Nightwood*.

Julie becoming what she has read presents the embedding movement of disavowal. Story and dream imagery simultaneously cover and depict Julie's sexual abuse. Her dreams, given shape, as the text suggests, by the fact that Wendell is concurrently molesting her, draw on multifarious images of femininity culled from "what she had read." In these dreams, spectrality, fragmentation, and falling represent the disavowal of this abuse.

The central story within story in "Julie Becomes What She Had Read" is the strangely sexualized death scene of little Arabella Lynn, who dies of guilt over momentarily doubting in God the Father (107). The deluge that accompanies Arabella Lynn's interment represents divine excrement, the effusion that disavows injustice, signaling the shittiness of the narrator's aestheticization and approval of Arabella's death: "Ah, what a picture for the beholder!" (108).[73] Arabella's death is not only beautiful, the narrator enthuses, but saves her from the "sin [that] might have battened on that edifice, dragging it down into inevitable ruin" (108). As Taylor suggests, the many details that ornament her death and burial draw attention to the sexual and voyeuristic elements of the sentimental genre that the scene parodies.[74] However, the language of haunting adds another layer of meaning to the uncomfortable complexity of affect, the strange mixture of sorrow and pleasure that Taylor notes. This surface affect is haunted as Arabella's spectral body haunts her gown: "See how she kneels in her figure-haunted gown!" (107). Likewise, Julie's violated body haunts the idealizing and sensual dreams that cover her violation and haunts *Ryder*'s many stories, layers, and juxtapositions.

After Arabella Lynn is fragmented, the narrator tells us, she dies while Julie becomes a sixteen-year-old girl whose image and idyllic, yet sinister, surroundings suggest the molestation in distorted form:

> Down she looses her hair as though it were the molten sluices from the gorged parapet melting in the noonday heat, flooding the garden, covering the roses with a web of brightness. A thousand birds sing in ecstasy for all she has yet to learn. Love shall be, never being, and life shall go ahead, a fine queen on a black-rumped mare, forging and breathing like a man; or in the dark of some forgotten close, life, like an idiot girl, smelling of neither puberty, shall finger the hem of her reverses, and count one, while, in the underbrush, and through the hot hedged day, a rabbit fleetly paws the earth, harkening the weather's inconstancy, and the changing of a leaf. (109)

Following this erotic dream, Julie is amidst a group of little girls who are "scourged and blasphemed," become mothers, and fall "this way and that, silent and soft and docile" (109). She then wakes to see Wendell looming over her and Sophia running. She becomes, in Sophia's curious phrase, not her daughter but her "no daughter ever," a formulation that echoes her dream that "love shall be, never being." Julie, first split and then nonexistent, is subsequently disowned by Wendell via two more negations: "she is none of mine. Did I not hear her deriding me greatly?" The molestation that she has just (not) experienced exists only insofar as Julie haunts her own splitting and disavowal.

Ryder does not offer a perspective from which incest appears as a true secret. It appears as precisely what, in Abraham and Torok's theory, creates a psychic crypt: a half-secret, an aporia in the discourse of a love object that surrounds the unspeakable half-known "secret" and secretes it into a psychic tomb. Sexualized relations are the *Ryder* family norm—perhaps because Wendell, who sees himself as "all things to all men, and all women's woman," sees no reason to refrain from having sex with anyone (164). Even Sophia's injunction to Wendell after his presumable molestation of Julie, "Do not strike her" (109), suggests that the sexual abuse is to her both permissible and unspeakable, since it is only the threat of physical violence that provokes her protective words. Suggestions of incestuous sexual relations in the Ryder family abound. For instance, Elisha and Wendell seem to get close in bed while talking of "woman": "In the dark Elisha wet his lips, and said softly, tell me, what is a woman?" (224) On falling asleep after having defined woman, Wendell, "his red hair spread like a girl's upon the pillow," and Elisha, whose mouth is now open, "nightlong played down his father's leg the second movement of the 'Sonata Pathetique,' his father's hand twitching in the midnight scale" while "dreaming things they never thought of" (226). In "Amelia and Kate Taken to Bed" Timothy may molest Julie (as argued by Ponsot) while she cries "'Wendell! Wendell!' as she lay on her bed of playful maternity, aged ten, holding to her breast the rag doll thrown from the door to the immediate left by the strong arm of Timothy, who was God and the Father" (95). Wendell observes of his own first sexual encounter that "every man . . . has been initiated into these matters either by a kitchen slut or an elder aunt, who remains a maiden for all of that" (167). Mere copulation, he implies, is not enough to remove the aunt's status as "maiden" without the company of a spoken acknowledgment. Julie's experience of incest is excluded from speech as a function of the text's, and the family's, narrative and social style.[75] Her response of silent counter-negation of family and speech leaves her, as her dreams reveal, with no foothold in the world.

VIII. INSIDE-OUT AND JUXTAPOSED WORDS

Ryder's mendacious representations cause splitting, aporias, and alienations between what is represented and what is elided in its structure, world, characters, images, and most obviously in its stories within stories. These stories within stories present us with a series of redoubled characters and double parts. Wendell's story of Arthur's story of Molly and Eva, Amelia's story of Felice and Alix, O'Connor's story or monologue on doctoring and the Judgment Seat, Anne's story of Horace Chubble and the lynch mob's verbal dismantling of the raped girl all show a preoccupation with dichotomies and the spaces between oppositional terms.

In every case, these terms and characters are split and doubled, it is implied, by some fetishistic ideal of a whole. One of *Ryder*'s most persistent dualisms is "woman." The male gaze on and entry into her body split woman by the idealized beauty, virtue, motherliness, and delicacy that she must see herself as representing.[76] *Ryder* expresses the fragmented being of women by splitting them in two: two sisters, a pregnant woman, a woman and her vagina or "woman within woman," a past and future with no present, a mother and child, a wife and mistress (153). These pairs are sometimes also subdivided.

Wendell's story of Arthur's story of Molly and Eva describes the splitting of women by patriarchal ideals—here the ideal of feminine virtue. The town's fixity on the question of who was the "holier" or more "wholesome" creates a hole, the story implies, that divides one woman into two. That Molly and

Eva, split by the ideal of virtue, are actually one woman is suggested by the fact that the bad one (Eva) is always seen going to, and the good one (Molly) coming from, church. Such a seemingly impossible feat would be impossible for two women, but simple for a woman repeatedly "cleansed" of her sins by the confessional. The argument that suspends the activities of the town so that "there they were a good full week later, never having changed their position, in kitchens and bedrooms, in garret and cellar, in house and in street, all rucked and rumpled with the heat of the matter, and no solution in sight" concerns the question of which is the "holier," or the more "wholesome" (217). As well as freezing the town in stasis, the argument fixes the separation of Molly/Eva, since it excludes the knowledge that they are not separate. Molly (the good sister) then dies in childbirth, and Eva is found with a baby by the "wise man" sent by the town to confront them. "The thing is reversed," Eva tells him. "Moll has gone to the Lord, and I have come from the Lord, so let them change their rag for another. Moll is dead, and I'm a mother, and be damned to you and the rest" (219). The death of Molly and birth of Eva's (or Molly's) child, a Christ figure, allegorizes the expulsion of the internalized ego-ideal that split one woman into "good" and "bad." Accordingly it kills the "good" woman, since good women, as *Ryder* suggests, are constitutively split by their superegos. With the death of Molly, Eva (a surly Virgin Mary figure) and her child form a whole. The townspeople must necessarily "change their rag"—that is, replace the discourse of "holiness" that splits one woman into two.

However happy this conclusion, it must be remembered that this story is told by "Arthur," a travelling salesman invented by Wendell to account for the additional mother and children in his household to a town delegation at his door. It carries Wendell's signature "mythemes" of idealized death in childbirth and motherhood, and the God-father/lover who unifies the woman's split subjectivity. In Wendell's story to the townspeople, the reason for Arthur's absence ("He is afraid that . . . the sleeve of his left cuff may be pissed upon") is "perfectly clear," but meaningless. Perhaps for this reason, Wendell's "explanation" has the desired effect of making the man with the cane "beg [Wendell's] pardon a thousand times for . . . [the] inconvenience" and leave (220).

Figures of the redoubled women, (w)hole(iness), (dying) mothers, and children abound in *Ryder*. Amelia's bedtime story also presents women who are fractured and destroyed by internalized ideals. "Felice and Alix," another sister duo, die in childbirth as a result of their hyper-aestheticized femininity. Each comparison of the two establishes Alix as Felice's ideal ego and uncanny double, and exposes her as lacking:

> Felice had little hands, Alix had smaller; Felice had a tiny waist and two breasts as delicate as the first setting of blanc mange. Alix's waist was only a hand's span and her bosom was no greater than two tears set low. Felice had golden hair, Alix's was fine and thin and curling.
>
> Felice had a little skeleton as chipped of angles as a Ming, and as light as ash. Alix's flesh covered her bones as thinly as ice on a tree. Felice's ankles were faultless, Alix's were as weightless as cuttlebone and as fragile. (155)

The dualism of Felice/Alix is accomplished through reflection and contrast, their hyperbolic femininity like a mirror that splits one woman in two by revealing her lack. But this ideal is itself an ideal of nonbeing, the failure to achieve it a failure to disappear. Alix's minuteness and daintiness outdistances Felice's in being closer to nothing at all, the ultimate feminine ideal for Amelia. Their death in childbirth, then, is the achievement of ideal femininity.

Ryder's primary as well as embedded stories figure the divided woman. Amelia and Kate are divided by the fetishistic "ideal" of Wendell: one fat, lazy, coarse, a mistress and enjoying herself, the other skinny, hard working, prudish, a wife and martyred. Each torments the other with what she is not to Wendell. Wendell reaps full enjoyment from their situation by putting them in bed together, "only a hate apart," himself the "bodkin" in the middle (172). Indeed, Barnes does her best to split the human referents of *Ryder*'s characters from their representations. As Andrew Field has suggested, Barnes names Amelia, based on her mother Elizabeth Chappell Barnes, after her father's mistress, Marguerite *Amelia* Alvarez de Rocafuerte, who he says is the prototype of Kate Careless. Likewise, Field notes, she names Sophia, based on her grandmother Zadel, after Zadel's replacement, the second wife of Axel Gustafson (*Ryder*'s Alex), *Sophia* Steele Billings (26). Elizabeth and Zadel, reading *Ryder*, are presumably alienated from their representations, which are nonetheless perhaps impossible to completely cast out.

Ryder's women's deadly fixation on, and internalization of, the wound of patriarchal discourse is allegorized by the number one cause of their death: childbirth, "the death that craws within" (77). Deadly childbirth is the outcome of the "splitting" entry of the fetishized penis, the phallus, into the woman.[77] The child in the mother's womb is a figure of the melancholic woman.[78] Women in *Ryder*, who internalize ideals of feminine beauty or saintliness, are destroyed by the bodily impossibility of accommodating them; their repressed parts come back out screaming. Wendell's unnamed mistress, Felice, Alix, and Molly (of Molly/Eva) die in childbirth, the raped girl is expected to, Amelia is certain that she will—and ends up being expelled from the family as a result of it. Wendell, tellingly, considers death in childbirth a woman's most saintly possible circumstance (202).

Not all of the women in *Ryder* internalize the male gaze. Some, like Sophia and Molly Dance, cross it with their own. Molly's self-identification as only her name, "Bottom up or head up . . . it's Molly Dance to the end, and that's more than most people can say" (199), allows her to remain particular, "hard to catch" or to define in general terms.[79] Women can also, like Julie, try to avoid internalizing patriarchal ideology by remaining silent or, like Anne, by incorporating this ideology only as a bunion: Anne's bunion, "the very weathercock of morals," throbs in empathy with social "impropriety" (112). Since to "have" the phallus (to father, for instance, "the great race of Ryders"), the man must have the (fetishized) woman, the woman can take away his control of meaning by asserting her own vision. She can make him aware, fleetingly, that she sees him as lacking.

Another mode of feminine fragmentation is suggested in "Rape and Repining," the monologue of a parochial English lynch mob who drive an unnamed raped girl to a neighboring country. In the eyes of the mob, and in the many eyes of the animals that are trained on her in their narrative (25), the raped girl's violation divides her from the virginal feminine ideal and, thus, makes her "counterfeit" (26), no longer "what she should be" (21). Since her virginal body emblematized authentic regional identity, her violated one splits it into two alienated parts: "the Annual Rent paid to the Queen . . . cannot make Tittencote smack of Tittencote, and you gone slipping down to hell" (23). She is hence banished to a "Neighboring Land," where (it is hoped) her body will be rid of "Uncertainty," made "Honest," as a patch for a hole:

> Get from our Country and over the Border and into some Neighboring Land, there to lie, until some Blithering Scabby Potsherd mends a Stewpan with you, or lays you between Hot Iron and Hot Iron, and so melts you down, to make a Cap for his Heel. So shaken loose, so cutpursed that the Uncertainty is out of you, so set you back as Current Coin . . . that you turn to Honest Flesh. (28)

Since her penetrated vagina splits certainty (the virginal ideal) and "Uncertainty" (the sullied flesh), she must be rehabilitated only as a part-object, a fragment of leather or a scrap of iron. She can thereafter be authentic only as a scrap, not as a woman, and only in the future, not in the present. "Certainty" allows no slippage between the female body and the feminine ideal. If perforated, nonidentical to the ideal, the body is no longer a woman but a future part-object. Accordingly, the raped girl's coming child will be always already disavowed, "set . . . backward upon the Beast of Time . . . and his Father and Mother will say, 'We resemble that hereafter, which was before, and is not.'" The temporal mechanism of disavowal denies the present; what is disavowed seems to exist on either side of the present, from which it constantly recedes. Like jam in *Through the Looking Glass*, it appears in the future and past of the moment in which it is invoked.

The vagina in *Ryder* represents women's split being. *Ryder* imagines it as a kind of psychic crypt where "full speech" emerges and disappears, eluding clarity by eluding the present. Anne gives it a chthonic status, calling it "woman within woman" (153). This image suggests the feminine melancholic disavowal of the "bad parts" of the self, the parts that discourse disowned, and their secretion into intrapsychic space.[80] Childbirth accordingly figures the re-emergence of these parts and the destabilization that accompanies it: the indirect, partial, or inexplicit movement toward a fuller meaning that Lacan calls "full speech," and Abraham and Torok "anasemia."[81]

The gender divide in social power, Anne suggests, is linked to the misleading appearance of anatomical difference: "This, now I do think on it, is the matter with the world, that a man's greatness do come right out bang upon us, a woman's is in her flesh and hidden. How can one expect the ways of men to go right when things are so mixed up?" (153) Man's unconscious, one might say, is right out there in the open—it is the very social structure—while woman's is "in her flesh," and its content emerges at her own expense. Like the psychic tomb, the vagina "is great at the core and dwindles as you reach her outer jacket, so that you see a monstrous little of a dire plot," just the odd fleeting ghost.

In *Ryder* femininity and melancholia, or cryptophoria, are not yet as conflated as they are in *Nightwood*.[82] *Ryder*'s women may externalize and thereby domesticate the shitty ideal before it kills them, as its more dirt-tolerant women show. While childbirth kills or torments women who are fully identified with ideals, it comes more lightly to women who "make a roadway" for meaning with their own shit, like Eva, Sophia, Molly Dance, Lady Terrance, and Kate Careless. Sophia has her chamber pots, Molly Dance lives in filth, her kitchen and outhouse wet with human effluents that "stunk and sounded. . . . There was not a dry plank in the two buildings that one could put foot to" (193). Liking "all things, of all kinds, all at once, in the same place," Molly has no need for dialectics. She has no concept of good and evil: "What would your good and evil have meant to her, or how could she have understood it?" (193) Lady Terrence's liking for the "rudiments and hidden parts" of animals also suggests this domestication of excrement. She is a gourmand of "malign concoction[s]" and "could remember to a tripe to what she was beholden" (208). What she eats cannot return to destroy her (as it does in childbirth), since it has never been elided. Kate Careless is likewise comfortable with excrement and childbirth, a potential emptier of chamber pots on the heads of fathers of the law, a noncleaner of Wendell's pigeons' shit (90). Thus, unlike the "other kind of woman," Kate cannot be counted on to clean up for Wendell by removing herself when woken up at night and asked to leave the family. It is the woman of "pale existence," Amelia, who cleans up Wendell's messes to protect him. Ultimately this includes herself. Women, *Ryder* suggests, are like ambulatory messes of refuse who trail into the past, into their own bodies. They may either "clean themselves up" by aspiring to an ideal of nonbeing, like Felice and Alix, or else celebrate themselves by celebrating dirt and excrement.

Like the vagina, the rectal hole marks an absent presence in *Ryder*'s symbolic field, but unlike the feminine reproductive system, which is aligned with feminine melancholia, the digestive system and particularly excrement are associated with manipulative modes of perversion, excremental speech that distorts the particular through its picturesque arrangements of signifiers. Barthes's theory of "mythology" and Abraham and Torok's of "antimetaphor" both describe this function of associating objects contiguously to overlay their (shameful) history with the "naturalness" of their present association.[83] The "mythic" association fills the historical one, which is "nothing erased but much submerged."

This picture, however, is haunted by traces of its secrets: "For of the banquet doth the turde tell/And rown in the belly's dark always/The secrets of the supper all bewray" (64–5). The "turde" leaves a trail into the disavowed past, if read dialogically (within its frame(s)) instead of monologically, as a "picture forever arranged" (*Nightwood*, 111). If we read the Cheerful's "choice" to die in childbirth (and not be spoken of) alongside *Ryder*'s—and history's—treatment of dying mothers, we will see it as imposing its "Wendellness" on them. Similarly, if we take Felice's and Alix's beauteous delicacy and death in childbirth into the Victorian context which the story's language suggests, we will note the relation of the social customs and medical practices that reinforced the ideal of feminine delicacy to high rates of death in childbirth at this time, and will wonder at Amelia's investment in her chilling myth of "feminine death-drivenness." It is a matter of contextualizing the mythemes of excremental speech.

As well as cynical, strict, and melancholic perverts and psychotics, we have Horace Chubble, the fetishist, and Anne de Grier, the phobic. Chubble, described in a letter of Anne's to Amelia, has a fixated relation to duality and its gap. However, for him these formations are predominantly external. "When I die," he tells Anne's employer, "I shall have a beautiful new pair of wings and a cambric nightgown, and with a goose-quill in my bottom, I'll brush round heaven looking under the angels' garments for *duplicity*" (74, emphasis added). The shocked Anne observes to Amelia that

> those bent on heaven and those bent on hell have got fearfully confused as to direction, so they do stumble into each other, learning things not fitting to their separate goals. Therefore imagine, dear sister, where we will all land in the

> end—somewhere in mid-air, no doubt, for that we are fit for neither place, and a dreadful sight is that space between two stools, where Mr. Chubble can be heard remarking on goose-quills to my lady. (74)

Duplicity here refers to the bifurcated lower parts of angels. Once again, the genital regions mark the space between what is spoken and what is true. The goose-quill in Chubble's anus suggests (as well as the obvious phallic symbolism) a pen in an inkwell dedicated to reportage on them. With this reportage he wishes to fill the anatomical space of "duplicity" that he may find. The places in "mid-air" between heaven and hell, and the "space between two stools" (the ones holding Chubble and her Ladyship, one hopes) are likewise aporic no-places between dualisms or "stools." Such spaces, for Anne, are "a dreadful sight" since they appear insufficient to render the individuals dedicated to one of their framing terms (heaven or hell) adequately separate. Anne's fear is warranted, for her wish to distinguish herself and her Lady from Chubble aligns her with him through their shared fixations on external "duplicity" and what lies between its divisions. As in feminine melancholia, holiness and doubleness are in each case accompanied by fixation. However, here the fixation is on a thing imagined as external to the character. The goose-quill dedicated to recording duplicity and the space in mid-air between heaven and hell create, Barnes suggests, the very separations that they mark as pre-existing. The fixation on this space—between good and bad, heaven and hell—creates the duality, as *Nightwood* also suggests.

In contrast to *Ryder*'s perverse characters, Matthew O'Connor uses language vaguely and idiosyncratically. Instead of creating divisions around a clear, fixed ideal, he unhinges signs from referents and makes ideals appear strange and potentially obscene, as indeed they are. O'Connor, too, has an image for the gap in meaning. It is probably an anus, but neither it, nor what it frames, are clear. "The Soliloquy of Dr. Matthew O'Connor (Family Physician to the Ryders) on the Way to and from the Confessional of Father Lucas," allusively links the Judgment Seat and Judgment to corresponding human bifurcations and gaps. Rather than imagining God as an object of knowledge, it gestures ambiguously and multivalently toward Him:

> It's a devil a bit of peace I'll get, says I, banging my head against the scrofula and the tapeworm and the syphilis and the cancer and the pectoris and the mumps and the gleet and the pox of mankind, I says, and me with my susceptible orbs staring down into and up through the cavities and openings and fissures and entrances of my fellowmen, and following some, and continuing others, and increasing many, and them swelling and opening and contracting and pinching like the tides of the sea, and me a mortal like the sea with my ebb and flow, and my good heart, and my thundering parts and my appetites and my hungers. . . . Visit me often, [Father Lucas] says, and I'll give you comfort and kind

> words and a little consolation that shall inch thee on thy way a bit, and bring thee nearer the Celestial Gate, slip by slop, cleansing your soul as you go, that you may not enter altogether dusty and dirty and mucked before the Judgment Seat, with its two in front and its two behind and the four sighing Holy! Holy! Holy! God save the behind, I said, and staggered out into the life and traffic of my days. (137–8)

This passage superimposes God with the human posterior, figuring both God and the anus as an empty space surrounded by doubled parts and lined with excrement. The image is nevertheless left vague—the reader can guess at, but not ascertain definitively, what is being described. O'Connor's "two in front" and "two behind" suggest cloven lower body parts, as well as the two cherubim who traditionally attended God's Mercy Seat. And O'Connor's "Holy! Holy! Holy!" suggests the holes situated between these parts, as well as the Seat's traditional appellation, "Holy of Holies." O'Connor's punning links the Judgment Seat with the anus through their common form as a gap between dualisms. However, what "holiness" really signifies remains unfixed, multivalent.

O'Connor stares into human and perhaps divine orifices with his "susceptible orbs" but does not fill them with determinate content. His gesture uses double entendre to unhinge itself from denotation, redoubling the figures of doubleness and holiness. His simultaneously "sacred" (religious) and "profane" (sexual) interest in holiness, though appearing self-contradictory, enables his gesture toward an empty space that remains undefined as something or nothing. His multivalent language allows "both sides" of the possible issue (for instance sacred and profane "holiness," being and nonbeing) to coexist, since neither is clear enough to distort the other.

O'Connor's soliloquy also contains an apocalypse story fraught with vague religious imagery. In his imagined church,

> The candles took root and grew and rose toward the ceiling, and bloomed and wilted and died, and the ceiling grew and mounted and bloomed and wilted and died, and came down. . . . The figures at the altar blurred, crossed, melted into each other; fornication of the mass, parted and bred Death, Death's wailing child in wax, lying in a bowl of wine, mouth open for the gushing breast of grief, pouring forth the Word in an even belt of wrath. . . . Sorrow burst and the seeds fell and took root, and climbed about the stations of the cross and bore Him down to earth, and climbed on and on and bore Matthew and Nora and [many others] down to earth, and climbed on and bore their children and their children's children down to earth, and the children of them begotten, and were not appeased, and climbed and bore man down utterly, and stretched out and took his works and bore them down also, and there was Nothing, and this, too, they reached for and closed on, trembling terribly and gently. (140)

This scene is reminiscent of the contemplative experiences of dissolution that I describe in my introduction. In it, sacred objects, structures, and nothing itself all wilt, melt, and are brought "down to earth." Nothing itself is brought down by the dehiscence of Sorrow, while the excremental Word "pour[s] forth in an even belt of wrath." This jumble of metaphysical images is an extreme example of *Ryder*'s characteristic approach to destabilizing meaning. It describes the process by which everything (and nothing) are brought down to earth, the horizontal on which life perilously erects itself. "Seeds of sorrow," little capsules perhaps of what is unspoken but not gone, eventually burst, grow and bear everything and nothing (the last dualism) as ghosts bring *Nightwood*'s characters down. Seeds of sorrow, like psychic crypts, cause characters, sublime objects, and negation itself, to go down.[84]

IX. THE PICTURE'S SHARP EDGE

The question of how to read Barnes's *tableaux* has often been posed. Precise and often repulsive, they startle with a luridness that, unconnected to anything, immediately passes away. Like the Barthesian "myth" that distorts a particular history by naturalizing it, the picture in *Ryder* represents, in distorted fashion, a half-remembered unspeakable history.[85] Barnes's writing gives us pictures and stories that show everything that her society usually hid: human anatomy and digestive cycles, excrement, family sexual abuse, lesbian, gay, and straight sex. Yet most of it (some of *Ryder* was excised) bypassed the censors, which surprised Barnes less, perhaps, than it surprises her readers. Like the Barthesian myth, the Barnesian image is a tableau of contiguous objects that distort and pacify their interrelations. The secret is arranged in a context that renders it "innocent," filling this arrangement with some other, often more general, meaning. The secret is on its way to the picture's sharp edge, where it vanishes. Perhaps Julie's dreams simply tell us something about the nature of little girls—that they are so sweet and delicate that they naturally die of guilt for doubting the existence of God. Or perhaps we are merely meant to enjoy their beautifully rendered deaths. Like the cryptophore's seemingly innocuous behavior, the Barnesian tableau hides the secret in full view.

By writing gaps and frames into *Ryder*'s narratives and images, Barnes imposes limits on the power of its narratives and its storytellers: father, mother, grandmother, and society. She exposes the lesions in stories where there were bland-faced contiguities. But these gaps and divisions in certainty are always being filled. God is left indeterminate by O'Connor, different from Wendell only in that he "does not tremble" in "the balance" (202). Elsewhere, however, He resembles Wendell or Sophia. *Ryder*'s God vacillates between

O'Connor's and "woman's" singular "God only," and the God of the doubled object, "God and the father," who releases the "mighty rains of Heaven"—whose creation is one more excremental narrative. The Other in *Ryder* is both (w)hole and split, like a reversible figure whose central shape resolves into two peripheral shapes, then back again as the viewer's cognition shifts in the fixed movement of disavowal.

NOTES

1. Lacan follows Freud's foundational discussions of disavowal, in which the emerging subject simultaneously believes in, and disbelieves, the mother's lack, or "castration" (her limited power over the subject) and is driven by anxiety to supplement that limit by reformulating it in a literalized way.
2. Lacan, *Seminar III, The Psychoses*, 204–5.
3. Fink, *Clinical Introduction*, 173.
4. Herring, *Djuna*, 54–5.
5. Emily Coleman Archives, University of Delaware library.
6. Barnes, 1935 letter to Coleman.
7. Neagoe, cited by Barnes in a 1935 letter to Coleman.
8. Eliot, "Introduction," *Nightwood*, xi.
9. As quoted by Herring in *Djuna*, 276.
10. Field, *Djuna*, 95.
11. Ibid., 90, 32.
12. Kannenstine, *Art*, xv.
13. Ibid.
14. Martins, "Gender," Marcus, "Laughing," Taylor, "Making Contact." For Martins, Robin "consciously becomes the 'cultural' ideal of 'natural,' 'bestial,' "prediscursive' Woman' to trouble this ideal'" (123). Marcus reads "the agency of [Robin's] desire and its refusal to be fixed by the desire of lesbian lovers or husband, contained in motherhood, or controlled by T.S. Eliot's or other critics'" reading of her as doomed, damned, or pathologically placed as a medical case study [as] a textual triumph" (237). Taylor reads a queer ethos in *Nightwood*'s implicit refusal of identity politics.
15. Stevenson, "Grotesque," 82.
16. Caselli, *Improper Modernism*, 214.
17. Taylor, *Affective*, 6; O'Neal, *Djuna Barnes*, 19; Herring, *Djuna*, 235
18. Setz, "Trees," 145.
19. Barnes, 1934–1935 letters to Coleman.
20. In an unpublished memoir Barnes writes, "My grandmother Zadel was my first mother and father. I did not accept my mother and father until later in life." Broe, "Introduction," 4).
21. See Broe, "Introduction," *Silence*, 4, 377; Herring, *Djuna*, 5, 10, 17–18, 43–7.
22. May 5, 1935, letter to Coleman.

23. Ibid., 84, 175; 87.
24. Ibid., 80–1.
25. O'Neal, *Djuna Barnes*, 62, 175.
26. Ibid., xv and *passim*; Field, *Djuna*, 231–4, Herring, *Djuna*, 296–304.
27. O'Neal, *Djuna Barnes*, 15.
28. Ibid., 182, 188, 191.
29. Ibid., 189, 194. For the Foreword see Appendix II, 213–15.
30. Herring, *Djuna*, 1, 313.
31. See ibid., 252–3, 274–8, 286–7, 299, and O'Neal, *Djuna Barnes*.
32. O'Neal, *Djuna Barnes*, 157, 191.
33. Ibid., 74.
34. Abraham and Torok, *Shell*, 155–6.
35. Goldberg, "Overview," 43–5.
36. *Ryder*'s form and content, Sanchez-Pardo argues, represent Kleinian paranoid-schizoid mechanisms. For Klein, melancholia/orality is associated with the feminine subject-position and sadism/anality with the masculine one (*Cultures*, throughout).
37. The image, writes Lacan, "reveals something in so far as it is distinct from what might be called an itself that is behind" (*Seminar XI*, 99).
38. Whitley, "Nations," 81–98.
39. Lacan, *Seminar I, Freud's Papers on Technique*, 45. Writes Lacan, "the more uncertain the text that the subject gives us, the more it is meaningful."
40. Lacan, "Response," 319.
41. Lacan, *Seminar I, Freud's Papers on Technique*, 46.
42. Barthes describes "mythologies" as systems of signs whose significations naturalize someone else's manipulative social agenda to the viewer/reader. Myths are contiguous: "The elements of the form . . . are related as to place and proximity: the mode of presence of the form is spatial. The concept, on the contrary, appears in a global fashion, it is a kind of nebula, the condensation, more or less hazy, of a certain knowledge. Its elements are linked by associative relations" (*Mythologies*, 126).
43. Writes Barthes: "if I clearly distinguish the meaning and the form, and consequently the distortion that one imposes on the other, I undo the signification of the myth" (ibid., 128).
44. Emily Coleman Archives, University of Delaware library. Writes Barnes in a 1935 letter to Coleman, "possibly none of the events of our life are real until the second event (like the meeting of sperm and ova) gives them body."
45. Caruth, *Experience*. Writes Caruth, "the trauma of the accident, its very unconsciousness, is borne by an act of departure. It is a departure that, in the full force of its historicity, remains at the same time in some sense absolutely opaque, both to the one who leaves and also to the theoretician, linked to the sufferer in his attempt to bring the experience to light. Yet at the same time, this very opacity generates the surprising force of a knowledge, for it is the accident, in German, *Unfall*, that reverberates in Freud's own theoretical insight drawn from the example, which is laced in the German with other forms of *fallen*, 'to fall.' . . . Between the *Unfall*, the accident, and the 'striking' of the insight, its *auffallen*, is the force of a fall, a falling that is

transmitted precisely in the unconscious act of leaving. It is this *unconsciousness of leaving* that bears the impact of history" (22).

46. Miller, "Havoc," 166. Miller has identified Barnes's illegibility with the epochal shift and disjuncture between the time she wrote *Ryder* and the time in her childhood it depicts.

47. Ibid., 175.

48. Taylor, *Affective*, 79.

49. Miller, "Havoc," 165.

50. Ibid., 164.

51. Lacan, like Barnes, compares the emergence and disappearance of full speech to vaginal "pulsation": "We find here [in the register of indestructible desire that escapes from time] the rhythmic structure of the pulsation of the slit. . . . The appearance/disappearance [of unconscious content] takes place between two points, the initial and the terminal of this logical time—between the instant of seeing, when something of the intuition itself is always elided, not to say lost, and that elusive moment when the apprehension of the unconscious is not, in fact, concluded" (*Seminar XI*, 32).

52. See Žižek, *For They Know*, 245. Žižek here describes three modes of perverse disavowal, "which could be called 'normal,' 'manipulative,' [or cynical], and 'fetishistic' *stricto sensu*." These modes are respectively exemplified in *Ryder* by Amelia, Sophia and Wendell. "Normal" disavowal and "melancholia" will be aligned in my usage, since in both, in *Ryder*, what is known and not known is preserved in the subject as other. Cryptophoria partakes of both, but with a specificity of detail that my chapter on *Nightwood* will be more concerned with describing, since it is more established there.

53. Sanchez-Pardo comes to a similar conclusion, writing that "*Ryder* questions the sacrificial logic that grounds language and the social upon the death of the mother, upon what Luce Irigary calls 'originary matricide'" (*Cultures*, 316). For Sanchez-Pardo, "In *Ryder* the symbolic equation that literally appears as the death drive compulsively reappears under the guise of reproductive anxiety, in the disruption and destabilization of forms that mimic the laboring female body and the irresolution of the work of mourning, emerging in the pervasive cadence of melancholia" (341).

54. Miller, "Havoc," 172.

55. Warren describes Sophia's palimpsestic pictures as a "reinscription of the domestic space as cultural pantheon [which] parallels Sophia's reworking of traditional femininity [and] develops the novel's polyphony, by including a remarkable range of figures whom she admires" (*Consuming*, 55). Warren notes only the culturally valued figures, and does not mention the newspaper clippings.

56. Though some critical responses have suggested that *Ryder* has one narrator, and that this is the adult Julie, its diversity of narrative voices and agendas suggests that they may not issue from a single fictional entity. *Ryder* itself does not suggest that its narrator is Julie.

57. Taylor, *Affective*, 106, 79.

58. As Kate tells Wendell, "you know not what you do, and leave it to me to find out and my father to guard" (*Ryder*, 159).

59. As Barthes discusses, myths are not necessarily bad: a mytheme in service of a progressive/subversive agenda is ethically different from one that naturalizes political oppression (*Mythologies*, 146–8).

60. Miller, "Havoc," 174.

61. Ibid., 174-5.

62. As Sanchez-Pardo observes, Sophia's maiden name, Grieves, suggests *grief* and *graves*, the death and burial of the maternal body as the foundation of patriarchy (*Cultures*, 315).

63. Abraham and Torok, *Shell*, 114. Barnes also uses the term "after life" for Sophia's life after her loss of Alex, who betrayed her with "a wench" (*Ryder*, 84): "In after life, Sophia looked upon [her will, stipulating that she be buried with Alex] with amazement" (80).

64. This positive assimilation of experience is what Abraham and Torok call "introjection." In contrast to Klein's (and my) use of the term, they use it to describe a process of ego expansion and maturation (*Shell*, 114).

65. Amelia, though in the act of cleaning Wendell's pigeons' excrement, is nonetheless for Warren presenting "a significant challenge to bourgeois morality" (*Djuna Barnes*, 67) with her story of the primeval life-web (*Ryder*, 115). Anne's observation that "there's no wit in woman's thinking one thing and doing another" may be weighed against this argument (*Ryder*, 73).

66. As Sanchez-Pardo notes, Wendell's myth of sufficiency exploits Sophia, who begs, and Amelia and Kate, who bear children in conditions of drudgery (*Cultures*, 311–16).

67. This "itself that is behind" a picture, writes Lacan, is the gaze of the other that renders the subject himself split, a picture as well as a being. In *Seminar XI* Lacan describes the gaze as "the *object a* in the visual field" (105). As such, it "serves as a symbol of the lack, that is to say, of the phallus . . . insofar as it is lacking" (103).

68. Though I have associated the quest to say everything with psychotic writing, Serge André links it to the imperative in "the pervert" to fulfill the lack in the Other ("Structure of Perversion," 119).

69. Caruth, *Experience*, 76.

70. Little Emily, too, relinquishes her sexuality and dies in aesthetic splendor: "'and here,' said Emily, 'take the needle from me, it is too heavy!' and she closed her sweet violet eyes and breathed no more'—And the darkness pulled at the lamp and at Julie and tore her away from her beloved [Sophia] while yet she lay upon her breast" (*Ryder*, 122).

71. Taylor, *Affective*, 96.

72. Ponsot and Dalton have discussed the implicit sexual abuse of Julie in *Ryder*. See "Escaping from Eden" and "A Reader's *Ryder*."

73. The deluge may also be a figure for Wendell's ejaculation, as it has been read by Dalton ("Escaping," 170). There is an indistinction between semen and excrement in *Ryder*.

74. Taylor, *Affective*, 99–101.

75. Lévi-Strauss argues in *The Elementary Structures of Kinship* that incest may be the source of language. Its unspeakability may found the need for the binary oppositions which structure language (8).

76. Žižek describes feminine melancholia as the "fascination towards the wound" of the male gaze (*Ticklish*, 248–9).

77. Sanchez-Pardo links feminine sexuality to melancholia since both, in Kleinian theory, are the products of excessive orality and introjection of the superego (*Cultures*, 73–93).

78. Just as the melancholic "saintly" mother cannot give birth without dying, the child "cannot cast out" the mother, as Sophia knows to her advantage (*Ryder*, 12).

79. Sanchez-Pardo interprets this passage in terms of Molly's resistance to "the splitting imposed by the law (into libertine, whore, thief, bad mother)." By constituting herself as "Molly Dance to the end," she writes, Molly "resists disintegration and remains whole" (*Cultures*, 334). I read also Molly's insistence on her particularity.

80. Klein reverses Freud's theory that women have laxer superegos than men, and maintains that the reverse is true. Writes Sanchez-Pardo, "for Klein, anatomical differences . . . stress the importance of oral impulses and introjective tendencies in the girl, resulting in the 'introjection of her superego [being] more extensive than the boys. . . . The processes of introjection and projection are also stronger in women, and this is of vital importance for the development of their egos'" (*Cultures*, 83).

81. Abraham and Torok describe "anasemia" as "the founding silence of any act of signification" (*Shell*, 84). It "designates the status of concepts which, though deliberately disruptive of a unifying, conscious self, outline the ultimate unconscious sense or source of the disruption" (77). Thus, anasemia advances "toward this nonpresence in us, the place from which all meaning ultimately springs" (85).

82. In *Nightwood*, feminine redoubling is reflected in lesbian sexuality, figured as an uncanny external redoubling of an internal crypt.

83. Barthes cites the picture of a French-African soldier saluting the French flag on the cover of a French magazine to exemplify how "mythology" seeks to eclipse the shameful history of French imperialism in Africa by naturalizing French nationalism in French-Africans (*Mythologies*, 116 –22). Abraham and Torok cite coprophagy as an example of "antimetaphor." It attempts to abolish the metaphorical associations of shit with the shameful secret by pretending that it is appetizing (*Shell*, 132–3).

84. Like Barnes, Lacan links both sexual reproduction and consciousness to "dehiscence" or the bursting of seed pods. Lacan writes that there is "a vital dehiscence constitutive of man" which "render[s] foreign" the "original organic chaos" that the child experiences before acquiring language, and enables "the Heraclitean notion of Discord . . . to shine once more" ("Aggressiveness," 94).

85. Freud's suggestion, in "Fetishism" (1927), that a fetish-object chosen for its proximity, in a repressed memory, to the parents' genitals (for instance, high-heeled shoes may be chosen for their proximity to the mother's genitals in the first encounter), must be modified when the trauma is remembered, because the fetish-object could not stand for something repressed, but could distort something remembered.

Chapter 4

Ghost Words

Nightwood's Cryptic Imperatives

I. HAUNTING OR POSSESSION

Djuna Barnes wrote *Nightwood* largely while living in Greenwich Village, New York, and Hayford Hall, England, but we can see from the notes she took during her prolonged breakup with Thelma Wood that she began the novel in Paris between 1927 and 1931. *Nightwood*'s five main characters (Felix Volkbein, Matthew O'Connor, Robin Vote, Nora Flood, and Jenny Petherbridge) live and love primarily in Paris, although some wander to Vienna and America toward the novel's end. It has long been accepted that the novel is a roman à clef and that the character Robin is based on Thelma Wood, the love of Barnes's life, Nora on Barnes, O'Connor on Dan Mahoney, Barnes's drinking buddy, and Jenny Petherbridge on Henriette Metcalf, who supplanted Barnes as Thelma's partner.[1] Their portraits are far from mimetic, however; rather they stage, with slight variations, Barnes's personal ghosts. The characters' ghosts spring from the unspeakable parts of their family histories—parts they cannot communicate to others directly because they transgress taboos of race, gender, and sexuality. Though each character's ghost has a distinguishable cause, each has a similar effect on the character that it haunts and comes to possess. These effects, iterated in *Nightwood's* syntax, character behavior, and scenes, suggest the ghosts' common origin and gesture persistently toward a single intrapsychically preserved object of the libido: a shameful love and secret, and the words that give it half-life. This preserved object, as I discussed in the introduction and previous chapter, may be the sexual relationship that Barnes had with her grandmother, Zadel Barnes Gustafson.[2] In this manner, Barnes's work may be read to invoke not only its own secrets, but also the author's own history.

We should, says Dr. Matthew O'Connor, doubt "everything seen, done, spoken, precisely because we have a word for it, and not its alchemy" (83).

This is particularly true in *Nightwood*, whose images and scenes encrypt other meanings. An image, in *Nightwood*, is "a stop the mind makes between uncertainties" (111). The visible image captures the mind, but the arrested movement necessary for clear visibility imposes a separation in time, and the image's connection to the past becomes oblique. The relations that constitute it are frozen, vague in their particulars yet naturalized to some extent, as Barthes suggests. The image provides an echo of its own lost past in the field of the visible, something with which it seems the viewer can reunite—though actually it is already gone.

In *Nightwood*, haunting signals the simultaneous presence and absence of the love object to the subject, who disavows this object. *Nightwood*'s frequent spectral tropes suggest the ghosts of rapacious and loved family members, unspeakable scenes and, by extension, race, religion, and gender. These ghosts are embedded in and staged by its language and characters. Both text and characters constantly cite "crypts" and "phantoms" but never clearly expose the meanings that they cite. Barnes visually depicts both this paradoxical double movement of disavowal and the disavowed content in a gesture distinctive to her characters, images, animals, and objects—a movement, descent, falling or departure that is paradoxically motionless.

Though Abraham and Torok write, "to stage a word . . . constitutes an attempt at exorcism, an attempt . . . to relieve the unconscious by placing the effects of the phantom in the social realm," *Nightwood* offers no exorcism of its ghost words (176). The words that hide the secret also *are* the secret. Yet, though there is nothing outside of language, there is the possibility of the direct encounter with what language disavows. Haunted language and subjectivity break down in *Nightwood* as its characters attempt to replace their ghosts and confusions with full presence—in Barnes's terminology, to "hold the memory too close."[3] This does not dispel the ghosts, but leads to "possession," or total control by them. The compulsive actions of *Nightwood*'s characters in the final scenes of the novel occur simultaneously with their attempted abolition of difference, and with a dearth of metaphor in the novel's language. At its end, *Nightwood*'s ghost words cease to "haunt" and, instead, take over character behavior, and present as madness.

A psychic phantom may be socially functional if it is adopted as conventional behavior.[4] In *Nightwood*, phantoms are literarily functional: the social fabric of the novel presents a collective staging of love and loss.[5] Ghosts of lost loves animate the characters' behavior in relation to phantasmatic institutional power (the nation, the nobility, the military, the church and the medical profession), as well as influencing their relations to human love objects. Therefore, though Abraham and Torok claim that "to stage a word . . . constitutes an attempt at exorcism, an attempt . . . to relieve the unconscious by placing the effects of the phantom in the social realm,"[6] I argue that *Nightwood* offers no exorcism through its ghost words because it is the social realm itself that haunts its characters. *Nightwood*'s characters, like its circus people, have no inner life separate from "public life" (11). Yet haunted language and subjectivity break down in *Nightwood* as its characters attempt to replace their ghosts and confusions with embodied presences and certainties. This does not dispel the ghosts but leads instead to possession, wherein the ghosts exert unusual control over the characters. The incongruous behavior of *Nightwood*'s characters in the final scenes of the novel—their words and acts that involve bowing or "going down" – coincide with their attempts to abolish difference and with a dearth of metaphor in the novel's language. At its end, *Nightwood*'s ghost words cease merely to haunt. The words "wolf" and "bow down" or "go down" seem to possess characters and result in behaviors such as helpless genuflection, bowing and going down before a loved or revered other. Such scenes appear so often that they suggest a traumatic return on the part of the author herself, and raise the possibility that the characters enact Barnes's own scenes of shame and abandonment.

Contrary to critics who read in *Nightwood*'s form and content an uncompromising resistance to clarity and explication, I argue that the syntax and form of *Nightwood*'s language and fictional scenes must be separated from their content to allow the novel's subtly encrypted meanings to emerge. Ghost words, "wolf" and "go down" or "bow down," though they appear in surreptitious forms and within the discourses of race and class (Felix), gender and sexuality (Robin, O'Connor, Nora), and species (Robin) haunt *Nightwood*'s language and narrative, seemingly influencing character behavior and consequently the action of the novel. I read Abraham and Torok's theory of cryptophoria through Lacan's discussion of "disavowal" to draw from *Nightwood* a cryptic, yet insistent, presentation of the novel's explicit and implicit secrets. Not only Nora, but also Robin, Felix, O'Connor, and *Nightwood*'s language itself are all haunted by what Abraham and Torok call psychic crypts and phantoms: internalized love objects and the secret, affect-charged words associated with them. Further, the behavior of *Nightwood*'s characters, the novel's suspended images, evocative word choices, and its unclear and indirect style may also invoke the author's own—likewise encrypted—secrets.

The ghosts that constitute subjectivity in *Nightwood* enact a shift from haunting to possession. Its characters' ghost words begin as absent presences (haunting) but solidify into fully embodied symptoms that capture their subjectivity (possession). Robin, Nora, Felix, and O'Connor all enact cryptic imperatives throughout the novel and finally go down under them as they lose all sense of the difference, as such, between words and identities. O'Connor, as Judith Lee has argued, attempts to remind his interlocutors of the figurativity of language and the possibility of difference.[7] However, Nora's denial of difference seems to break his hold on it and to underwrite the novel's slide into ametaphorical language use and possessed character behavior: Nora and Robin's going down before each other, Felix's helpless bowing, and O'Connor's insistence on a selfsame identity with his dead brother in the chapter, "Go Down, Matthew" (160).

The shift of these ghostly power figures from haunting to possession is suggested at the novel's outset in the death scene of Felix's father, Guido, whose secrets are then embodied in Hedvig. In her life with the secretly Jewish Guido, Hedvig believed the false story of his baronetage, "as a soldier 'believes' a command" (5). She responds to his inability to "be one with her" by "moving toward him in recoil" in a doubled movement of inclusion and exclusion that cannot wholly include but must also alienate him (3). Though Guido, "in life . . . had done everything to span the impossible gap" that his secret maintained between Hedvig and himself, at his death "her body . . . became the barrier and Guido died against that wall, troubled and alone" (3). In death, at the end of language, the "impossible gap" of the secret solidifies into a love object that remains inaccessible.

Hedvig is a mother who also embodies the military and sovereign powers of "Old Europe" (9) and presents, as Rachel Potter discusses, "an image of nationalist belonging."[8] Giving birth to Felix "with the gross splendor of a general saluting the flag, she . . . thrust him from her, and died" (1). Her gesture and death represent the withdrawal of maternal, institutional, and national power figures from *Nightwood*'s postwar social fabric. The maternal figure—the subject's primary identification—and Europe's institutional centers of power exist in the imagined past—if at all—after *Nightwood*'s first pages. Yet its characters are driven down before their apparitions throughout the novel, "going down before the impending and inaccessible as before a great heat" (2–3). The lost love that *Nightwood*'s characters entomb reappears in the outside world as a beloved person, nation, or institution that impels them in pursuit of a "great past" that is both embodied and withheld (9). Each character descends before this phantasm, as though humanity could return to the past by yielding a little of our recently attained vertical stature. Each seeks the time before abandonment, but there is no such time—ironically, the sense of a time before subsists only in the encoded repetition of the abandonment: the curiously immobile descent. This descent cites the moment when unity with the beloved, first apprehended as lost, seemed almost still attainable. *Nightwood*'s "détraqués" (crazies) concoct images and titles that, taken at face value, contradict their "estrangement" from the (m)other and her law, whereas their animality (the circus people), bowing (Felix and Guido Sr.), and going down (O'Connor, Nora and Robin) affirm it (11). These ghosts take hold as the novel nears its end. O'Connor finally loses his "power of speech"[9] and identifies as his dead brother, and Felix unwillingly bows in "mortal shame" to the imagined Grand Duke of Russia (123). Robin transforms into a wolf, a symbol in modernity for the grandmother,[10] the "degenerate" [11] and the outlaw, the life that is in a legal sense already dead.[12]

Since *Nightwood* envisions subjectivity as a product of haunting or possession by an institutional or familial other, the novel's subversive import is thrown into question. Though the theoretical approaches of Foucault and Butler have been used to read Barnes's work as opening space for new modes of agency and articulation, *Nightwood* does not render agency as distinct from biopower (Foucault) or compelled citation (Butler). For *Nightwood*'s characters, as for Barnes, the loss of the first love object—the (grand)mother figure—does not enable an impartial and consistent (however harsh) social order in which limited autonomy can be claimed. Rather, *Nightwood*'s specters haunt a perverse universe and compel fetishistic behavior. Its characters' behaviors, though depicted as involuntary, bestial and "abandoned," remain enigmatic. They depict not repression, not the unconscious, but disavowal—the half-known that is at once accepted and rejected by being staged within another ostensible meaning. *Nightwood*'s cryptic tableaux attempt to create a textual unconscious by presenting, yet forbidding, knowledge to the reader—an action meant to shore up personal boundaries. While this strategy may have supplemented Barnes's sense of the difference between her ghosts and herself, the fates of *Nightwood*'s characters suggest the opposite. Though their behaviors may establish interpsychic boundaries by mystifying other characters (and *Nightwood*'s readers), intrapsychically, such behavior has the reverse effect: it undermines the autonomy that interpsychic boundaries are meant to secure, becoming so compulsive that the ghost words can be said to possess the characters.

Barnes defends herself against the phantom possession that she envisions for her characters by staging her ghost words in *Nightwood*'s suspended images, innocent-seeming phrases and bizarre character behaviors that seem incongruous or incidental to their situation. The fragmentation, resistance to interpretation, and repetition notable in the novel's tableaux and character behaviors are characteristic of cryptophoric, or fetishistic modes of expression, which fix meanings (here, the shameful and exciting connotations of significant words) in opaque, repetitive patterns. *Nightwood*'s narrative voice and characters draw on, but deny, the imperative charge of these words by staging their other, literal meanings. Thus, though I do read these cryptic words and behaviors figuratively, I also argue that they are staged literally in the novel in a way that withholds their figurative dimension from the reader. This simultaneous invocation and concealment, the double movement of disavowal, seems to supplement Barnes's sense of separation from what she invokes and hides.

As discussed in the introduction, in cryptophoria, words reminiscent of the fetish word(s) are spoken or acted out repeatedly by the cryptophore, with the apparent intention to communicate something other than the meaning associated with the shameful secret. This both invokes the secret and its erotic charge and keeps it at a distance. These fetishized objects or scenes gesture toward the intrapsychically preserved object of the libido: the shameful love and secret, and the word(s) that give it half-life. With this cryptic style, *Nightwood* establishes a difference between knowing and not knowing that acts as both invocation and boundary for the ghostly grandmother.

II. ROBIN AND NORA, PARENTS AND CHILDREN

As critics such as Victoria Smith and Merrill Cole have noted, Robin represents the lost past for both Felix and Nora. Julie Taylor notes that Robin "carries traces of both a disavowed past and the positive affect initially invested in that past (or, put differently, of both shame and the pleasure before the shame)."[13] While I agree, I also maintain that Robin evokes this past not because she is somehow free from the social order, as critics suggest, but because her foreclosure of her own abandonment by her mother embodies her as the novel's phantasmatic maternal figure. As the materfamilias of dream, Robin contains an unseen populace, "a company unaware" (57) of "unclean spirits" (168), the spirits and ghost words of others. Robin's movements and gestures, such as departing and returning, going down, and dashing dolls (147) and—almost—her son (48) to the ground, recall both the abandoning mother figure that she appears to have incorporated and the abandoned child self that goes down before that figure.

Since Robin's "picture forever arranged" (37) deceives the viewer into imagining eternal value, O'Connor says that the defense against her is an excremental trail between night and day that attaches the "detach[ed]" value to the particular instance, to the body's "nighttime" history (89). Similarly, in *Ryder*, the offal that history leaves can be preserved to maintain history's particularity: "of the banquet doth the turde tell" (65). O'Connor counsels the melancholic Nora to use dung "to make a roadway for" the past—"The brawl of the Beast leaves a path for the Beast" (84). In both novels, this trail of dirt is imagined to allow both the subject's past and the beast to come into the present without excessive agony. The trail of dirt left by the past love is a defense against the torment of being "too sharply reminded" of it by its sudden appearance in the outside world (89). Robin herself is this reminder—come upon, in Nora's case, "heavily, like an engine stalling against your chest" (84). Those, like Nora, who do not make a "roadway" come upon her and "all the things you can't bear and love . . . all at once" (135).

Nightwood's cryptophoric style attempts to defend against this too-sudden return of the past, with its words and images that bring the past surreptitiously into the present. This presentation of the past, perhaps, made *Nightwood* more an artistic than a therapeutic success for Barnes; its language seems too opaque for the reasonably clear articulations that talk therapy requires. O'Connor's and Nora's talks fail so spectacularly as therapy that they have been read as deliberately parodic.[14] *Nightwood* is less hopeful than *Ryder*, with its sloppy happy women, about the effectiveness of this presentation/abjection of the past. O'Connor, who attempts to bridge night and day, past and present, subject and object, fails to do so in *Nightwood*. *Nightwood*'s ghosts remain unreconciled, instead becoming ever more present and tormenting.

Critical readings of Robin that extrapolate from her an alternative realm to *Nightwood*'s, which informs Robin's behavior and makes her silence meaningful, overlook the ghosts that always already influence her. In these readings, Robin's supposed indeterminacy is conflated with an agency that the novel itself denies her. Robin's psychology, the relation of her behavior to the social world in which she lives, receives short shrift. The refusals and intentions that critics ascribe to her ignore *Nightwood*'s own descriptions of her as "lost" and "possessed" (48, 113). True, Robin is not possessed as a partner by her husband or lovers for long, as Susannah Martins points out, but the title of the book's last section, "The Possessed," surely includes her—and especially her final prostration—in its referential field (167).[15] Toward *Nightwood*'s conclusion, Robin erases the metaphorical dimension from the novel's description of her as a "beast" (37). Rather than refusing or subverting patriarchal determinations, her final descent to her hands and knees stages her and Nora's psychic phantoms—which have come to possess her—painfully literally. It is in this sense that it depicts, in Potter's words, a narrative "falling away from law, tradition, and history" and from "the humanist narrative of subjective self-realization."[16]

Robin neither has agency herself, nor does she enable it in other characters. She does not permit her lovers to mourn their original losses, as Gary Sherbert argues.[17] He suggests that Nora identifies Robin with her grandmother because of their lesbian relationship; thus, "Robin's entombment consciously repeats Nora's unconscious entombment of her grandmother and therefore offers a means of healing Nora's psychic wound."[18] This reading would support Jonathan Flatley's argument that ghosts enable a subjects' fuller engagement with present reality. By Flatley's and Sherbert's logic, perhaps, Robin's evocation of Nora's grandmother may have enabled Djuna Barnes, as author, fuller presence to these characters' prototypes—and perhaps even to the ghostly sociohistorical forces that estrange her characters and that are deeply though enigmatically imbricated in the interpersonal dynamics of her characters. The power of *Nightwood*'s affective map for readers is evident in the many stories of women, heartbroken over other women, crying on Barnes's doorstep at Patchin Place. However, the mourning, for Sherbert, or empowered melancholia, for Flatley, that *Nightwood* enabled for readers may not have been enabled for Barnes: the disidentification necessary to this may have been vexed, as *Nightwood*'s logic suggests.

I maintain that Nora conflates Robin and her grandmother because of Robin's homosexual "identity," not because of their lesbian relationship.[19] Robin's androgynous appearance and correlative exclusion from subjectivity (by *Nightwood*'s logic) allows her lovers to deny that their losses ever occurred. Robin's androgyny, as O'Connor tells Nora, makes her the image of a time before loss and separation "where what we never had stands waiting" (137). In *Nightwood*, the term "invert" is not used in relation to Nora or Jenny—who merely, as they say, have sex with women. Instead, "invert" refers only to O'Connor and to Robin, who "resembles a boy" (136). Further, the novel's ending suggests the reverse of a successful therapeutic outcome for Nora.

As Foucault discusses, modernity was characterized by the transformation of sexuality and sexual object choice from a practice (as *Nightwood* implies it is for Nora and Jenny) to an identity, as seen in Robin's inversion. Inversion—imagined as childish, androgynous underdevelopment—is a characteristic of modern sexology's cretin, who lacks the power of speech.[20] Robin, the cretinous (silent, childish) "invert," is "the living lie of our centuries," which "our miscalculated longing has created" (136–7), a formulation that suggests the miscalculations and luxurious abhorrence of modern pseudoscientific disciplines. Robin stages the social specter of homosexual "subhumanity," and the power relation that creates it.

Robin is available to become her lovers' and modern sexology's fetish because her androgyny recalls a time before sexual difference. She has no "volition for refusal" and, thus, no gender (43). Robin, the invert, represents the lost homosexual love on whose disavowal, Butler suggests, heterosexual identity is premised.[21] Nora's melancholic claim, "a woman is yourself, caught as you turn in panic," invokes this model (143). Robin, accordingly, appears as the lost love object both in particular (Nora's grandmother) and in general (the same-sex parent figure that every heterosexual "never loved" and "never grieved").[22] In O'Connor's words,

> What is this love we have for the invert, boy or girl? . . . They go far back in our lost distance where what we never had stands waiting; it was inevitable that we should come upon them, for our miscalculated longing has created them. They are our answer to what our grandmothers were told love was, and what it never came to be; they, the living lie of our centuries. (136–7)

The love that "our grandmothers" were told of, which "never came to be," is answered from without as the "invert." Robin represents "the sweetest lie of all" to her lovers because she embodies what is disavowed by this lie: the same-sex lost love that they "never had." Her "'aside' voice of the actor" speaks of what is always peripheral to "the scene" as cryptophoric subjects present it, the spectral margin in which their disavowed relationships are maintained (38). It is "enchanted with the gift of postponed abandon," the postponement of the love object's abandonment of the subject. O'Connor tells Nora that Robin has power over her because Nora is unable to "make a roadway" for "the night," her disavowed secret, that would allow her to remember it by day (84). Thus, it "come[s] upon [her] heavily—an engine stalling itself upon [her] chest," in the form of Robin (84). Far from offering Nora and Felix a means of mourning their losses, Robin functions as a fetish-object to reinforce their melancholic disavowal of lost love.

Of all the characters, Robin is the least able to mourn through language, and is, therefore, the most preoccupied. Inasmuch as language is ametaphorical for Robin, literal enactment becomes her only source of meaning. Hence, she looks for herself through reproduction and travel. Similarly, physical violence from Nora and Jenny renders her docile and prone, whereas she is indifferent to their pleading (144, 76). Nonetheless, Robin is an "infected carrier of the past," which can be seen in her use of, and seeming subjection to, the particular words associated with it, like "wolf" and "go down" (37). Her appearance, itself, recalls cryptophoric incorporation, which Abraham and Torok claim involves a fantasy that the lost, unnamable object is literally taken into the subject via the mouth.[23] She seems at once edible ("we feel that we could eat her"), eaten ("eaten death returning"), and voracious ("human hunger pressing its breast to its prey") (37). This hunger that she embodies and invokes is for the imagined return to "a forgotten experience" of pre-subjective unity, "a mirage of an eternal wedding" (37). Robin's passive acquiescence to motherhood and her conversion to Catholicism also imply that she, herself, is the mother whom she "never lost":

> Strangely aware of some lost land in herself, she took to going out; wandering the countryside . . . she wandered to thoughts of women, women that she had come to connect with women. Strangely enough, these were women in history. . . . She prayed, and her prayer was monstrous because there was no margin left in it for damnation or forgiveness, for praise or for blame. . . . She only told of herself in a preoccupation that was its own predicament. (45–7)

Robin's preoccupation is "its own predicament" because it makes her unable to represent and mourn any loss or separation. "She herself is the only 'position'" (146) in an imaginary unity in which the desires of others are indistinguishable from her own and thus irresistible. Her "very lack of identity makes [her] ourselves" (88). Robin "had come to connect with women," but she "only told of herself" (47). There is no other in her prayer, and hence, there is "no margin left for damnation or forgiveness, for praise or for blame." Robin's cryptophoric lovers, searching in her for the "one sole condition" that they have forfeited, instead encounter the loss of symbolic language, which is predicated on difference (112). The melancholy that Robin awakens in others mirrors her own difficulty in distinguishing her subjectivity by "thinking herself alone" (167). To Felix, it seems that "her attention . . . had already been taken by something not yet in history" (44). This thing not yet in history is Robin herself: her entry into subjectivity through the loss of imaginary unity with her mother. Felix's demand for a child, "Wo ist das kind?" echoes Robin's own search for herself (45). In response, she "conceived herself pregnant" in a strange autofertilization, mimicking her mother by conceiving herself (45). She occupies the positions of both her mother and herself, her mother's object.

Robin's childlike behavior and her adoption of "boy's clothes" (147) with Nora—previously, with Felix, she had favored old dresses and skirts (42)—also suggests the melancholic incorporation of her abandoned son, Guido. As the abandoning mother, she "didn't want him," but after giving birth to him she was "lost" (48). As an abandoned child, Robin cries "like a child who has walked into the commencement of a horror." However, she is, in the manner of the cryptophore, "secret about [Guido]. . . . Why talk?" (49). Instead, she symptomizes her loss of her son by dressing in "boy's clothes" and playing with toys for hours. Her abandonment by her own mother is restaged with Guido, whom she almost dashes down to the ground before her (48). Robin's "going down" before the Madonna on Catholic altars also stages this abandonment in more traditional terms, with herself as the child and the Madonna as mother (46). Though she "long[s] to be kept" (58), Robin repeatedly abandons as the mother and is "lost" as the child (55).

In these scenes, Robin's "monstrous" life interchanges the roles of parent and child, power and outcast, betrayer and betrayed (47). With Nora, Guido, and Jenny's foster child, Sylvia, Robin occupies the subject positions of both abandoning mother and abandoned child. Because Nora has a psychic crypt of her own, Robin can play the role of Nora's grandmother while she plays her own mother. Her inhabitation of these roles is evident in the way that she seduces and subsequently abandons Sylvia (115). Like Nora falling "in one place" (51), and like the poor cow during an air raid that "had gone somewhere very fast . . . yet was still standing there" (22), Sylvia is pictured as both departing and staying still in response to horror. When Jenny, a repulsive grandmother figure, attacks Robin, an attractive one, and simultaneously a child figure, they fall forward into each other as if uniting (76). O'Connor describes Sylvia, who is with Jenny and Robin, as "running away from something grown up . . . she was sitting still and she was running" (106). These double movements (falling forward in marred union, running away while being still) implicate Sylvia in "something grown up" from which she cannot separate herself. She, too, "flung herself down" and even her plea, "Let me go!" is "controlled with terror" (76). Sylvia is cast in the role of Nora in her childhood of brutalized innocence. Sylvia has "fallen in love" with Robin, who wakes her up throughout the night to ask her to confirm this (115). However, Robin then forgets Sylvia, whose response is shame: "[S]hame went all over her" (116). "Who is Sylvia?" asks O'Connor, innocently, of Nora, naming the title of a popular song.

Robin's attraction to Jenny Petherbridge, an aged and predatory "squatter," can also be read as a response to Nora's psychic crypt (65). The ravening Jenny fascinates both Nora (131) and Robin (144), as do elderly prostitutes, and these may represent Nora's desire for an older woman encrypted. A crypt, Abraham and Torok write, walls off and protects a guilty pleasure to maintain the expectation that it may be resumed.[24] In *Nightwood*, Nora's encrypted expectation is suggested by Dr. O'Connor's success in commanding her "attention for the first time" with his description of the zombielike Tuppeny Upright. A Tuppeny is a whore whose price has been reduced by age to tuppence, who stands while "letting you do it, as silent and indifferent as the dead, as if . . . waiting for something that they had been promised when they were little girls" (130 – 1). Nora's dead grandmother, he implies, is indifferent. It is Nora's desire for her that causes her to go "slowly along in the dark" (130). Nora's claim to O'Connor that "it is only through me, of all my family, that my grandmother dies, over and over" (149) avows her sense of her grandmother as victim, damned to a cycle of life and death by Nora's love and disavowal, just as Nora's letters "raise" Robin from her "sleep" (125) "as cannons bring up the dead from deep water" (150). However, the leering, waistcoated grandmother in Nora's dream, "symbolizing her life out of her life" that "now appeared to Nora as something being done to Robin," testifies to Nora's simultaneous sense of her grandmother as a predator (63). "Steaming in the vapors of someone else about to die" and living "among her own things like a visitor to a room kept 'exactly as it was when'" (65–6), Jenny incarnates the grandmother in her predatory, "ridiculous," yet sexualized, aspect (63). Together, Robin and Jenny make a tableau vivant of Nora's cryptophoria: "eternally separated, in a cataleptic frozen gesture of abandon," they "presented two halves of a movement" of advance and withdrawal (69).

Nora falls in response to Robin, as well as falling "continually and forever" through the "gap in 'world pain'" (64). Such falling may be read as a reference to her own encrypted memories and also, perhaps, to Robin's; the two are not fully distinguished (169). Nora's psychic crypt, like Robin's, is signaled by the "preoccupation" in which she is "endlessly embroiled" (53). However, unlike Robin, Nora is not silent. Through language, she has at least partially entered the social order, which excludes and masks knowledge of her encrypted grandmother; "the world" itself is hence partitioned off from her, "like a ship in a bottle" (53). Nora's love for Robin is also crypt-like: it is encapsulated and preserved, a "deposit of the heart, analogous in all degrees to the 'findings' in a tomb" (56). Nora herself suggests that a lack of understanding and a "want[ing] to forget" create this sealed structure that contains, but excludes, what "we have loved": "All that we have loved becomes the 'forbidden' when we have not understood it all, as the pauper is the rudiment of the city, knowing something of the city, which the city, for its own destiny, wants to forget" (156).

Along with the expected images of sealed structures and containers, images of motionless movement and descent or departure allude not only to the contents of Nora's psychic crypt, but to Nora's crypt-like presentation, as such. The image of Nora "eternally moving downward" through the "gap in 'world pain,'" but "in one place, and perpetually before the eye" (51) again describes the relation between Nora and the world that her secret of incestuous love and loss entails. As the world appears visible, immobile and separate to Nora, so she appears conspicuous and suspended to the world.

Nora's "grandmother's bedroom" dream describes the intrapsychic correlative of her perpetual motionless fall before the world's eye, and represents her psychic crypt as the saturating "lost presence" of her grandmother in the continuous act of departing:

> This chamber that had never been her grandmother's, which was, on the contrary, the absolute opposite of any known room her grandmother had ever moved or lived in, was nevertheless saturated with the lost presence of her grandmother, who seemed to be in the continual process of leaving it. The architecture of dream had rebuilt her everlasting and continuous, flowing away in a long gown of soft folds and chin laces, the pinched gatherings that composed the train taking an upward line over the back and hips in a curve that not only bent age but fear of bent age demands. (63)

In a parallel to Nora's dream, the architecture of *Nightwood*, itself, rebuilds the grandmother as "everlasting and continuous" but constantly "flowing away," apprehended only in her departure, and recalled in Robin's departure. The grandmother subsists most fully for Nora in her actual loss of Robin. This loss was prefigured even while they lived together. For Nora, whose eyes "report not so much the object as the movement of the object" (52), Robin's behavior and desire "to go and yet to stay" (140) always already recalls the ever departing presence, the fleeting, but recurring, connotation of the psychic crypt. The only way to annul this postponed abandonment would be to abolish time and space itself, perhaps in death, so that the division of past from future, connotation from denotation, might be impossible. This is the wish O'Connor describes in the bereft lover:

> face down, with that terrible longing of the body that would, in misery, be flat with the floor; lost lower than burial, utterly blotted out and erased so that no stain of her could ache upon the wood, or snatched back to nothing without aim—going backward through the target, taking with her the spot where she made one. (95)

Descending, going down, is going back in time to reinstate a time prior to the losses inflicted by life. Thus, the girls in the toilets, going down on their lovers, cry, "I'm an angel on all fours, with a child's feet behind me, seeking my people who have never been made, going down face foremost" (95). Their descent, described in the most sordid possible terms, seeks to recapture the only time before loss and shame: the time before subjectivity. But this pre-time is surrounded on all sides by past, future, and damnation: "God damned you before me, and after me you shall be damned, kneeling and standing away till we vanish!" To go down on the "damned and betraying" loved one is to come as near as possible to the time before the betrayal: "In the acceptance of depravity," says O'Connor, "the sense of the past is most fully captured" (118).

This substitution of the staged loss for the lost object appears in Robin's movements and their effects on Nora and Felix. Robin's endless cycle of desertions and returns, which proceed from her desire "to leave and not to go" (140), circumvents time and separation by this logic of substitution. Nora cannot avoid falling victim to Robin's desertion because it recalls an imagined past in which Nora and her grandmother were one: "As an amputated hand cannot be disowned because it is experiencing a futurity, of which the victim is its forebear, so Robin was an amputation that Nora could not renounce" (59). Robin also experiences separation from her mother substitute, Nora, as something that has yet to happen; loss is always a form of futurity for her.

Barnes stages Robin's relation to Nora as her failed attempt to enter into subjectivity. It appears that Robin's failure to enact the first separation (which Butler speculates is a ritual of guilt and acquittal) bars her attempt to become human, so she substitutes Nora for the law and trusts that Nora's inability to renounce her will bring her partly into the human fold.[25] Since Robin can neither feel, nor be absolved of, guilt, she seeks subjectivity through her secret betrayals of her mother substitute Nora, and through Nora's condemnation and forgiveness. Robin's privacy consists in her life away from Nora because she can experience herself as a separate subject only through Nora's experience of the separation between herself and Robin. O'Connor makes a remark to Nora which suggests that cryptophoria is involved in Robin's "making [Nora] the Madonna" (146): "Night people do not bury their dead, but on the neck of you, their beloved and waking, sling the creature, husked of its gestures" (89). Nora's suffering and forgiveness are Robin's salvation and, inseparably, her damnation; Nora is both "the Madonna" and "a devil" that "make[s] everything dirty" (143). "Only you," Robin tells Nora, "mustn't be gay or happy, not like that, it's not for you, only for everyone else in the world" (155).

On seeing a whore dozing in her room next to an altar to the Madonna, Nora realizes that she was "a fixed dismay" to Robin, "the space between the human and the holy head" (157). The Madonna, Nora suggests, does not absolve the whore but divides her: their relation creates guilt, but it is the Madonna who is "indecent" by being "fixed" and "eternal." The whore, arms akimbo "as if half of her slept, and half of her suffered," is incompletely interpellated by the Madonna, the suffering half of her perhaps knowing that she is guilty, the sleeping half yet believing that she is innocent. Likewise, Robin is "innocent because she can't do anything in relation to anyone but herself" (146) but is simultaneously "driv[en] . . . out of her wits" by Nora's "shadow" (155).

The subjectivity that Robin gains through Nora, Nora's "grandmother's bedroom" dream suggests, is inscribed by the phantom grandmother. In this dream, her grandmother's "life out of her life" appears as something "being done to Robin, Robin disfigured and eternalized by the hieroglyphics of sleep and pain" (63). Nora's break with Robin "befoul[s]" Robin because it reiterates an earlier split in Nora's conscious relation to her grandmother, when the grandmother could no longer be imagined as "innocent" and sleeping but began instead to be seen as "corrupt" and predatory (146). As Nora claims, no "rot had touched [Robin] until then, and there before my eyes I saw her corrupt all at once and withering because I had struck her sleep away" (145). Robin loses her "innocen[ce]," her experience of loss as a futurity, and suddenly resembles something ruined and re-encountered, "something once beautiful found in a river" (142). On seeing Robin ametaphorically embody her grandmother, Nora "went mad and [has] been mad ever since" (145).

In her madness, Nora appeals first to Robin and then to O'Connor to speak, as though speech might restore a symbolic universe, and thus sanity, to a psyche threatened with dissolution, "Matthew, for God's sake, say something, you're awful enough to say it, say something!" (145). Nora wishes O'Connor to take on the role of the parent figure who (re)instates language—for Lacan, the father, whose function as a guarantor of meaning is later ceded to God or some other authority figure, for Abraham and Torok, the mother, who must teach the child language so that it may begin "mourning" her (128). Nora asks

O'Connor to decode and verbalize her dreams, the "hieroglyphics of sleep and pain" (63) that "disfigured" Robin, "What was that dream saying, for God's sake, what was that dream?" To this, O'Connor indirectly articulates Robin's unspoken desire, which he shares: "Mother of God! It's my mother without argument I want" (149). He implies that the loss of unity with the mother figure, her desire, and the desire for her, must be articulated before Nora's dream can symbolize anything. But Nora denies her separateness from Robin and thus implicitly denies O'Connor's power to reinstate figurative language by naming Robin's demand for Nora, and Nora's for Robin, as desire. In words that foreshadow the end of individuation and figurativity in *Nightwood*, Nora tells O'Connor that if she and Robin had slept in the whore's bed, they (Nora and Robin) would have "molted our parts, as figures in the waxworks are molted down to their story, so we would have broken down to our love" (158). However instead of coming together like melting wax figures, or even like regular human lovers, they finally reunite only in mutual prostration before the ghosts that possess them: the mother and grandmother figures, whose return each represents to the other. This is neither union nor separation, but possession, the compulsive, anti-metaphorical citation of the ghost words "wolf" and "go down."

Given also the discussions of the significance of "Red Riding Hood and the wolf in bed" in critical interpretations of *Nightwood*, and Barnes's remarks about Thelma Wood's "wolf's blood," it is surprising that Robin's final going down has not yet been read as lycanthropy.[26] Such a reading would be consistent with Abraham and Torok's theory of the phantom and allow for an assessment of Robin's wolfishness as a symptom of Nora's psychic crypt. Accordingly, Robin's escape into an alternate mode of being—one critics have presumed to be free of the desires of others—during her reunion with Nora, in fact, represents her capture by the phantom of Nora's crypt, and is a testimony to its grandmotherly content. Robin's attempt to become the wolf for real by going down on all fours with Nora's dog may be read as an attempt to neutralize Nora's shameful secret by staging the fetish word, "wolf," associated with it. In an English folk tradition that is still alive, the touching of wood neutralizes the power of language to invoke what has been left out or denied by a statement.[27] It is, therefore, significant that Nora's body strikes "the wood" at the same moment that Robin stages the grandmother-wolf (169). The action simultaneously suggests the final nullification of the figurative power of language and Nora's desire for the grandmother, which emerges anti-metaphorically in Robin.

III. GOING DOWN AND THE WOLF

The final descents and genuflections of Felix, O'Connor, Nora and Robin suggest their takeover by ghost words. Such descents and genuflections are figurative in O'Connor's case, but literal for the others. Though scenes of prostration have appeared earlier, the characters' behavior in their closing scenes appears less voluntary and even less appropriate to social context. Robin's "transformation" into a wolf, Felix's helpless bowing, and O'Connor and Nora's "going down" symptomize relations of abandonment between both parent and child and power and outlaw or "sacred life." Felix cites his "racial memory" of anti-Semitic persecution; O'Connor cites a triangulation with his mother and brother; Nora, the most transparently Barnes-based character, cites her grandmother and her child self; and Robin cites her own mother and child self, as well as Nora's grandmother. Concomitantly, these characters stage social specters (Jewish, homosexual, and transgendered identities) in prostrations that anti-metaphorically enact the "symmetry of *homo sacer* and sovereign"—that is, the symmetry of the law (or rather, the ravening power), which governs their desire, and the social outlaw (*wargus*), who is both bound and abandoned by this law.[28] Their prostrations suggest sadomasochistic theatre's mimesis of the relation of power to outlaw or "sacred life," as Agamben describes it. In *Nightwood*, as in sadomasochistic theatre, this social relation appears in a context in which it is not "in the picture."

Nora's insistence to O'Connor that "[Robin] is myself" is rooted in Robin's "anonymity" (55), the "great passionate indifference" or nondifferentiation that she "treat[s] her lovers to" (139). Aptly, *Nightwood*'s phrasing makes it impossible to conclude whether it is Nora and Robin or the "spirits" of "love and anonymity" that are "haunted of" one another (55). In their haunted state, Nora and Robin present to each other the missing "half of the story that both forgot" (138), embodying each other's lost encrypted loves and lost selves interchangeably; however, once separated, Nora seeks to reunite with Robin by becoming her. She traces Robin's steps, sleeps with her lovers, "haunt[s] the cafés where Robin had lived her night-life" (156). Robin, who also searches for herself, recommences her visits to chapel Madonnas and searches the faces of wild animals for images of a life free from the desires of others (168–9). Ironically, Robin's search for herself is determined by others' desires: by discourses of degeneracy and primitivism, by Nora's encrypted grandmother, and by the phantom word "wolf." Because of Nora's insistence on their unity and Robin's inability to achieve subjectivity, they end, as O'Connor predicts, "locked together, like the poor beasts that get their antlers mixed and are found dead that way" (100). Nora and Robin's last scene takes place before an altar to the Madonna, the "impending and inaccessible" mother before whom Robin descends, while Nora goes down before the grandmother-wolf who possesses Robin. Not only, as Potter argues, does Robin's "crawling on all fours with a dog" represent "the culmination of a narrative falling away from the humanist narrative of subjective self-realization," it represents the triumph of anti-metaphorical, non-narrative, and dehumanizing meaning.[29]

In Abraham and Torok's work, in European folktale, and in *Nightwood*, itself, the wolf is an uncanny figure for both the "unhomely" sexual predator and the "homely" grandmother.[30] Martins interprets Nora's thought, on seeing Dr. O'Connor in a nightgown, "Children . . . like Red Riding Hood and the wolf in bed" (79) as a recasting of the Freudian primal scene in which the horizontal position of the wolf feminizes it. Martins argues that "the prostrate wolf is associated with the passive female object of desire—the mother, in the primal scene."[31] The story of Red Riding Hood, itself, however, as well as the strong presence of the grandmother in *Nightwood*, suggest the wolf as grandmother. That this thought occurs to Nora upon seeing O'Connor in drag, lying "beside himself" (80), implies to Martins that "the wolf and Red Riding Hood are the same person."[32] In Nora's subjective economy, then, she and the grandmother are "the same person." Further, Nora's thought is "only the sensation of a thought" (79). Nora does not fully articulate the idea of the wolf, even in thought, because "wolf," as something that children like to have in bed with Red Riding Hood, is a fetish word, a key to the psychic crypt containing her grandmother.

Except for Nora's "sensation of a thought," the text circles the grandmother-wolf in its many references to dogs, unspecified "beasts," prostrate women, and "bitches." However, the wolf was a popular trope in modernity. It could stand for mental illness, as with Freud's Wolf Man,[33] and, consecutively, for the degeneracy attributed to homosexuality.[34] It also troped predatory humans (Red Riding Hood), man in the "state of nature" (Thomas Hobbes), and *homo sacer* (as Agamben discusses). Sacred life, writes Agamben, has been symbolized by the werewolf by political writers throughout history because "the transformation into a werewolf corresponds perfectly to the state of exception. . . . What had to remain in the collective unconscious as a monstrous hybrid of human and animal [is] at its origin the figure of the man who has been banned from the city, [in] a zone of indistinction between the human and the animal" (106). Thus, Agamben argues, the figure of the banned werewolf who dwells within the city, in proximity to the sovereign, tropes the truth that "[s]overeign violence is . . . founded not on a pact but on the exclusive inclusion of bare life in the state" (107).

Barnes was something of a Hobbesian, as O'Neal discusses in his memoir. Its title, "*Life is painful, nasty, and short . . . in my case it has only been painful and nasty*," comes from a conversation with Barnes, who applied Hobbes's famous description of life in the "state of nature" to herself. Barnes also advocated for Hobbes's oft-quoted statement that all human relations are market relations, according to O'Neal, who said, "She told me hundreds of times that the only reason anyone does anything is for money" (174). The Hobbs family in *The Antiphon* represents the Hobbesian "state of nature" in the form of parental lawlessness. The Barnes-figure's father, the rapacious Titus Hobbs, is dead, and "his beasts, the girls" (128) are gone. But her brothers are clearly upholding family tradition in attempting to "stand her on four feet" (176), and her mother, Augusta Hobbs, finally murders her with a large curfew bell (222), seemingly for resisting her brothers' advances. In both *The Antiphon* and *Nightwood*, Hobbes's "*homo hominis lupus*" (the state in which "man is a wolf to men") tropes family and sexual abuse.

IV. FELIX'S AND O'CONNOR'S ANTIMETAPHORS

Like Robin and Nora, Felix and O'Connor symptomize abandoning maternal figures in their strange words, behaviors, and descents, which I read in my introduction as antimetaphors, or anti-symbolic renderings of symbolic content. Felix wants to reunite with the past in his love for Robin, the image of this past. To Felix, Robin seems to bring together his "broken fate" by uniting "an image and its reflection," the representation of his great past that he labors to construct, and what is, he imagines, represented (38). He is drawn to Robin, he tells O'Connor, by her "undefinable disorder, a sort of 'odor of memory'" that gave her the "quality of one sole condition" shared by his aunt's story of his family: the "condition" of never having lost that Robin suggests to her lovers. He describes this as "a fluid sort of possession . . . what then appeared to me to be security, and which was, in reality, the most formless loss" (112–13). That Robin's "loss" is "formless," that her "possession" is "fluid," that her "memory" is only an "odor," suggests that this loss is unformulated in language. Felix ascribes his love for Robin to his fabricated past. "My family is preserved because I have it only from the memory of one single woman, my aunt; therefore it is single, clear, and unalterable. . . . Through this I have a sense of immortality. Our basic idea of eternity is a condition that *cannot vary*" (112).

Felix, whose people embodied "sacred life" throughout European history, believes that the "great past" he has lost is the splendor of a noble family. Robin, whose "fluid sort of possession" is actually a "formless loss" that "cannot vary," represents the real loss that he does not know but that subsists for him in the gaps, or "formless loss[es]," in his aunt's narrative.

Though Felix does not know these losses, he symptomizes them. In his mother, Hedvig, who gives birth to him on a bed with a "valance stamped with the bifurcated wings of the House of Hapsburg" (1), the novel represents the "Old Europe" (9) of Felix's obsession (especially Austria, Germany and the military) as a maternal figure. Felix, like his father, Guido, pays homage to the powers that Hedvig embodies, "going down . . . as before a great heat" (2–3). Their spasmodic "genuflexion that the hunted body makes from muscular contraction" (2) suggests the transgenerational phantom of anti-Semitism, the genuflexions of hunted bodies compulsively repeated in the hunter's absent presence. "Thrust[ing] him from her and dy[ing]," Hedvig represents Felix's abandonment by "Old Europe" (1). His choices of Robin and of Frau Mann evoke his disavowed loss: "Again in the ambit of his father's futile attempts to encompass the rhythm of his wife's stride" (44–5), Felix iterates modernity's anti-Semitic discourses on the feminine Jew's futile mimicry of the manly Aryan.[35] He also makes strange remarks; confronting Robin's indifference to his stories of the "great past" in which their marriage has "included" her, he adds, "I am deceiving you!" and wonders what he means (45). Most tellingly, he stages the "racial memories" of persecution encrypted in his aunt's narrative of his past. These memories, "binding . . . about" Felix's father, were testified to only by his clutching of a yellow and black handkerchief "that cried aloud of the ordinance of 1468 . . . demanding that, with a rope about its neck, Guido's race should run in the Corso for the amusement of the Christian populace" (2). Not dispelled by their articulation by the handkerchief, these phantoms cause Felix to "Bow Down" in (re) citations of the dehumanization of his people by European Christians (1). Taylor has noted the compulsion underlying Felix's bowing, writing, "Felix is so thoroughly shaped by shame that the interest-excitement that forms the basis for his 'bowing down'" transforms his shame response itself into "an affect invested with interest." She suggests that this affect-charged performance "illustrates the potential closeness of pleasure to the painful experience of shame" because it suggests "Felix's initial interest is already bound up with shameful attachments."[36] However, Felix's final "abandoned" bow of a "madman" toward the imagined Grand Duke Alexander of Russia suggests not so much conscious investments of interest as "possession" by the unknown memories that haunt him (122–3). Felix, "his head making a complete half-swing, as an animal will turn its head away from a human, as if in mortal shame" (123), compulsively cites a bestial history he does not know.

However, Felix's last moments with the young Guido, "the shadow of his anxiety," offer a more functional, if still compelled, reiteration and suggest more productive affects than shame (120). "Carrying a pocket full of medicines, and a little flask of oil for the chapping hands of his son," he invokes the stereotype of the Jewish peddler, equipped with medicines and concerned with the vicissitudes of corporeality (122). His "Come . . . you are cold" (123), recalls the "cold yet hysterical abandon" with which "the Christian populace" applauded the torture of Jews (2). But Guido, though "cold," is not "abandoned." Felix, rubbing oil into his son's hands, cites a "Jewishness" that, though stereotypical, suggests a more empowered reappropriation of the past.

O'Connor, the standard-bearer of language and difference throughout the novel, knows better than to take Robin's "formless loss" as "security." When speaking of the night to Nora, O'Connor speaks chiefly of things' difference from one another, and from themselves at one time and another time, of the importance of understanding this difference, and of the pain that it causes the lover who would be her beloved's only object—and who tries, therefore, to deny difference. O'Connor suggests that it is the heterogeneity and mutability of the night, and the change it makes "to a person's identity" and to "things" that Nora must learn to accept (81, 85). Like Barnes, herself, O'Connor attempts to use language to shore up identity while gesturing at its inadequacy, since a "word" for a thing is not its "alchemy" (83). His stories, he admits, are "lies" motivated by his friends' appeals to him to "say something" (135). However, his final monologues suggest that he himself has denied difference and loss and internalized lost objects.

In "Go Down, Matthew," O'Connor presents a psychic crypt that contains his brother, "as if my memory of him were himself" (152). Nora, who "believed in the word" (51), insists to him that Robin "is myself" (127). Her insistence on this point brings O'Connor to "confused and unhappy silence" (158) and the conclusion that all his speech was "for nothing" (165). Drunk in a bar after his escape from Nora, O'Connor insists on his literal identity with his dead brother:

> Is not a brother his brother also, the one blood cut up in lengths, one called Michael and the other Matthew? . . . Who's to say that I'm not my brother's wife's husband and that her children were not fathered in my lap? Is it not to his honor that he strikes me as myself? (160)

If it was his mother that O'Connor "want[ed]" and his brother whom she loved, then his object choice of men, identification as a woman and claims of identity with his brother suggest a childhood triangulation and "shameful secret" involving mother and brother.[37] O'Connor's once taboo, now acknowledged, desire for his mother was first incorporated as his adoption of female gender. Once O'Connor identifies as female, I argue that the brother then replaces the mother as love object about which a psychic crypt was formed.[38] Nora's thought on seeing O'Connor in a nightgown that "he dresses to lie beside himself" also suggests this double possession (80). Brimming with feminine accessories, the room "was also muscular, a cross between a *chambre à coucher* and a boxer's training camp," and contained an abdominal brace that "gave the impression that the feminine finery had suffered venery"

(79). The room represents O'Connor's layered identity: the feminine surface (drag) that yet, "giving back evidence" of the brother occupying it, is "mauled as the last agony" (80).

Not only O'Connor's female gender, but also his profession of performing illegal abortions at a convent may be read as cryptophoric references to his mother and brother (114). O'Connor's description of wombs as the prisons of damned convicts (97), his wish that we could be born in the grave and crawl into the uterus to die (99) and his cryptic "I began to wail for all the little beasts in their mothers" (105) all raise the question of his motivation for his profession. His interventions change the womb from a place of life to a place of death, suggesting perhaps a desire to retroactively eliminate his unborn brother—and, consecutively, himself—in utero. Since he incorporates his mother, the first identification, this reversal of his brother's and his own birth would transform the male physiology of his body surface, as well as eliminate his encrypted brother from his psyche. By cryptophoric logic, he would become "entirely" a woman, "with a womb as big as a king's kettle," instead of having "a face . . . like an old child's bottom" (91). O'Connor's profession may cryptophorically express his wish to have his mother "all to [him]self," a wish that Barnes might have echoed, since as Herring documents she resented having to share Zadel's affection with her father, Wald Barnes, and with proliferating siblings and half-siblings.[39] An early draft of *Nightwood* shares this vision: in one of O'Connor's excised stories of serving in the First World War, a sergeant about to handcuff him, "gave up the ghost," and instead took his hand to lead him to prison. O'Connor then felt that he "had a mother. . . . I had always wanted one *all to myself*!"[40] His anticipated incarceration reminds O'Connor of his mother: "in our mother's wombs we are close prisoners all" (97). For him, the crypt-like structure of the womb contains and excludes the child as a prison both contains and excludes the outlaw within "the people."

Tellingly, O'Connor's work of abortion reformulates the relation between law and outlaw, as Agamben describes it, by giving the mother the power to "take life or let live" in relation to the fetus.[41] O'Connor, who wishes to exorcise his brother and so to have his mother "all to [him]self," works at the vanguard of modern advances in technology and the disciplines that increasingly expose life to death. Yet given the usually shattering and lethal effects of childbearing in Barnes's work, O'Connor's cryptophoric profession in *Nightwood* suggests a defense by the subject against the other that invades it, a power to destroy rather than be destroyed. But this choice is only possible when the other is corporeal, the forebear rather than the futurity of its own amputation. That O'Connor's job stages his encrypted desires suggests also that it may be a predetermined "choice," another repetition of the moment when unity with the beloved, first apprehended as lost, seemed almost attainable.

V. EXORCISM AND EXCISION

Excised from *Nightwood*'s final version is a fragment rendering Barnes's rape at age 17 by 52-year-old Percy Faulkner.[42] The Barnes character, then Catherine, "had gone down on the floor and hugged my grandmother by her knees, dropping my head down, saying, 'Don't let it happen!' and she said, 'It had to happen.'"[43] Also cut was the narrative of Barnes's betrayal by and prostration before her second great love, Ernst Hanfstengl (1887–1975), to whom she was engaged from 1914–1916. He broke off their engagement because she wasn't German and went on to become the chief minister of the foreign press for the Nazi party from 1932–1937, according to Phillip Herring. In an early version of *Nightwood*, "Catherine" describes their final, violent sex scene:

> And he took me by the wrist and began turning my wrist. . . . I began to go down with the pain in my arm. And he said "Down, and say that there is nothing that I do not understand about you!" And I said "You understand nothing, now I know you understand nothing!" And I kept saying "Nothing!"[44]

Almost entirely absent from *Nightwood*, too, is the controlling behavior of Robin's prototype, Thelma Wood, who seemingly demanded sexual freedom for herself and Barnes's virtual house arrest.[45] *Nightwood* alludes to Robin's possessiveness once:

> All the time she was watching me to see that no one called, that the bell did not ring, that I got no mail, nor anyone hallooing in the court, though she knew that none of these things could happen. My life was hers. . . . And one time, at about three in the morning when she came in, she was angry because for once I had not been there all the time, waiting. (147)

However, this passage, unconnected to anything else in Robin's characterization or the novel's action, is quickly buried by the many suggestions that Nora was the possessive one and it is this story that critical readings have adopted. Scenes of Nora clearly victimized by anyone but herself are cut because Nora stands too obviously for Barnes. *Nightwood*'s other characters, mainly, enact the scenes of abjection and abandonment.

For each character, as for Barnes, the ghost must be exorcised, but paradoxically, it is likewise in each attempted exorcism that the ghost subsists. Ghosts are named, called into being, but never directly and they never melt in the clear light of day. The ghost moves and flickers in the night. It departs to come near, beneath the skin. Contrary to most accounts, what agency may appear in *Nightwood* does not constitute a refusal (associated with Robin) that is distinct from an imperative. Agency appears instead as a haunted, nearly predetermined volition that retains a trace of difference. Fetish words like “wolf” and “go down” supplement Barnes’s sense of separation from the person and scenes to which they cryptically refer. Drafted while the slow loss of Thelma recalled Zadel’s betrayal in all its horror, *Nightwood* both calls and banishes Barnes’s beloved ghost with words whose figurative, personal meanings are depicted literally and bind Barnes’s characters to their most startling behaviors.

VI. IDEOLOGY IN *RYDER* AND *NIGHTWOOD*

Criticism on *Ryder* has often seen in its overt dualisms two ideological narratives at war: homophonic versus polyphonic, patriarchal versus feminist, or conservative versus libertine, though this purported content was rarely, until recently, considered closely in relation to its own fragmented form. Esther Sanchez-Pardo is an exception, reading both *Ryder*’s form and content as staging a failure to move from a “paranoid economy” of part-objects to a depressive vision of whole objects.[46]

Though the opposition that Sanchez-Pardo finds between whole and part-objects is illuminating, this distinction is itself at issue in *Ryder*. To a certain extent, the Kleinian dichotomy of whole and part-objects can be transposed onto the dichotomy I will draw between particulars and generals. The general, counter-intuitively, would be the part-object, a misrepresented fragment of the particular. The particular—were it accessible—would be the whole object, the whole story. However, the particular in Barnes’s work is a hole rather than a whole: an aporia that when represented is immediately general. In both *Ryder* and *Nightwood*, spectrality is associated with the fleeting particular whose elision is necessary to the general image, sign, or narrative. Barnes’s contrast of particulars and generals prefigures Caruth’s observation that “it is the necessary betrayal of a particular past in the understanding of a history” that allows the history to be told.[47]

This preoccupation with what is necessarily elided by the whole orients *Ryder* toward the deconstruction, not the re-articulation, of any ideology or any “mythology” in the Barthes-inflected sense. *Ryder*’s narrators and characters suggest alternate modes of agency not chiefly through the liberated sex or counter-hegemonic narratives that have drawn critical attention, but through subversions of language’s meaning-making. *Ryder*’s subversions of discourses of spiritualism, prophetic vision, and social manners undermine authority less with “countermyth” than with “antimyth”: ambiguity, multivalence, framing, bathos, anachronism, and idiosyncratic or holophrastic language that exposes all narrative as myth. While *Ryder*’s women do revise cultural narratives to "suit themselves" with empowered roles, their stories are myths among others, that secure them some discursive ground to stand on, but do not eradicate the gaps that perforate this ground and its inhabitants. As Ann Martin argues, Barnes imagines oppression not as two unequal camps (for instance, patriarchy's repression of the feminine and/or queer), but as a network in which aggressors are simultaneously victims, and in which all language has a hidden agenda.

Diane Warren reads *Ryder* intertextually as a challenge to homophonic hegemony by feminine polyphony, with its women's multifarious capacities, desires, and stories spilling over the clear social boundaries of patriarchy. Warren presents the "stiltsman's" remark that "[e]verything is true that is honored" as the ideological principle behind *Ryder*'s subversions (20). Given *Ryder*'s themes of rape and incest, however, the question arises whether if something or someone is dishonored, they are, by this logic, rendered false. The lynch mob in "Rape and Repining" would then give voice to *Ryder*'s own ethical stance (28). Moreover, *Ryder*'s polyphony does not include all women's voices: Julie and the unnamed rape victim are silent, apart from Julie's "You, you, you!"—meant for her father but voiced through teeth clamped in the flesh of his mistress—as if even an accusation without content cannot be spoken to him directly (143).

As well as aligning feminism with the most thoroughgoing relativism possible and positing this as an unequivocal social good and *Ryder*'s "unifying concept" (Warren), critics discussing agency in *Ryder* have found distinctly feminine modes of carnivalesque grotesquerie that overturn patriarchal narratives. Stevenson, for instance, uses Molly's account of the biblical Eden story, in which the man "snapped . . . up" the apple, as an example of Molly's counter mythology, although it is not included in Molly's creation story, but multiply framed as a story (Molly's) of a story (Mary's) of a story (the calf's foot's). Susan Edmunds has noted the inconsistency between critics for whom Wendell represents the forces of oppression (particularly the arguments concerned with establishing his sexual abuse of Julie) and the critics who see him as subversive. By contrast Edmunds sees a more historically specific binary opposition between two different groups of social reformers, conservative and libertine, and a critique of both.

Ryder not only resists all certainty and closure, as Miller and Caselli have recently argued, but mocks narrative knowledge and injunctions—counter myths and manifestos to "reach not beyond the image" included.[48] With the character Kate Careless, for instance, *Ryder* parodies women's alternative stories and spiritualist practices:

> [Kate] had strange wisdom, because she needed a recompense, for that she went off into trances, seeing men at war, and her will-of-the-wisp sister in a

> long white gown—the dead do not supply colors. Right buxom was that sister when she died, folding her hands over a well-turned breast, but she came back maiden, death and the maiden. Who doubts this matter? Who doubts the word and testimony of the common woman? . . . Who doubts the word of the mother who sees that which compensates the condition? Not I! (223)

Kate Careless's stories, like Molly Dance's, are described as "ignorant," "vulgar," idiosyncratic, and open to doubt, but this does not put them at the cutting edge of *Ryder*'s subversive project. *Ryder* does not suggest that we should read Amelia's, Mary's, or Molly's stories any differently than we do Kate's "strange wisdom"; it parodies the figure of the "wise fool" and resists aligning it unequivocally with an anti-patriarchal perspective, since Wendell, the patriarch, uses the trope of the wise fool, too. "Education," says he, "makes [the child] a monologuist in the presence of God, instead of a disciple" (130). Such a claim places him among Warren's champions of polyphony. But Wendell's mission is avowedly the multiplication of himself, both by "becoming" and by impregnating others (165). *Ryder* suggests the dysfunctional aspects of this mandate not only through the deaths in childbirth that it portrays, but also by Wendell's incapacity to support the life and well-being of his proliferating "selves"—his families—and his eventual decision to abandon one of his two families. The biological or textual drives toward multiplicity, this outcome suggests, might result in the eventual inability to maintain and relate to the vast creative proliferation of stories, alternatives, or people.

Further, *Ryder*'s characters emblematize the battling ideological positions that critics have often described, with the favored battleground in critical writing, the heterosexual bed, where only sexually "liberated" females like Molly Dance have been held to exemplify female agency. Even Sanchez-Pardo falls into this trap: "There are four exceptional women in *Ryder* who rebel against the patriarchal imperative and take pleasure in sex" (334).[49] In these readings, *Ryder*'s rebel woman must first have sex with the narcissistic man. Only then can she deflate him with her independent particularities, and the vicissitudes they present to him: the disappearance of his wallet, her post-menopausal sterility, or the possibility that she has already conceived with Dan the policeman. The question of agency in women who do not have sex with men (e.g., Julie and Anne) has not been posed. Sex is *Ryder*'s most spectacular mode of subversion; it gives the man a reflection of himself that can be taken away. But Anne and Julie do have agency, if agency is a space of separation from an imperative, a space in which something might emerge. The space of separation from *Ryder*'s narratives that make its sexual encounters subversive can also be created without them. This occurs, for instance, in Julie's dreams and negations, in Anne's weird fixation on smut and propriety, and in Matthew

O'Connor's vague monologues. What emerges is "full speech," not recreations of the social world with different power relations in place.

Barnes's linking of Julie's sexual abuse to *Ryder*'s dualistic and fractured images, stories and language suggests that her relentless deposition of clear language stems from an early experience of its power to distort. While *Ryder* may be read as making "universal" claims about language, its debunking of language may also be read as a response to the particular, incommunicable experience of incestuous familial abuse. *Ryder*'s "full speech," perhaps, should not be filled with too general a significance. Its "unnaturalness" lurks beneath the façades of stories that appear natural until "framed."

Interpretations of *Nightwood*, like those of *Ryder*, have tended to read feminine and queer empowerment into it, often by way of silence rather than polyphony. Jane Marcus and Susannah Martins have read *Nightwood* through the theories of Judith Butler and Michel Foucault in order to portray its most silent character, Robin Vote, as an exemplar of queering the subject. Merrill Cole reads Robin as figuring an "excluded interior" of historicity "that is most intimate to it, even if disavowed,"[50] and thus "leaves space for something not yet in history, something not yet realized, to emerge."[51] Though what this thing that *Nightwood* "leaves space for" might be, or how it might "emerge," is unspecified, it is associated with marginal subjectivity and desire. For Christine Coffman, it is the space of "another symbolic," the realm of the "people that have never been made," where the "angel on all fours" (*Nightwood* 95) and Robin, belong.[52] Silence, particularly Robin's, is seen as opening or leaving "space for" something beyond the social order. O'Connor's warning, "Don't learn anything, for it is always learned on another person's body," suggests the bodily subjection involved in "learning" through language, a subjection inapplicable to the silent Robin (147). But like Robin's lovers, *Nightwood* critics have sometimes persisted in longings of their own, reading in the character's silence a place of potential articulation outside the linguistic and social boundaries of the work without, until recently, also considering less empowering implications of this silence. Potter considers the relationship of humanness to narrative in *Nightwood*, writing that its characters and narrative "refuse to develop," but that it self-reflexively portrays, especially in Robin, "the implications of suggesting that the relationship between subjectivity and narration might be blocked."[53] We concur that what agency there is in *Nightwood* is created and maintained by language and narrative, however fragmentary and indirect. Where Potter suggests, however, that *Nightwood*'s silences and "nonlinguistic vocal noise" gestures toward the humanness "of those on the outside of the law, the state, or the family," I would argue that what emerges in its silence is the total determination of the subject by the social world. The silent Robin is, of all the characters, the most "possessed" by language.[54]

While *Ryder* describes the mechanisms by which "psychic crypts" and "phantoms" are formed, *Nightwood* more explicitly describes their effects on characters. *Ryder* repeats a pattern of splitting into two and many (that are also one) in its imagery, structure and narrative. This "anasemic" (as per Abraham and Torok) or "full" (as per Lacan) expression mimics the splitting and psychic encryption that may have been attendant on Barnes's early experience of meaningfulness. *Ryder* charts the growth of crypts by gesturing toward the aporias in its own narratives and the ways that they swallow up or bury the experience of the particular body. *Nightwood* shows us the end of this process, a graveyard where words and behaviors act as tombstones to mark what lies buried. If we accept, as many critics do, that *Ryder*'s Julie is intended to represent Barnes, the characters encrypted by Nora (*Nightwood*'s Barnes character) can be transposed to a certain extent on to the still living Ryder family. The aporias that will bury them are discernable in *Ryder*'s structure, narrative, and imagery. Sophia's lies to Julie, and the open secrets of the Ryder family, can be imagined as re-emerging as a full-blown psychic crypt containing her grandmother in *Nightwood*'s Nora. In *Nightwood* (whose working title was "Bow Down") genuflection stages the subject's simultaneous expulsion and capture by the other. Its characters cite scenes of shame, abandonment, and possible sexual abuse by bowing down not to invisible depths, but always visibly, before a loved or revered, usually standing, other. Going down can be read in Barnes's work in terms of compulsive reenactments of the words associated with what Abraham and Torok call "shameful secrets," as Taylor's reading also suggests:

> "go down" is, I think, a phrase that neatly captures Barnes's exploration of the ways in which sexual pleasure is inscribed within scenes of debasement. In the extant drafts of *Nightwood* there are at least two allusions to the performance of oral sex that Barnes grande-dameishly denies as a referent for the phrase "go down."[55]

This observation supports my reading of "go down" as a cryptonymic citation of one or more originary traumatic scenes from Barnes's early life. I do not suggest that this reading is necessarily true, or truer than any other reading of Barnes's creative negotiations of trauma and agency, but that rather than being reductive, it too can exist alongside them in—to borrow from *Ryder*—conglomerate juxtaposition (14).

To read Barnes's work with recourse to biography has been seen, with reason, as counter-productive, given its intentional opacity and its implicit challenge to the "true story." As Caselli observes, for Barnes, "The secret, rather than producing obscurity, preserves clarity of vision, which would be lost once the secret goes public."[56] Because of the need, in reading Barnes's work, to eschew the search for "the true story," Caselli argues that "biography and autobiography are . . . problems rather than solutions in Barnes."[57] Further, Caselli points out, Barnes herself denigrated the whole notion of biographies as explanatory: "The complexity found in the published work is not compensated by a clearer, less obscure, less (or more) disturbing dimension which we call 'life'; the idea that there can be a formula to make sense of it is presented in both published texts and letters as ludicrous."[58]

Taylor extends these observations in her discussion of Barnes's polyvalent (both pleasurable and painful) representations of sexual trauma. For Taylor, emphases on polyvalent affect and antiphony (understood as ritualistic, repetitive, collective, and performative textual characteristics) allow Barnes to "dramatize the testimony of sexual trauma without reifying victimhood or producing a simplified moralistic narrative."[59] In her analysis of Barnes's 1958 play, *The Antiphon*, generally understood as depicting family sexual abuse the most unmistakably of all Barnes's work, Taylor notes an inverse correlation between biographical transparency and textual characteristics that suggest trauma. Writes Taylor, "excision of several of the play's balder statements about the Hobbs family's history of sexual violence is matched by an increased emphasis on characteristics I relate to the trauma response: performativity and performance, stylized ritual, and affective complexity."[60] Taylor reads the trauma response in Barnes's works' complex interplay of surface and performative textual effects, and argues that situating these effects alongside one another rather than privileging some over others enables Barnes to establish agency beyond that constructed by conventional sexual abuse narratives. Barnes's work suggests to Taylor that trauma responses do not proceed from biographical depths; none of its various affective responses, she argues, are or should be privileged over another by a depth-model of trauma that seeks a narrative of its origin. Rather, the witnessing in present time of affect-charged scenes or spectacles where pleasure and pain combine in "remarkable and unexpected" ways produces trauma responses.[61] Because it highlights how affects like pain and pleasure co-exist, Taylor concludes, Barnes's work allows us to find "traces of bliss *within* trauma and other kinds of negative experiences and feelings."[62] For Taylor, through this focus on polyvalent and embodied affect as well as "a self-conscious representation of the performative nature of testimony and witnessing, Barnes ultimately gets beyond categories of victimhood and *ressentiment*."[63]

I agree with Taylor that Barnes emphasizes intersubjective, embodied affect, and performativity, and like Taylor, I read these stylistic choices as creating productive ambivalence in place of individualized depth-narratives and perpetrator-victim categories. I would note that this co-existence of positive and negative affects in sexual trauma is not surprising from a psychoanalytic perspective (it is explicit in Abraham and Torok's discussion of cryptophoria and Lacan's discussion of *jouissance*) nor was it considered as productive of happiness or empowerment. Psychoanalysis may be wrong in this, and Taylor may be right in suggesting, if I read her correctly, that it is Barnes's creative presentation of these polyvalent affects that is empowering. However, though Barnes's stylistic choices may defy the voyeurism of readers, conventional moralism, and the limiting roles of victim and perpetrator, they may also reflect and reinforce less empowering psychic and social effects. I don't wish to seem conventionally moralistic, or as reifying categories of perpetrator and victim, but since Taylor is after all referring to the sexual abuse of a child and her later strategies for empowerment and recovery, I would note that it is widely understood as therapeutic for sexual abuse survivors to recognize that they were not responsible for their abuse—that is, to establish categories of abuser and victim, notwithstanding any pleasure or positive affect they might or might not have felt in the experience or in its traumatic return. This is not to suggest that they reify themselves as victims, but that at some point they recognize that they were not responsible for what took place and thus let go of shame, pleasurable or otherwise.

For Taylor, Barnes's rendering of shame exemplifies her traversing of victimhood and resentment through the complexity and open-endedness of affect in her work. Taylor reads shame through the theory of psychologist Silvan Tomkins as "a negative affect that is itself dependent on the pre-existence of a positive affect, specifically interest, excitement, or enjoyment," and finds in this positive affect a source of empowerment and happiness in Barnes's work.[64] I agree with Taylor that the shame evoked by Barnes's scenes involves pleasure as well as pain, but I'm less convinced that Barnes's work suggests the positive correlation of this pleasure-pain to happiness. The downward movement that appears so often in Barnes's work, and that Taylor aptly identifies with the pleasure-pain of shame, is also associated in Barnes's writing with despair, loss of will, and death wish: "that terrible longing of the body that would [be] utterly blotted out and erased."[65] In *Ryder*, likewise, "seeds of sorrow" bear the many voices and performances that Barnes's work showcases down to a state that is not empowered, not happy, but quiescent—to earth, to nothingness, and to not even nothingness.[66] Further, shame or other polyvalent affects are not represented in the text as better alternatives for survivors of childhood sexual abuse than "simplified moralistic narratives" in which the responsibility for the sexual relationship is placed squarely on the adult perpetrator. I respect Taylor's wish to "honor the complexities of traumatic experience without pathologizing the subject."[67] However, her insistence on a nonpathologizing reading of Barnes's sexual trauma opens the question for me of whether it can be acceptable in literary studies to argue that a subject's trauma response to sexual abuse is not healthy and empowering. If to do so is unacceptable, it becomes difficult to engage with much of trauma studies, especially with self-identified trauma survivors who wish to heal, rather than cultivate, trauma. The question of whether it is permissible to suggest that trauma responses have unhealthy components deserves attention.

Another important question that Caselli's scholarship raises is whether we should read texts as their authors seem to ask us to. Barnes's claims to dislike biographical readings and her tendency to both invoke and deny her life as a referent for her creative work can be read biographically. Without reducing Barnes to the role of victim or denying her works' broader relevance, such a reading might consider other possible dimensions of her affective complexity, alternative structuring principles, and resistance to the idea of a "true story."

Rather than portraying any kind of discourse, even their own, as reliably anti-patriarchal or subversive, *Ryder* and *Nightwood* suggest that all articulation, since it is abstracted from particulars, is implicated in oppression. As critics note, these works offer much mimicry, parody, indecency, proliferation, polyphony, ambiguity, and radical relativism. However, there is nothing else in the text for all this to undermine. It is as if the gestures of subversion themselves conjure a vision, for scholarly readers, of univocal language and patriarchal power that does not appear in the works except as a ghost of these subversive gestures. It is questionable whether Barnes herself renders subversive language as distinct from patriarchal language, or personal agency as distinct from hegemony, given the extent to which her narrative action and character behavior are influenced by language patterns that invoke and bar her personal ghosts. Ghosts of unspeakable scenes haunt and possess *Nightwood*'s very syntax and *Nightwood* suggests little alternative to haunted identity and language. By the logic of disavowal that dominates it, the exorcism of the ghost is also its invocation.

I do not see Barnes as replacing clear meaning with withheld meaning or affective intensity, simply to resist patriarchal constructions. Barnes's style also has a less socially functional dimension. I reconsider the biographical implications of *Ryder* and *Nightwood* in order to question the empowering or counter-hegemonic status given to ambiguity, polyvalence, performativity, and the trauma response in readings of Barnes's work, and to point to the potentially disempowering aspects of what Taylor calls the "circular affect in which disavowed pleasures may erupt once more," which I identify with disavowal itself.

The work that Taylor places last in her book and which she most draws on to make her argument about the happiness attendant on polyvalent affect is Barnes's early work, *Ladies Almanack* (first published in 1928), while Barnes's last, unrelentingly bleak long work, *The Antiphon*, appears first in Taylor's book. *The Antiphon*, while most exhibiting characteristics that

Taylor aptly identifies with the trauma response, carries no trace of a positive outcome that might be consistent with her argument. Indeed Barnes's work, from early to late, becomes less humorous and more fraught with horror and despair. Barnes's aesthetics may, arguably, have allowed her to represent the ahistorical and multivalent experience of trauma in truer ways than singular narratives afford, but I don't see evidence that these circular affects and fragmented and antiphonic style enabled her to "get beyond" less sophisticated responses to childhood trauma. In the aesthetic register, of course, she triumphs. However, the tendency Taylor notes to accumulate versions, details and narratives, and to both invite and repudiate other people's attempts to represent her, can appear compelled as well as pleasurable and empowering.

This accumulation without selection, of versions of herself and her work, may have become rampant as she grew older. According to Taylor, and to O'Neal, who was close to Barnes between 1978 and 1981, she became very disorganized, endlessly rewriting *The Antiphon* and later poems, generating mountains of unsorted fragments of various works, often interspersed among other fragments such as shopping lists.[68] O'Neal's description of her process recalls Abraham and Torok's descriptions of cryptophoria as well as Taylor's and Caselli's discussions of Barnes's textual proliferation and antiphony. Writes O'Neal,

> Ideas and key phrases poured forth over and over again as she created more and more drafts of fairly similar material. . . . A phrase may have been new, or a combination of words fresh, but the themes had been formulated decades earlier. What she needed to edit was now nearly as old as I, and she was simply overwhelmed by the mass of her own creation.[69]

Barnes's later isolation and disorganization was much exacerbated by illness and heartbreak, and is not surprising or unusual given the circumstances faced by modernity's aging population. However, it may also highlight potential disadvantages in her habitual ways of writing and of relating to her experience and to others, and these disadvantages may co-exist with the advantages that Taylor and Caselli highlight.

Barnes endeavored to guard difference and particularity, her own, from language itself. To emphasize the difference between the symbol and the thing it refers to, Barnes makes the distortions and gaps of language visible as such. Her writing therefore subjects the narratives of power figures and narrators less to counter-narratives, as critics have claimed, than to a gaze that sees ghosts and aporias in them. For Barnes, absence, holes, fractures, graves, ghosts, and wounds figure precarious spaces that are elided by the disavowals of a fluctuating universe in which the only law is that of enjoyment. These liminal spaces suggest a boundary to the power of language and parent figures. However, these spaces are themselves formed of words: they can pour forth shameful innuendo, disgorge rotting ideals and call up predatory love objects. Words not only veil the secret; they are the very life and substance of the secret. They are corrupt, but there is nothing else—or if there is, it is silent.

NOTES

1. See Field, *Djuna*; Castle, *Literature*, 4; Benstock, *Women*, 233–57; Faderman, "Djuna Barnes (1892–1982)," 411–12; and Weiss, *Paris*, 168.

2. See Herring, *Djuna*, 54–9; and "Zadel Barnes," 107–16.

3. Writes Barnes in a 1934 letter to Coleman, "I suppose one lives by lack of ability to hold the memory too close—otherwise none of us would reach maturity." Emily Coleman Archives, University of Delaware library.

4. Abraham and Torok, *Shell*, 176.

5. See Žižek, *Sublime*. Žižek describes political disavowal as the mechanism by which the internal antagonisms of a political body are projected onto a subcategory within it, whose exclusive inclusion allows the political body to misrecognize itself as an organic whole corrupted only by the subcategory (Jews, homosexuals, and so on). See also Agamben's discussion of the sovereign exception in *Homo Sacer*, 37–8.

6. Abraham and Torok, *Shell*, 176.

7. Lee, "Nightwood," 217. O'Connor's and other characters' "power of speech," writes Lee, "is associated with the experience of separation and difference" (216).

8. Potter, "Nightwood's Humans," 68.

9. Lee, "Nightwood," 216.

10. Torok states that "the 'wolf' is chosen [in fairytales] precisely for its implicit reference to the grandmother" (*Shell*, 181).

11. The ending of the popular modern novel *Vandover and the Brute*, argues Seitler, could be a model for the ending of *Nightwood*, with the sexually indiscriminate Vandover on all fours barking "Wolf-wolf!" ("Down on All Fours," 556).

12. Agamben describes "homo sacer" as a category of life that is contained in the political order but has no legal status in it (*Homo Sacer*, 82). He reads the ancient, cross-cultural figure of the wolf man as a trope for homo sacer (104–11).

13. Taylor, *Affective*, 113.

14. Martins, "Gender," 111.

15. Ibid., 126.

16. Potter, 68, 66.

17. Sherbert, "Hieroglyphics," *passim*.

18. Ibid., 117.

19. Foucault, *History of Sexuality Vol. I*, 43. By the end of the nineteenth century, writes Foucault, "The . . . medical category of homosexuality was constituted . . . less by a type of sexual relations than by a certain quality of sexual sensibility, a certain way of inverting the masculine and feminine in oneself. Homosexuality . . .

was transposed from the practice of sodomy onto a kind of interior androgyny, a hermaphroditism of the soul."

20. See Gilman, *Difference*, 193.

21. Butler, *Psychic*. Gender, Butler speculates, may be a repetitive behavior resulting from melancholic inward "turns" from the lost same-sex Other, thus "formed and consolidated through identifications which are in part composed of disavowed grief" (139).

22. Ibid., 147.

23. Abraham and Torok, *Shell*, 128–32.

24. Ibid., 114.

25. Butler, *Psychic*, 113–16. Guilt and acquittal first "interpellate" the subject in Butler's adaption of Althusserian "ideological interpellation." Writes Butler, "[T]he very possibility of subject formation depends on a passionate pursuit of a recognition which . . . is inseparable from a condemnation" (113).

26. Herring, *Djuna*, 157.

27. See Simpson and Roud, *English Folklore*, 365.

28. Agamben finds this "symmetry of sovereign and homo sacer [in] the complicity that ties the masochist to the sadist, the victim to the executioner" (*Homo Sacer*, 135).

29. Potter, 66.

30. For a discussion of the wolf as a trope in folklore and modernism for the social predator, see Martin, *Red Riding Hood*.

31. Martins, "Gender," 120.

32. Ibid.

33. Freud's study of the Wolf Man, "Infantile Neurosis," is taken up by Abraham and Torok in *The Wolf Man's Magic Word*. However, here the significance of the wolf proceeds from the Wolf Man's multilingualism: "wolf" homophonically resembles the Russian "fly" (zipper); so it is not relevant to my study of Barnes's cryptonymy.

34. See Cole, "Backwards," 405; Coffman, *Insane*, 135; and Seitler, "Down on All Fours," 554. Writes Seitler, "becoming animal represents a sexual subjectivity . . . that takes place . . . between the flaps of the nature-culture, sex-gender binary, and through a series of spaces in which the characters of *Nightwood* gather and meet in nocturnal, degenerate, and wretched festivity" (554).

35. See Gilman, *Freud, Race, and Gender*.

36. Taylor, *Affective*, 117.

37. Butler suggests that queer identity may not lack gender melancholy, but involve "an effort to disavow a constitutive relationship to heterosexuality" (*Psychic*, 148).

38. Though the novel's narrative voice refers to O'Connor in the masculine and Barnes scholars still do so, in today's (and his own) terminology O'Connor is a heterosexual woman.

39. Herring documents Barnes's avowed "resentment" of her father and grandmother's close relationship in "Zadel" (117).

40. Barnes, *Nightwood: The Original Version and Related Drafts*, 278.

41. Agamben, *Homo Sacer*, 87.

42. See Field, *Djuna*, 43, 49–53.

43. Barnes, *Nightwood: The Original Version and Related Drafts*, 299–300.

44. Ibid., 303.
45. Field, *Djuna*, 157.
46. Sanchez-Pardo, *Cultures*, 339. Miller is another exception, reading *Ryder*'s form and content as expressing the disjuncture of the time Barnes wrote it and the time in her youth that it is chiefly set ("Havoc," 171.)
47. Caruth, *Experience*, 30.
48. Caselli, "Strong"; Miller, "Havoc."
49. Sanchez-Pardo's list does not include Laura Twelvetree and Kate Careless, who are both portrayed as enjoying sex, but not otherwise much rebelling against the patriarchal imperative.
50. Although Cole suggests that Robin's last name, "Vote," ironizes her lack of volition ("Backwards," 406), he also maintains that Robin is "the novel's sovereign power" (408–9). For Cole, *Nightwood* "celebrates . . . alterity's escape" in Robin (392).
51. Ibid., 405.
52. Coffman writes that by reversing the symbolic's terms of "beast turning human" to "human turning beast" Robin "opens a space for its displacement" (*Insane*, 135). Though for Coffman, Robin is psychotic because of her "refusal to accept the foundational condemnation through which the Western symbolic would install guilt," the novel suggests that "she might, within another symbolic, be otherwise" (120).
53. Potter, 66.
54. Ibid., 66, 73.
55. Taylor, *Affective*, 118.
56. Caselli, *Improper Modernism*, 196.
57. Ibid., 194.
58. Ibid., 193.
59. Taylor, *Affective*, 37.
60. Taylor, "Revising the Antiphon,"128.
61. Taylor, *Affective*, 182.
62. Ibid., 182.
63. Ibid., 40. Taylor describes *ressentiment* as "the reactive state in which suffering is reworked in negative forms of action (such as revenge)" (39).
64. Ibid., 102.
65. Barnes, *Nightwood*, 95.
66. Barnes, *Ryder*, 140.
67. Taylor, *Affective*, 5.
68. For discussion of Barnes's disorganized approach to writing in later years, and her view of other people's motivations, see especially O'Neal, *Djuna Barnes*, and Taylor, *Affective*.
69. O'Neal, *Djuna Barnes*, 87.

Conclusion

I have traced Djuna Barnes's and H.D.'s particular ways of relating to loved others, power figures, and meaning itself, to their patterns of thought and writing. I hope in doing so to broaden frameworks of intelligibility in literary studies for modes of consciousness that are concurrent with asymbolic thought and writing. H.D.'s and Barnes's enigmatic styles, and their visions of martyrdom or of possession, can and have been read as intentional commentary on, or re-envisioning of, their sociohistorical contexts; however, H.D.'s depictions of the sexualized attack of heroic or divine males upon herself, or Barnes's depictions of eroticized possession, also represent lived experiences—of embodied union with the divine, the dissolution of boundaries, power relations in modernity, the transcultural and transhistorical violence of patriarchy to feminine or queer power, the cosmic clash of opposite energies or drives. I have read H.D.'s and Barnes's work as testifying to transpersonal experiences that are yet fraught with unresolved conflicts.

By aligning the family and relationship dynamics that appear in H.D.'s and Barnes's biographies with their language patterns and social and cosmological visions, I have interpreted writing that has often been considered intentionally uninterpretable in terms of psychic processes. I hope to have also suggested ways of opening out the discursive boundaries between the pathological, the modernist, and the spiritual text, and the categories of "madness," "literature," and "spirituality" that are contested within these texts and in the scholarship surrounding them. The relations between writing, hegemonic discourse, and madness have been examined in thoughtful and exploratory ways in scholarship on writers such as Antonin Artaud, Louis-Ferdinand Céline, Friedrich Hölderlin, and of course (though not always) Schreber.[1] The literary languages of James Joyce, Jean Rhys, Henry James, Vladimir Nabokov, and Gustave Flaubert, who were not in their lives institutionalized or defined as mad by "experts," have also been scrutinized for symptoms of abnormality. I believe that literary studies is evolved enough to hold a space where writers,' even women writers,' admitted brushes with madness need not detract from the high esteem in which they are held. Nuanced inquiry into the relations of marginalized modes of subjectivity, the discourses that marginalize them, literary movements and works, and perhaps literary criticism itself, might indeed contribute to our understanding of how the academic disciplines impact the ways that texts, and people, are received and understood, and thus enhance our capacity to communicate across the disciplines and their constructions. Perhaps divisions between legitimate texts—and people—and illegitimate ones run as deep as language and the kinds of faith and meaning that it enables in various readerships. These divisions may elide the ways of commenting on the world, relating to others, and constructing meaning that texts share across the disciplines.

H.D.'s and Barnes's writing is not only haunted by the perceived imperative of the other that, in Lacan's view, dominates psychotic and perverse language, but it is also haunted by the question of the desire of the other that, for Lacan, constitutes neurotic subjectivity. It thus demonstrates, as Lacan also insists, that his psychic structures are not fixed limits for psychic life, but rather patterns of thought and affect that can predominate interchangeably. Psychoanalyst Jean Laplanche (1924–2012), who like Abraham and Torok theorized more individualized early formations of object relations, points out that in Lacan's theory of psychosis we cannot after all say exactly what is meant by the connection or disconnection of signifiers to signifieds. In doing so he references Schreber, since the *Memoirs* are the most influential source text in the early study of psychosis. Writes Laplanche, "If language is intentionality right from the beginning, it is only on the basis of this intentionality that one can distinguish the signifier and signified as having a certain autonomy; the idea of a signifier "as such" may represent only an extreme moment of abstraction that psychosis approaches but never reaches. *That which is missing* when Schreber says the word father, which he certainly does say, has yet to be determined."[2] As Laplanche suggests, since for Lacan the castrated subject is *mistaken* in imagining a real connection between signifier and signified, it is difficult to say exactly what constitutes their connection or lack thereof. The intention when using a word such as "father" to communicate something that has been vividly, directly, and not too traumatically experienced perhaps has some effect, as I have speculated, in calling the signified into being, for the communicator and perhaps also for those who receive the communication. This vividness and intention may come from the awareness of something—anything—not in reference to anything else, but in itself. In disavowal too, there is a distortion in the intention to communicate something vividly experienced, since speech, objects or actions are meant rather to supplement psychic boundaries. However, the ability to experience something directly and vividly, and the intention to communicate it, is subject to change in everyone.

I share H.D.'s view that individual psychic integration is a requisite for positive social change and also note that great turmoil can attend this integration.

However, her writing evidences a belief that in order to (variously) stop the war, or bring about a new era, this psychic integration is only requisite for herself and not, noticeably, for others. This appears as a key misunderstanding. Early transpersonal theorist Roberto Assagioli (1888–1974) speculates that "spiritual awakening" may sometimes involve a "confusion between levels," where the ego mistakes itself as the "higher Self," and thus as universally important, and this seems plausible.[3] Similarly, the iconic spiritual teacher Ram Dass (1931–2019), a psychology professor at Harvard before he became a mystic (a practitioner of Buddhist meditation and a devotee of the Hindu guru, Neem Karoli Baba), writes that psychotic and mystical experiences touch the same innate truth of unity with, or identity as, the divine.[4] Ram Dass suggests that the only practical difference is that the mystic, as well as recognizing their own identity with the divine, also recognizes that everyone else is also identical with the divine. He illustrates this theory by recounting a visit to his brother, then an inpatient in a psychiatric ward. He, his brother, and his brother's doctor met together, his brother arguing that he was Christ. Writes Ram Dass,

> I say to him: "Sure man you're Christ and I'm Christ too." He says: "You don't understand.". . . So they lock him up. And he says, "I don't know . . . me . . . I'm a responsible member of society, I go to church, me they put in a mental hospital. You, you've got a beard, you wear a dress, you, you're out free." Sure because as far as I'm concerned we're all God, that's the difference. That's the difference. And if you really think another guy is God he doesn't lock you up. He's funny about that.[5]

While this vision is far from the psychoanalytic canon, it resonates with Lacan's theory that psychosis proceeds from the foreclosure of difference. For H.D. and Schreber, the idea of playing a unique role as God's consort in determining the fate of the world involves anxiety and a fierce sense of an imperative that they personally be martyred. A mystical vision in which the healing and integration of the world was understood to involve personal healing and integration, but not to be the responsibility of one subject in a unique relation to God, might not only elicit a different response from other people, as Ram Dass suggests—but might also reflect a psychic process more fully attuned to the difference, importance, and depth of others.

Lacan himself suggested that the other type of person besides "the psychotic" who directly encountered the Other's *jouissance* was the mystic.[6] Contemporary critical discussion as to what separates mental illness from religiosity or spirituality is ongoing, and transpersonal psychology, anti-psychiatry, some contemporary psychoanalysis, and the mad pride movement all suggest that the conventional distinction between the two is untenable, and that conventionally accepted categories of madness are really contingent, and indistinct from what "ordinary" people experience in contemplative or mystical states.[7] The texts I study share discursive patterns with countless others. Any distinctions to be made among them proceed from mysterious increments of awareness, agency, and intention, as well as the genres in which they are received. George Atwood holds the view that subjects in "the abyss" (as he re-languages what is labeled as madness) experience the symbols of their subjective annihilation by actual others who see them as mad as if they were literal events: personal attacks, invasions, soul murders. This view is consonant with Lacan's idea that "what is refused in the symbolic order re-emerges in the real," as well as Abraham and Torok's understanding of antimetaphor. However, Atwood offers a model in which the abyss is a universal possibility contingent on life circumstances, and in which the thought and behavior patterns that whirl through it are completely permeable to therapeutic intervention.[8] Atwood describes the abyss in terms reminiscent of contemplatives' descriptions of the dissolution and groundlessness that can occur as a result of practice, such as meditation teacher Shinzen Young's description of the pit of "the void."[9] Writes Atwood, "Phenomenologically, going mad is a matter of a fragmentation of the soul, of a fall into nonbeing, of becoming subject to a sense of erasure and annihilation. . . . The abyss is a possibility inhering in every human life."[10] Indeed, for Atwood, therapeutic intervention consists simply in understanding the traumatic experiences that are ametaphorically expressed by the so-called delusions. Such understanding and mirroring, itself, restores the subject, quickly or slowly, from the abyss to safe ground.

Certain ways of suffering, such as melancholy, alienation, dissociation, anxiety, and post-traumatic stress disorder are flagged as characteristically modern and contemporary, and these have often been correlated with the fragmentation, repetition, indeterminacy, and incompleteness of modernism's aesthetic forms.[11] But how particular formal qualities in the texts might correlate to the individual writer's particular ways of relating to others and to the social world has rarely been explored in detail in Anglophone literary studies. Such a methodology could be used to examine the way that institutions—for example, religious or academic institutions—produce and engage with particular kinds of texts. What modes of negation do we bring to texts, and how are these determined by discipline-specific patterns of thought and interpretation?

In reclaiming H.D. and Barnes into modernist literary studies, where they had been all but erased, critics have emphasized their ways of affirming feminine or queer empowerment, expression, and agency, and understandably discouraged arguments that they saw as potentially enabling their remarginalization. There is a high degree of accord among H.D. scholars that her writing transcends patriarchal narratives through its mode of meaning, which is variously intersubjective,[12] indeterminate,[13] syncretic,[14] and heterodox.[15] These modes of meaning, it is argued, oppose the "traditional" modes of meaning that underpin inherently violent interpretative decisions,[16] concepts,[17] common knowledge,[18] authorized meanings,[19] and destructive binaries.[20] H.D.'s way of writing is hence associated with pacifism, anti-authoritarianism and syncretic pluralism (Friedman), anti-imperialism (Vetter), anti-hegemony (Baccolini), modernism (Scanlon), queer sexuality (McCabe), racial politics (Walsh) and transcendental mystical experiences and awareness (Augustine, Hollenberg, Friedman, Rado). Critics have, however, tended to elide the problematic or contradictory elements of these representations, and to reproduce and naturalize a vision of polarized "masculine" and "feminine" principles, with various particulars associated with them (patriarchy, univocity, violence, imperialism, nationalism, oppression, rational certainty, Christian dogmatism, hyper-rationalism, war, death, as opposed to subversion, queerness, nurture, polyphony, freedom, transnationalism, anti-imperialism, religious syncretism, pluralism, mysticism), in the discourse around H.D.'s and Barnes's work.[21] It thus depends on the very dualistic vision that these critics insist is subverted in H.D.'s and Barnes's writing. Can her work not also inspire us as respondents to move toward transcending destructive binaries?

The very prevalent use of binary oppositions in critical readings of H.D.'s and Barnes's work appears to me as a response, in part, to its symbolic disorder, and to the concomitant necessity that *something else besides it* be invoked in order for it to make sense. Patriarchy,[22] imperialism and nationalism,[23] war and male violence,[24] repression and sterile reason,[25] clear language and univocity,[26] dogmatic Christianity,[27] heteronormativity,[28] or a composite of these, are opposed to the texts and conceptual meaning and, thereby, construed *in distinction from this other thing*. This echoes H.D.'s literary invocations of a masculine principle that opposes the feminine one that her heroines embody, and her attempt to locate meaning in their (non)relationships. Since words are not taking meaning from a differentiated system of concepts, imagined sexual difference and (dis)union are sometimes taken by critics as productive of a meaning that remains unclear, yet unassailable.

Psychoanalysis furnishes critical distance but imposes its own ideological baggage; for instance, it arguably privileges the symbolic order and the castrated subject, and suggests that people, words, and meanings are indeed separate and that to think and act otherwise is crazy. However, the idea of the truth as the reunification of all beings and/or the reunification of words and their referents is ancient, surfacing in various religious texts, Eastern and Western, as well as in literary theory. "Reversing castration" has not only a palpable appeal to many nonpsychotics, but also a crucial place in Western academic thought. Much literary criticism finds its closure in a gesture toward some experience or truth outside of language or symbol.

One approach to H.D.'s and Barnes's work, or similar texts, might be to enter into the authors' own frames of reference as much as possible while also retaining radically different frames, not mere negative terms like "patriarchy" or "madness," but systems that can be applied provisionally in order to create a dyad between authorial and critical perspectives. I have used the models of psychic life suggested by Lacan, Klein, and Abraham and Torok very differently in regard to Barnes and to H.D., and suggest that these models would likewise be applicable to other literary or critical texts in very different ways. Nevertheless, such applications might enable new examinations of the questions of agency, meaning, and difference that emerge in these texts.

Though it is a cliché to claim that great writers and other artists are mad and that this is crucial to their gifts, the writing and other creative work of most people who are considered mad are given serious attention on only rare occasions, usually as case studies. Characteristics that are taken to disqualify the works and their authors from having authority (such as delusions, loosening of associations, and conceptual destitution) are present in *Sword* and, to a lesser extent, in *Helen*; *Ryder* and *Nightwood* can also be read for psychic trouble. Yet all of these works are considered to be worthy of serious study by many people who arbitrate culture. More attention to asymbolic modes of meaning in works labeled in various disciplines and institutions as "literary," "pathological," and "mystical" could advance the discussion of what is at issue in them, what they share, and how their reception has been impacted by the beliefs, investments, and projections of their readers.

NOTES

1. The "symbolic oppositions" to the "name of the father" that triggered their breakdowns have been read by modern theorists in a variety of scenarios comparable to the repudiations that H.D. suffered, from Schreber's failed political candidacy, childlessness, and later appointment as *Senatspräsident* (Lacan, Santner, Weber) to Hölderlin's failure to impress Schiller with the originality of his writing and his mother with the legitimacy of his poetic vocation. Laplanche, *Hölderlin*, 80–1, 91–2.

2. Laplanche, *Hölderlin*, 140.

3. Assagioli, "Self-Realization and Psychological Disturbances," 34–5.

4. Ram Dass, *Be Here Now*, 16–18. Writes Ram Dass, "That psychosis business is an interesting business. If you go through the doorway too fast and you're not ready for it you're bound hand and foot and thrown into Outer darkness. You may land anywhere and lots of people end up in mental hospitals. The reason they do is: they went through the door with their ego on . . . they go on a Huge ego trip and it's called the Messianic Complex. It's called paranoia, delusions of grandeur." (98–9)

5. Ibid., 99.

6. Lacan, *Seminar XX*, 61–77.

7. See, for instance, R.D. Laing, Tomás Agosin, "Mysticism and Psychosis"; Roberto Assagioli, "Self-Realization"; John Weir Perry, "Spiritual Emergence"; Paris Williams, *Rethinking Madness;* David Lukoff, "Diagnosis"; and George Atwood, *Abyss*. Writes Laing, "if we can begin to understand sanity and madness in existential social terms, we . . . will be enabled to see more clearly the extent to which we confront common problems and share common dilemmas" ("Transcendental Experience," 53).

8. Writes Atwood, "In Schreber, I see a child locked into a power struggle with a parent—there is evidence (Shatzman, 1773; Orange, 1995) that it was his father—a struggle for existence itself. The ideas of unmanning and being made into a woman involve a stripping away of what makes this male child who he is . . . the child to whom all of this has happened and is happening is telling the story in the so-called delusions and hallucinations, and if that story is heard, that might make all the difference for Schreber. . . . I would want to let him know that I was listening . . . I certainly would not inform him of his diagnosis of dementia praecox or schizophrenia. . . . I am quite sure his psychiatrist [Professor Emile Flechsig], whom he considered his mortal enemy, spoke to him in precisely such a way, and contributed greatly to his destruction. . . . Schreber was utterly brilliant. . . . If someone were really paying attention, it would not be lost upon him" (*Abyss*, 37–9).

9. Young, "Dark Night." Writes Young, "Within the Buddhist tradition, [the experience of ego dissolution] is sometimes referred to as 'falling into the Pit of the Void.' It entails an authentic and irreversible insight into Emptiness and No Self. Instead of being empowering and fulfilling . . . it turns into the opposite. In a sense, it's Enlightenment's Evil Twin. This is serious but still manageable through intensive . . . guidance under a competent teacher."

10. Atwood, *Abyss*, 32–3.

11. See Walter Benjamin's *The Origins of German Tragic Drama* and *The Writer of Modern Life*, Theodor Adorno, Walter Benjamin, Ernst Bloch, Bertolt Brecht, and Georg Lukács's *Aesthetics and Politics*, Fredric Jameson's *Marxism and Form*, Julia Kristeva's *Black Sun*, Esther Sanchez-Pardo's *Cultures of the Death Drive*, Jonathan Flatley's *Affective Mapping*, Jean-Michel Rabaté's *The Ghosts of Modernity*, and Shoshanna Felman's *Writing and Madness*.

12. Thomas, "Creative," 158.

13. Debo and Vetter, *Approaches*, 6.

14. Ibid., 7; Baccolini, "War Literature," 123; Friedman, "Teaching Trilogy," 140.

15. Debo and Vetter, *Approaches*, 25.

16. Hirsh, "God," 76.

17. Morris, "Ticking," 60.

18. Keeling, "British Modernist," 117.

19. Hirsh, "God," 74.

20. Baccolini, "War Literature," 124.

21. See for instance Lara Vetter, *A Curious Peril*; and Anette Debo and Lara Vetter, *Approaches*.

22. See Friedman, *Psyche*.

23. See Vetter, *Curious*.

24. See especially Friedman, *Psyche* and "Teaching"; Baccolini, "War Literature"; Hogue and Vandivere, "Introduction."

25. See Chisholm, *H.D.'s Freudian Poetics*.

26. See Gelpi, "H.D."; Warren, *Consuming;* Kloepfer, Caselli, *Improper Modernisms*.

27. See Kannenstine, *The Art of Djuna Barnes*.

28. See Friedman, *Psyche*; McCabe, "Teaching Sex"; Coffman, *Insane*; Marcus, *Laughing*; Martins, "Gender."

Bibliography

Abraham, Nicolas, and Maria Torok. *The Shell and the Kernel: Renewals of Psychoanalysis*. Edited and translated by Nicholas T. Rand. Chicago: University of Chicago Press, 1994.

———. *The Wolf Man's Magic Word: A Cryptonymy*. Translated by Nicholas T. Rand. Minneapolis: University of Minnesota Press, 1986.

Adorno, Theodor. *Aesthetic Theory*, edited by Gretel Adorno, Rolf Tiedemann, and Robert Hullot-Kentor, translated by Robert Hullot-Kentor. London: Althone, 1997.

______, Walter Benjamin, Ernst Bloch, Bertolt Brecht, and Georg Lukács. *Aesthetics and Politics*. London: NLB, 1977.

Adyashanti. *The End of Your World: Uncensored Straight Talk on the Nature of Enlightenment*. Boulder: Sounds True, 2008.

———. *The Way of Liberation: A Practical Guide to Spiritual Enlightenment*. Campbell: Open Gate Sangha, 2012.

Agamben, Giorgio. *Homo Sacer: Sovereign Power and Bare Life*. Translated by Daniel Heller-Roazen. Stanford: Stanford University Press, 1998.

Agosin, Tomás. "Mysticism and Psychosis." *Seeds of Unfolding* 6, no. 4 (Fall 1989), page range unavailable. http://www.seedsofunfolding.org/issues/11_08/feature_english.htm (accessed December 2020).

Almaas, A. H. *The Unfolding Now: Realizing Your True Nature through the Practice of Presence*. Boston: Shambhala Publications, 2008.

Ambelain, Robert. *The Practical Kabbalah, Parts I and II*. Translated by Piers A. Vaughan. Part I: www.markfoster.net/rn/texts/practicalkabbalah-part1.pdf; Part II: www.thule-italia.net/esoterismo/Theurgia%20pratica%20cabalistica.pdf (accessed December 2020).

American Psychiatric Association. *Diagnostic and Statistical Manual of Mental Disorders, Fifth Edition*. Arlington: American Psychiatric Association, 2013.

Anderson, Elizabeth. *H.D. and Modernist Religious Imagination*. London: Bloomsbury Academic, 2013.

André, Serge. "The Structure of Perversion: A Lacanian Perspective." In *Perversion: Psychoanalytic Perspectives, Perspectives on Psychoanalysis*, edited by Danny Nobus and Lisa Downing, 109–26. London: Karnac, 2006.

Angyal, Adras. "Disturbances of Thinking in Schizophrenia." In *Language and Thought in Schizophrenia*, edited by J.S. Kasanin, 115–23. New York: Norton, 1964.

Apollon, Willy, Danielle Bergeron, and Lucie Cantin, eds. *After Lacan: Clinical Practice and the Subject of the Unconscious*. Introduction by Robert Hughes and Kareen Ror Malone. Albany: State University of New York Press, 2002.

Assagioli, Roberto. "Self-Realization and Psychological Disturbances." In *Spiritual Emergency: When Personal Transformation Becomes a Crisis*, edited by Stanislav and Christina Grof, 27-48. Los Angeles: Jeremy P. Tarcher, 1989.

Atwood, George E. *The Abyss of Madness*. New York and London: Routledge, Taylor & Francis Group (Psychoanalytic Inquiry Book Series), 2011.

Augustine, Jane. Introduction to *The Gift*, edited by Jane Augustine. Gainesville: University Press of Florida, 1998.

———."Preliminary Comments on the Meaning of H.D.'s *The Sword Went Out to Sea*." *Sagetrieb* 15, nos 1–2 (1996): 121–32.

———. "Teaching H.D. and Spirituality." In *Approaches to Teaching H.D.'s Poetry and Prose*, edited by Anette Debo and Lara Vetter, 63–9. New York: MLA, 2011.

Aurobindo, Sri. *Savitri: A Legend and a Symbol*. http://www.auro-ebooks.com/savitri/ (accessed December, 2020).

Baccolini, Raffaella. "Teaching H.D.'s Work in a War Literature Course." In *Approaches to Teaching H.D.'s Poetry and Prose*, edited by Anette Debo and Lara Vetter, 120–6. New York: MLA, 2011.

Baker, Caroline, and Guy MacPherson. *The Extinction Dialogues*. Oakland: Tayen Lane Publishing, 2014.

Barthes, Roland. *Mythologies*. Translated by Annette Lavers. New York: Hill & Wang, 1972.

Barnes, Djuna. *The Antiphon*. In *Selected Works of Djuna Barnes*, 43–55. New York: Farrar, Straus and Cudahy, 1962.

______. 1934–1935 letters to Emily Holmes Coleman. Series I.2, Djuna Barnes letters to Coleman, 1934-1974. In the Emily Holmes Coleman papers 1952-1988, University of Delaware Library, Museums and Press, Newark, Del.

———. *Nightwood*. New York: New Directions, 1937.

———. *Nightwood: The Original Version and Related Drafts*. Edited by Cheryl J. Plumb. Champaign: Dalkey Archive Press, 1995.

———. *Ryder*. Illinois: Dalkey Archive Press, 1995, c. 1928.

Benjamin, Walter. *The Origins of German Tragic Drama*. London: Verso, 1998.

———. *The Writer of Modern Life: Essays on Charles Baudelaire*. Edited by Michael W. Jennings, translated by Howard Eiland, Edmund Jephcott, Rodney Livingstone, and Harry Zonn. Cambridge, MA: Belknap Press, 2006.

Benstock, Shari. *Women of the Left Bank: Paris, 1900–1940*. Austin: University of Texas Press, 1986.

Bhagavata Purana: Selected Translations, edited and translated by Ravi M. Gupta and Kenneth R. Valpey. New York: Columbia University Press, 2016.

Bleuler, Eugen. "The Basic Symptoms of Schizophrenia." In *Organization and Pathology of Thought*, edited by David Rapaport, 581–649. New York: Columbia University Press, 1965.

Bowlby, John. *The Making and Breaking of Affectional Bonds*. London: Tavistock Publications, 1979.

Britton, Willoughby. *The Dangers of Meditation*. https://buddhism-controversy-blog.com/2014/03/11/the-dangers-of-meditation-advice-for-meditators-an-interview-with-leigh-brasington-by-willoughby-britton/ (accessed December 2020).

———. "The Messy Truth About Mindfulness." *Mindful*. www.mindful.org/willoughby-britton-the-messy-truth-about-mindfulness/ (accessed December 2020).

Broe, Mary Lynn. "Introduction." In *Silence and Power: A Reevaluation of Djuna Barnes*, edited by Mary Lynn Broe, 3-26. Carbondale: Southern Illinois University Press, 1991.

______. "My Art Belongs to Daddy: Incest as Exile—The Textual Economics of Hayford Hall." In *Women's Writing in Exile*, edited by Mary Lynn Broe and Angela J.C. Ingram, 41–86. Chapel Hill: University of North Carolina, 1989.

Buddhaghosa, Ven. Badantácariya. *Visuddimagga: The Path of Purification*, translated by Bhikku Ñánamoli. Kandy: Buddhist Publication Society, 2011. https://www.accesstoinsight.org/lib/authors/nanamoli/PathofPurification2011.pdf (accessed July 2019).

Butler, Judith. *Bodies That Matter: On the Discursive Limits of "Sex."* New York: Routledge, 1993.

———. *The Psychic Life of Power: Theories in Subjection*. Stanford: Stanford University Press, 1997.

Cameron, Norman. "Experimental Analysis of Schizophrenic Thinking." In *Language and Thought in Schizophrenia*, edited by J. S. Kasanin, 50–63. Proceedings of the Chicago 1939 American Psychiatric Association Conference. New York: Norton, 1964.

Caruth, Cathy. *Unclaimed Experience: Trauma, Narrative, and History*. Baltimore: The Johns Hopkins University Press, 1996.

Caselli, Daniela. *Improper Modernism: Djuna Barnes's Bewildering Corpus*. Farnham: Ashgate, 2009.

———. "'If Some Strong Woman': Djuna Barnes's Great Capacity for All Things Uncertain." In *Shattered Objects: Djuna Barnes's Modernism*, edited by Elizabeth Pender and Cathryn Setz, 147-62. University Park: Pennsylvania State University Press, 2020.

Castle, Terry. *The Literature of Lesbianism: A Historical Anthology from Ariosto to Stonewall*. New York: Columbia University Press, 2003.

Charan, Gunada. *Srimadbhagavatum: A Concise Narrative,* translated by Amalendu Sen. New Dehli: Munishram Manoharlal, 1986.

Chisholm, Dianne. *H.D.'s Freudian Poetics: Psychoanalysis in Translation*. Ithaca: Cornell University Press, 1992.

Coffman, Christine. *Insane Passions: Lesbianism and Psychosis in Literature and Film*. Connecticut: Wesleyan University Press, 2006.

Cole, Merrill. "Backwards Ventriloquy: The Historical Uncanny in Djuna Barnes's *Nightwood*." *Twentieth-Century Literature* 52, no. 4 (Winter 2006): 391–412.

Coleman, Emily Holmes. *Rough Draft: The Modernist Diaries of Emily Holmes Coleman, 1929–1937*. Edited by Elizabeth Podnieks. Newark: University of Delaware Press, 2012.

Dalton, Anne B. "Escaping from Eden: Djuna Barnes' Revision of Psychoanalytic Theory and Her Treatment of Father-Daughter Incest in *Ryder*." *Women's Studies* 22 (1993): 163–79.

Dean, Tim. "Lacan Meets Queer Theory." In *Perversion: Psychoanalytic Perspectives, Perspectives on Psychoanalysis*, edited by Danny Nobus and Lisa Downing, 261–322. London: Karnac, 2006.

Debo, Anette, and Lara Vetter. "Introduction: Biographical Contexts." In *Approaches to Teaching H.D.'s Poetry and Prose*, edited by Anette Debo and Lara Vetter, 25-31. New York: MLA, 2011.

Deleuze, Gilles. *The Logic of Sense*. Edited by Constantin V. Boundas, translated by Mark Lester with Charles Stivale. New York: Columbia, 1990.

Deleuze, Gilles, and Félix Guattari. *Anti-Oedipus: Capitalism and Schizophrenia*. Translated by Robert Hurley, Mark Seem, and Helen R. Lane. New York: Viking Press, 1977.

Detloff, Madelyn. "Burnt Offerings or Incendiary Devices? Ambivalence, Trauma, and Cultural Work in *The Gift* and *Trilogy*." In *Approaches to Teaching H.D.'s Poetry and Prose*, edited by Anette Debo and Lara Vetter, 127–34. New York: MLA, 2011.

———. *The Persistence of Modernism: Loss and Mourning in the Twentieth Century*. Cambridge: Cambridge University Press, 2009.

Dobson, Sylvia. "'Shock Knit Within Terror': Living Through World War II." *The Iowa Review* 16, no. 3 (Fall 1986): 232–45.

Duncan, Robert. *The H.D. Book*. Edited and introduced by Michael Boughn and Victor Coleman. Berkeley: University of California Press, 2011.

DuPlessis, Rachel Blau. *H.D.: The Career of That Struggle*. Brighton: Harvester, 1986.

Edmunds, Susan. *Out of Line: History, Psychoanalysis, Montage in H.D.'s Long Poems*. Stanford: Stanford University Press, 1994.

Eliot, Thomas Stearns. "Introduction." In *Nightwood*, xi-xvii. New York: New Directions, 1937.

Epstein, Mark. *Thoughts Without a Thinker: Psychotherapy from a Buddhist Perspective*. New York: Basic Books, 1995.

_____. *The Trauma of Everyday Life*. New York: Penguin, 2013.

Faderman, Lillian. "Djuna Barnes (1892–1982)." In *Chloe Plus Olivia: An Anthology of Lesbian Literature from the Seventeenth Century to the Present*, 411–12. New York: Viking Press, 1994.

Farber, Seth. *The Spiritual Gift of Madness: The Failure of Psychiatry and the Rise of the Mad Pride Movement*. Rochester: Inner Traditions, 2012.

Feldstein, Richard, Bruce Fink, and Maire Jaanus. *Reading Seminars I and II: Lacan's Return to Freud*. Albany: State University of New York Press, 1996.

Felman, Shoshanna. *Writing and Madness*. Translated by Martha Noel Evans. Ithaca: Cornell University Press, 1985, c. 1978.

Field, Andrew. *Djuna: The Formidable Miss Barnes*. Austin: University of Texas Press, 1985.

Fink, Bruce. *A Clinical Introduction to Lacanian Psychoanalysis: Theory and Technique*. Cambridge, MA: Harvard University Press, 1999.

Flatley, Jonathan. *Affective Mapping: Melancholia and the Politics of Modernism*. Cambridge, MA: Harvard University Press, 2008.

Foucault, Michel. *The History of Sexuality Vol. I*. Translated by Robert Hurley. New York: Random House, 1990.

Freud, Sigmund. *Beyond the Pleasure Principle*. Edited and translated by James Strachey. New York: Norton, 1961.

———. *Civilization and Its Discontents*. Translated by David McLintock. New York: Penguin, 2002.

———. "Dreams and Occultism." In *The Complete Psychological Works of Sigmund Freud Vol. XXII (1932–36)*, edited and translated by James Strachey, 31–56. London: Hogarth, 1964.

———. "Fetishism." In *The Complete Psychological Works of Sigmund Freud Vol. XXI (1927–1931)*, edited and translated by James Strachey, 149–57. London: Hogarth, 1961.

———. "History of an Infantile Neurosis." In *The Complete Psychological Works of Sigmund Freud Vol. XVII (1917-1919)*, edited and translated by James Strachey, 7-122. London: Hogarth, 1955.

———. *The Interpretation of Dreams*. 3rd ed. Edited and translated by James Strachey. New York: Hogarth, 2010.

———. "The Loss of Reality in Neurosis and Psychosis." In *The Essentials of Psycho-Analysis*, edited by Clifford Yorke, translated by James Strachey. London: Hogarth, 1986.

———. *The Schreber Case*. Translated by Andrew Webber. New York: Penguin, 2003.

———. *Totem and Taboo*. In *The Complete Psychological Works of Sigmund Freud Vol. XIII (1913–14)*, edited and translated by James Strachey. London: Hogarth, 1955.

Friedman, Susan Stanford, ed. *Analyzing Freud: Letters of H.D., Bryher, and Their Circle*. New York: New Directions, 2002.

———. *Psyche Reborn: The Emergence of H.D*. Bloomington: Indiana University Press, 1981.

———. "Teaching *Trilogy*: H.D.'s War and Peace." In *Approaches to Teaching H.D.'s Poetry and Prose*, edited by Anette Debo and Lara Vetter, 135–41. New York: MLA, 2011.

Friedman, Susan Stanford, and Rachel Blau DuPlessis. *Signets: Reading H.D.* Madison: University of Wisconsin Press, 1990.

Gelpi, Albert. "H.D.: Hilda in Egypt." In *H.D.*, edited by Harold Bloom, 123–39. New York: Chelsea House, 1989.

Gifford, James. "H.D.'s *Hirslanden Notebooks* & Durrell's Claudia: Occult Modernism Across the Curtain & in the Mirror." *ANQ: A Quarterly Journal of Short Articles, Notes, & Reviews* 30.3 (2017): 145–149.

Gilman, Sander L. *Difference and Pathology: Stereotypes of Sexuality, Race, and Madness*. Ithaca: Cornell University Press, 1985.

———. *Freud, Race, and Gender*. Princeton: Princeton University Press, 1993.

Goldberg, Arnold. "An Overview of Perverse Behavior." In *Perversion: Psychoanalytic Perspectives, Perspectives on Psychoanalysis*, edited by Danny Nobus and Lisa Downing, 39–58. London: Karnac, 2006.

Gottesman, Irving. *Schizophrenia Genesis: The Origins of Madness*. New York: W. H. Freeman and Company, 1991.

Grof, Stanislav, and Christina Grof. *The Stormy Search for the self: A Guide To Personal Growth Through Transformative Crisis*. New York, Jeremy P. Tarcher, 1992.

"Spiritual Emergency: Understanding Evolutionary Crisis." In *Spiritual Emergency: When Personal Transformation Becomes a Crisis*, edited by Stanislav and Christina Grof, 1-26. Los Angeles: Jeremy P. Tarcher, 1989.

Guest, Barbara. *Herself Defined: The Poet H.D. and Her World*. New York: Doubleday, 1984.

H.D./Delia Alton. *The Gift*: *The Complete Text*. Edited and annotated by Jane Augustine. Gainesville: University of Florida Press, 1998.

———. "H.D. by Delia Alton." *The Iowa Review* 16, no. 3 (Fall 1986): 180–221.

———. *Helen in Egypt*. New York: New Directions, 1974, c. 1961.

———. *Hermetic Definition*. New York: New Directions, 1971, c. 1958.

———. *HERmione*. New York: New Directions, 1981.

———. *Hippolytus Temporizes & Ion*. Edited by Carol Camper. New York: New Directions, 2003.

———. *Hirslanden Notebooks*. Edited and introduced by Matte Robinson and Demetres P. Tryphonopoulos. Victoria: ELS Editions, 2015.

———. *Magic Mirror, Compassionate Friendship, Thorn Thicket: A Tribute to Erich Heydt*. Edited by Nephie Christodoulides, with a preface by Demetres Tryphonopoulos and Matte Robinson. Victoria: ELS Editions, 2012.

———. *Majic Ring*. Edited and introduced by Demetres P. Tryphonopoulos. Gainesville: University Press of Florida, 2009.

———. *The Mystery*. Edited by Jane Augustine. Gainesville: University Press of Florida, 2009.

———. *Notes on Thought and Vision* and *The Wise Sappho*. San Francisco: City Lights Books, 1982.

———. *The Sword Went Out to Sea (Synthesis of a Dream)*. Edited by Cynthia Hogue and Julie Vandivere. Gainesville: University Press of Florida, 2007.

———. *Tribute to Freud*. New York: New Directions, 1984.

———. *Trilogy*. *[The Walls Do Not Fall; Tribute to the Angels; The Flowering of the Rod]*. New York: New Directions, 1973, c. 1945.

Heffernan, Teresa. *Post-apocalyptic Culture: Modernism, Postmodernism, and the Twentieth-century Novel*. Toronto: University of Toronto Press, 2008.

Hejazi, Michael. "After Illness." *The Networker* 20, no. 3 (spring 2016), 13.

Herring, Phillip. *Djuna: The Life and Work of Djuna Barnes*. New York: Viking Press, 1995.

———. "Zadel Barnes: Journalist." *Review of Contemporary Fiction* 13, no. 3 (1993): 107–16.

Hickman, Miranda B. "'Uncanonically Seated': H.D. and Literary Canons." In *The Cambridge Companion to H.D.*, edited by Miranda Hickman, 9–22. New York: Cambridge University Press, 2012.

Hirsh, Elizabeth. "God or Goods? Teaching *Tribute to Freud* in an Undergraduate Course on Critical Theory." In *Approaches to Teaching H.D.'s Poetry and Prose*, edited by Anette Debo and Lara Vetter, 70–6. New York: MLA, 2011.

Hobson, Suzanne. "Credulous Readers: H.D. and Psychic Research Work." In *Incredible Modernism: Literature, Trust, and Deception*, Edited by John Attridge and Rod Rosenquist. London: Routledge, 2013.

Hogue, Cynthia, and Julie Vandivere. Introduction to *The Sword Went Out to Sea (Synthesis of a Dream)*, edited by Cynthia Hogue and Julie Vandivere, xv-liii. Gainesville: University Press of Florida, 2007.

Hokanson, Robert O'Brien. "'Is it all a Story?': Questioning Revision in H.D.'s *Helen in Egypt*." *American Literature* 64, no. 2 (June 1992): 331–46.

Holland, Norman N. "H.D.'s Analysis with Freud." *PsyArt* 6 (2002): no pagination. http://psyartjournal.com/article/show/n_holland-hds_analysis_with_freud (accessed July 2019).

Hollenberg, Donna Krolik, ed. *Between History and Poetry: The Letters of H.D. and Norman Holmes Pearson*. Iowa: University of Iowa Press, 1997.

———. "'She Showed a Way to Penetrate Mystery': Teaching H.D. and Denise Levertov." In *Approaches to Teaching H.D.'s Poetry and Prose*, edited by Anette Debo and Lara Vetter, 142–7. New York: MLA, 2011.

Jaffe, Nora Crow. "'She Herself is the Writing': Language and Sexual Identity in H.D." *Literature and Medicine* 4 (1985): 86–111.

Jameson, Fredric. *Marxism and Form: Twentieth-Century Dialectical Theories of Literature*. Princeton: Princeton University Press, 1971.

James, William. "Final Impressions of a Psychical Researcher." *Memories and Studies*. https://ebooks.adelaide.edu.au/j/james/william/memories/chapter8.html. (accessed November 2018).

Johnson, Sue M. "Couple and Family Therapy: An Attachment Perspective." In *Handbook of Attachment: Theory, Research and Clinical Applications*, edited by Cassidy J. Shaver, 811–29. New York: Guilford Press, 2008.

Kannenstine, Louis F. *The Art of Djuna Barnes: Duality and Damnation*. New York: New York University Press, 1977.

Keeling, Bret L. "H.D. and the British Modernist Tradition: *Kora and Ka*, Mythopoesis, and England's Great War." In *Approaches to Teaching H.D.'s Poetry and Prose*, eduted by Anette Debo and Lara Vetter, 114–19. New York: MLA, 2011.

Kermode, Frank. *The Sense of an Ending: Studies in the Theory of Fiction with a New Epilogue*. Oxford: Oxford University Press, 2000.

Klein, Melanie. *Love, Guilt and Reparation and Other Works 1921–1945*. New York: The Free Press, 1984.

———. "Notes on Some Schizoid Mechanisms." In *Envy and Gratitude and Other Works 1946–1963*, 1–24. London: Hogarth Press, 1975.

———. "A Study of Envy and Gratitude." In *The Selected Melanie Klein*, edited by Juliet Mitchell, 211–29. New York: The Free Press, 1987.

Kloepfer, Deborah Kelly. *The Unspeakable Mother: Forbidden Discourse in Jean Rhys and H.D.* Ithaca: Cornell University Press, 1989.

Kornfield, Jack. *A Lamp in the Darkness: Illuminating the Path Through Difficult Times*. Boulder: Sounds True, 2014.

Kristeva, Julia. *Black Sun: Depression and Melancholia*. Translated by Leon S. Roudiez. New York: Columbia University Press, 1989.

Lacan, Jacques. "Aggressiveness in Psychoanalysis." In *Écrits: The First Complete Edition in English*, translated by Bruce Fink in collaboration with Héloïse Fink and Russell Grigg, 82–101. New York: Norton, 2006.

———. "The Direction of the Treatment and the Principles of Its Power." In *Écrits: The First Complete Edition in English*, translated by Bruce Fink in collaboration with Héloïse Fink and Russell Grigg, 489–542. New York: Norton, 2006.

———. "The Function and Field of Speech and Language in Psychoanalysis." In *Écrits: The First Complete Edition in English*, translated by Bruce Fink in collaboration with Héloïse Fink and Russell Grigg, 197–268. New York: Norton, 2006.

———. "The Instance of the Letter in the Unconscious." In *Écrits: The First Complete Edition in English*, translated by Bruce Fink in collaboration with Héloïse Fink and Russell Grigg, 412–44. New York: Norton, 2006.

———. "Introduction to Jean Hyppolite's Presentation of Freud's 'Verneinung'." In *Écrits: The First Complete Edition in English*, translated by Bruce Fink in collaboration with Héloïse Fink and Russell Grigg, 308–17. New York: Norton, 2006.

———. "Logical Time and the Assertion of Anticipated Certainty." In *Écrits: The First Complete Edition in English*, translated by Bruce Fink in collaboration with Héloïse Fink and Russell Grigg, 161–75. New York: Norton, 2006.

———. "On Freud's '*Trieb*'." In *Écrits: The First Complete Edition in English*, translated by Bruce Fink in collaboration with Héloïse Fink and Russell Grigg, 722–5. New York: Norton, 2006.

______. "On A Purpose." In *Écrits: The First Complete Edition in English*, translated by Bruce Fink in collaboration with Héloïse Fink and Russell Grigg, 303-7. New York: Norton, 2006.

———. "On a Question Prior to Any Possible Treatment of Psychosis." In *Écrits: The First Complete Edition in English*, translated by Bruce Fink in collaboration with Héloïse Fink and Russell Grigg, 445–88. New York: Norton, 2006.

______. "Position of the Unconscious." In *Écrits: The First Complete Edition in English*, translated by Bruce Fink in collaboration with Héloïse Fink and Russell Grigg, 703-21. New York: Norton, 2006.

———. "Response to Jean Hyppolite's Commentary on Freud's 'Verneinung'." In *Écrits: The First Complete Edition in English*, translated by Bruce Fink in collaboration with Héloïse Fink and Russell Grigg, 318–33. New York: Norton, 2006.

———. *The Seminar of Jacques Lacan: Book I, Freud's Papers on Technique, 1953–1954*. Edited by Jacques-Alain Miller, translated by John Forrester. New York: Norton, 1988.

———. *The Seminar of Jacques Lacan: Book II, The Ego in Freud's Theory and in the Technique of Psychoanalysis, 1954–1955*. Edited by Jacques-Alain Miller, translated by Sylvana Tomaselli. New York: Norton, 1991.

———. *The Seminar of Jacques Lacan: Book III, The Psychoses, 1955–1956*. Edited by Jacques-Alain Miller, translated by Russell Grigg. New York: Norton, 1993.

———. *The Seminar of Jacques Lacan: Book VIII, Transference, 1960–1961*. Edited by Jacques-Alain Miller, translated by Bruce Fink. Cambridge: Polity, 2015.

———. *The Seminar of Jacques Lacan: Book XI, The Four Fundamental Concepts of Psychoanalysis*. Edited by Jacques-Alain Miller, translated by Bruce Sheridan. New York: Norton, 1981.

———. *The Seminar of Jacques Lacan: Book XX, On Feminine Sexuality, the Limits of Love and Knowledge (Encore), 1977–1978*. Edited by Jacques-Alain Miller, translated by Bruce Fink. New York: Norton, 1998.

———. "The Signification of the Phallus." In *Écrits: The First Complete Edition in English*, translated by Bruce Fink in collaboration with Héloïse Fink and Russell Grigg, 575–84. New York: Norton, 2006.

———. "The Subversion of the Subject and the Dialectic of Desire in the Freudian Unconscious." In *Écrits: The First Complete Edition in English*, translated by Bruce Fink in collaboration with Héloïse Fink and Russell Grigg, 671–702. New York: Norton, 2006.

LaChance, Charles. "The Sexual Sublime and Hilda Doolittle." *English* 53 (2004): 31–58.

Laing, R.D. "Transcendental Experience in Relation to Religion and Psychosis." In *Spiritual Emergency: When Personal Transformation Becomes a Crisis*, edited by Stanislav and Christina Grof, 49-62. Los Angeles: Jeremy P. Tarcher, 1989.

Laplanche, Jean. *Hölderlin and the Question of the Father*. Edited and translated by Luke Carson. Victoria: ELS, 2007.

Lee, Judith. "*Nightwood*: 'The Sweetest Lie'." In *Silence and Power: A Reevaluation of Djuna Barnes*, edited by Mary Lynn Broe, 207–20. Carbondale: Southern Illinois University Press, 1991.

Lemaire, Anika. *Jacques Lacan*. Translated by David Macey. Boston: Routledge, 1977.

Lévi-Strauss, Claude. *The Elementary Structures of Kinship*. Translated by James Bell, John von Sturmer, and Rodney Needham. Boston: Beacon Press, 1969.

Lewis, Bradley. *Moving Beyond Prozac, DSM, and the New Psychiatry: The Birth of Postpsychiatry*. Ann Arbor: University of Michigan Press, 2010.

Leys, Ruth. *Trauma: A Genealogy*. Chicago: University of Chicago Press, 2000.

Lifton, Robert Jay. *The Protean Self: Human Resilience in an Age of Fragmentation*. Chicago: University of Chicago Press, 1993.

Loy, David R. *Lack and Transcendence: The Problem of Death and Life in Psychotherapy, Existentialism, and Buddhism*. Somerville: Wisdom Publications, 2018.

_____. *Nonduality: A Study in Comparative Philosophy*. New Jersey: Humanities Press International, 1998. http://www.davidloy.org/downloads/Loy_Nonduality.pdf. (accessed July 2019).

Lukoff, David. "The Diagnosis of Mystical Experiences with Psychotic Features." *The Journal of Transpersonal Psychology* 17, no 2 (1985): 155–81.

Marcus, Jane. "Laughing at Leviticus: *Nightwood* as Woman's Circus Epic." In *Silence and Power: A Reevaluation of Djuna Barnes*, edited by Mary Lynn Broe, 195–206. Carbondale: Southern Illinois University Press, 1991.

Martin, Ann. *Red Riding Hood and the Wolf in Bed: Modernism's Fairy Tales*. Toronto: University of Toronto Press, 2006.

Martins, Susanna S. "Gender Trouble and Lesbian Desire in Djuna Barnes's *Nightwood*." *Frontiers: A Journal of Women's Studies* 20 (1999): 108–26.

Masters, Robert A. *Spiritual Bypassing*. Berkeley: North Atlantic Books, 2010.

Materer, Timothy. *Modernist Alchemy: Poetry and the Occult*. Ithaca: Cornell University Press, 1995.

Maynard, James. "Robert Duncan's *The H.D. Book*." In *Approaches to Teaching H.D.'s Poetry and Prose*, edited by Anette Debo and Lara Vetter, 148–52. New York: MLA, 2011.

McCabe, Susan. "Teaching Sex and Sexuality in H.D.: 'I Had Two Loves Separate'." In *Approaches to Teaching H.D.'s Poetry and Prose*, edited by Anette Debo and Lara Vetter, 92–9. New York: MLA, 2011.

MacCabe, Colin. Introduction to *The Schreber Case*, translated by Andrew Webber, vi-xxii. New York, Penguin, 2003.

McMahan, David L. "Buddhist Modernism." In *Buddhism in the Modern World*, edited by David L. McMahan, 159-76. London: Routledge, 2012.

———. *The Making of Buddhist Modernism*. London: Oxford University Press, 2008.

Miller, Tyrus. "'The Havoc of Nicety'": Djuna Barnes's *Ryder* and the Catastrophe of Epochal Change." In *Shattered Objects: Djuna Barnes's Modernism*, edited by Elizabeth Pender and Cathryn Setz, 163-77. University Park: Pennsylvania State University Press, 2020.

Moody, A. David. *Tracing T.S. Eliot's Spirit: Essays on his Poetry and Thought*. Cambridge: Cambridge University Press, 1996.

Morris, Adalaide. "The Concept of Projection: H.D.'s Visionary Powers." In *Signets: Reading H.D.*, edited by Susan Stanford Friedman and Rachel Blau Du Plessis, 273–96. Madison: University of Wisconsin Press, 1990.

———. "H.D. by Delia Alton." *The Iowa Review* 16, no. 3 (Fall 1986): 174–9.

———. *How To Live/What to Do: H.D.'s Cultural Poetics*. Chicago: University of Illinois Press, 2003.

———. "Ticking Differently: H.D.'s Time in Philadelphia." In *Approaches to Teaching H.D.'s Poetry and Prose*, edited by Anette Debo and Lara Vetter, 56–62. New York: MLA, 2011.

Morton, Timothy. *Hyperobjects: Philosophy and Ecology After the End of the World.* Minneapolis: University of Minnesota Press, 2013.

Nasser, Mervat. "The Rise and Fall of Anti-Psychiatry." *Psychiatric Bulletin* 19 (1995): 743–6.

New, Caroline. *Agency, Health and Social Survival: The Ecopolitics of Rival Psychologies*. New York: Routledge, 2015.

O'Neal, Hank. *"Life is painful, nasty and short . . . in my case it has only been painful and nasty": Djuna Barnes 1978–1981*. New York: Paragon House, 1990.

Pappas, Robin. "H.D. and Havelock Ellis: Popular Science and the Gendering of *Thought and Vision*." *Women's Studies* 38 (2009): 151–82.

Payne, Richard K. "Buddhism and the Powers of the Mind." In *Buddhism in the Modern World*, edited by David L. McMahan, 234–55. London: Routledge, 2012.

Pender, Elizabeth, and Cathryn Setz. "Introduction." In *Shattered Objects: Djuna Barnes's Modernism*, edited by Elizabeth Pender and Cathryn Setz, 1-25. University Park: Pennsylvania State University Press, 2020.

Perry, John Weir. "Spiritual Emergence and Renewal." In *Spiritual Emergency: When Personal Transformation Becomes a Crisis*, edited by Stanislav and Christina Grof, 63–76. Los Angeles: Jeremy P. Tarcher, 1989.

———. *Trials of the Visionary Mind: Spiritual Emergency and the Renewal Process*. Albany: State University of New York Press, 1999.

Pondrom, Cyrena N. "Approaches to Teaching *Helen in Egypt*." In *Approaches to Teaching H.D.'s Poetry and Prose*, edited by Anette Debo and Lara Vetter, 84–91. New York: MLA, 2011.

Ponsot, Marie. "A Reader's *Ryder*." In *Silence and Power: A Reevaluation of Djuna Barnes*, edited by Mary Lynn Broe, 94–136. Carbondale: Southern Illinois University Press, 1991.

Prendergast, Catherine. "The Unexceptional Schizophrenic: A Post-Modern Introduction." In *The Disability Studies Reader*, 4th ed., edited by Lennard J. Davis, 236–45. New York: Routledge, 2013.

Potter, Rachel. "*Nightwood's* Humans." In *Shattered Objects: Djuna Barnes's Modernism*, edited by Elizabeth Pender and Cathryn Setz, 61-74. University Park: Pennsylvania State University Press, 2020.

Rabaté, Jean-Michel. *The Ghosts of Modernity*. Gainesville: University Press of Florida, 1996.

Rado, Lisa. "Portraits of an Artist: Introducing Students to H.D.'s Poetry." In *Approaches to Teaching H.D.'s Poetry and Prose*, edited by Anette Debo and Lara Vetter, 49–55. New York: MLA, 2011.

Ragland, Ellie. *Essays on the Pleasures of Death: From Freud to Lacan*. New York: Routledge, 1995.

Rainey, Lawrence S. "Canon, Gender, and Text: The Case of H.D." *College Literature* 18, no. 3 (Fall 1991): 106–25.

Ram Dass. *Be Here Now*. Taos: Lama Foundation, 1978.

Rappaport, David. *Organization and Pathology of Thought*. New York: Columbia University Press, 1951.

Robinson, Matte. *The Astral H.D.* London: Bloomsbury Academic, 2016.

———. "Introduction." In *Hirslanden Notebooks: An Annotated Scholarly Edition*, edited by Matte Robinson and Demetres P. Tryphonopoulos, ix-xxxi. Victoria: ELS, 2015.

Rust, John. "Schizotypal Thinking Among Members of Occult Sects." *Social Behavior and Personality* 20, no. 2 (1992): 121–9.

Samyutta Nikaya (Grouped Discourses attributed to the Buddha from the *Tipitaka*, or Pali Canon) 56.11 (Dhammacakkappavattana Sutta), in Suta Pitaka, trans. Thānissaro Bhikkhu. *Access to Insight*, 2005. https://www.accesstoinsight.org/tipitaka/sn/sn56/sn56.011.than.html (accessed July 2019).

Sanchez-Pardo, Esther. *Cultures of the Death Drive: Melanie Klein and Modernist Melancholia*. Durham, NC: Duke University Press, 2003.

Santner, Eric L. *My Own Private Germany: Daniel Paul Schreber's Secret History of Modernity*. Princeton: Princeton University Press, 1996.

Schreber, Daniel Paul. *Memoirs of My Nervous Illness*. Edited and translated by Ida Macalpine and Richard A. Hunter. Introduction by Samuel M. Weber. Cambridge, MA: Harvard University Press, 1988.

Scott, Bonnie Kime. *Refiguring Modernism, Vol. 1: The Women of 1928*. Bloomington: Indiana University Press, 1996.

Seitler, Dana. "Down on All Fours: Atavistic Perversions and the Science of Desire from Frank Norris to Djuna Barnes." *American Literature: A Journal of Literary History, Criticism and Bibliography* 73 (2001): 544–56.

Setz, Cathryn. "Trees of Heaven": Djuna Barnes's Late Metaphysical Verse. In *Shattered Objects: Djuna Barnes's Modernism*, edited by Elizabeth Pender and Cathryn Setz, 130-46. University Park: Pennsylvania State University Press, 2020.

Sherbert, Gary. "Hieroglyphics of Sleep and Pain: Djuna Barnes's Anatomy of Melancholy." In *Response to Death: The Literary Work of Mourning*, edited by Christian Riegel, 117–44. Edmonton: University of Alberta Press, 2005.

Shimrat, Irit. "Meeting With Hilda Fernandez." *The Networker* 17, no. 2 (summer 2012): 7.

Simpson, Jacqueline, and Steve Roud. *A Dictionary of English Folklore*. New York: Oxford University Press, 2000.

Smith, Victoria L. "A Story Beside(s) Itself: The Language of Loss in Djuna Barnes's *Nightwood*." *PMLA* 114, no. 2 (March 1999): 194–206.

Stevenson, Sheryl. "Writing the Grotesque Body." In *Silence and Power: A Reevaluation of Djuna Barnes*, edited by Mary Lynn Broe, 81–93. Carbondale: Southern Illinois University Press, 1991.

Surette, Leon. *The Birth of Modernism: Ezra Pound, T.S. Eliot, W.B. Yeats, and the Occult*. Montreal: McGill-Queen's University Press, 1993.

Sword, Helen. *Ghostwriting Modernism*. Ithaca: Cornell University Press, 2002.

Taylor, Julie. *Djuna Barnes and Affective Modernism*. Edinburgh: Edinburgh University Press, 2012.

_____. "Revising the Antiphon, Restaging Trauma; or, Where Sexual Politics Meet Textual History." *Modernism/modernity* 18, no. 1 (January 2011): 125–47.

_____. "Making Contact: Affect, Queer Historiography, and 'Our Djuna.'" In *Shattered Objects: Djuna Barnes's Modernism*, edited by Elizabeth Pender and

Cathryn Setz, 193-206. University Park: Pennsylvania State University Press, 2020.

Thānissaro Bhikkhu (Geoffrey DeGraff). *The Shape of Suffering: A Study of Dependent Co-Arising*, 2008. https://www.dhammatalks.org/books/ShapeOfSuffering/Contents.html (accessed December 2020).

Thomas, Heather H. "Teaching H.D. in the Creative Writing Classroom." In *Approaches to Teaching H.D.'s Poetry and Prose*, edited by Anette Debo and Lara Vetter, 153–9. New York: MLA, 2011.

Tolle, Eckhart. *A New Earth*. New York: Dutton, 2005.

Tonning, Erik, Matthew Feldman, and David Addyman. *Modernism, Christianity, and Apocalypse: Studies in Religion and the Arts*. Boston: Brill Press, 2014.

Trigilio, Tony. *"Strange Prophecies Anew": Rereading Apocalypse in Blake, H.D., and Ginsberg*. New Jersey: Fairleigh Dickinson University Press, 2000.

Tryphonopoulos, Demetres P. *The Celestial Tradition: A Study of Ezra Pound's* The Cantos. Waterloo: Wilfred Laurier University Press, 1992.

Trungpa, Chogyam. *Cutting through Spiritual Materialism*. Boston: Shambhala Publications, 2002.

Turkle, Sherry. "French Anti-psychiatry." In *Critical Psychiatry: The Politics of Mental Health*, edited by David Ingleby, 150–83. London: Free Association Books, 2004.

Vervaeke, John, Timothy Lillicrap, and Blake Richards. "Relevance Realization and the Emerging Framework in Cognitive Science." *Journal of Logic & Computation* 22, no. 1 (February 2012): 79–99.

_____ and Leo Ferraro. "Relevance, Meaning, and the Cognitive Science of Wisdom." In *The Scientific Study of Personal Wisdom: From Contemplative Traditions to Neuroscience*, edited by Michael Ferrari and Nic Westrate, 21-51. New York: Springer, 2012.

_____, Christopher Mastropietro, and Filip Miscevic. *Zombies in Western Culture: A Twenty-First-Century Crisis.* Cambridge: Open Book Publishers, 2017. https://www.openbookpublishers.com/product.php/602/zombies-in-western-culture--a-twenty-first-century-crisis?602/zombies-in-western-culture--a-twenty-first-century-crisis. (accessed July 2019).

Vetter, Lara. *Modernist Writings and Religio-Scientific Discourse*. New York: Palgrave Macmillan, 2010.

Vetter, Lara. *A Curious Peril: H.D.'s Late Modernist Prose*. Gainesville: University Press of Florida, 2017.

Von Domarus, Eilhard. "The Specific Laws of Logic in Schizophrenia." In *Language and Thought in Schizophrenia*, edited by Jacob S. Kasanin, 104–14. Proceedings of the Chicago 1939 American Psychiatric Association Conference. New York: Norton. 1964.

Warren, Diane. *Djuna Barnes's Consuming Fictions*. Burlington: Ashgate, 2008.

Weber, Samuel M. Introduction to *Memoirs of My Nervous Illness*, edited and translated by Ida Macalpine and Richard A. Hunter, vii-liv. Cambridge, MA: Harvard University Press, 1988.

Warren, Henry Clarke. *Buddhism in Translations*. New York: Atheneum, 1963.

Weiss, Andrea. *Paris Was a Woman: Portraits from the Left Bank*. San Francisco: Harper San Francisco, 1995.

West, Paul. "Afterword: The Havoc of this Nicety." In *Ryder*, 243-50. Illinois: Dalkey Archive Press, 1995. c. 1928.

Wheeler, Lesley. "Mapping *Sea Garden*." In *Approaches to Teaching H.D.'s Poetry and Prose*, edited by Anette Debo and Lara Vetter, 40-8. New York: MLA, 2011.

White, Robert W. *The Abnormal Personality: A Textbook*. 2nd ed. New York: Ronald Press, 1948.

Whitley, Catherine. "Nations and the Night: Excremental History in James Joyce's *Finnegan's Wake* and Djuna Barnes's *Nightwood*." *Journal of Modern Literature* 24, no. 1 (fall 2000): 81–98.

Williams, Paris. *Rethinking Madness: Towards a Paradigm Shift in Our Understanding and Treatment of Psychosis*. San Francisco: Sky's Edge, 2012.

Willis, Elizabeth. "A Public History of the Dividing Line: H.D., the Bomb, and the Roots of the Postmodern." *Arizona Quarterly* 63, no. 1 (spring 2007): 81–108.

Young, Shinzen. "Dark Night." *Shinzen's Blog*. http://shinzenyoung.blogspot.ae/2011/11/dark-night.html (accessed September 2018).

Žižek, Slavoj. *For They Know Not What They Do: Enjoyment as a Political Factor*. London: Verso, 1991.

———. "Kant and Sade: The Ideal Couple" *Lacanian Ink* 13, 1998. https://www.lacan.com/zizlacan4.htm (accessed July 2019)

———. *The Sublime Object of Ideology*. New York: Verso, 1989.

———. The Ticklish Subject: The Absent Centre of Political Ontology. London: Verso, 1999.

Index

About the Author

Lheisa Dustin is an independent scholar. Born in Winnipeg, Canada, she majored in English, religious studies, and creative writing for her bachelor's and master's at Concordia University, Montreal, and in English literature for her PhD at the University of Victoria. She has taught English in Mexico, India, Saudi Arabia, Qatar, and the United Arab Emirates, as well as in Canada and Oman. She has published articles on Theravada Buddhism and T.S. Eliot's *The Waste Land*, in *Notes and Queries*, H.D.'s *The Sword Went Out to Sea*, in *Genre*, and Djuna Barnes's *Nightwood*, in *Criticism*.

www.ingramcontent.com/pod-product-compliance
Lightning Source LLC
LaVergne TN
LVHW091533200926
848483LV00002B/384
* 9 7 8 1 6 8 3 9 3 2 3 0 7 *